Disorders Index

Epidermolysis bullosa acquisita, 574
Epidermolysis bullosa simplex, 576
Erysipelas, 273
Erysipeloid, 287
Erythema ab igne, 694
Erythema elevatum diutinum, 653
Erythema infectiosum, 468
Erythema multiforme, 626
Erythema nodosum, 635
Erythema toxicum neonatorum, 582
Erythrasma, 419
Erythrodermic psoriasis, 213
Erythroplasia of Queyrat, 749
Erythropoietic protoporphyria 680
Exanthem subitum, 471
Exercise-induced anaphylaxis, 145
Exfoliative erythroderma, 491
External otitis, 294
Extramammary Paget's disease, 764
Fifth disease, 468
Fire ant stings, 538
Folliculitis decalvans, 860
Folliculitis, 279
Furuncles (boils), 284
Gardner's syndrome, 913
Genital warts, 336
German measles, 467
Gonorrhea, 330
Granuloma annulare, 898
Granuloma inguinale, 329
Guttate psoriasis, 212
Hairy leukoplakia, 363
Halo nevi, 781
Hand eczema, 50
Hand, foot, and mouth disease, 462
Henoch-Schönlein purpura, 645
Herpes simplex, 381
Herpes zoster, 394
Herpetic whitlow, 873
Hidradenitis suppurativa, 202
Hirsutism, 846
Hypersensitivity vasculitis, 642
Ichthyosis vulgaris, 115
Idiopathic guttate hypomelanosis, 689
Intertrigo, 418
Irritant contact dermatitis, 82
Isotretinoin, 186
Junction nevus, 774
Kaposi's sarcoma, 827
Kawasaki syndrome, 474
Keloids, 709
Keratoacanthoma, 711
Keratoderma blennorhagicum, 216
Keratolysis exfoliativa, 55
Keratolysis, pitted, 416
Keratosis pilaris, 116

Labial melanocytic macule, 782
Lentigo (liver spots), 691
Lentigo maligna, 794
Leukocytoclastic vasculitis, 642
Leukonychia, 882
Leukoplakia, 751
Lichen planopilaris, 861
Lichen planus, 250
Lichen sclerosis et atrophicus, 257
Lichen simplex chronicus, 54, 63, 66
Linear IgA bullous dermatosis, 556
Lupus erythematosus, 592
Lyme disease, 517
Lymphangioma circumscriptum, 825
Male-pattern baldness, 842
Malignant melanoma, 786
Mastocytosis, 156
Measles, 460
Meningococcemia, 299
Methotrexate 229
Milia, 194
Miliaria rubra, 205
Morphea, 620
Mucha-Habermann disease, 261
Muir-Torre syndrome, 914
Mycosis fungoides, 754
Myiasis, 534
Necrobiosis lipoidica, 897
Neurotic excoriations, 68
Nevoid basal cell carcinoma syndrome, 731
Nevus flammeus (port-wine stains), 819
Nevus sebaceous, 715
Nummular eczema, 54
Onycholysis, 880
Onychomycosis 875
Otitis externa, 294
Paronychia, 867
Parvovirus B-19 infection, 468
Pearly penile papules, 339
Pediculosis, 506
Pemphigoid, 567
Pemphigus, 559
Perioral dermatitis, 30, 195
Perlèche, 450
Pilar cyst, 719
Pilar cysts, 719
Pitted keratolysis, 416
Pityriasis alba, 118, 689
Pityriasis lichenoides chronica, 261
Pityriasis rosea, 246
Pityriasis rubra pilaris, 240
Plantar warts, 374
PLEVA 261
Poikiloderma vasculare atrophicans, 756
Poikiloderma, 609
Poison ivy, 85

Continued

Disorders Index

Polyarteritis nodosa, 640
Polymorphous light eruptions, 671
Pompholyx (dyshidrosis), 58
Porphyria cutanea tarda, 675
Port-wine stains, 819
Postherpetic neuralgia, 400
Pressure urticaria, 144
Prurigo nodularis, 68,
PUPPP, 152
Pseudofolliculitis barbae, 280
Pseudomonas folliculitis, 290
Pseudopelade, 860
Pseudoporphyria, 679
Pseudoxanthoma elasticum, 916
Psoriasis, 209
Pustular psoriasis
Pyoderma gangrenosum, 653
Pyogenic granuloma, 826, 889
Rocky Mountain spotted fever, 524
Rosacea, 198
Roseola infantum, 471
Rubella, 467
Scabies, 497
Scarlet fever, 464
Schamberg's disease, 656
Scleroderma, 613
Seabather's eruption, 540
Sebaceous hyperplasia, 720
Seborrheic dermatitis, 242
Seborrheic keratosis, 698
Senile comedones, 194
Serum sickness, 155
Sézary syndrome, 760
Shingles, 394
Skin tags, 706
Small-vessel vasculitis, 642
Speckled lentiginous nevus, 778
Spider angioma, 830
Spider bites, 512
Spitz nevus, 781
Squamous cell carcinoma, 744
Staphylococcal scalded skin syndrome, 288
Stasis dermatitis, 72
Stasis ulcers, 14
Steroid acne, 33, 191
Steroid atrophy, 34
Steroid rosacea, 30
Stevens-Johnson syndrome, 630
Stinging insects, 531
Strawberry hemangiomas, 815
Striae, 15
Stucco keratosis, 705
Sturge-Weber syndrome, 822
Sunburn, 233
Superficial basal cell carcinoma, 726
Superficial spreading melanoma, 788

Sweet's syndrome, 650
Swimmer's itch, 539
Sycosis barbae, 282
Syphilis, 315
Syringoma, 721
Systemic lupus erythematosus, 600
T-cell lyphoma, cutaneous, 754
Telangiectasia macularis eruptiva perstans, 157
Telangiectasia, 830
Telogen effluvium, 841
Tendinous xanthoma, 904
Terry's nails, 885
Tick bite paralysis, 526
Tinea amiantacea, 243
Tinea barbae, 434
Tinea capitis, 427
Tinea corporis, 420
Tinea cruris, 417
Tinea gladiatorum, 422
Tinea incognito, 38, 417, 426
Tinea pedis, 413
Tinea unguium, 874
Tinea versicolor, 451
Toxic epidermal necrolysis, 491, 627
Toxic shock syndrome, 479
Transient neonatal pustular melanosis, 582
Trichomonas vaginalis, 440
Trichomycosis axillaris, 862
Trichotillomania, 858
Tuberous sclerosis, 909
Tuberous xanthoma, 904
Tufted folliculitis, 860
Unilateral nevoid telangiectasia syndrome, 832
Urethritis, 309
Urticaria pigmentosa, 156
Urticaria, 129
Urticarial vasculitis, 154
Vaginal lichen planus, erosive, 255
Vaginosis, bacterial, 313t
Varicella, 389
Venous lake, 825
Venous ulcers, 73
Verrucous carcinoma, 752
Verrucous epidermal nevus, 714
Viral exanthems, 473
Virilization, 846
Vitiligo, 684
Von Recklinghausen's neurofibromatosis, 905
Warts, 368
Wegener's granulomatosis, 640, 648
White superficial onychomycosis, 876
Xanthelasma, 903
Xanthoma, 902
Xerosis, 60
Yellow nails syndrome, 884
Zoster sine herpete, 402

CORTICOSTEROIDS (TOPICAL)* Complete list on Page 958

Group	Brand name	%	Generic name	Tube size (gm; unless noted)
I	Cormax cream	0.05	Clobetasol propionate	15, 30, 45
	Cormax ointment	0.05		15, 30, 45
	Cormax scalp solution	0.05		25 ml, 50 ml
	Ultravate cream	0.05	Halobetasol propionate	15, 50
	Ultravate ointment	0.05		15, 50
	Diprolene lotion	0.05	Augmented betamethasone dipropionate	30 ml, 60 ml
	Diprolene ointment	0.05		15, 50
	Diprolene gel	0.05		15, 50
	Psorcon ointment	0.05	Diflorasone diacetate	15, 30, 60
II	Cyclocort ointment	0.1	Amcinonide	15, 30, 60
	Diprolene AF cream	0.05	Augmented betamethasone dipropionate	15, 50
	Diprosone ointment	0.05	Betamethasone dipropionate	15, 45
	Elocon ointment	0.1	Mometasone furoate	
	Lidex cream	0.05	Fluocinonide	15, 30, 60, 120
	Lidex gel	0.05		15, 30, 60
	Lidex ointment	0.05		30, 60
	Lidex solution	0.05		20, 60 ml
	Psorcon-E cream	0.05	Diflorasone diacetate	15, 30, 60
	Psorcon-E ointment	0.05		15, 30, 60
	Topicort cream	0.25	Desoximetasone	15, 60
	Topicort gel	0.05		15, 60
	Topicort ointment	0.25		15, 60
III	Betatrex ointment	0.1	Betamethasone valerate	45
	Cutivate ointment	0.005	Fluticasone propionate	15, 30, 60
	Diprosone cream	0.05	Betamethasone dipropionate	15, 45
	Diprosone lotion	0.05	Betamethasone dipropionate	20, 60 ml
	Elocon ointment	0.1	Mometasone furoate	15, 45
IV	Aristocort A ointment	0.1	Triamcinolone acetonide	15, 60
	Cyclocort cream	0.1	Amcinonide	15, 30, 60
	Dermatop-E ointment	0.1	Prednicarbate	15, 60
	Elocon cream	0.1	Mometasone furoate	15, 45
	Elocon lotion	0.1		30, 60 ml
	Kenalog ointment	0.1	Triamcinolone acetonide	15, 60
	Synalar ointment	0.025	Fluocinolone acetonide	15, 60
	Westcort ointment	0.2	Hydrocortisone	15, 45, 60
V	Betatrex cream	0.1	Betamethasone valerate	45
	Cutivate cream	0.05	Fluticasone propionate	15, 30, 60
	Dermatop-E cream	0.1	Prednicarbate	15, 60
	DesOwen ointment	0.05	Desonide	15, 60
	Kenalog cream	0.1	Triamcinolone acetonide	15, 60, 80
	Locoid cream	0.1	Hydrocortisone butyrate	15, 45
	Locoid ointment	0.1		15, 45
	Locoid solution			20, 60 cc
	Synalar cream	0.025	Fluocinolone acetonide	15, 60
	Westcort cream	0.2	Hydrocortisone valerate	15, 45, 60
VI	Aclovate cream	0.05	Prednicarbate	15, 45, 60
	Aclovate ointment	0.05	Prednicarbate	15, 45, 60
	DesOwen cream	0.05	Desonide	15, 60, 90
	DesOwen lotion	0.05		2, 4 oz
VII	Hytone cream	2.5	Hydrocortisone	1, 2 oz
	Hytone lotion	2.5		2 oz
	Hytone ointment	2.5		1 oz
		1.0	Hydrocortisone	Many brands

*Listed by potency group: group I is the most potent.

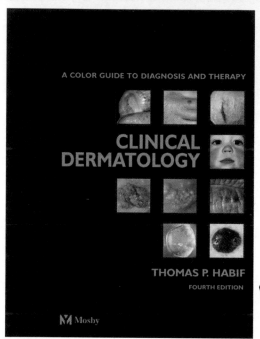
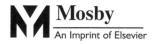
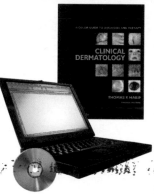
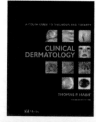
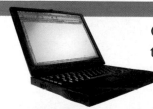

Clinical Dermatology
FOURTH EDITION
A COLOR GUIDE TO DIAGNOSIS AND THERAPY

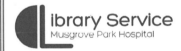

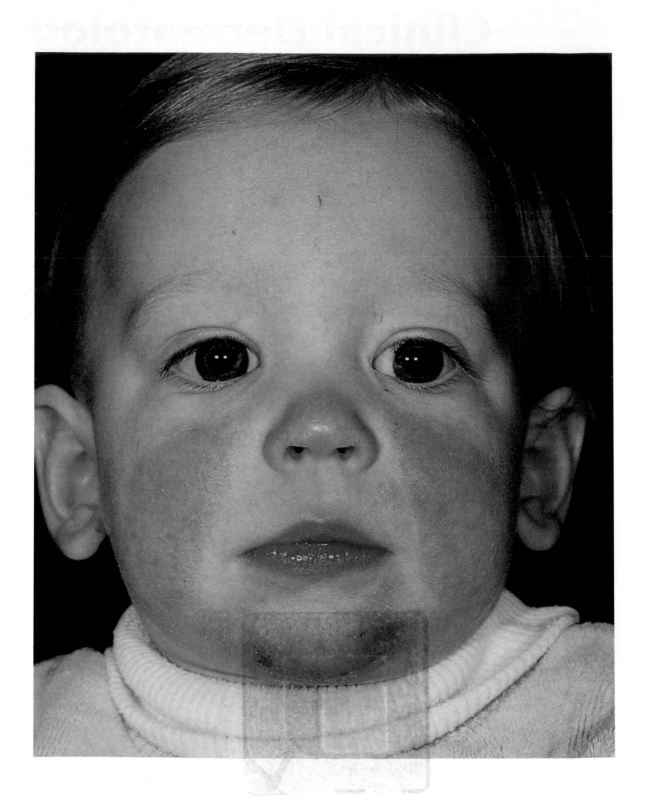

Clinical Dermatology
FOURTH EDITION
A COLOR GUIDE TO DIAGNOSIS AND THERAPY

Thomas P Habif MD

Adjunct Professor of Medicine (Dermatology)
Dartmouth Medical School
Hanover, NH, USA

Commissioning Editor: **Sue Hodgson**
Project Development Editor: **Louise Cook**
Publishing Services Manager: **Melissa Lastarria**
Layout Design: **Jeanne Genz**
Design Coordinator: **Jayne Jones**
Illustration Coordinator: **Michael Ruddy**

Project Organization: **Laura A. McCann**
Medical Photography: **Alan N. Binnick, MD**, and
 Thomas P. Habif, MD

Photographs: **Barry M. Austin, MD, Richard D. Baughman,
 MD, Daniel W. Collison, MD, Warren M. Pringle, MD,
 Cameron L. Smith, MD**, and **Steven K. Spencer, MD**

Technical Advice: **David V. Habif, Jr, MD**
Moral Support: **Dorothy, Tommy, and David**

Mosby Edinburgh London New York Oxford Philadelphia St Louis Sydney Toronto 2004

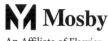

Mosby

An Affiliate of Elsevier

The Curtis Center
Independence Square West
Philadelphia, Pennsylvania 19106

CLINICAL DERMATOLOGY: A COLOR GUIDE TO
DIAGNOSIS AND THERAPY

Previous editions copyrighted 1985, 1990, 1996.

International Standard Book Number 0-323-01319-8

Printed in Chile

Last digit is the print number: 9 8 7 6 5 4 3 2 1

Preface

Clinical Dermatology is intended to be a practical resource for the busy clinician. Over 1000 illustrations are combined with disease descriptions and current and comprehensive therapeutic information. Bold headings are used to facilitate rapid access to information. Diseases can be accessed in many ways.

The classic method of organizing skin diseases is used. Common diseases are covered in depth. Illustrations of classic examples of these disorders and photographs of variations seen at different stages are included. Basic dermatologic surgical techniques are covered in detail. Specialized techniques such as Mohs' micrographic surgery are described so that the physician can be better prepared to suggest referral. Theoretical information, disease mechanisms, and rare disease are found in comprehensive textbooks.

Rapid Access to the Text

1. List of disorders with page references—inside front cover.
2. List of common topical steroids—follows disorders pages.
3. List of diseases by region with page references—inside back cover.
4. List of diseases by lesion type with page references—page 3.
5. Formulary is located on pages 945 to 973.

How to Use This Book

Students in the classroom

Students should learn the primary and secondary lesions and the distribution of diseases in Chapter 1 and study the differential diagnosis of each lesion. Select a few familiar diseases from each list and read about them. Study the close-up pictures carefully. Obtain an overview of the text. Turn the pages, look at the pictures, and read the captions.

Students in the clinic

You see skin abnormalities every day in the clinic. Try to identify these diseases, or ask for assistance. Study all diseases, especially tumors, with a magnifying glass or ocular lens. Read about what you see and you will rapidly gain a broad fund of knowledge.

Study Chapters 20 (Benign Skin Tumors), 21 (Premalignant and Malignant Nonmelanoma Skin Tumors), and 22 (Nevi and Malignant Melanoma). Skin growths are common, and it is important to recognize their features.

House officers are responsible for patient management. Read Chapter 2 carefully, and study all aspects of the use of topical steroids. These valuable agents are used to treat a great variety of inflammatory skin conditions. It is tempting to use these agents as a therapeutic trial and ask for a consultation only if therapy fails. Topical steroids mask some diseases, make some diseases worse, and create other diseases. Do not develop bad habits; if you do not know what a disease is, do not treat it.

The diagnosis of skin disease is deceptively easy. Do not make hasty diagnoses. Take a history, study primary lesions and the distribution, and be deliberate and methodical. Ask for help. With time and experience you will feel comfortable managing many common skin diseases.

The practicing clinician

Most skin diseases are treated by practitioners other than dermatologists. This includes primary care physicians, nurse practitioners and physician assistants. Clinicians involved in direct patient care should read the above guidelines for using this book. Learn a few topical steroids in each potency group. There are a great number of agents in the Formulary. Many in each table contain similar ingredients and have the same therapeutic effect. Develop an armamentarium of agents and gain experience in their use.

Inflammatory conditions are often confusing, and sometimes biopsies are of limited value in their diagnosis. Eczema is common, read Chapters 2 and 3. Acne is seen everyday, read Chapter 7. Managing acne effectively will provide a great service to many young patients who are very uncomfortable with their appearance. The clinical diagnosis of pigmented lesions is complicated. A dermatologist can often make a specific diagnosis without the need for a biopsy.

The dermatologist

Many dermatologists use the pictures as an aid to reassure patients. Examine the patient, make a diagnosis, and then show them an illustration of their disease. Many patients see the similarity and are reassured.

This book is designed to be a practical resource. All of the most current descriptive and therapeutic information that is practical and relevant has been included. All topics are researched on Medline. Details about basic science and complex mechanisms of disease can be found elsewhere. Rare diseases are found in larger textbooks.

Photography

The photographs were taken with medium format cameras, 35-mm macro cameras, and digital macro cameras. The digital images for this edition were taken by me with a Nikon D1 digital camera fitted with a 60 mm macro lens and a Canfield TwinFlash. The macro camera takes pictures that simulate the view through a hand lens. Therefore the distribution of the disease and the primary lesion can be accurately illustrated. Over 4000 new digital images were acquired in preparation for this edition. Alan N. Binnick, MD, Adjunct Assistant Professor of Medicine (Dermatology), Dartmouth Medical School, provided all of the new images taken with transparency film. He has 25 years of experience as a clinician, teacher, and expert photographer. His entire collection was available for this edition.

Production

The author writes the manuscript. The publishing company makes the book. Manufacturing a book is a complicated process. The key people involved in this effort are listed on the title page. As my first editor said 20 years ago, "if people ever realized what was involved in making a book, they would not believe that it could ever get done."

The layout and design of each page in this book is done the "old fashion way," by cutting and pasting images and strips of text by the layout artist. Page layout design is a science and an art. Jeanne Genz has designed all four editions of this book. This older, slower, noncomputerized technique created by an expert produces pages that are balanced and of maximum clarity. Computer layout programs are not capable of this art. The final "pasted" book is then converted to a digital file and printed on high-grade glossy paper on a sheetfed press. Glossy paper retains ink at the surface to enhance definition. Sheetfed presses print slowly and allow ink to be laid down precisely so that exceptional sharpness and color balance are achieved.

Thomas P. Habif
2003

Contents

1 **Principles of Diagnosis and Anatomy 1**
Skin anatomy 1
Epidermis 1
Dermis 1
Dermal nerves and vasculature 1
Diagnosis of skin disease 2
A methodical approach 2
Examination technique 2
Approach to treatment 2
Primary lesions 2
Secondary lesions 2
Special skin lesions 16
Regional differential diagnoses 18

2 **Topical Therapy and Topical Corticosteroids 23**
Topical therapy 23
Emollient creams and lotions 23
Severe dry skin (xerosis) 23
Wet dressings 24
Topical corticosteroids 25
Strength 25
Vehicle 26
Steroid-antibiotic mixtures 27
Amount of cream to dispense 27
Application 28
Adverse reactions 30

3 **Eczema and Hand Dermatitis 41**
Stages of eczematous inflammation 43
Acute eczematous inflammation 43
Subacute eczematous inflammation 44
Chronic eczematous inflammation 48
Hand eczema 50
Irritant contact dermatitis 51
Atopic hand dermatitis 53
Allergic contact dermatitis 54
Nummular eczema 54
Lichen simplex chronicus 54
Recurrent focal palmar peeling 55
Hyperkeratotic eczema 55
Fingertip eczema 57
Pompholyx 59
Id reaction 59

Eczema: various presentations 60
Asteatotic eczema 60
Nummular eczema 61
Chapped fissured feet 62
Self-inflicted dermatoses 63
Lichen simplex chronicus 63
Prurigo nodularis 68
Neurotic excoriations 68
Psychogenic parasitosis 70
Stasis dermatitis and venous ulceration: postphlebitic syndromes 72
Stasis dermatitis 72
Types of eczematous inflammation 72
Venous leg ulcers 74

4 **Contact Dermatitis and Patch Testing 81**
Irritant contact dermatitis 82
Allergic contact dermatitis 84
Systemically induced allergic contact dermatitis 84
Clinical presentation 84
Rhus dermatitis 88
Natural rubber latex allergy 90
Shoe allergy 92
Metal dermatitis 93
Cement dermatitis and burns 95
Further examples of allergic contact dermatitis 95
Patients with leg ulcers 97
Cosmetic and fragrance allergy 97
Diagnosis of contact dermatitis 98
Patch testing 98

5 **Atopic Dermatitis 105**
Pathogenesis and immunology 106
Clinical aspects 107
Infant phase (birth to 2 years) 108
Childhood phase (2 to 12 years) 111
Adult phase (12 years to adult) 114
Associated features 115
Dry skin and xerosis 115
Ichthyosis vulgaris 115
Keratosis pilaris 116
Hyperlinear palmar creases 118
Pityriasis alba 118

Atopic pleats 118
Cataracts and keratoconus 118
Triggering factors 120
Temperature change and sweating 120
Decreased humidity 120
Excessive washing 120
Contact with irritating substances 120
Contact allergy 120
Aeroallergens 120
Microbic agents 120
Food 120
Emotional stress 120
Treatment 120
Dry skin 122
Inflammation and infection 122
Infants 123
Children and adults 123
Tar 124
Hospitalization for severely resistant cases 125
Lubrication 125
Sedation and antihistamines 125
Phototherapy 126
Diet restriction and breast-feeding 126

6   Urticaria and Angioedema 129
Clinical aspects 130
Pathophysiology 133
Initial evaluation of all patients with urticaria 134
Acute urticaria 134
Chronic urticaria 136
Treatment of urticaria 139
Antihistamines 140
Epinephrine 141
Oral corticosteroids 141
Immunotherapy 141
Physical urticarias 142
Dermographism 142
Pressure urticaria 144
Cholinergic urticaria 145
Exercise-induced anaphylaxis 145
Cold urticaria 146
Solar urticaria 147
Heat, water, and vibration urticarias 147
Aquagenic pruritus 147
Angioedema 147
Acquired forms of angioedema 148
Hereditary angioedema 151
Contact urticaria syndrome 152
Pruritic urticarial papules and plaques of pregnancy 152
Urticarial vasculitis 154
Serum sickness 155
Mastocytosis 156

7   Acne, Rosacea, and Related Disorders 162
Acne 162
Classification 163

Overview of diagnosis and treatment 163
Etiology and pathogenesis 169
Approach to acne therapy 170
Acne treatment 171
Therapeutic agents for treatment of acne 178
Acne surgery 190
Other types of acne 190
Perioral dermatitis 195
Treatment 197
Rosacea (acne rosacea) 198
Skin manifestations 198
Ocular rosacea 200
Treatment 200
Hidradenitis suppurativa 202
Clinical presentation 202
Pathogenesis 202
Management 203
Miliaria 205
Miliaria crystallina 205
Miliaria rubra 205
Miliaria profunda 205

8   Psoriasis and Other Papulosquamous Diseases 209
Psoriasis 209
Clinical manifestations 210
Histology 211
Clinical presentations 211
Chronic plaque psoriasis 212
Guttate psoriasis 212
Generalized pustular psoriasis 213
Erythrodermic psoriasis 213
Light-sensitive psoriasis 214
Psoriasis of the scalp 214
Psoriasis of the palms and soles 214
Pustular psoriasis of the palms and soles 214
Keratoderma blennorrhagicum (Reiter's syndrome) 216
Psoriasis of the penis and Reiter's syndrome 216
Pustular psoriasis of the digits 216
Psoriasis inversus (psoriasis of the flexural or intertriginous areas) 217
Human immunodeficiency virus (HIV)-induced psoriasis 217
Psoriasis of the nails 218
Psoriatic arthritis 220
Treatment of psoriasis 222
Topical therapy 224
Systemic therapy 228
Biologic therapy for psoriasis 238
Pityriasis rubra pilaris 240
Seborrheic dermatitis 242
Infants (cradle cap) 242
Young children (tinea amiantacea and blepharitis) 242
Adolescents and adults (classic seborrheic dermatitis) 245
Acquired immunodeficiency syndrome 245
Pityriasis rosea 246
Lichen planus 250
Localized papules 250

Hypertrophic lichen planus 252
Generalized lichen planus and lichenoid drug eruptions 252
Lichen planus of the palms and soles 252
Follicular lichen planus 252
Oral mucous membrane lichen planus 254
Erosive vaginal lichen planus 255
Nails 255
Diagnosis 255
Treatment 256
Lichen sclerosus et atrophicus 257
Lichen sclerosus et atrophicus of the penis 258
Pityriasis lichenoides 261

9   **Bacterial Infections 267**
Skin infections 267
Impetigo 267
Ecthyma 272
Cellulitis and erysipelas 273
Cellulitis of specific areas 274
Necrotizing fasciitis 278
Folliculitis 279
Staphylococcal folliculitis 279
Keratosis pilaris 280
Pseudofolliculitis barbae (razor bumps) 280
Sycosis barbae 282
Acne keloidalis 283
Furuncles and carbuncles 284
Location 284
Bacteria 284
Predisposing conditions 284
Clinical manifestations 284
Differential diagnosis 285
Treatment of furuncles 285
Recurrent furunculosis 286
Erysipeloid 287
Clinical manifestation 287
Diagnosis 287
Treatment 287
Blistering distal dactylitis 287
Staphylococcal scalded skin syndrome 288
Epidermolytic toxin 288
Incidence 288
Clinical manifestations 288
Pathophysiology 289
Diagnosis 289
Treatment 289
***Pseudomonas aeruginosa* infection 290**
Pseudomonas folliculitis 290
Pseudomonas hot-foot syndrome 290
Pseudomonas cellulitis 292
External otitis 294
Malignant external otitis 297
Toe web infection 298
Ecthyma gangrenosum 298
Meningococcemia 299
Transmission 299
Incidence 299
Pathophysiology 299

Clinical manifestations 299
Diagnosis 301
Differential diagnosis 301
Management 301
Nontuberculous mycobacteria 304
M. ulcerans, M. fortuitum, M. chelonei, and *M. avium-intracellulare* 304

10   **Sexually Transmitted Bacterial Infections 307**
Sexually transmitted disease presentations 307
Genital ulcers 307
Syphilis 315
Incidence 315
Stages 315
Risk of transmission 317
T. pallidum 317
Primary syphilis 317
Secondary syphilis 318
Latent syphilis 320
Tertiary syphilis 320
Syphilis and human immunodeficiency virus 320
Congenital syphilis 320
Syphilis serology 321
Treatment of syphilis 323
Posttreatment evaluation of syphilis 324
Rare sexually transmitted diseases 325
Lymphogranuloma venereum 325
Chancroid 327
Granuloma inguinale (donovanosis) 329
Diseases characterized by urethritis and cervicitis 330
Gonorrhea 330
Neisseria gonorrhoeae 330
Nongonococcal urethritis 334

11   **Sexually Transmitted Viral Infections 336**
Genital warts 336
Human papillomavirus 336
Incidence 336
Transmission 336
Clinical presentation 337
Diagnosis 340
Treatment 340
Bowenoid papulosis 343
Molluscum contagiosum 344
Clinical manifestations 344
Diagnosis 344
Treatment 345
Genital herpes simplex 346
Prevalence 346
Risk factors 346
Rate of transmission 348
Primary and recurrent infections 348
Prevention 350
Laboratory diagnosis 350
Serology 351
Psychosocial implications 352
Treatment of genital herpes (Centers for Disease Control Guidelines) 352

Genital herpes simplex during pregnancy 354

Neonatal herpes simplex virus infection 355

Acquired immunodeficiency syndrome 356

Human immunodeficiency virus pathogenesis 356

Diagnosis 356

Viral burden 356

Assessment of immune status (CD4 + T-cell determinations) 357

Revised Centers for Disease Control and Prevention classification and management 357

Dermatologic diseases associated with human immunodeficiency virus infection 358

12 Warts, Herpes Simplex, and Other Viral Infections 368

Warts 368

Common warts 371

Filiform and digitate warts 372

Flat warts 373

Plantar warts 374

Subungual and periungual warts 378

Genital warts 378

Molluscum contagiosum 379

Herpes simplex 381

Oral-labial herpes simplex 384

Cutaneous herpes simplex 386

Eczema herpeticum 388

Varicella 389

Chickenpox in the immunocompromised patient 391

Chickenpox and HIV infection 391

Chickenpox during pregnancy 391

Congenital and neonatal chickenpox 392

Herpes zoster 394

Herpes zoster after varicella immunization 398

Herpes zoster and HIV infection 398

Herpes zoster during pregnancy 398

Syndromes 398

Prevention of postherpetic neuralgia: early combined antiviral drugs and antidepressants 404

Treatment of postherpetic neuralgia 404

13 Superficial Fungal Infections 409

Dermatophyte fungal infections 409

Tinea 413

Tinea of the foot 413

Pitted keratolysis 416

Tinea of the groin 417

Tinea of the body and face 420

Tinea of the hand 425

Tinea incognito 426

Tinea of the scalp 427

Tinea of the beard 434

Treatment of fungal infections 434

Candidiasis (Moniliasis) 440

Candidiasis of normally moist areas 440

Candidiasis of large skin folds 446

Candidiasis of small skin folds 449

Chronic mucocutaneous candidiasis 450

Tinea versicolor 451

Pityrosporum folliculitis 454

14 Exanthems and Drug Eruptions 457

Exanthems 460

Measles 460

Hand, foot, and mouth disease 462

Scarlet fever 464

Rubella 467

Erythema infectiosum (parvovirus B19 infection) 468

Roseola infantum (human herpes virus 6 and 7 infection) 471

Enteroviruses: echovirus and coxsackievirus exanthems 473

Kawasaki syndrome 474

Superantigen toxin-mediated illnesses 478

Toxic shock syndrome 479

Cutaneous drug reactions 482

Drug eruptions: clinical patterns and most frequently causal drugs 485

Exanthems (maculopapular) 485

Urticaria 488

Pruritus 489

Drug eruptions 490

Acute generalized exanthemous pustulosis 490

Acneiform (pustular) eruptions 490

Eczema 490

Blistering drug eruptions 491

Erythema multiforme and toxic epidermal necrolysis 491

Exfoliative erythroderma 491

Fixed drug eruptions 492

Lichenoid (lichen planus-like drug eruptions) 493

Lupus erythematosus-like drug eruptions 493

Photosensitivity 493

Pigmentation 494

Vasculitis 494

Lymphomatoid drug eruptions 494

Chemotherapy-induced acral erythema 494

Skin eruptions associated with specific drugs 494

15 Infestations and Bites 497

Scabies 497

Anatomic features, life cycle, and immunology 499

Clinical manifestations 500

Diagnosis 503

Treatment and management 504

Scabies in long-term care facilities 505

Pediculosis 506

Biology and life cycle 506

Clinical manifestations 507

Diagnosis 508

Treatment 509

Caterpillar dermatitis 510

Clinical manifestations 510

Diagnosis 512

Treatment 512

Spiders 512

Black widow spider 512

Brown recluse spider 514
Ticks 516
Lyme disease and erythema migrans 517
Rocky mountain spotted and spotless fever 524
Tick bite paralysis 526
Removing ticks 527
Cat-scratch and related diseases 528
Clinical manifestations 528
Neurologic complications 528
Bacillary angiomatosis 528
Diagnosis of cat-scratch disease 529
Treatment 529
Animal and human bites 529
Management 529
Stinging insects 531
Toxic reactions 531
Allergic reactions 531
Diagnosis 532
Indications for venom skin testing and immunotherapy 532
Treatment 532
Biting insects 533
Papular urticaria 533
Fleas 533
Myiasis 534
Mosquitoes 536
Creeping eruption 537
Management 537
Ants 538
Fire ants 538
Dermatitis associated with swimming 539
Swimmer's itch (fresh water) 539
Nematocyst stings 539
Florida, Caribbean, Bahamas 541
Echinoderms (sea urchins and starfish) 543

16 Vesicular and Bullous Diseases 547
Blisters 547
Autoimmune blistering diseases 547
Major blistering diseases 547
Classification 550
Diagnosis of bullous disorders 551
Dermatitis herpetiformis and linear IgA bullous dermatosis 554
Gluten-sensitive enteropathy 556
Lymphoma 556
Diagnosis of dermatitis herpetiformis 556
Bullae in diabetic persons 559
Pemphigus 559
Pathophysiology 561
Pemphigus vulgaris 561
Pemphigus foliaceus, IgA pemphigus, and pemphigus erythematosus 562
Diagnosis of pemphigus 564
Treatment 565
Pemphigus in association with other diseases 566
The pemphigoid group of diseases 567
Bullous pemphigoid 567

Localized pemphigoid 571
Benign chronic bullous dermatosis of childhood 572
Herpes gestationis (pemphigoid gestationis) 573
Pemphigoid-like disease 574
Epidermolysis bullosa acquisita 574
Benign familial chronic pemphigus 575
Epidermolysis bullosa 576
The newborn with blisters, pustules, erosions, and ulcerations 577

17 Connective Tissue Diseases 587
Diagnosis 587
Antinuclear antibody testing 587
Lupus erythematosus 592
Clinical classification 592
Subsets of cutaneous lupus erythematosus 593
Chronic cutaneous lupus erythematosus 596
Subacute cutaneous lupus erythematosus 598
Systemic lupus erythematosus 600
Other cutaneous signs of lupus erythematosus 602
Drug-induced lupus erythematosus 603
Neonatal lupus erythematosus 604
Diagnosis and management of cutaneous lupus erythematosus 605
Treatment 605
Dermatomyositis and Polymyositis 607
Polymyositis 607
Dermatomyositis 607
Scleroderma 613
Systemic sclerosis 613
Chemically induced scleroderma 613
CREST syndrome 617
Localized scleroderma 620

18 Hypersensitivity Syndromes and Vasculitis 626
Hypersensitivity syndromes 626
Erythema multiforme 626
The Stevens-Johnson syndrome/toxic epidermal necrolysis spectrum of disease 630
Stevens-Johnson syndrome 630
Toxic epidermal necrolysis 632
Erythema nodosum 635
Vasculitis 637
Vasculitis of small vessels 642
Hypersensitivity vasculitis 642
Henoch-Schönlein purpura 645
Antinuclear cytoplasmic antibody-associated small-vessel vasculitis 648
Wegener's granulomatosis 648
Churg-Strauss syndrome 649
Microscopic polyangiitis 649
Antinuclear cytoplasmic antibody-negative small-vessel vasculitis 649
Neutrophilic dermatoses 650
Sweet's syndrome (acute febrile neutrophilic dermatosis) 650
Erythema elevatum diutinum 653
Pyoderma gangrenosum 653
Schamberg's disease 656

19 Light-Related Diseases and Disorders of Pigmentation 661
Photobiology 661
Sun-damaged skin 662
Suntan and sunburn 668
Sun protection 668
Polymorphous light eruption 671
Hydroa aestivale and hydroa vacciniforme 674
Porphyrias 675
Porphyria cutanea tarda 675
Pseudoporphyria 679
Erythropoietic protoporphyria 680
Phototoxic reactions 681
Photoallergy 683
Disorders of hypopigmentation 684
Vitiligo 684
Idiopathic guttate hypomelanosis 689
Pityriasis alba 689
Nevus anemicus 690
Tuberous sclerosis 690
Disorders of hyperpigmentation 691
Freckles 691
Lentigo in children 691
Lentigo in adults 691
Melasma 692
Café-au-lait spots 694
Diabetic dermopathy 694
Erythema ab igne 694

20 Benign Skin Tumors 698
Seborrheic keratoses 698
Stucco keratoses 705
Dermatosis papulosa nigra 706
Cutaneous horn 706
Skin tags (acrochordon) and polyps 706
Dermatofibroma 708
Hypertrophic scars and keloids 709
Keratoacanthoma 711
Epidermal nevus 713
Nevus sebaceous 715
Chondrodermatitis nodularis chronica helicis 716
Epidermal cyst 717
Pilar cyst (wen) 719
Senile sebaceous hyperplasia 720
Syringoma 721

21 Premalignant and Malignant Nonmelanoma Skin Tumors 724
Basal cell carcinoma 724
Pathophysiology 725
Histologic characteristics 726
Clinical types 726
Management and risk of recurrence 732
Actinic keratosis 736
Squamous cell carcinoma 744
Squamous cell carcinoma of the extremities (Marjolin's ulcer) 747

Bowen's disease 748
Erythroplasia of Queyrat 750
Leukoplakia 751
Verrucous carcinoma 753
Arsenical keratoses and other arsenic-related skin diseases 753
Cutaneous T-cell lymphoma 754
Paget's disease of the breast 763
Extramammary Paget's disease 764
Cutaneous metastasis 765

22 Nevi and Malignant Melanoma 773
Melanocytic nevi 773
Common moles 774
Special forms 776
Atypical nevi 782
Malignant melanoma 786
Superficial spreading melanoma 789
Nodular melanoma 792
Lentigo maligna melanoma 794
Acral lentiginous melanoma 796
Benign lesions that resemble melanoma 797
Dermoscopy 798
Classification of atypical melanocytic nevi 799
Pregnancy, oral contraceptives, prognosis, and risk 806
Management 806
Biopsy 806
Initial diagnostic workup 808
Follow-up examinations 808
Staging and prognosis 810
Melanoma staging system 810
Medical treatment 810
Treatment of lentigo maligna 811

23 Vascular Tumors and Malformations 814
Congenital vascular lesions 814
Hemangiomas of infancy 815
Malformations 819
Acquired vascular lesions 824
Cherry angioma 824
Angiokeratomas 824
Venous lake 825
Lymphangioma circumscriptum 825
Pyogenic granuloma (lobular capillary hemangioma) 826
Kaposi's sarcoma 827
Telangiectasias 830
Spider angioma 830
Hereditary hemorrhagic telangiectasia 831
Unilateral nevoid telangiectasia syndrome 832
Scleroderma 832
Generalized essential telangiectasia 832

24 Hair Diseases 834
Anatomy 834
Physiology 836
Evaluation of hair loss 838
Generalized hair loss 841

Localized hair loss 842
Androgenic alopecia in men (male-pattern baldness) 842
Adrenal androgenic female-pattern alopecia 844
Hirsutism 846
Alopecia areata 855
Trichotillomania 858
Traction (cosmetic) alopecia 859
Scarring alopecia 860
Trichomycosis 862

25 **Nail Diseases 864**
Anatomy and physiology 864
Normal variations 868
Nail disorders associated with skin disease 869
Acquired disorders 871
Bacterial and viral infections 871
Fungal nail infections 874
Trauma 880
The nail and internal disease 884
Congenital anomalies 886
Color and drug-induced changes 886
Tumors 888

26 **Cutaneous Manifestations of Internal Disease 893**
Internal cancer and skin disease 893
Cutaneous paraneoplastic syndromes 893
Cutaneous manifestations of diabetes mellitus 896
Necrobiosis lipoidica 896
Granuloma annulare 898
Acanthosis nigricans 900
Xanthomas and dyslipoproteinemia 902
Neurofibromatosis 905
Tuberous sclerosis 909
Cancer-associated genodermatoses 912
Cowden's disease (multiple hamartoma syndrome) 912
Muir-Torre syndrome 914
Gardner's syndrome 915

Pseudoxanthoma elasticum 916
Guide to information for families with inherited skin disorders 917

27 **Dermatologic Surgical Procedures 921**
Local anesthesia 922
Hemostasis 922
Wound healing 923
Postoperative wound care 925
Skin biopsy 926
Punch biopsy 926
Shave biopsy and shave excision 926
Simple scissor excision 928
Electrodesiccation and curettage 929
Techniques 929
Curettage 930
Techniques—curettage 930
Techniques—electrodesiccation and curettage of basal cell carcinoma 930
Blunt dissection 931
Technique 931
Cryosurgery 931
Technique 932
Extraction of cysts 933
Technique 933
Mohs' micrographic surgery 934
Technique 934
Chemical peels 936
Filling materials 936
Liposuction 936
Lasers 937
Botulinum toxin 938

Appendix 940

Dermatologic Formulary 945

Index 975

SKIN ANATOMY

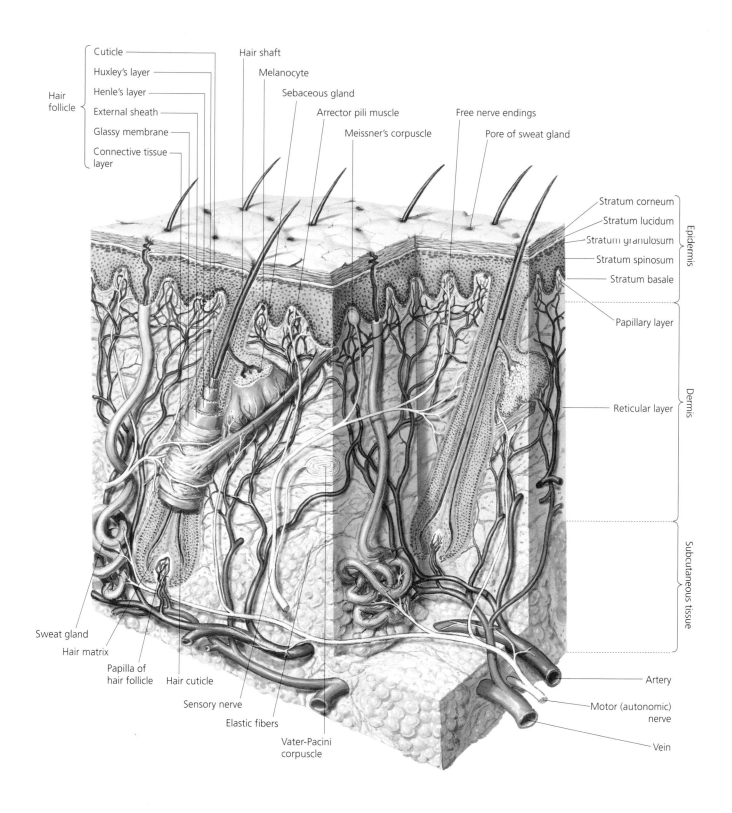

Hair follicle
- Cuticle
- Huxley's layer
- Henle's layer
- External sheath
- Glassy membrane
- Connective tissue layer

Hair shaft

Melanocyte

Sebaceous gland

Arrector pili muscle

Meissner's corpuscle

Free nerve endings

Pore of sweat gland

Stratum corneum
Stratum lucidum
Stratum granulosum
Stratum spinosum
Stratum basale

Epidermis

Papillary layer

Reticular layer

Dermis

Subcutaneous tissue

Sweat gland

Hair matrix

Papilla of hair follicle

Hair cuticle

Sensory nerve

Elastic fibers

Vater-Pacini corpuscle

Artery

Motor (autonomic) nerve

Vein

Principles of Diagnosis and Anatomy

❑ **Skin anatomy**
  Epidermis
  Dermis
  Dermal nerves and vasculature

❑ **Diagnosis of skin disease**
  A methodical approach
  Examination technique
  Approach to treatment
  Primary lesions
  Secondary lesions
  Special skin lesions

❑ **Regional differential diagnoses**

Skin Anatomy

The skin is divided into three layers: the epidermis, the dermis, and the subcutaneous tissue. The skin is thicker on the dorsal and extensor surfaces than on the ventral and flexor surfaces.

Epidermis

The epidermis is the outermost part of the skin; it is stratified squamous epithelium. The thickness of the epidermis ranges from 0.05 mm on the eyelids to 1.5 mm on the palms and soles. The microscopic anatomy of the epidermal-dermal junction is complex; it is discussed in detail in Chapter 16. The innermost layer of the epidermis consists of a single row of columnar cells called basal cells. Basal cells divide to form keratinocytes (prickle cells), which comprise the spinous layer. The cells of the spinous layer are connected to each other by intercellular bridges or spines, which appear histologically as lines between cells. The keratinocytes synthesize insoluble protein, which remains in the cell and eventually becomes a major component of the outer layer (the stratum

corneum). The cells continue to flatten, and their cytoplasm appears granular (stratum granulosum); they finally die as they reach the surface to form the stratum corneum. There are three types of branched cells in the epidermis: the melanocyte, which synthesizes pigment (melanin); Langerhans' cell, which serves as a frontline element in immune reactions of the skin; and Merkel's cell, the function of which is not clearly defined.

Dermis

The dermis varies in thickness from 0.3 mm on the eyelid to 3.0 mm on the back; it is composed of three types of connective tissue: collagen, elastic tissue, and reticular fibers. The dermis is divided into two layers: the thin upper layer, called the papillary layer, is composed of thin, haphazardly arranged collagen fibers; the thicker lower layer, called the reticular layer, extends from the base of the papillary layer to the subcutaneous tissue and is composed of thick collagen fibers that are arranged parallel to the surface of the skin. Histiocytes are wandering macrophages that accumulate hemosiderin, melanin, and debris created by inflammation. Mast cells, located primarily about blood vessels, manufacture and release histamine and heparin.

Dermal nerves and vasculature

The sensations of touch and pressure are received by Meissner's and the Vater-Pacini corpuscles. The sensations of pain, itch, and temperature are received by unmyelinated nerve endings in the papillary dermis. A low intensity of stimulation created by inflammation causes itching, whereas a high intensity of stimulation created by inflammation causes pain. Therefore scratching converts the intolerable sensation of itching to the more tolerable sensation of pain and eliminates pruritus.

The autonomic system supplies the motor innervation of the skin. Adrenergic fibers innervate the blood vessels (vasoconstriction), hair erector muscles, and apocrine glands. Autonomic fibers to eccrine sweat glands are cholinergic. The sebaceous gland is regulated by the endocrine system and is not innervated by autonomic fibers. The anatomy of the hair follicle is described in Chapter 24.

Diagnosis of Skin Disease

What could be easier than the diagnosis of skin disease? The pathology is before your eyes! Why then do nondermatologists have such difficulty interpreting what they see?

There are three reasons. First, there are literally hundreds of cutaneous diseases. Second, a single entity can vary in its appearance. A common seborrheic keratosis, for example, may have a smooth, rough, or eroded surface and a border that is either uniform or as irregular as a melanoma. Third, skin diseases are dynamic and change in morphology. Many diseases undergo an evolutionary process: herpes simplex may begin as a red papule, evolve into a blister, and then become an erosion that heals with scarring. If hundreds of entities can individually vary in appearance and evolve through several stages, then it is necessary to recognize thousands of permutations to diagnose cutaneous entities confidently. What at first glance appeared to be simple to diagnose may later appear to be simply impossible.

Dermatology is a morphologically oriented specialty. As in other specialties, the medical history is important; however, the ability to interpret what is observed is even more important. The diagnosis of skin disease must be approached in an orderly and logical manner. The temptation to make rapid judgments after hasty observation must be controlled.

A methodical approach

The recommended approach to the patient with skin disease is as follows:

HISTORY. Obtain a brief history, noting duration, rate of onset, location, symptoms, family history, allergies, occupation, and previous treatment.

DISTRIBUTION. Determine the extent of the eruption by having the patient disrobe completely.

PRIMARY LESION. Determine the primary lesion. Examine the lesions carefully; a hand lens is a valuable aid for studying skin lesions. Determine the nature of any secondary or special lesions.

DIFFERENTIAL DIAGNOSIS. Formulate a differential diagnosis.

TESTS. Obtain a biopsy and perform laboratory tests, such as skin biopsy, potassium hydroxide examination for fungi, skin scrapings for scabies, Gram stain, fungal and bacterial cultures, cytology (Tzanck test), Wood's light examination, patch tests, dark field examination, and blood tests.

Examination technique

DISTRIBUTION. The skin should be examined methodically. An eye scan over wide areas is inefficient. It is most productive to mentally divide the skin surface into several sections and carefully study each section. For example, when studying the face, examine the area around each eye, the nose, the mouth, the cheeks, and the temples.

During an examination, patients may show small areas of their skin, tell the doctor that the rest of the eruption looks the same, and expect an immediate diagnosis. The rest of the eruption may or may not look the same. Patients with rashes should receive a complete skin examination to determine the distribution and confirm the diagnosis. Decisions about quantities of medication to dispense require visualization of the big picture. Many dermatologists now advocate a complete skin examination for all of their patients. Because of an awareness that some patients are uncomfortable undressing completely when they have a specific request such as treatment of a plantar wart, other dermatologists advocate a case-by-case approach.

PRIMARY LESIONS AND SURFACE CHARACTERISTICS. Lesions should be examined carefully. Standing back and viewing a disease process provides valuable information about the distribution. Close examination with a magnifying device provides much more information. Often the primary lesion is identified and the diagnosis is confirmed at this step. The physician should learn the surface characteristics of all the common entities and gain experience by examining known entities. A flesh-colored papule might be a wart, sebaceous hyperplasia, or a basal cell carcinoma. The surface characteristics of many lesions are illustrated throughout this book.

Approach to treatment

Most skin diseases can be managed successfully with the numerous agents and techniques available. If a diagnosis has not been established, medications should not be prescribed; this applies particularly to prescription of topical steroids. Some physicians are tempted to experiment with various medications and, if the treatment fails, to refer the patient to a specialist. This is not a logical or efficient way to practice medicine.

Primary lesions

Most skin diseases begin with a basic lesion that is referred to as a primary lesion. Identification of the primary lesion is the key to accurate interpretation and description of cutaneous disease. Its presence provides the initial orientation and allows the formulation of a differential diagnosis. Definitions of the primary lesions and their differential diagnoses are listed and illustrated on pp. 3 to 11.

Secondary lesions

Secondary lesions develop during the evolutionary process of skin disease or are created by scratching or infection. They may be the only type of lesion present, in which case the primary disease process must be inferred. The differential diagnoses of secondary lesions are listed and illustrated on pp. 12 to 16.

Primary Lesions—Macules

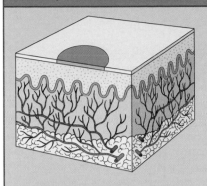

Macule

A circumscribed, flat discoloration that may be brown, blue, red, or hypopigmented

Brown

Becker's nevus (p. 780)
Café-au-lait spot (p. 694)
Erythrasma (p. 419)
Fixed drug eruption (p. 492)
Freckle (p. 691)
Junction nevus (p. 774)
Lentigo (p. 691)
Lentigo maligna (p. 794)
Melasma (p. 692)
Photoallergic drug eruption (p. 683)
Phototoxic drug eruption (p. 681)
Stasis dermatitis (p. 73)
Tinea nigra palmaris

Blue

Ink (tattoo)
Maculae ceruleae (lice) (p. 508)
Mongolian spot
Ochronosis

Red

Drug eruptions (p. 485)
Juvenile rheumatoid arthritis
   (Still's disease)
Rheumatic fever
Secondary syphilis (p. 318)
Viral exanthems (p. 473)

Hypopigmented

Idiopathic guttate hypomelanosis (p. 689)
Nevus anemicus (p. 690)
Piebaldism
Postinflammatory psoriasis (p. 222)
Radiation dermatitis
Tinea versicolor (p. 451)
Tuberous sclerosis (p. 690)
Vitiligo (p. 684)

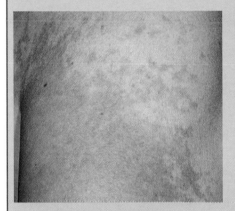

Becker's nevus

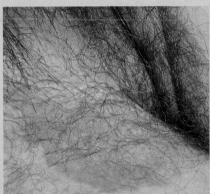

Erythrasma

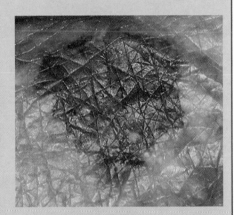

Lentigo

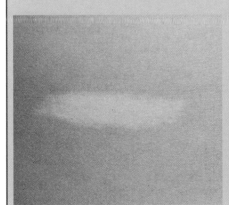

Tuberous sclerosis

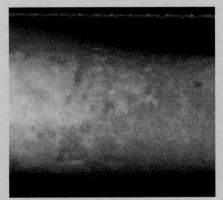

Phototoxic drug eruption

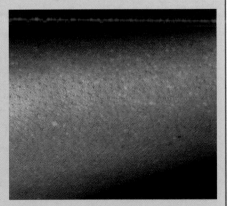

Idiopathic guttate hypomelanosis

Primary Skin Lesions—Papules

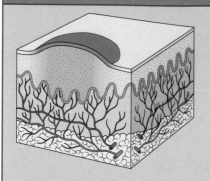

Papule

An elevated solid lesion up to 0.5 cm in diameter; color varies; papules may become confluent and form plaques

Flesh colored, yellow, or white
Achrochordon (skin tag) (p. 706)
Adenoma sebaceum (p. 909)
Basal cell epithelioma (p. 724)
Closed comedone (acne) (p. 171)
Flat warts (p. 373)
Granuloma annulare (p. 898)
Lichen nitidus
Lichen sclerosis et atrophicus (p. 257)
Milium (p. 194)
Molluscum contagiosum (p. 379)
Nevi (dermal) (p. 776)
Neurofibroma (p. 906)
Pearly penile papules (p. 339)
Pseudoxanthoma elasticum (p. 916)
Sebaceous hyperplasia (p. 720)
Skin tags (p. 706)
Syringoma (p. 721)
Brown
Dermatofibroma (p. 708)
Keratosis follicularis
Melanoma (p. 786)
Nevi (p. 774)
Seborrheic keratosis (p. 698)
Urticaria pigmentosa (p. 156)
Warts (p. 371)

Red
Acne (p. 172)
Atopic dermatitis (p. 107)
Cat-scratch disease (p. 528)
Cherry angioma (p. 824)
Cholinergic urticaria (p. 145)
Chondrodermatitis helicis (p. 716)
Eczema (p. 414)
Folliculitis (p. 279)
Insect bites (p. 534)
Keratosis pilaris (p. 116)
Leukocytoclastic vasculitis (p. 643)
Miliaria (p. 205)
Polymorphic light eruption (p. 672)
Psoriasis (p. 212)
Pyogenic granuloma (p. 826)
Scabies (p. 500)
Urticaria (p. 130)
Blue or violaceous
Angiokeratoma (p. 824)
Blue nevus (p. 782)
Lichen planus (p. 250)
Lymphoma
Kaposi's sarcoma (pp. 365, 827)
Melanoma (p. 786)
Mycosis fungoides (p. 754)
Venous lake (p. 825)

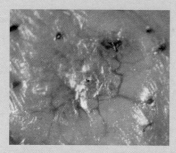

Sebaceous hyperplasia

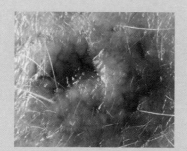

Basal cell epithelioma

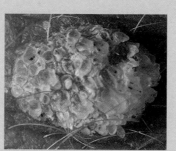

Wart (cylindrical projections)

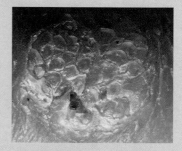

Wart (mosaic surface)

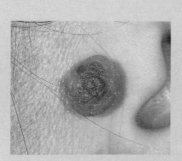

Nevi (dermal)

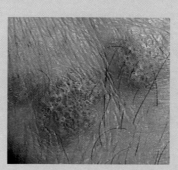

Lichen planus

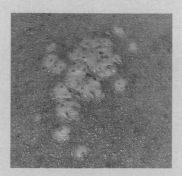

Lichen sclerosis et atrophicus

Primary Skin Lesions—Papules

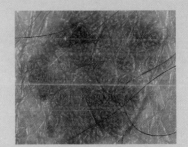

Seborrheic keratosis

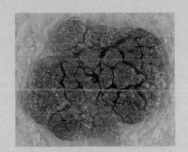

Seborrheic keratosis

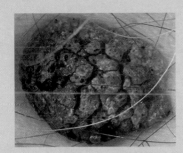

Seborrheic keratosis

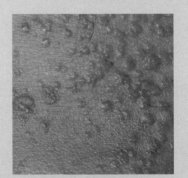

Melanoma

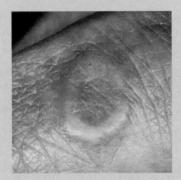

Granuloma annulare

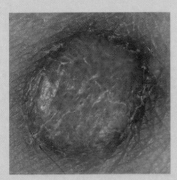

Dermatofibroma

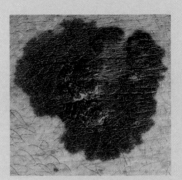

Flat warts

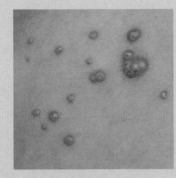

Molluscum contagiosum

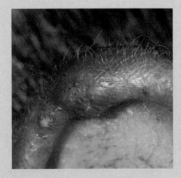

Chondrodermatitis nodularis chronica helicis

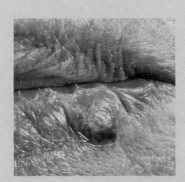

Venous lake

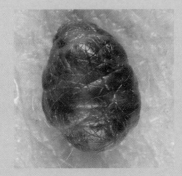

Cherry angioma

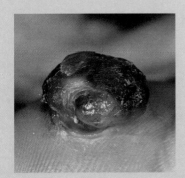

Pyogenic granuloma

Primary Skin Lesions—Plaques

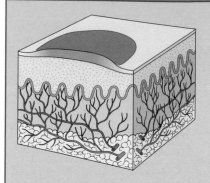

Plaque

A circumscribed, elevated, superficial, solid lesion more than 0.5 cm in diameter, often formed by the confluence of papules

Eczema (p. 45)

Cutaneous T-cell lymphoma (p. 754)

Paget's disease (p. 763)

Sweet's syndrome (p. 650)

Papulosquamous (papular and scaling) lesions (p. 209)

Discoid lupus erythematosus (p. 596)

Lichen planus (p. 250)

Pityriasis rosea (p. 246)

Psoriasis (p. 210)

Seborrheic dermatitis (p. 245)

Syphilis (secondary) (p. 318)

Tinea corporis (p. 420)

Tinea pedis (p. 413)

Tinea versicolor (p. 451)

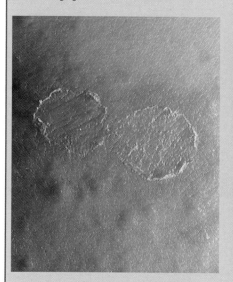

Pityriasis rosea

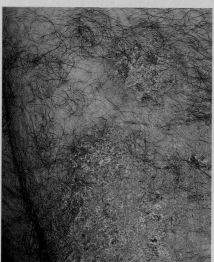

Eczema

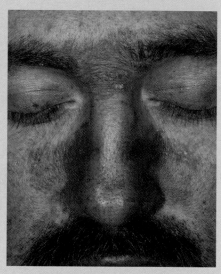

Seborrheic dermatitis

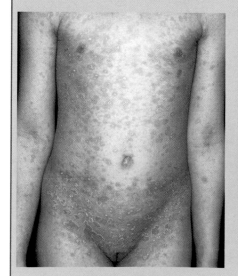

Pityriasis rosea

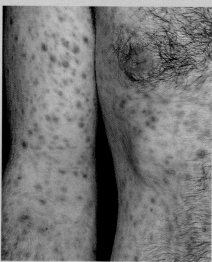

Syphilis (secondary)

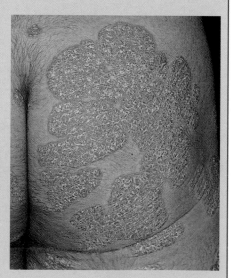

Psoriasis

Primary Skin Lesions—Plaques

Lichen planus

Discoid lupus erythematosus

Cutaneous T-cell lymphoma

Tinea corporis

Tinea pedis

Tinea versicolor

Psoriasis

Paget's disease

Sweet's syndrome

Primary Skin Lesions—Nodules

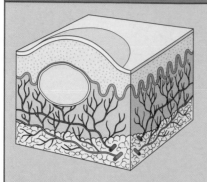

Nodule
A circumscribed, elevated, solid lesion more than 0.5 cm in diameter; a large nodule is referred to as a tumor

Basal cell carcinoma (p. 724)
Erythema nodosum (p. 635)
Furuncle (p. 284)
Hemangioma (p. 815)
Kaposi's sarcoma (pp. 365, 827)
Keratoacanthoma (p. 711)
Lipoma
Lymphoma
Melanoma (p. 786)
Metastatic carcinoma (p. 766)
Cutaneous T-cell lymphoma (p. 754)
Neurofibromatosis (p. 906)
Prurigo nodularis (p. 68)
Sporotrichosis
Squamous cell carcinoma (p. 744)
Warts (p. 371)
Xanthoma (p. 904)

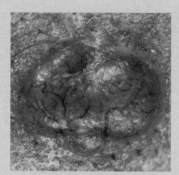

Basal cell carcinoma

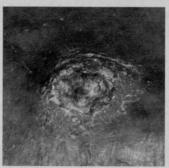

Squamous cell carcinoma

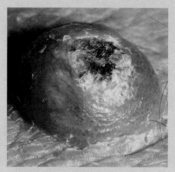

Keratoacanthoma

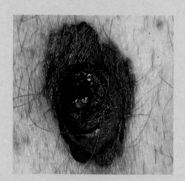

Melanoma

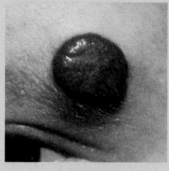

Hemangioma

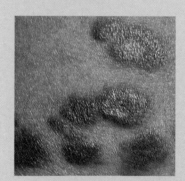

Kaposi's sarcoma

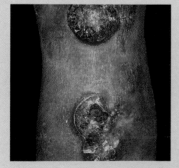

Cutaneous T-cell lymphoma

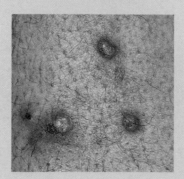

Prurigo nodularis

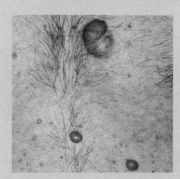

Neurofibromatosis

Primary Skin Lesions—Pustules

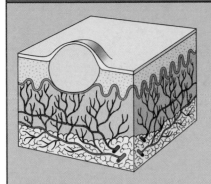

Pustule

A circumscribed collection of leuko-cytes and free fluid that varies in size

Acne (p. 172)
Candidiasis (p. 446)
Chicken pox (p. 39)
Dermatophyte infection (p. 417)
Dyshidrosis (p. 58)
Folliculitis (p. 279)
Gonococcemia (p. 333)
Hidradenitis suppurativa (p. 202)
Herpes simplex (p. 382)
Herpes zoster (p. 395)
Impetigo (p. 268)
Keratosis pilaris (p. 116)
Pseudomonas folliculitis (p. 290)
Psoriasis (p. 213)
Pyoderma gangrenosum (p. 653)
Rosacea (p. 198)
Scabies (p. 500)
Varicella (p. 390)

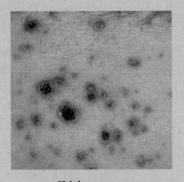

Chicken pox

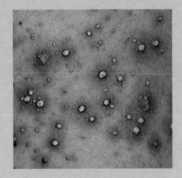

Folliculitis

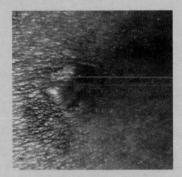

Gonococcemia

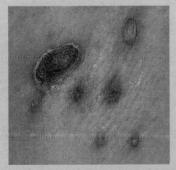

Impetigo

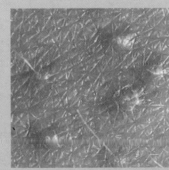

Keratosis pilaris

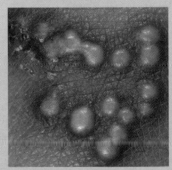

Herpes simplex

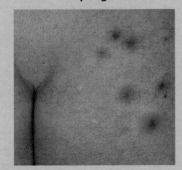

Pseudomonas folliculitis

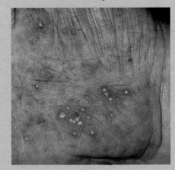

Dyshidrosis

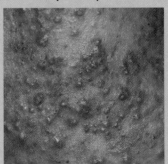

Acne

Primary Skin Lesions—Vesicles and Bullae

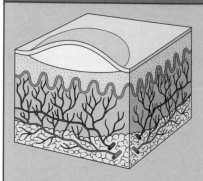

Vesicle
A circumscribed collection of free fluid up to 0.5 cm in diameter

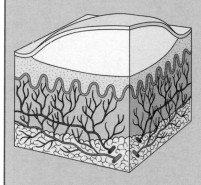

Bulla
A circumscribed collection of free fluid more than 0.5 cm in diameter

Vesicles
Benign familial chronic pemphigus (p. 575)
Cat-scratch disease (p. 528)
Chicken pox (p. 390)
Dermatitis herpetiformis (p. 554)
Eczema (acute) (p. 42)
Erythema multiforme (p. 629)
Herpes simplex (p. 382)
Herpes zoster (p. 395)
Impetigo (p. 268)
Lichen planus
Pemphigus foliaceus (p. 568)
Porphyria cutanea tarda (p. 678)
Scabies (p. 500)

Bullae
Bullae in diabetics (p. 559)
Bullous pemphigoid (p. 568)
Cicatricial pemphigoid (p. 571)
Epidermolysis bullosa acquisita (p. 574)
Fixed drug eruption (p. 492)
Herpes gestationis (p. 573)
Lupus erythematosus
Pemphigus (p. 561)

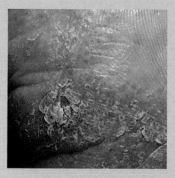

Eczema (acute)

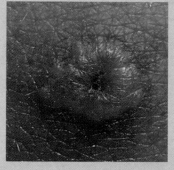

Chicken pox

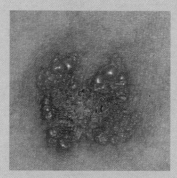

Dermatitis herpetiformis

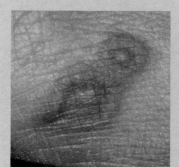

Erythema multiforme

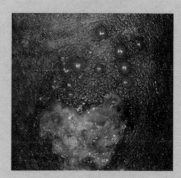

Herpes simplex

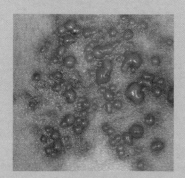

Herpes zoster

Primary Skin Lesions—Wheals (Hives)

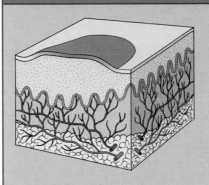

Angioedema (p. 147)
Dermographism (p. 142)
Hives (p. 130)
Cholinergic urticaria (p. 145)
Urticaria pigmentosa (mastocytosis) (p. 156)

Wheal (hive)

A firm edematous plaque resulting from infiltration of the dermis with fluid; wheals are transient and may last only a few hours

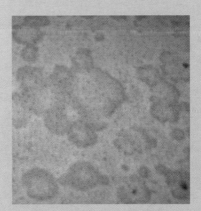

Angioedema

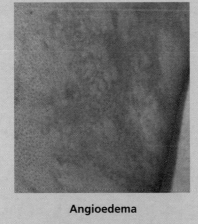

Angioedema

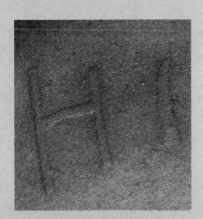

Dermographism

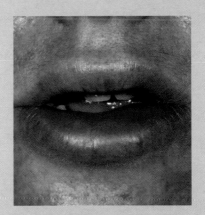

Hives

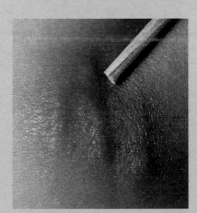

Urticaria pigmentosa

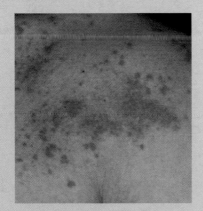

Cholinergic urticaria

Secondary Skin Lesions—Scales

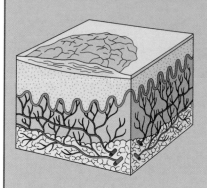

Scales
Excess dead epidermal cells that are produced by abnormal keratinization and shedding

Fine to stratified
Erythema craquele (p. 60)
Ichthyosis—dominant (quadrangular) (p. 115)
Ichthyosis—sex-linked (quadrangular) (p. 115)
Lupus erythematosus (carpet tack) (p. 596)
Pityriasis rosea (collarette) (p. 247)
Psoriasis (silvery) (p. 210)
Scarlet fever (fine, on trunk) (p. 465)
Seborrheic dermatitis (p. 245)
Syphilis (secondary) (p. 318)
Tinea (dermatophytes) (p. 410)
Tinea versicolor (p. 451)
Xerosis (dry skin) (p. 23)
Scaling in sheets (desquamation)
Kawasaki syndrome (p. 476)
Scarlet fever (hands and feet) (p. 466)
Staphylococcal scalded skin syndrome (p. 288)
Toxic shock syndrome (p. 479)

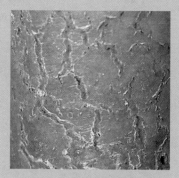

**Erythema craquele
(dense scale)**

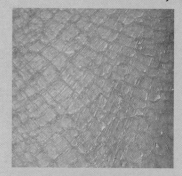

**Ichthyosis—dominant
(quadrangular)**

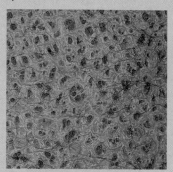

**Ichthyosis—sex-linked
(quadrangular)**

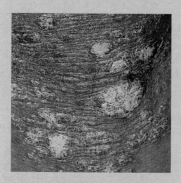

Psoriasis (silvery)

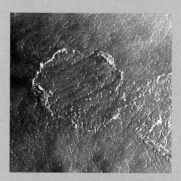

Pityriasis rosea (collarette)

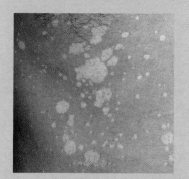

Tinea versicolor (fine)

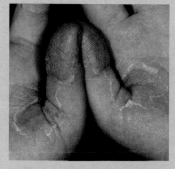

Scarlet fever (desquamation)

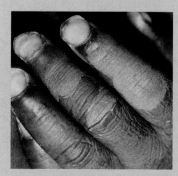

**Kawasaki syndrome
(desquamation)**

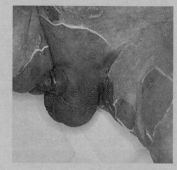

**Staphylococcal scalded
skin syndrome (desquamation)**

Secondary Skin Lesions—Crusts

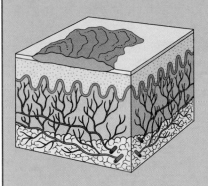

Acute eczematous inflammation (p. 42)
Atopic (face) (p. 109)
Impetigo (honey colored) (p. 270)
Pemphigus foliaceus (p. 563)
Tinea capitis (p. 431)

Crust
A collection of dried serum and cellular debris; a scab

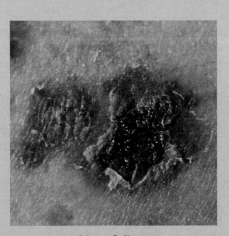

Atopic (lips)

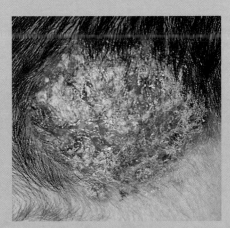

Impetigo (honey colored)

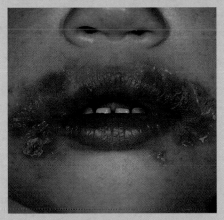

Pemphigus foliaceus

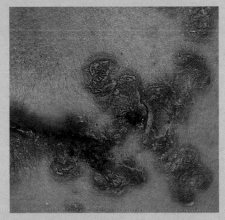

Tinea capitis

Secondary Skin Lesions—Erosions and Ulcers

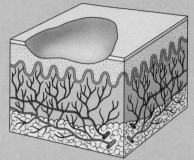

Erosion

A focal loss of epidermis; erosions do not penetrate below the dermoepidermal junction and therefore heal without scarring

Candidiasis (p. 445)

Dermatophyte infection (p. 413)

Eczematous diseases (p. 63)

Herpes simplex (p. 381)

Intertrigo (p. 447)

Neurotic excoriations (p. 69)

Perlèche (p. 450)

Senile skin (p. 665)

Tinea pedis (p. 413)

Toxic epidermal necrolysis (p. 633)

Vesiculobullous diseases (p. 547)

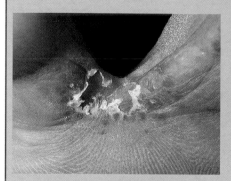

Tinea Pedis

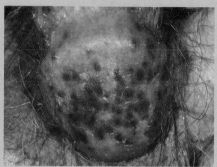

Candidiasis

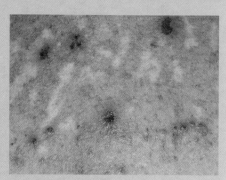

Neurotic excoriations

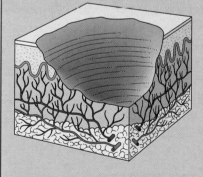

Ulcer

A focal loss of epidermis and dermis; ulcers heal with scarring

Aphthae

Chancroid (p. 327)

Decubitus

Factitial (p. 69)

Ischemic

Necrobiosis lipoidica (p. 897)

Neoplasms (p. 728)

Pyoderma gangrenosum (p. 653)

Radiodermatitis

Syphilis (chancre) (p. 316)

Stasis ulcers (p. 74)

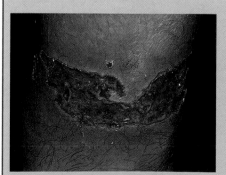

Ulcer

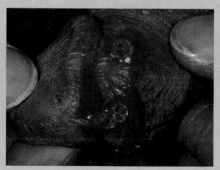

Chancroid

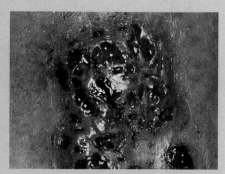

Pyoderma gangrenosum

Secondary Skin Lesions—Fissures and Atrophy

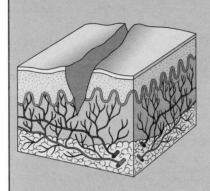

Chapping (hands, feet) (p. 51)
Eczema (fingertip) (p. 56)
Intertrigo (p. 447)
Perlèche (p. 450)

Fissure
A linear loss of epidermis and dermis with sharply defined, nearly vertical walls

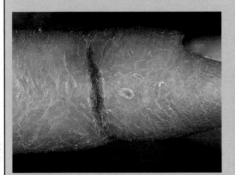

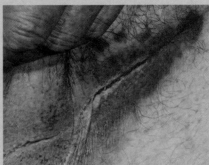

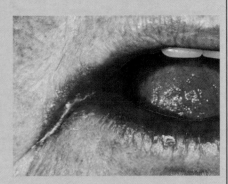

| Eczema | Intertrigo | Perlèche |

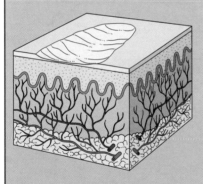

Aging (p. 665)
Dermatomyositis (p. 608)
Discoid lupus erythematosus (p. 97)
Lichen sclerosis et atrophicus (p. 257)
Morphea (p. 621)
Necrobiosis lipoidica (p. 897)
Radiodermatitis
Striae (p. 37)
Topical and intralesional steroids (p. 35)

Atrophy
A depression in the skin resulting from thinning of the epidermis or dermis

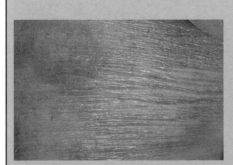

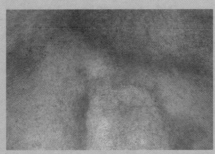

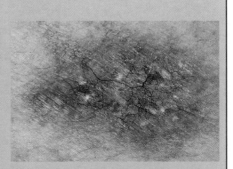

| Lichen sclerosis et atrophicus | Morphea | Topical and intralesional steroids |

Secondary Skin Lesions—Scars

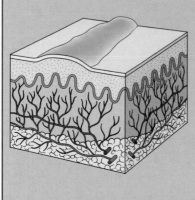

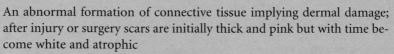

Acne (p. 174)

Burns

Herpes zoster (p. 397)

Hidradenitis suppurativa (p. 202)

Keloid (p. 709)

Porphyria (p. 678)

Varicella (p. 390)

Scar

An abnormal formation of connective tissue implying dermal damage; after injury or surgery scars are initially thick and pink but with time become white and atrophic

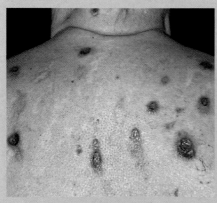

Keloid

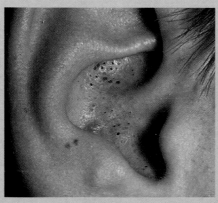

Herpes zoster

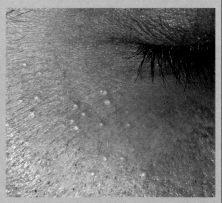

Porphyria

Special Skin Lesions

EXCORIATION

An erosion caused by scratching; excoriations are often linear

COMEDONE

A plug of sebaceous and keratinous material lodged in the opening of a hair
   follicle; the follicular orifice may be dilated (blackhead) or narrowed
   (whitehead or closed comedone)

MILIA

A small, superficial keratin cyst with no visible opening

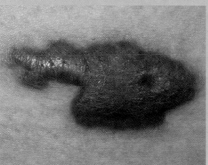

Excoriation

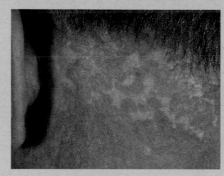

Comedones

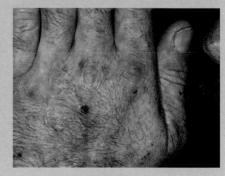

Milia

Special Skin Lesions—cont'd

CYST

A circumscribed lesion with a wall and a lumen; the lumen may contain fluid or solid matter

BURROW

A narrow, elevated, tortuous channel produced by a parasite

LICHENIFICATION

An area of thickened epidermis induced by scratching; the skin lines are accentuated so that the surface looks like a washboard

TELANGIECTASIA

Dilated superficial blood vessels

PETECHIAE

A circumscribed deposit of blood less than 0.5 cm in diameter

PURPURA

A circumscribed deposit of blood greater than 0.5 cm in diameter

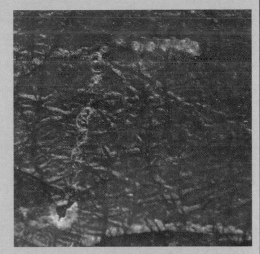

Scabies burrow

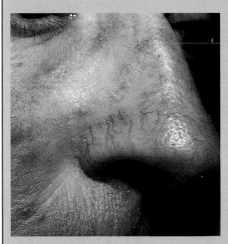

Telangiectasia rosacea

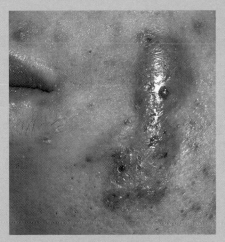

Acne cyst

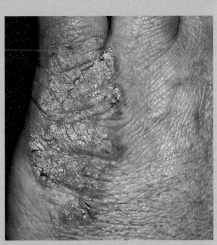

Lichenification

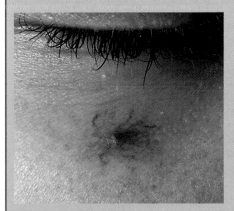

T. spider angioma

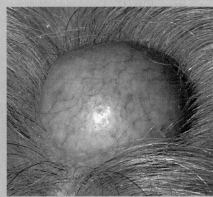

Pilar cyst

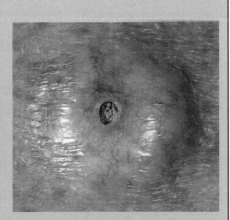

Epidermal cyst

Regional Differential Diagnoses

Most skin diseases have preferential areas of involvement. Disease locations are illustrated below; diseases are listed alphabetically by location on pp. 19 to 22. Common diseases that are obvious to most practitioners are not included.

Diseases such as contact dermatitis and herpes zoster that can be found on any skin surface have also been left out of most of the lists.

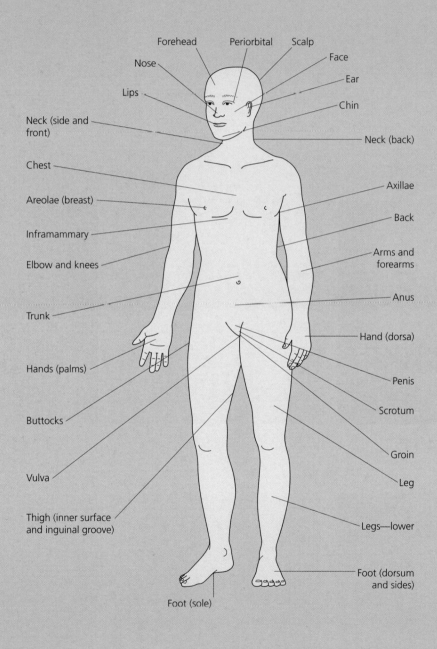

Forehead Periorbital Scalp
Nose Face
Lips Ear
Chin
Neck (side and front) Neck (back)
Chest Axillae
Areolae (breast) Back
Inframammary Arms and forearms
Elbow and knees Anus
Trunk Hand (dorsa)
Hands (palms) Penis
Buttocks Scrotum
Vulva Groin
Thigh (inner surface and inguinal groove) Leg
Legs—lower
Foot (dorsum and sides)
Foot (sole)

Regional Differential Diagnoses—cont'd

Anus
Candidiasis 445
Condyloma lata (secondary syphilis) 318
Extramammary Paget's disease 764
Gonorrhea 332
Herpes simplex/zoster 381
Hidradenitis suppurativa 202
Lichen sclerosis et atrophicus 257
Lichen simplex chronicus 54
Psoriasis (gluteal pinking) 211
Streptococcal cellulitis 277
Syphilis (primary—chancre) 317
Vitiligo 684
Warts 364

Areolae (breast)
Eczema 45
Fox-Fordyce spots 169
Paget's disease 763
Seborrheic keratosis 702

Arms and forearms
Acne 192
Atopic dermatitis 111
Cat-scratch disease 528
Dermatitis herpetiformis (elbows) 554
Dermatomyositis 607
Eruptive xanthoma 904
Erythema multiforme 626
Granuloma annulare 898
Herpes zoster 394
Insect bite 533
Keratoacanthoma 711
Keratosis pilaris 116
Leukocytoclastic vasculitis 642
Lichen planus 250
Lupus erythematosus 600
Neurotic excoriations 68
Nummular eczema 54
Pigmentary demarcation lines
Pityriasis alba (white spots) 118
Polymorphic light eruption 671

Prurigo nodularis 68
Purpura (in sun-damaged skin) 662
Scabies 497
Scleroderma 613
Seborrheic keratosis (flat) 664
Sporotrichoid spread
Squamous cell carcinoma 744
Stellate pseudo scars 665
Sweet's syndrome 650
Swimming pool granuloma (mycobacteria) 304
Tinea 420

Axillae
Acanthosis nigricans 900
Acrochordons 706
Candidiasis 447
Contact dermatitis 85
Erythrasma 419
Fox-Fordyce spots 169
Freckling-Crowe's Sign (von Recklinghausen's disease) 906
Furunculosis 286
Hailey-Hailey disease 551
Hidradenitis suppurativa 202
Impetigo 267
Lice 506
Pseudoxanthoma elasticum 916
Scabies 497
Striae distensae 37
Tinea 420
Trichomycosis axillaris 862

Back
Acne 174
Amyloidosis 894
Atrophoderma
Becker's nevus 780
Cutaneous T cell lymphoma 754
Dermatographism 142
Erythema ab igne 694
Keloids—acne scars 709
Lichen spinulosis
Melanoma 790
Nevus anemicus 690
Notalgia paresthetica

Pityriasis lichenoides et varioliformis acuta (PLEVA) 261
Seborrheic keratosis 698
Striae distensae 37
Tinea versicolor 451
Transient acantholytic dermatosis (Grover's disease)

Buttocks
Cutaneous T cell lymphoma 754
Erythema ab igne 694
Furunculosis 286
Herpes simplex (females) 386
Hidradenitis suppurativa 202
Psoriasis 212
Scabies 497
Striae distensae 37
Tinea 421

Chest
Acne 174
Actinic keratosis 736
Darier's disease
Eruptive syringoma 4
Eruptive vellus hair cyst
Keloids 16
Nevus anemicus 3
Seborrheic dermatitis 242
Steatocystoma multiplex 451
Tinea versicolor 451
Transient acantholytic dermatitis (Grover's disease)

Chin
Acne 172
Atopic dermatitis 108
Basal cell carcinoma 720
Dental sinus
Epidermal cyst 717
Impetigo 267
Perioral dermatitis 30
Warts (flat) 373

Ear
Actinic keratosis 736
Atypical fibroxanthoma
Basal cell carcinoma 720

Bowen's disease 748
Cellulitis 294
Chondrodermatitis nodularis chronica helicis 716
Eczema (infected) 296
Epidermal cyst 717
Hydroa vacciniforme 674
Keloid (lobe) 709
Lupus erythematosus (discoid) 596
Lymphangitis 294
Melanoma 795
Ochronosis 3
Pseudocyst
Psoriasis 218
Ramsey-Hunt syndrome (herpes zoster) 399
Relapsing polychondritis
Seborrheic dermatitis 242
Squamous cell carcinoma 744
Tophi (gout)
Venous lake 825

Elbows and knees
Calcinosis cutis/CREST 617
Dermatitis herpetiformis 554
Erythema multiforme 491
Gout
Granuloma annulare 898
Lichen simplex chronicus 54
Psoriasis 210
Rheumatoid nodule
Scabies 497
Xanthoma 902

Face
Actinic keratosis 742
Adenoma sebaceum 4
Alopecia mucinosa 894
Angioedema 129
Atopic dermatitis 108
Basal cell carcinoma 720
Cowden's disease 912
CREST 617
Dermatosis papulosa nigra 706
Eczema 85
Erysipelas 273

Continued

Regional Differential Diagnoses—cont'd

Face—cont'd

Favre Racouchot (senile
  comedones) 194
Granuloma faciale
Herpes simplex 381
Herpes zoster 394
Impetigo 267
Keratoacanthoma 711
Lentigo maligna 794
Lupus erythematosus
  (discoid) 596
Lupus erythematosus
  (systemic) 600
Lymphocytoma cutis
Melasma 3
Molluscum contagiosum
  344
Nevus sebaceous 715
Pemphigus erythematosus
  559
Perioral dermatitis 30
Pilomatrixoma
Pityriasis alba (white spots)
  118
Psoriasis 214
Rosacea 198
Scleroderma 613
Sebaceous hyperplasia 720
Seborrheic dermatitis 242
Seborrheic keratosis 698
Secondary syphilis 318
Spitz's nevus 781
Squamous cell carcinoma
  744
Steroid rosacea 30
Sweet's syndrome 627
Sycosis barbae
  (folliculitis-beard) 282
Tinea 434
Trichoepitheliomas 909
Warts (flat) 373
Wegener's granulomatosis
  640

Foot (dorsum and sides)

Calcaneal petechiae
  (black heel) 374
Contact dermatitis 85
Cutaneous larva migrans
  537
Erythema multiforme 491
Granuloma annulare 898

Hand, foot, and mouth
  disease 462
Keratoderma blennorrhag-
  ica (Reiter's disease) 216
Lichen planus 250
Lichen simplex chronicus
  54
Painful fat herniation
  (piezogenic papules)
Pernio
Pyogenic granuloma 826
Scabies 497
Stucco keratosis 705
Tinea 413

Foot (sole)

Arsenical keratosis 753
Corn (clavus) 374
Cutaneous larva migrans
  537
Dyshidrotic eczema
Epidermolysis bullosum
  576
Erythema multiforme 491
Hand, foot, and mouth
  disease 462
Hyperkeratosis 580
Immersion foot
Juvenile plantar dermatosis
Keratoderma
Keratoderma blennorrhag-
  ica (Reiter's disease) 216
Lichen planus 252
Melanoma 796
Nevi 774
Pitted keratolysis 416
Pityriasis rubra pilaris
  240
Psoriasis (pustular) 214
Pyogenic granuloma 826
Rocky Mountain spotted
  fever 524
Scabies (infants) 502
Syphilis (secondary) 318
Tinea 413
Tinea (bullous) 414
Verrucous carcinoma 753
Wart

Forehead

Actinic keratosis 736
Basal cell carcinoma 720
Flat warts 373

Herpes zoster 394
Psoriasis 214
Scleroderma (en coup
  de sabre) 622
Sebaceous hyperplasia 720
Seborrheic dermatitis 242
Seborrheic keratosis 698
Sweet's syndrome 627

Groin

Acrochordons (skin tags)
  706
Candidiasis 440
Condyloma 338
Erythrasma 419
Extramammary Paget's
  disease 764
Hailey-Hailey disease 551
Hidradenitis suppurativa
  202
Histiocytosis X 580
Intertrigo 15
Lichen simplex chronicus
  54
Molluscum contagiosum
  344
Pemphigus vegetans 561
Psoriasis (without scale) 211
Seborrheic keratosis 698
Striae (topical steroids) 15
Tinea 417

Hand (dorsa)

Acquired digital
  fibrokeratoma 888
Acrosclerosis 617
Actinic keratosis 736
Atopic dermatitis 105
Atypical mycobacteria 304
Blue nevus 782
Calcinosis cutis/CREST 617
Cat-scratch disease 528
Contact dermatitis 85
Cowden's disease 912
Dermatomyositis 607
Erysipeloid 287
Erythema multiforme 491
Gonorrhea 330
Granuloma annulare 898
Herpes simplex/zoster 381
Impetigo 267
Keratoacanthoma 711
Lentigo 691

Lichen planus 250
Lupus erythematosus
  (systemic) 600
Mucous cyst (finger) 888
Orf (finger)
Paronychia (acute, chronic)
  871, 872
Pityriasis rubra pilaris 240
Polymorphic light eruption
  671
Porphyria cutanea tarda
  675
Pseudo PCT (porphyria
  cutanea tarda) 675
Psoriasis 215
Pyogenic granuloma 826
Scabies 497
Scleroderma 613
Seborrheic keratosis 664
Sporotrichosis 8
Squamous cell carcinoma
  745
Stucco keratosis 705
Sweet's syndrome 651
Swimming pool granuloma
  744
Tinea 425
Tularemia (ulcer)
Vesicular "id reaction" 59
Xanthoma 902

Hands (palms)

Basal-cell nevus syndrome
  (pits) 731
Calluses/corns 374
Contact dermatitis 85
Cowden's disease 912
Dyshidrotic eczema 58
Eczema 50
Erythema multiforme 491
Hand, foot, and mouth
  disease 462
Keratoderma 894
Keratolysis exfoliativa 55
Lichen planus (vesicles) 250
Lupus erythematosus 592
Melanoma
Pityriasis rubra pilaris 240
Pompholyx 59
Psoriasis 214
Pyogenic granuloma 826
Rocky Mountain spotted
  fever 524

Regional Differential Diagnoses—cont'd

Scabies (infants) 502
Syphilis (secondary) 318
Tinea 425
Vesicular "id reaction" 59
Wart 371

Inframammary
Acrochordon (skin tags) 707
Candidiasis 440
Contact dermatitis 85
Intertrigo 418
Psoriasis (without scale)
Seborrheic keratoses 702
Tinea versicolor 451

Leg
Basal cell carcinoma 728
Bites 533
Bowen's disease 748
Dermatofibroma 708
Disseminated superficial actinic porokeratosis
Ecthyma 272
Ecthyma gangrenosum 298
Eruptive xanthomas 904
Kaposi's sarcoma 827
Livedo reticularis
Lupus panniculus
Majocchi's granuloma (tinea) 422
Melanoma 791
Nummular eczema 54
Panniculitis 75
Pityriasis lichenoides et varioliformis acuta (PLEVA) 261
Porokeratosis of Mibelli
Prurigo nodularis 68
Pyoderma gangrenosum 653
Squamous cell carcinoma 744
Urticarial vasculitis 154
Vasculitis (nodular lesions) 637
Wegener's granulomatosis 640
Churg-Strauss syndrome 640
Polyarteritis nodosa 640
Weber-Christian disease

Legs—lower
Bites 533
Cellulitis 273
Dermatofibroma 708
Diabetic bullae 559
Diabetic dermopathy (shin spots) 694
Erysipelas 273
Erythema induratum
Erythema nodosum 635
Flat warts 373
Folliculitis 279
Granuloma annulare 898
Henoch-Schönlein purpura 640
Ichthyosis vulgaris 115
Idiopathic guttate hypomelanosis 689
Leukocytoclastic vasculitis 642
Lichen planus 250
Lichen simplex chronicus 54
Majocchi's granuloma (tinea) 422
Myxedema (pretibial)
Necrobiosis lipoidica 14
Purpura 17
Schamberg's purpura 656
Stasis dermatitis 72
Subcutaneous fat necrosis (associated with pancreatitis)
Sweet's syndrome 652
Vasculitis (nodular lesions) 637
Weber-Christian disease
Xerosis 60

Lips
Actinic cheilitis 738
Allergic contact dermatitis 84
Angioedema 129
Aphthous ulcer
Fordyce spots (upper lips) 169
Herpes simplex 381
Labial melanotic macule 782
Leukoplakia 751
Mucous cyst
Perlèche 450
Pyogenic granuloma 826

Squamous cell carcinoma 744
Venous lake 825
Wart

Neck (side and front)
Acanthosis nigricans 900
Acne 171
Acrochordon (skin tags) 706
Atopic dermatitis 112
Berloque dermatitis 683
Contact dermatitis 85
Dental sinus
Elastosis perforans serpiginosa
Epidermal cyst 717
Folliculitis 279
Impetigo 267
Pityriasis rosea 246
Poikiloderma of Civatte 663
Pseudofolliculitis 280
Pseudoxanthoma elasticum 916
Sycosis barbae (fungal, bacterial) 282
Tinea 421
Wart 372

Neck (back)
Acne 171
Acne keloidalis 283
Actinic keratosis 736
Cutis rhomboidalis nuchae 664
Epidermal cyst 717
Folliculitis 279
Furunculosis
Herpes zoster 394
Lichen simplex chronicus 54
Neurotic excoriations 68
Salmon patch 823
Tinea 421

Nose
Acne 171
Actinic keratosis 736
Adenoma sebaceum 910
Basal cell carcinoma 720
Discoid lupus erythematosus 861

Fissure (nostril) 15
Granulosa rubra nasi
Herpes simplex 381
Herpes zoster 394
Impetigo 267
Lupus erythematosus 600
Nasal crease
Nevus 775
Rhinophyma 200
Rosacea 198
Seborrheic dermatitis 242
Squamous cell carcinoma 744
Telangiectasias 199
Trichofolliculoma
Wegener's granulomatosis 640

Penis
Aphthae (Behcet's syndrome) 14
Balanitis circinata (Reiter's syndrome) 216
Bite (human) 529
Bowenoid papulosis 343
Candidiasis (under foreskin) 445
Chancroid 327
Condyloma (warts) 337
Contact dermatitis (condoms) 85
Erythroplasia of Queyrat (Bowen's disease) 750
Factitious
Fixed drug eruption 492
Giant condyloma (Buschke-Lowenstein) 749
Granuloma inguinale 329
Herpes simplex/zoster 381
Lichen nitidus 4
Lichen planus 255
Lichen sclerosis et atrophicus (balanitis xerotica obliterans) 258
Lymphogranuloma venereum 325
Molluscum contagiosum 344
Nevus
Pearly penile papules 339
Pediculosis (lice) 506
Penile melanosis

Continued

Regional Differential Diagnoses—cont'd

Penis—cont'd
Psoriasis 216
Scabies 501
Sclerosing lymphangitis
   (nonvenereal)
Seborrheic keratosis 700
Squamous cell carcinoma
   744
Syphilis (chancre) 316
Zoon's (plasma cell)
   balanitis

Periorbital
Acrochordons (skin tags)
   706
Angioedema 129
Atopic dermatitis 114
Cat-scratch disease 528
Colloid degeneration
   (milium)
Contact dermatitis 85
Dermatomyositis 607
Milia 4
Molluscum contagiosum
   344
Nevus of Ota
Seborrheic dermatitis 242
Senile comedones 194
Syringoma 721
Xanthelasma 903

Scalp
Acne necrotica
Actinic keratosis 736
Alopecia neoplastica
   (metastases) 766
Atypical fibroxanthoma
Basal cell carcinoma
Contact dermatitis 85
Cylindroma
Dermatitis occipital
   (excoriation) 69
Eczema
Folliculitis 279
Herpes zoster 394
Kerion (inflammatory
   tinea) 430
Lichen planopilaris 861
Lupus erythematosus
   (discoid) 596
Melanoma
Neurotic excoriations 69

Nevi 775
Nevus sebaceous 715
Pediculosis capitis 507
Pilar cyst (wen) 719
Prurigo nodularis 68
Psoriasis 214
Seborrheic dermatitis 242
Seborrheic dermatitis
   (histiocytosis X)
Seborrheic keratosis 702
Tinea 427

Scrotum
Angiokeratoma (Fordyce)
   824
Condyloma 337
Epidermal cyst 717
Extramammary Paget's
   disease 764
Henoch-Schönlein
   syndrome 640
Lichen simplex chronicus
   54
Nevus 775
Scabies 501
Seborrheic keratosis 700

Thigh (inner surface and inguinal groove)
Acrochordons (skin tags)
   706
Candidiasis 447
Eczema
Erythrasma 419
Extramammary Paget's
   disease 764
Fissures 418
Granuloma inguinale 329
Hidradenitis suppurativa
   202
Intertrigo 418
Keratosis pilaris (anterior)
   116
Lichen sclerosis et
   atrophicus 257
Striae distensae 37
Tinea 417

Trunk
Accessory nipple
Anetoderma

Ash leaf spot 911
Atopic dermatitis 110
Capillary hemangiomas 826
Chickenpox 389
CTCL (mycosis fungoides)
   754
Drug eruption
   (maculopapular) 485
Epidermal cyst 717
Erythema annulare
   centrifugum
Familial atypical mole
   syndrome 784
Fixed drug eruption 492
Folliculitis (classical and
   hot tub) 290
Granuloma annulare
   (generalized) 898
Hailey-Hailey disease 551
Halo nevus 781
Herpes zoster 394
Keloids 16
Lichen planus (generalized)
   252
Lichen sclerosis et
   atrophicus 257
Lupus erythematosus
   (subacute cutaneous) 598
Measles 460
Miliaria 205
Nevus anemicus 690
Nevus spilus 779
Parapsoriasis 756
Pediculosis (lice) 506
Pemphigus foliaceous 562
Pityriasis rosea 246
Pityriasis rubra pilaris 240
Pityrosporum folliculitis
   454
Poikiloderma vasculare
   atrophicans 756
Psoriasis (guttate) 212
Sarcoid
Scabies 802
Scleroderma (localized,
   morphea) 620
Seborrheic dermatitis 242
Steatocystoma multiplex
Syphilis (secondary) 318
Tinea 420
Tinea versicolor 451

Transient acantholytic
   dermatosis (Grover's
   disease)
Unilateral nevoid
   telangiectasia 832
Urticaria pigmentosa 156
Viral exanthem 473
von Recklinghausen's neu-
   rofibromatosis 906

Vulva
Allergic contact dermatitis
   85
Angiokeratoma
   (of Fordyce) 824
Behcet's syndrome
Bowen's disease 748
Candidiasis 440
Chancroid 327
Cicatricial pemphigoid 548
Epidermal cyst 718
Erythrasma 419
Extramammary Paget's
   disease 764
Fibroepithelial polyp 707
Folliculitis 279
Fox-Fordyce spots 169
Furunculosis 284
Granuloma inguinale 329
Herpes simplex/zoster 381
Hidradenitis suppurativa
   202
Intertrigo 418
Leukoplakia 751
Lichen planus 255
Lichen sclerosis et
   atrophicus 258
Lichen simplex chronicus
   54
Melanoma 788
Molluscum contagiosum
   344
Nevus 775
Pediculosis 506
Psoriasis 211
Squamous cell carcinoma
   744
Stevens-Johnson syndrome
   627
Verrucous carcinoma 753
Warts 338

Topical Therapy and Topical Corticosteroids

❏ **Topical therapy**
   Emollient creams and lotions
   Severe dry skin (xerosis)
   Wet dressings

❏ **Topical corticosteroids**
   Strength
   Vehicle
   Steroid-antibiotic mixtures
   Amount of cream to dispense
   Application
   Adverse reactions

Topical Therapy

A wide variety of topical medications are available for treating cutaneous disease (see Dermatologic Formulary, p. 945). Specific medications are covered in detail in the appropriate chapters, and the basic principles of topical treatment are discussed here.

The skin is an important barrier that must be maintained to function properly. Any insult that removes water, lipids, or protein from the epidermis alters the integrity of this barrier and compromises its function. Restoration of the normal epidermal barrier is accomplished with the use of mild soaps and emollient creams and lotions. There is an old and often-repeated rule: "If it is dry, wet it; if it is wet, dry it."

DRY DISEASES. Dry skin or dry cutaneous lesions have lost water and, in many instances, the epidermal lipids and proteins that help contain epidermal moisture. These substances are replaced with emollient creams and lotions.

WET DISEASES. Exudative inflammatory diseases pour out serum that leaches the complex lipids and proteins from the epidermis. A wet lesion is managed with wet compresses that suppress inflammation and debride crust and serum. Repeated cycles of wetting and drying eventually make the lesion dry. Excessive use of wet dressings causes severe drying and chapping. Once the wet phase of the disease has been controlled, the lipids and proteins must be restored with the use of emollient creams and lotions, and wet compressing should stop.

Emollient creams and lotions

Emollient creams and lotions restore water and lipids to the epidermis (see Dermatologic Formulary, pp. 945). Preparations that contain urea (e.g., Carmol 10, 20, 40, vanamide), or lactic acid (e.g., Lac-Hydrin, AmLactin) have special lubricating properties and may be the most effective. Creams are thicker and more lubricating than lotions; petroleum jelly and mineral oil contain no water.

Lubricating creams and lotions are most effective if applied to moist skin. After bathing is an ideal time to apply moisturizers. Wet the skin, pat dry, and immediately apply the moisturizer. Emollients should be applied as frequently as necessary to keep the skin soft. Chemicals such as menthol and phenol (e.g., Sarna Lotion) are added to lubricating lotions to control pruritus (see Dermatologic Formulary, p. 945).

Severe dry skin (xerosis)

Dry skin is more severe in the winter months when the humidity is low. "Winter itch" most commonly affects the hands and lower legs. Initially the skin is rough and covered with fine white scales; later, thicker tan or brown scales may appear. The most severely affected skin may be criss-crossed with shallow red fissures. Dry skin may itch or burn. Preparations listed in the Formulary on p. 945 should be used for mild cases; severe dry skin responds to 12% lactate lotion (Lac-Hydrin, AmLactin).

Wet dressings

Wet dressings, also called *compresses*, are a valuable aid in the treatment of exudative (wet) skin diseases (see Box 2-1). Their importance in topical therapy cannot be overstated. The technique for wet compress preparation and application is described in the list below.

1. Obtain a clean, soft cloth such as bedsheeting or shirt material. The cloth need not be new or sterilized. Compress material must be washed at least once daily if it is to be used repeatedly.

2. Fold the cloth so there are at least four to eight layers and cut to fit an area slightly larger than the area to be treated.

3. Wet the folded dressings by immersing them in the solution, and wring them out until they are sopping wet (neither running nor just damp).

4. Place the wet compresses on the affected area. Do not pour solution on a wet dressing to keep it wet because this practice increases the concentration of the solution and may cause irritation. Remove the compress and replace it with a new one.

5. Dressings are left in place for 30 minutes to 1 hour. Dressings may be used two to four times a day or continuously. Discontinue the use of wet compresses when the skin becomes dry. Excessive drying causes cracking and fissures.

Wet compresses provide the following benefits:

- Antibacterial action: Aluminum acetate, acetic acid, or silver nitrate may be added to the water to provide an antibacterial effect (Table 2-1).
- Wound debridement: A wet compress macerates vesicles and crust, helping to debride these materials when the compress is removed.
- Inflammation suppression: Compresses have a strong antiinflammatory effect. The evaporative cooling causes constriction of superficial cutaneous vessels, thereby decreasing erythema and the production of serum. Wet compresses control acute inflammatory processes, such as acute poison ivy, faster than either topical applied or orally administered corticosteroids.
- Drying: Wet dressings cause the skin to become dry. Wetting something to make it dry seems paradoxical, but the effects of repeated cycles of wetting and drying are observed in lip chapping, caused by lip licking; irritant hand dermatitis, caused by repeated washing; and the soggy sock syndrome in children, caused by perspiration.

The temperature of the compress solution should be cool when an antiinflammatory effect is desired and tepid when the purpose is to debride an infected, crusted lesion. Covering a wet compress with a towel or plastic inhibits evaporation, promotes maceration, and increases skin temperature, which facilitates bacterial growth.

Box 2-1 Diseases Treated With Wet Compresses
Acute eczematous inflammation (poison ivy)
Eczematous inflammation with secondary infection (pustules)
Bullous impetigo
Herpes simplex and herpes zoster (vesicular lesions)
Infected exudative lesions of any type
Insect bites
Intertrigo (groin or under breasts)
Nummular eczema (exudative lesions)
Stasis dermatitis (exudative lesions)
Stasis ulcers
Sunburn (blistering stage)
Tinea pedis (vesicular stage or macerated web infections)

Table 2-1 Wet Dressing Solutions		
Solution	**Preparation**	**Indications**
Water	Tap water does not have to be sterilized.	Poison ivy, sunburn, any noninfected exudative or inflamed process
Burrow's solution (aluminum acetate) Domeboro astringent powder packets Effervescent tablets	Dissolve one, two, or three packets of Domeboro powder in 16 ounces of water.	Mildly antiseptic; for acute inflammation. Poison ivy, insect bites, athlete's foot
Silver nitrate, 0.1%-0.5% (prepared by some pharmacists and some hospitals)	Supplied as a 50% aqueous solution; stains skin dark brown and metal black.	Bactericidal, for exudative infected lesions (e.g., stasis ulcers and stasis dermatitis)
Acetic acid, 1%-2.5%	Vinegar is 5% acetic acid. Make a 1% solution by adding ½ cup of vinegar (white or brown) to 1 pint of water.	Bactericidal: for certain gram-negative bacteria (e.g., *Pseudomonas aeruginosa*), otitis externa, *Pseudomonas intertrigo*

Topical Corticosteroids

Topical corticosteroids are a powerful tool for treating skin disease. Understanding the correct use of these agents will result in the successful management of a variety of skin problems. Many products are available, but all have basically the same antiinflammatory properties, differing only in strength, base, and price.

Strength

POTENCY: GROUPS I THROUGH VII. The antiinflammatory properties of topical corticosteroids result in part from their ability to induce vasoconstriction of the small blood vessels in the upper dermis. This property is used in an assay procedure to determine the strength of each new product. These products are subsequently tabulated in seven groups, with group I the strongest and group VII the weakest (see the Formulary and the inside front cover of this book). The treatment sections of this book recommend topical steroids by group number rather than by generic or brand name because the agents in each group are essentially equivalent in strength.

Lower concentrations of some brands may have the same effect in vasoconstrictor assays as much higher concentrations of the same product. One study showed that there was no difference in vasoconstriction between Kenalog 0.025%, 0.1%, or 0.5% creams.[1]

CHOOSING THE APPROPRIATE STRENGTH. Guidelines for choosing the appropriate strength and brand of topical steroid are presented in Box 2-2 and the diagram at the right. The best results are obtained when preparations of adequate strength are used for a specified length of time. Weaker, "safer" strengths often fail to provide adequate control. Patients who do not respond after 1 to 4 weeks of treatment should be reevaluated.

CHOOSING A TOPICAL STEROID

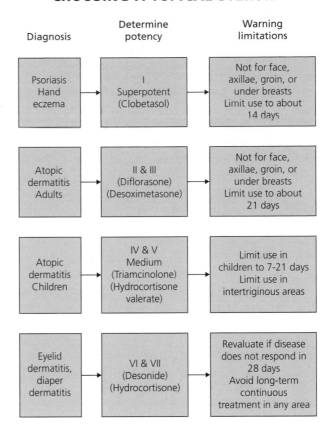

Diagnosis	Determine potency	Warning limitations
Psoriasis Hand eczema	I Superpotent (Clobetasol)	Not for face, axillae, groin, or under breasts Limit use to about 14 days
Atopic dermatitis Adults	II & III (Diflorasone) (Desoximetasone)	Not for face, axillae, groin, or under breasts Limit use to about 21 days
Atopic dermatitis Children	IV & V Medium (Triamcinolone) (Hydrocortisone valerate)	Limit use in children to 7-21 days Limit use in intertriginous areas
Eyelid dermatitis, diaper dermatitis	VI & VII (Desonide) (Hydrocortisone)	Revaluate if disease does not respond in 28 days Avoid long-term continuous treatment in any area

Box 2-2 Suggested Strength of Topical Steroids to Initiate Treatment*

Groups I-II	Groups III-V	Groups VI-VII
Psoriasis	Atopic dermatitis	Dermatitis (eyelids)
Lichen planus	Nummular eczema	Dermatitis (diaper area)
Discoid lupus†	Asteatotic eczema	Mild dermatitis (face)
Severe hand eczema	Stasis dermatitis	Mild anal inflammation
Poison ivy (severe)	Seborrheic dermatitis	Mild intertrigo
Lichen simplex chronicus	Lichen sclerosis et atrophicus (vulva)	
Hyperkeratotic eczema	Intertrigo (brief course)	
Chapped feet	Tinea (brief course to control inflammation)	
Lichen sclerosis et atrophicus (skin)	Scabies (after scabicide)	
Alopecia areata	Intertrigo (severe cases)	
Nummular eczema (severe)	Anal inflammation (severe cases)	
Atopic dermatitis (resistant adult cases)	Severe dermatitis (face)	

*Stop treatment, change to less potent agent, or use intermittent treatment once inflammation is controlled.
†Use on the face may be justified.

MEGAPOTENT TOPICAL STEROIDS (GROUP I). Cormax (clobetasol propionate), Ultravate (halobetasol propionate), Diprolene (betamethasone dipropionate), and Psorcon (diflorasone diacetate) are the most potent topical steroids available. Cormax and Ultravate are the most potent, and Psorcon and Diprolene are equipotent.

In general no more than 45 to 60 gm of cream or ointment should be used each week (see Table 2-2). Side effects are minimized and efficacy increased when medication is applied once or twice daily for 2 weeks followed by 1 week of rest. This cyclic schedule (pulse dosing) is continued until resolution occurs.[2] Intermittent dosing (e.g., once or twice a week) can lead to a prolonged remission of psoriasis if used after initial clearing.[3] Alternatively, intermittent use of a weaker topical steroid can be used for maintenance. Psorcon can be used with plastic dressing occlusion; Cormax, Ultravate, and Diprolene should not be used with occlusive dressings.

Patients must be monitored carefully. Side effects such as atrophy and adrenal suppression are a real possibility, especially with unsupervised use of these medications.[4] Refills should be strictly limited.

CONCENTRATION. The concentration of steroid listed on the tube cannot be used to compare its strength with other steroids. Some steroids are much more powerful than others and need be present only in small concentrations to produce the maximum effect. Nevertheless, it is difficult to convince some patients that Lidex cream 0.05% (group II) is more potent than hydrocortisone 1% (group VII).

It is unnecessary to learn many steroid brand names. Familiarity with one preparation from groups II, V, and VII gives one the ability to safely and effectively treat any steroid-responsive skin disease. Most of the topical steroids are fluorinated (i.e., a fluorine atom has been added to the hydrocortisone molecule). Fluorination increases potency and the possibility of side effects. Products such as Westcort Cream have increased potency without fluorination; however, side effects are possible with this midpotency steroid.

COMPOUNDING. Avoid having the pharmacist prepare or dilute topical steroid creams. The active ingredient may not be dispersed uniformly, resulting in a cream of variable strength. The cost of pharmacist preparation is generally higher because of the additional labor required. High-quality steroid creams, such as triamcinolone acetonide (Kenalog, Aristocort), are available in large quantities at a low cost.

GENERIC VERSUS BRAND NAMES. Many generic topical steroid formulations are available (e.g., betamethasone valerate, betamethasone dipropionate, fluocinolone acetonide, fluocinonide, hydrocortisone, and triamcinolone acetonide). In many states, generic substitutions by the pharmacist are allowed unless the physician writes "no substitution." Vasoconstrictor assays have shown large differences in the activity of generic formulations compared with brand-name equivalents: many are inferior,[5] a few are equivalent,[6] and a few are more potent than brand-name equivalents. Many generic topical steroids have vehicles with different ingredients (e.g., preservatives) than brand-name equivalents.[7]

Vehicle

The vehicle, or base, is the substance in which the active ingredient is dispersed. The base determines the rate at which the active ingredient is absorbed through the skin. Components of some bases may cause irritation or allergy.

CREAMS. The cream base is a mixture of several different organic chemicals (oils) and water, and it usually contains a preservative. Creams have the following characteristics:
- White color and somewhat greasy texture
- Components that may cause irritation, stinging, and allergy
- High versatility (i.e., may be used in nearly any area); therefore creams are the base most often prescribed
- Cosmetically most acceptable, particularly emollient bases (e.g., Aristocort-A, Cyclocort)

Table 2-2 Restriction on the Use of Group I Topical Steroids*	Length of therapy	Grams per week	Use under occlusion
Cormax (clobetasol propionate)[†]	14 days	60	No
Cormax scalp solution[†]	14 days	50 ml	No
Olux foam	14 days	50	No
Ultravate (halobetasol propionate)	14 days	60	No
Diprolene (betamethasone dipropionate)[†]	Unrestricted	45	No
Psorcon (diflorasone diacetate)[†]	Unrestricted	Unrestricted	Unrestricted

*Restrictions are listed in the package inserts.
[†]Generic form available.

- Possible drying effect with continued use; therefore best for acute exudative inflammation
- Most useful for intertriginous areas (e.g., groin, rectal area, and axilla)

OINTMENTS. The ointment base contains a limited number of organic compounds consisting primarily of greases such as petroleum jelly, with little or no water. Many ointments are preservative-free. Ointments have the following characteristics:

- Translucent (look like petroleum jelly)
- Greasy feeling persists on skin surface
- More lubrication, thus desirable for drier lesions
- Greater penetration of medicine than creams and therefore enhanced potency (see inside front cover; Synalar Cream in group V and Synalar Ointment in group IV)
- Too occlusive for acute (exudative) eczematous inflammation or intertriginous areas, such as the groin

GELS. Gels are greaseless mixtures of propylene glycol and water; some also contain alcohol. Gels have the following characteristics:

- A clear base, sometimes with a jellylike consistency
- Useful for acute exudative inflammation, such as poison ivy, and in scalp areas where other vehicles mat the hair

SOLUTIONS AND LOTIONS. Solutions may contain water and alcohol, as well as other chemicals. Solutions have the following characteristics:

- Clear or milky appearance
- Most useful for scalp because they penetrate easily through hair, leaving no residue
- May result in stinging and drying when applied to intertriginous areas, such as the groin

FOAMS. A foam preparation of betamethasone valerate (Luxiq) and clobetasol propionate (Olux) is available. Olux contains a superpotent steroid. Treatment beyond 2 consecutive weeks is not recommended, and the total dosage should not exceed 50 gm per week because of the potential for the drug to suppress the hypothalamic-pituitary-adrenal (HPA) axis. Use in children under 12 years of age is not recommended. Foams spread between the strands of hair until they reach the scalp, where the foam melts and delivers the active drug. Foams are useful for treatment of scalp dermatoses and in other areas for acute eczematous inflammation such as poison ivy and plaque psoriasis.

Steroid-antibiotic mixtures

LOTRISONE CREAM AND LOTION. Lotrisone cream contains a combination of the antifungal agent clotrimazole and the corticosteroid betamethasone dipropionate. It is indicated for the topical treatment of tinea pedis, tinea cruris, and tinea corporis. This product is used by many physicians as their topical antiinflammatory agent of first choice. Most inflammatory skin disease is not infected or contaminated by fungus. Lotrisone is a marginal drug for cutaneous fungal infections. Brand-name Lotrisone cream is no longer available; it has been replaced by a brand-name lotion. The generic cream costs approximately $25.00 for 15 gm and $45.00 for 45 gm. Generic betamethasone dipropionate cream costs approximately $12.00 for 15 gm and $18.00 for 45 gm. Generic clotrimazole costs approximately $10.00 for 30 gm.

OTHER ANTIBIOTICS AND CORTICOSTEROID MIXTURES. Mycolog II (Nystatin; Triamcinolone Acetonide) is indicated for the treatment of cutaneous candidiasis. Nystatin does not treat fungi that cause tinea pedis. The majority of steroid-responsive skin diseases can be managed successfully without topical antibiotics.

Amount of cream to dispense

The amount of cream dispensed is very important. Patients do not appreciate being prescribed a $90.00, 60-gm tube of cream to treat a small area of hand dermatitis. Unrestricted and unsupervised use of potent steroid creams can lead to side effects. Patients rely on the physician's judgment to determine the correct amount of topical medicine. If too small a quantity is prescribed, patients may conclude that the treatment did not work. It is advisable to allow for a sufficient amount of cream, and then to set limits on duration and frequency of application. Many steroids (e.g., triamcinolone, hydrocortisone) are available in generic form. They are purchased in bulk by the pharmacist and can be dispensed in large quantities at considerable savings.

The amount of cream required to cover a certain area can be calculated by remembering that 1 gm of cream covers 100 square cm of skin.[8] The entire skin surface of the average-sized adult is covered by 20 to 30 gm of cream.

The fingertip unit and the rule of hand provide the means to assess how much cream to dispense and apply.

FINGERTIP UNIT. A fingertip unit (FTU) is the amount of ointment expressed from a tube with a 5-mm diameter nozzle, applied from the distal skin crease to the tip of the index finger. One FTU weighs approximately 0.5 gm.[9]

THE RULE OF HAND. The hand area can be used to estimate the total area of involvement of a skin disease and to assess the amount of ointment required. The area of one side of the hand is defined as one hand area. One hand area of involved skin requires 0.5 FTU or 0.25 gm of ointment, or four hand areas equal 2 FTUs equal 1 gm. The area of one side of the hand represents approximately 1% of body surface area so it requires 1 FTU (2 hand units) to cover 2% of the body surface. Approximately 282 gm is required for twice-daily applications to the total body surface (except the scalp) for 1 week.[10]

Application
Frequency

TACHYPHYLAXIS. Tachyphylaxis refers to the decrease in responsiveness to a drug as a result of enzyme induction. The term is used in dermatology in reference to acute tolerance to the vasoconstrictive action of topically applied corticosteroids. Experiments have revealed that vasoconstriction decreases progressively when a potent topical steroid is applied to the skin three times a day for 4 days.[11] The vasoconstrictive response returned 4 days after termination of therapy. These experiments support years of complaints by patients about initially dramatic responses to new topical steroids that diminish with constant use. It would therefore seem reasonable to instruct patients to apply creams on an interrupted schedule.

INTERMITTENT DOSING

Group I topical steroids. Optimum dosing schedules for the use of potent topical steroids have not been determined. Studies show that steroid-resistant diseases, such as plaque psoriasis and hand eczema, respond most effectively when clobetasol (Cormax) is applied twice a day for 2 to 3 weeks.[12,13] Treatment is resumed after 1 week of rest. The schedule of 2 weeks of treatment followed by 1 week of rest is repeated until the lesions have cleared.

Intermittent treatment of healed lesions can lead to prolonged remission. Psoriatic patients with lingering erythema remained clear with applications three times a day on 1 day a week.[3] Twice-weekly applications of clobetasol kept 75% of psoriatic patients[7] and 70% of hand eczema patients[14] in remission.

Short weekly bursts of topical corticosteroids may play a role in keeping an adult's atopic dermatitis under control. Weekly applications of fluticasone ointment (Cutivate), applied once daily for 2 consecutive days each week maintained the improvements achieved after the initial treatment phase and delayed relapse.[13]

Groups II through VII topical steroids. The optimum frequency of application and duration of treatment for topical steroids have not been determined. Adequate results and acceptable patient compliance occur when the following steps are taken:

1. Apply groups II through VI topical steroids twice each day.
2. Limit the duration of application to 2 to 6 weeks.
3. If adequate control is not achieved, stop treatment for 4 to 7 days and begin another course of treatment.

Excellent control can be achieved with pulse dosing. These are general guidelines; specific instructions and limitations must be established for each individual case.

Methods

SIMPLE APPLICATION. Creams and ointments should be applied in thin layers and slowly massaged into the site one to four times a day. It is unnecessary to wash before each application. Continue treatment until the lesion is clear. Many patients decrease the frequency of applications or stop entirely when lesions appear to improve quickly. Other patients are so impressed with the efficacy of these agents that they continue treatment after the disease has resolved in order to prevent recurrence; adverse reactions may follow this practice.

Different skin surfaces vary in the ability to absorb topical medicine. The thin eyelid skin heals quickly with group VI or VII steroids, whereas thicker skin on palms and soles offers a greater barrier to the penetration of topical medicine and requires more potent therapy. Intertriginous (skin touches skin) areas (e.g., axilla, groin, rectal area, and underneath the breasts) respond more quickly to creams that are weaker in strength. The apposition of two skin surfaces performs the same function as an occlusive dressing, which greatly enhances penetration. The skin of infants and young children is more receptive to topical medicine and responds quickly to weaker creams. A baby's diaper has the same occlusive effect as covering with a plastic dressing. Penetration of steroid creams is greatly enhanced; therefore, only group V, VI, or VII preparations should be used under a diaper. Inflamed skin absorbs topical medicines much more efficiently. This explains why red, inflamed areas generally have such a rapid initial response when treated with weaker topical steroids.

OCCLUSION. Occlusion with a plastic dressing (e.g., Saran Wrap) is an effective method for enhancing absorption of topical steroids. The plastic dressing holds perspiration against the skin surface, which hydrates the top layer of the epidermis, the stratum corneum. Topical medication penetrates a moist stratum corneum from 10 to 100 times more effectively than it penetrates dry skin. Eruptions that are resistant to simple application may heal quickly with the introduction of a plastic dressing. Nearly any area can be occluded; the entire body may be occluded with a vinyl exercise suit, available at most sporting goods stores.

Discretion should be used with occlusion. Occlusion of moist areas may encourage the rapid development of infection. Occlusive dressings are used more often with creams than with ointments, but ointments may be covered if the lesions are particularly dry. Weaker, less expensive products (e.g., triamcinolone cream, 0.1%) provide excellent results. Large quantities of this medicine may be purchased at a substantial savings.

METHOD OF OCCLUSION. The area should be cleaned with mild soap and water. Antibacterial soaps are unnecessary. The medicine is gently rubbed into the lesions, and the entire area is covered with plastic (e.g., Saran Wrap, Handi-Wrap, plastic bags, or gloves; Figures 2-1 to 2-3). The plastic dressing should be secured with tape so that it is close to the skin and the ends are sealed; an airtight dressing is unnecessary. The plastic may be held in place with an Ace bandage or a sock. The best results are obtained if the dressing remains in place for at least 2 hours. Many patients find that bedtime is the most convenient time to wear a plastic dressing and therefore wear it for 8 hours. More medicine is applied shortly after the dressing is removed and while the skin is still moist.

Dressings should not remain on the area continuously because infection or follicular occlusion may result. If an occluded area suddenly becomes worse or pustules develop, infection, usually with staphylococci, should be suspected (Figure 2-4). Oral antistaphylococcal antibiotics should be given (e.g., cephalexin [Keflex] 500 mg 2 to 4 times a day).

A reasonable occlusion schedule is twice daily for a 2-hour period or for 8 hours at bedtime, with simple application once or twice during the day.

Occluded areas often become dry, and the use of lubricating cream or lotion should be encouraged. Cream or lotion may be applied shortly after medicine is applied, when the plastic dressing is removed, or at other convenient times.

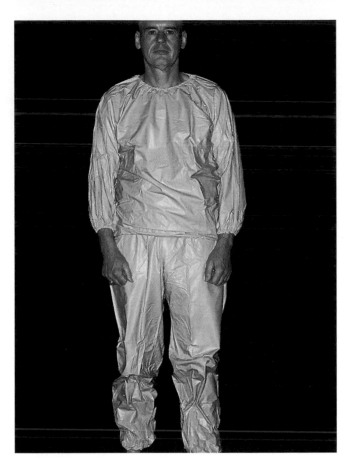

Figure 2-3 Occlusion of the entire body. A vinyl exercise suit is a convenient way to occlude the entire body.

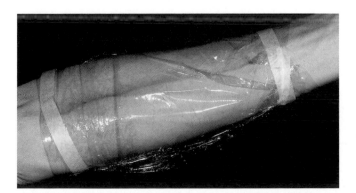

Figure 2-1 Occlusion of the hand. A plastic bag is pulled on and pressed against the skin to expel air. Tape is wound snugly around the bag.

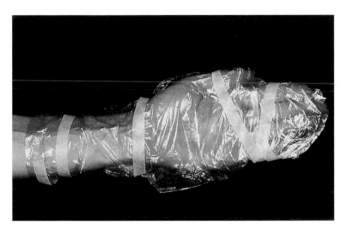

Figure 2-2 Occlusion of the arm. A plastic sheet (e.g., Saran Wrap) is wound about the extremity and secured at both ends with tape. A plastic bag with the bottom cut out may be used as a sleeve and held in place with tape or an Ace bandage.

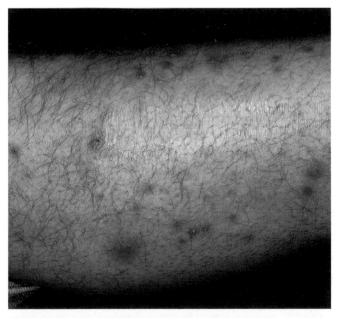

Figure 2-4 Infection following occlusion. Pustules have appeared at the periphery of an eczematous lesion. Plastic dressing had been left in place for 24 hours.

Systemic absorption

The possibility of producing systemic side effects from absorption of topical steroids is of concern to all physicians who use these agents. A small number of case reports have documented systemic effects after topical application of glucocorticoids for prolonged periods. Cataracts, retardation of growth, failure to thrive, and Cushing's syndrome have all been reported.

AVOID WEAKER, "SAFE" PREPARATIONS. In an attempt to avoid complications, physicians often choose a weaker steroid preparation than that indicated; these weaker preparations all too frequently fall short of expectations and fail to give the desired antiinflammatory effect. The disease does not improve, but rather becomes worse because of the time wasted using the ineffective cream. Pruritus continues, infection may set in, and the patient becomes frustrated. Treatment of intense inflammation with hydrocortisone cream 0.5% is a waste of time and money. Generally, a topical steroid of adequate strength (see Box 2-2) should be used 2 to 4 times daily for a specific length of time, such as 7 to 21 days, in order to obtain rapid control. Even during this short interval adrenal suppression may result when groups I through III steroids are used to treat wide areas of inflamed skin. This suppression of the hypothalamic-pituitary-adrenal axis is generally reversible in 24 hours and is very unlikely to produce side effects characteristic of long-term systemic use.[15]

CHILDREN. Many physicians worry about systemic absorption and will not use any topical steroids stronger than 1% hydrocortisone on infants. The group V topical steroid, fluticasone propionate cream 0.05% (Cutivate) appears to be safe for the treatment of severe eczema for up to 4 weeks in children 3 months of age and older. Children between 3 months and 6 years with moderate to severe atopic dermatitis (> or equal to 35% body surface area; mean body surface area treated, 64%) were treated with fluticasone propionate cream, 0.05% twice daily for 3 to 4 weeks. Mean cortisol levels were similar at baseline and at the end of treatment.[16] The relative safety of moderately strong topical steroids and their relative freedom from serious systemic toxicity despite widespread use in the very young has been clearly demonstrated. Patients should be treated for a specific length of time with a medication of appropriate strength. Steroid creams should not be used continually for many weeks, and patients who do not respond in a predictable fashion should be reevaluated.

Group I topical steroids should be avoided in prepubertal children. Use only group VI or VII steroids in the diaper area and for only 3 to 10 days. Monitor growth parameters in children on chronic topical glucocorticoid therapy.

ADULTS. Suppression may occur during short intervals of treatment with group I or II topical steroids, but recovery is rapid when treatment is discontinued. Physicians may prescribe strong agents when appropriate, but the patient must be cautioned that the agent should be used only for the length of time dictated.

Adverse reactions

Because information concerning the potential dangers of potent topical steroids has been so widely disseminated, some physicians have stopped prescribing them. Topical steroids have been used for approximately 30 years with an excellent safety record. They do, however, have the potential to produce a number of adverse reactions. Once these are understood, the most appropriate-strength steroid can be prescribed confidently. The reported adverse reactions to topical steroids are listed below.

Rosacea, perioral dermatitis, acne

Skin atrophy with telangiectasia, stellate pseudoscars (arms), purpura, striae (from anatomic occlusion, e.g., groin)

Tinea incognito, impetigo incognito, scabies incognito

Ocular hypertension, glaucoma, cataracts

Allergic contact dermatitis

Systemic absorption

Burning, itching, irritation, dryness caused by vehicle (e.g., propylene glycol)

Miliaria and folliculitus following occlusion with plastic

Skin blanching from acute vasoconstriction

Rebound phenomenon (i.e., psoriasis becomes worse after treatment is stopped)

Nonhealing leg ulcers; steroids applied to any leg ulcer retard healing process

Hypopigmentation

Hypertrichosis of face

A brief description of some of the more important adverse reactions is presented in the following pages.

Steroid rosacea and perioral dermatitis

Steroid rosacea[17] is a side effect frequently observed in fair-skinned females who initially complain of erythema with or without pustules, the "flusher blusher complexion." In a typical example, the physician prescribes a mild topical steroid, which initially gives pleasing results. Tolerance (tachyphylaxis) occurs, and a new, more potent topical steroid is prescribed to suppress the erythema and pustules that may reappear following the use of the weaker preparation. This progression to more potent creams may continue until group II steroids are applied several times each day. Figure 2-5, A, shows a middle-aged woman who has applied a group V steroid cream once each day for 5 years. Intense erythema and pustulation occurs each time attempts are made to discontinue topical treatment (Figure 2-5, B, C). The skin may be atrophic and red with a burning sensation.

Perioral dermatitis (see Chapter 7) is sometimes caused by the chronic application of topical steroids to the lower face; pustules, erythema, and scaling occur about the nose, mouth, and chin.

STEROID ROSACEA

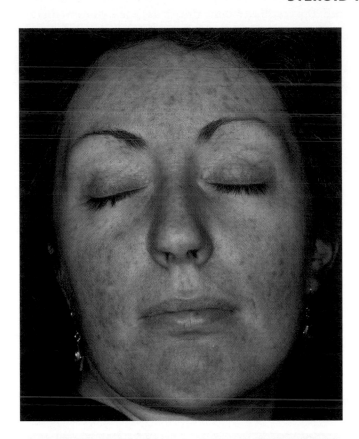

A, Numerous red papules formed on the cheeks and forehead with constant daily use of a group V topical steroid for more than 5 years.

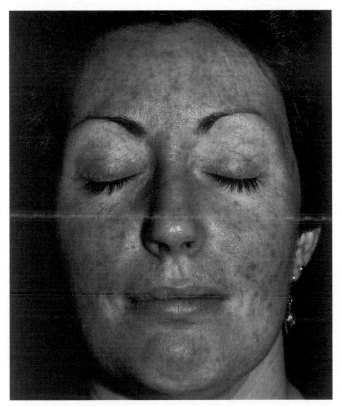

B, Ten days after discontinuing use of group V topical steroid.

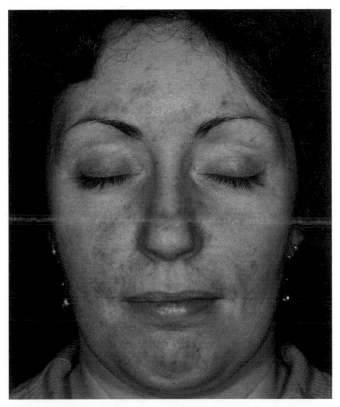

C, Two months after use of topical steroids was discontinued. Telangiectasia has persisted; rosacea has improved with oral antibiotics.

Figure 2-5

MANAGEMENT. Strong topical steroids must be discontinued. Doxycycline (100 mg twice a day) or erythromycin (250 mg four times a day) may reduce the intensity of the rebound erythema and pustulation that predictably occur during the first 10 days (Figures 2-6, 2-7, 2-8, and 2-9). Occasionally, cool, wet compresses, with or without 1% hydrocortisone cream, are necessary if the rebound is intense. Thereafter, mild noncomedogenic lubricants (those that do not induce acne, such as Curel lotion) may be used for the dryness and desquamation that occur. Erythema and pustules are generally present at a low level for months. Low dosages of doxycycline (50 mg twice a day) or erythromycin (250 mg two or three times a day) may be continued until the eruption clears. The pustules and erythema eventually subside, but some telangiectasia and atrophy may be permanent.

STEROID ROSACEA

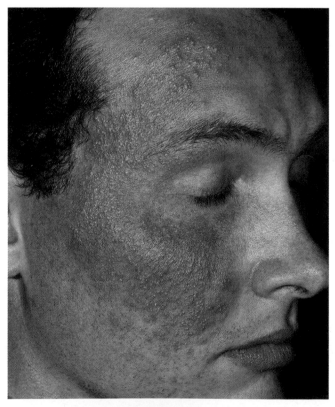

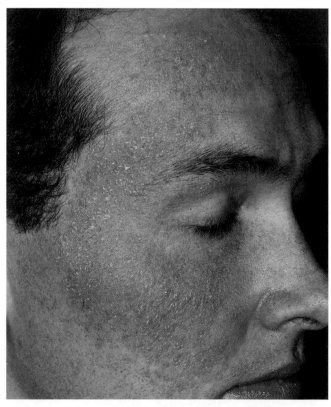

A, Intense erythema and pustulation appeared 10 days after discontinuing use of a group V topical steroid. The cream had been applied every day for 1 year.

B, Patient shown in *A* 24 days after discontinuing the group V topical steroid. Pustules have cleared without any treatment. Gradual improvement followed over the next several months.

Figure 2-6

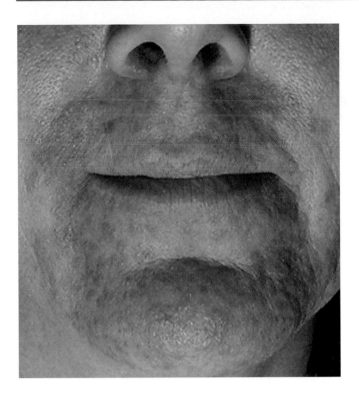

Figure 2-7 Perioral dermatitis. Pustules and erythema have appeared in a perioral distribution following several courses of a group III topical steroid to the lower face. The inflammation flares shortly after the topical steroid is discontinued.

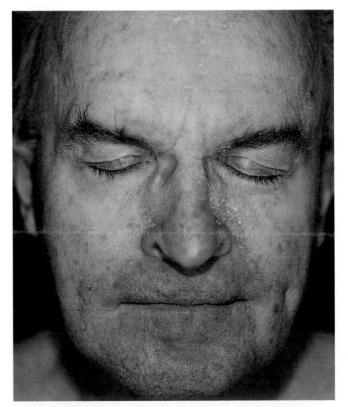

Figure 2-8 Steroid rosacea. A painful, diffuse pustular eruption occurred following daily application for 12 weeks of the group II topical steroid fluocinonide.

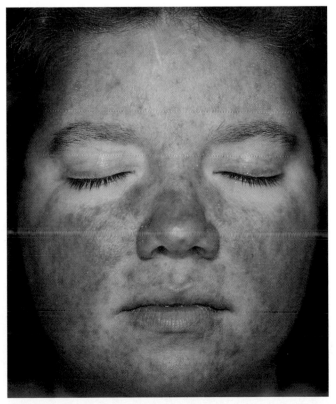

Figure 2-9 Steroid acne. Repeated application to the entire face of a group V topical steroid resulted in this diffuse pustular eruption. The inflammation improved each time the topical steroid was used but flared with increasing intensity each time the medication was stopped.

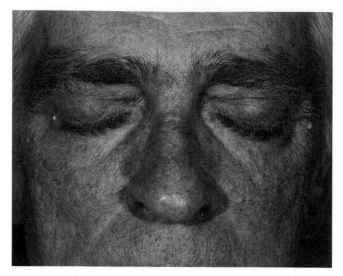

Figure 2-10 Steroid-induced telangiectasia. The patient in Figure 2-12 stopped all topical steroids. One year later he has permanent telangiectasia on the cheeks. His intraocular pressure was elevated but returned to near normal levels 3 months after stopping the fluocinonide.

Atrophy

Long-term use of strong topical steroids in the same area may result in thinning of the epidermis and regressive changes in the connective tissue in the dermis. The affected areas are often depressed slightly below normal skin and usually reveal telangiectasia, prominence of underlying veins, and hypopigmentation. Purpura and ecchymosis result from minor trauma. The skin becomes lax, wrinkled, and shiny. The face (Figures 2-10, 2-11, 2-12, and 2-13), dorsa of the hands (Figure 2-14), extensor surfaces of the forearms and legs, and intertriginous areas are particularly susceptible. In most cases atrophy is reversible and may be expected to disappear in the course of several months.[18] Diseases (such as psoriasis) that respond slowly to strong topical steroids require weeks of therapy; some atrophy may subsequently be anticipated (Figure 2-15).

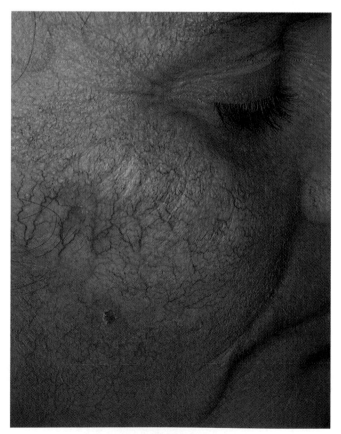

Figure 2-11 Atrophy and telangiectasia after continual use of a group IV topical steroid for 6 months. Atrophy may improve after the topical steroid is discontinued, but telangiectasia often persists.

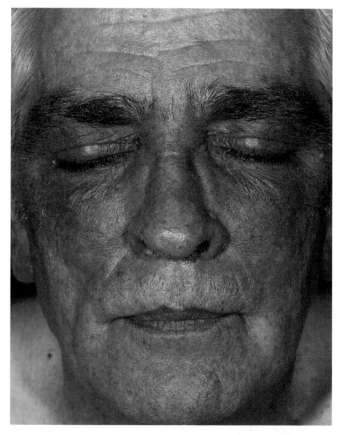

Figure 2-12 Steroid-induced erythema. This patient used the group II topical steroid fluocinonide almost constantly for 12 years. Erythema rather than pustules occurred each time the medication was stopped.

STEROID ATROPHY

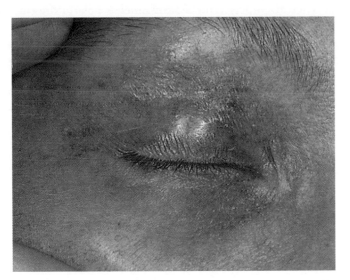

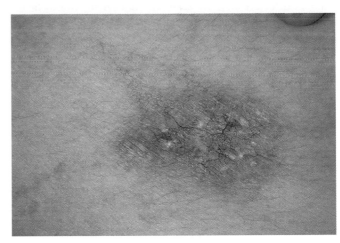

Figure 2-13

A, Daily application of the group II topical steroid desoximetasone to the lids resulted in almost complete atrophy of the dermis. The lids bleed spontaneously when touched. The intraocular pressure was elevated. There was marked improvement in the atrophy and intraocular tension 8 weeks after stopping the topical steroid.

B, Daily application for months of a group II topical steroid to the skin on the abdomen produced severe atrophy with telangiectasia.

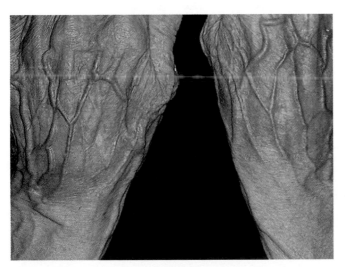

Figure 2-14 Severe steroid atrophy after continual occlusive therapy over several months. Significant improvement in the atrophy occurs after topical steroids are discontinued.

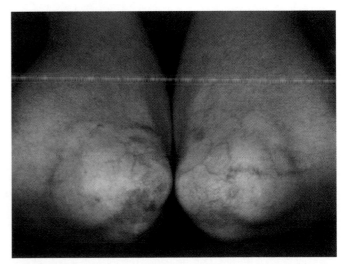

Figure 2-15 Steroid atrophy. Atrophy with prominence of underlying veins and hypopigmentation following use of Cordran Tape applied daily for 3 months to treat psoriasis. Note that small plaques of psoriasis persist. Atrophy improves after topical steroids are discontinued, but some hypopigmentation may persist.

OCCLUSION. Occlusion enhances penetration of medicine and accelerates the occurrence of this adverse reaction. Many patients are familiar with this side effect and must be assured that the use of strong topical steroids is perfectly safe when used as directed for 2 to 3 weeks. Patients must also be assured that if some atrophy does appear, it resolves in most cases when therapy is discontinued.

MUCOSAL AREAS. Atrophy under the foreskin (Figure 2-16) and in the rectal and vaginal areas may appear much more quickly than in other areas.[19] The thinner epidermis of-fers less resistance to the passage of corticosteroids into the dermis. These are intertriginous areas where the apposition of skin surfaces acts in the same manner as a plastic dressing, retaining moisture and greatly facilitating absorption. These delicate tissues become thin and painful, sometimes exhibiting a susceptibility to tear or bleed with scratching or intercourse. The atrophy seems to be more enduring in these areas. Therefore careful instruction about the duration of therapy must be given (e.g., twice a day for 10 days). If the disease does not resolve quickly with topical therapy, reevaluation is necessary.

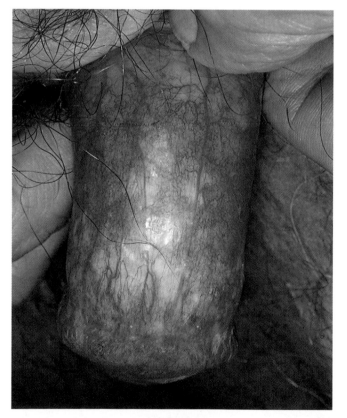

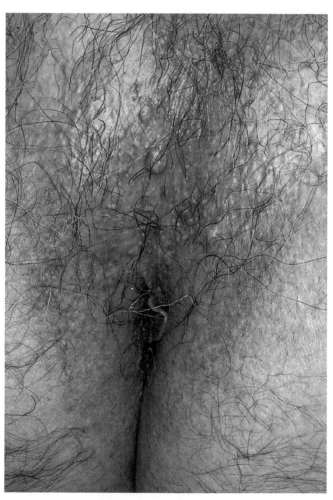

Figure 2-16

A, Steroid atrophy under the foreskin. Application of the group V topical steroid triamcinolone acetonide under the foreskin each day for 8 weeks produced severe atrophy and prominent telangiectasia of the shaft of the penis. The foreskin acted like an occlusive dressing to greatly enhance penetration of the steroid. Bleeding occurred with the slightest trauma. There was marked improvement 3 weeks after the medication was stopped.

B, Erythema, atrophy, and pain occured after the daily application of a group V topical steroid for 3 months.

STEROID INJECTION SITES. Atrophy may appear very rapidly after intralesional injection of corticosteroids (e.g., for treatment of acne cysts or in attempting to promote hair growth in alopecia areata). The side effect of atrophy is used to reduce the size of hypertrophic scars and keloids. When injected into the dermis, 5 mg/ml of triamcinolone acetonide (Kenalog) may produce atrophy; 10 mg/ml of triamcinolone acetonide almost always produces atrophy. For direct injection into the skin, stronger concentrations should probably be avoided.

LONG-TERM USE. Long-term use (over months) of even weak topical steroids on the upper inner thighs or in the axillae results in striae similar to those on the abdomens of pregnant women (Figure 2-17). These changes are irreversible. Pruritus in the groin area is common, and patients receive considerable relief when prescribed the less potent steroids. Symptoms often recur after treatment is terminated. It is a great temptation to continue topical treatment on an "as needed" basis but every attempt must be made to determine the underlying process and discourage long-term use.

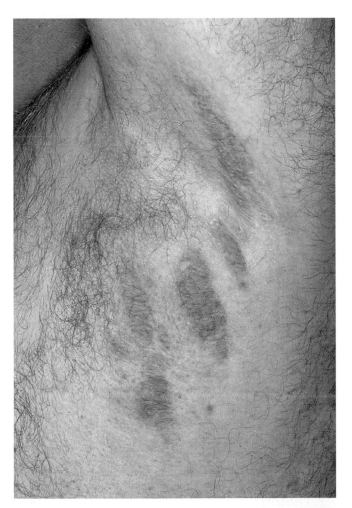

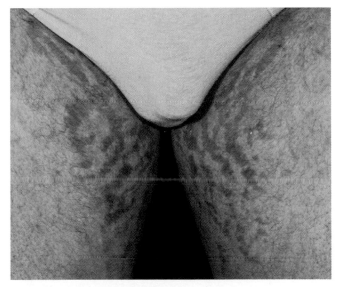

Figure 2-17

A, Striae of the axillae appeared after using Lotrisone cream continuously for 3 months.

B, Striae of the groin after long-term use of group V topical steroids for pruritus. These changes are irreversible.

Alteration of infection

Cortisone creams applied to cutaneous infections may alter the usual clinical presentation of those diseases and produce unusual atypical eruptions.[20,21] Cortisone cream suppresses the inflammation that is attempting to contain the infection and allows unrestricted growth.

TINEA INCOGNITO. Tinea of the groin is characteristically seen as a localized superficial plaque with a well-defined scaly border (Figure 2-18). A group II corticosteroid applied for 3 weeks to this common eruption produced the rash seen in Figure 2-19. The fungus rapidly spreads to involve a much wider area, and the typical sharply defined border is gone. Untreated tinea rarely produces such a florid eruption in temperate climates. This altered clinical picture has been called tinea incognito.

Figure 2-20 shows a young girl who applied a group II cream daily for 6 months to treat "eczema." The large plaques retain some of the characteristics of certain fungal infections by having well-defined edges. The red papules and nodules are atypical and are usually observed exclusively with an unusual form of follicular fungal infection seen on the lower legs.

Boils, folliculitis, rosacea-like eruptions, and diffuse fine scaling resulting from treatment of tinea with topical steroids have been reported. If a rash does not respond after a reasonable length of time or if the appearance changes, the presence of tinea, bacterial infection, or allergic contact dermatitis from some component of the steroid cream should be considered.

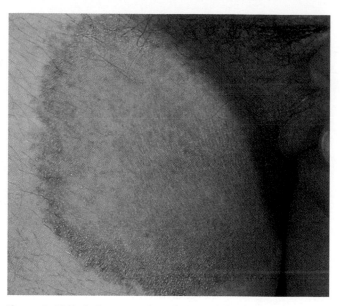

Figure 2-18 Typical presentation of tinea of the groin before treatment. Fungal infections of this type typically have a sharp, scaly border and show little tendency to spread.

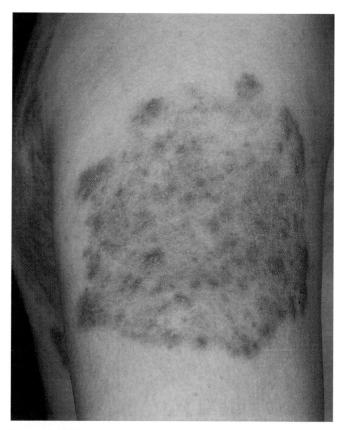

Figure 2-20 Tinea incognito. A plaque of tinea initially diagnosed as eczema was treated for 6 months with a group II topical steroid. Red papules have appeared where only erythema was once present.

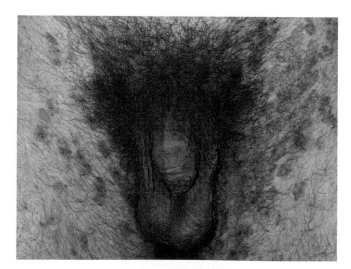

Figure 2-19 Tinea incognito. A bizarre pattern of widespread inflammation created by applying a group II topical steroid twice daily for 3 weeks to an eruption similar to that seen in Figure 2-18. A potassium hydroxide preparation showed numerous fungi.

INFESTATIONS AND BACTERIAL INFECTIONS. Scabies and impetigo may initially improve as topical steroids suppress inflammation. Consequently, both diseases become worse when the creams are discontinued (or, possibly, continued). Figure 2-21 shows numerous pustules on a leg; this appearance is characteristic of staphylococcal infection after treatment of an exudative, infected plaque of eczema with a group V topical steroid.

Contact dermatitis

Topical steroids are the drugs of choice for allergic and irritant contact dermatitis, but occasionally topical steroids cause such dermatitis.[22] Allergic reactions to various components of steroid creams (e.g., preservatives [parabens], vehicles [lanolin], antibacterials [neomycin], and perfumes) have all been documented. Figure 2-22 shows allergic contact dermatitis to a preservative in a group II steroid gel. The cream was prescribed to treat seborrheic dermatitis. Allergic reactions may not be intense. Inflammation created by a cream component (e.g., a preservative) may be suppressed by the steroid component of the same cream and the eruption simply smolders, neither improving nor worsening, presenting a very confusing picture.

Topical steroid allergy

Of patch-tested patients with dermatitis, 4% to 5% are allergic to corticosteroids. Patients affected by chronic dermatoses are at high risk for the development of sensitization to corticosteroids. Patients with any condition that does not improve or that deteriorates after administration of a topical steroid may be allergic to a component of the base or to the medication itself. Patients with stasis dermatitis and leg ulceration who are apt to use several topical medications for extended periods are more likely to be allergic to topical steroids. The over-the-counter availability of hydrocortisone makes long-term, unsupervised use possible. Allergy to topical steroids is demonstrated by patch or intradermal testing.

MANAGEMENT. When a patient does not respond as predicted or becomes worse while using topical corticosteroids, all topical treatment should be stopped. If corticosteroid therapy is absolutely necessary, one of the corticosteroids with a low sensitizing potential (e.g., mometasone furoate [Elocon], fluticasone propionate [Cutivate], betamethasone esters) could be used, and then only in an ointment base to avoid other allergens.[23]

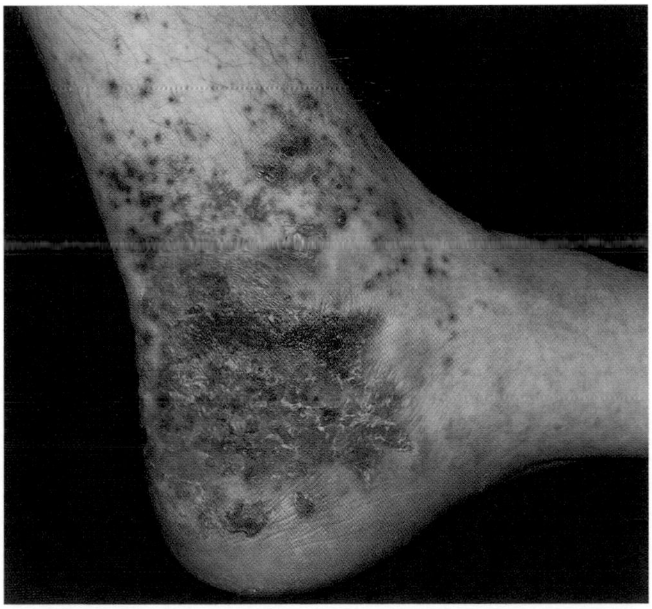

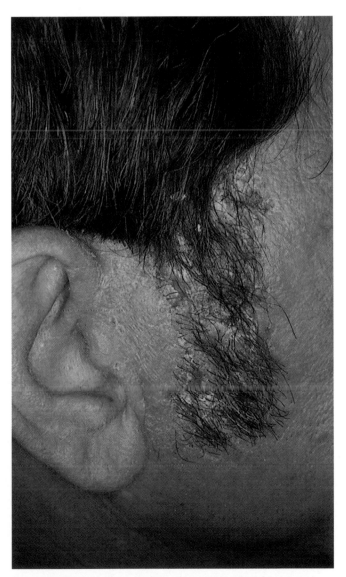

Figure 2-21 Impetiginized eczema with satellite pustules after treatment of exudative, infected eczema with a group V topical steroid.

Figure 2-22 Acute contact allergy to a preservative in a group II steroid gel.

PATCH TESTING. Allergy to a component of the vehicle or the steroid molecule may occur. Patch testing for steroid cream allergy is complicated and usually performed by patch-test experts.

Four groups of corticosteroids are recognized, where substances from the same group may cross-react.[23] The four groups are: group A (hydrocortisone type), group B (triamcinolone acetonides), group C (betamethasone type-nonesterified) and group D (hydrocortisone-17-butyrate type). The latter group is subclassified into two groups, group D1 (halogenated and with C16 substitution) and group D2 (the "labile" prodrug esters without the latter characteristics).

Tixocortol pivolate, hydrocortisone-17 butyrate, and budesonide are the screening agents of choice.[24] Patients should be patch tested to screen for corticosteroid allergy. If a corticosteroid sensitivity is detected, a more extensive corticosteroid series should be tested to determine cross-reactivity patterns. Cross-reactivity among topically administered corticosteroids is frequent.

Glaucoma

There are isolated case reports of glaucoma occurring after the long-term use of topical steroids about the eyes. Glaucoma induced by the chronic use of steroid-containing eyedrops instilled directly into the conjunctival sac is encountered more frequently by ophthalmologists. The mechanism by which glaucoma develops from topical application is not understood, but presumably, cream applied to the lids seeps over the lid margin and into the conjunctival sac. It also seems possible that enough steroid could be absorbed directly through the lid skin into the conjunctival sac to produce the same results.

Inflammation about the eye is a common problem. Offending agents that cause inflammation may be directly transferred to the eyelids by rubbing with the hand, or they may be applied directly, as with cosmetics. Women who are sensitive to a favorite eye makeup often continue using that makeup on an interrupted basis, not suspecting the obvious source of allergy. Patients have been known to alternate topical steroids with a sensitizing makeup. Unsupervised use of over-the-counter hydrocortisone cream might also induce glaucoma.

No studies have yet determined what quantity or strength of steroid cream is required to produce glaucoma. The patient shown in Figure 2-13 used a group II topical steroid on the eyelids daily for 3 years. Severe atrophy and bleeding with the slightest trauma occurred, and ocular pressure was elevated.

It is good practice to restrict the use of topical steroids on the eyelids to a 2- to 3-week period and use only groups VI and VII preparations.

References

1. Stoughton RB: Are generic formulations equivalent to brand name topical glucocorticosteroids? Arch Dermatol 1987; 121:1312.

2. Gammon WR et al: Intermittent short courses of clobetasol propionate ointment 0.05% in the treatment of psoriasis, Curr Ther Res 1987; 42:419.

3. Hardil E, Lindstrom C, Moller H: Intermittent treatment of psoriasis with clobetasol propionate, Acta Dermatol Venereol (Stockh) 1978; 58:375.

4. Katz HI et al: Superpotent topical steroid treatment of psoriasis vulgaris: clinical efficacy and adrenal function, J Am Acad Dermatol 1987; 16:804.

5. Olsen EA: A double-blind controlled comparison of generic and trade-name topical steroids using the vasoconstriction assay, Arch Dermatol 1991; 127:197.

6. Stoughton RB: Are topical glucocorticosteroids equivalent to the brand name? J Am Acad Dermatol 1988; 18:138.

7. Fisher AA: Problems associated with "generic" topical medications, Cutis 1988; 41:313.

8. Schlagel CA, Sanborn ED: The weights of topical preparations required for total and partial body inunction. J Invest Dermatol 1964; 42:252.

9. Long CC, Finlay AY: The finger-tip unit—a new practical measure, Clin Exp Dermatol 1991; 16:444.

10. Long CC, Averill RW: The rule of hand: 4 hand areas-2 FTU = 1 g, Arch Dermatol 1992; 128:1129.

11. duVivier A: Tachyphylaxis to topically applied steroids, Arch Dermatol 1976; 112:1245.

12. Svartholm H, Larsson L, Frederiksen B: Intermittent topical treatment of psoriasis with clobetasol propionate ('Dermovate'), Curr Med Res Opin 1982; 8:154.

13. Van DMJ et al: The management of moderate to severe atopic dermatitis in adults with topical fluticasone propionate: the Netherlands Adult Atopic Dermatitis Study Group, Br J Dermatol 1999; 140(6):1114.

14. Moller H, Svartholm H, Dahl G: Intermittent maintenance therapy in chronic hand eczema with clobetasol propionate and flupredniden acetate, Curr Med Res Opin 1983; 8:640.

15. Gomez EC, Kaminester L, Frost P: Topical halcinonide cream and betamethasone valerate: effects on plasma cortisol, Arch Dermatol 1977; 113:1196.

16. Friedlander S, Hebert A, Allen D: Safety of fluticasone propionate cream 0.05% for the treatment of severe and extensive atopic dermatitis in children as young as 3 months, J Am Acad Dermatol 2002; 46(3):387.

17. Leyden JJ, Thew M, Kligman AM: Steroid rosacea, Arch Dermatol 1974; 110:619.

18. Sneddon IB: The treatment of steroid-induced rosacea and perioral dermatitis, Dermatologica 1976; 152(suppl 1):231.

19. Goldman L, Kitzmiller KW: Perianal atrophoderma from topical corticosteroids, Arch Dermatol 1973; 107:611.

20. Ive FA, Mark SR: Tinea incognito, Br Med J 1968; 3:149.

21. Burry J: Topical drug addiction: adverse effects of fluorinated corticosteroid creams and ointments, Med J Aust 1973; 1:393.

22. Fisher AA, Pascher F, Kanof N: Allergic contact dermatitis due to ingredients of vehicles, Arch Dermatol 1971; 104:286.

23. Goossens A, Matura M, Degreef H: Reactions to corticosteroids: some new aspects regarding cross-sensitivity, Cutis 2000; 65(1):43.

24. Isaksson M et al: Patch testing with corticosteroid mixes in Europe: a multicentre study of the EECDRG, Contact Dermatitis 2000; 42(1):27.

❏ **Stages of eczematous inflammation**
Acute eczematous inflammation
Subacute eczematous inflammation
Chronic eczematous inflammation

❏ **Hand eczema**
Irritant contact dermatitis
Atopic hand dermatitis
Allergic contact dermatitis
Nummular eczema
Lichen simplex chronicus
Recurrent focal palmar peeling
Hyperkeratotic eczema
Fingertip eczema
Pompholyx
Id reaction

❏ **Eczema: various presentations**
Asteatotic eczema
Nummular eczema

❏ **Chapped fissured feet**

❏ **Self-inflicted dermatoses**
Lichen simplex chronicus
Prurigo nodularis
Neurotic excoriations

❏ **Psychogenic parasitosis**

❏ **Stasis dermatitis and venous ulceration:
postphlebitic syndromes**
Stasis dermatitis
Types of eczematous inflammation
Venous leg ulcers

Eczema (eczematous inflammation) is the most common inflammatory skin disease. Although the term *dermatitis* is often used to refer to an eczematous eruption, the word means inflammation of the skin and is not synonymous with eczematous processes. Recognizing a rash as eczematous rather than psoriasiform or lichenoid, for example, is of fundamental importance if one is to effectively diagnose skin disease. Here, as with other skin diseases, it is important to look carefully at the rash and to determine the primary lesion.

It is essential to recognize the quality and characteristics of the components of eczematous inflammation (erythema, scale, and vesicles) and to determine how these differ from other rashes with similar features. Once familiar with these features, the experienced clinician can recognize a process as eczematous even in the presence of secondary changes produced by scratching, infection, or irritation. With the diagnosis of eczematous inflammation established, a major part of the diagnostic puzzle has been solved.

THREE STAGES OF ECZEMA. There are three stages of eczema: *acute, subacute,* and *chronic.* Each represents a stage in the evolution of a dynamic inflammatory process (Table 3-1). Clinically, an eczematous disease may start at any stage and evolve into another. Most eczematous diseases, if left alone (i.e., neither irritated, scratched, nor medicated), resolve in time without complication. This ideal situation is almost never realized; scratching, irritation, or attempts at topical treatment are almost inevitable. Some degree of itching is a cardinal feature of eczematous inflammation.

Table 3-1 Eczematous Inflammation

Stage	Primary and secondary lesions	Symptoms	Etiology and clinical presentation	Treatment
Acute	Vesicles, blisters, intense redness	Intense itch	Contact allergy (poison ivy), severe irritation, id reaction, acute nummular eczema, stasis dermatitis, pompholyx (dyshidrosis), fungal infections	Cold wet compresses, oral or intramuscular steroids, topical steroids, antihistamines, antibiotics
Subacute	Redness, scaling, fissuring, parched appearance, scalded appearance	Slight to moderate itch, pain, stinging, burning	Contact allergy, irritation, atopic dermatitis, stasis dermatitis, nummular eczema, asteatotic eczema, fingertip eczema, fungal infections	Topical steroids with or without occlusion, lubrication, antihistamines, antibiotics, tar
Chronic	Thickened skin, skin lines accentuated (lichenified skin), excoriations, fissuring	Moderate to intense itch	Atopic dermatitis, habitual scratching, lichen simplex chronicus, chapped fissured feet, nummular eczema, asteatotic eczema, fingertip eczema, hyperkeratotic eczema	Topical steroids (with occlusion for best results), intralesional steroids, antihistamines, antibiotics, lubrication

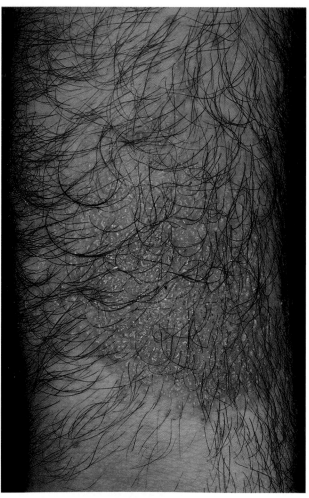

Figure 3-1 Acute eczematous inflammation. Numerous vesicles on an erythematous base. The vesicles may become confluent with time.

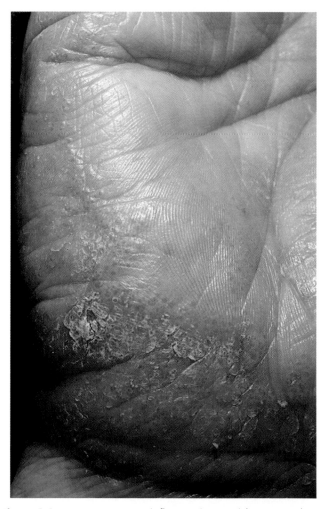

Figure 3-2 Acute eczematous inflammation. Vesicle appeared during a 24-hour period in this patient with chronic hand eczema. Episodes of acute inflammation had occurred several times in the past.

Stages of Eczematous Inflammation

Acute eczematous inflammation

ETIOLOGY. Inflammation is caused by contact with specific allergens such as *Rhus* (poison ivy, oak, or sumac) and chemicals. In the id reaction, vesicular reactions occur at a distant site during or after a fungal infection, stasis dermatitis, or other acute inflammatory processes.

PHYSICAL FINDINGS. The degree of inflammation varies from moderate to intense. A bright red, swollen plaque with a pebbly surface evolves in hours. Close examination of the surface reveals tiny, clear, serum-filled vesicles (Figures 3-1 and 3-2). The eruption may not progress or it may go on to develop blisters. The vesicles and blisters may be confluent and are often linear. Linear lesions result from dragging the offending agent across the skin with the finger during scratching. The degree of inflammation in cases caused by allergy is directly proportional to the quantity of antigen deposited on the skin. Excoriation predisposes to infection and causes serum, crust, and purulent material to accumulate.

SYMPTOMS. Acute eczema itches intensely. Patients scratch the eruption even while sleeping. A hot shower temporarily relieves itching because the pain produced by hot water is better tolerated than the sensation of itching; however, heat aggravates acute eczema.

COURSE. Lesions may begin to appear from hours to 2 to 3 days after exposure and may continue to appear for a week or more. These later-occurring, less inflammatory lesions are confusing to the patient, who cannot recall additional exposure. Lesions produced by small amounts of allergen are slower to evolve. They are not produced, as is generally believed, by contact with the serum of ruptured blisters, because the blister fluid does not contain the offending chemical. Acute eczematous inflammation evolves into a subacute stage before resolving.

TREATMENT

Cool wet dressings. The evaporative cooling produced by wet compresses causes vasoconstriction and rapidly suppresses inflammation and itching. Burrow's powder, available in a 12-packet box, may be added to the solution to suppress bacterial growth, but water alone is usually sufficient. A clean cotton cloth is soaked in cool water, folded several times, and placed directly over the affected areas. Evaporative cooling produces vasoconstriction and decreases serum production. Wet compresses should not be held in place and covered with towels or plastic wrap because this prevents evaporation. The wet cloth macerates vesicles and, when removed, mechanically debrides the area and prevents serum and crust from accumulating. Wet compresses should be removed after 30 minutes and replaced with a freshly soaked cloth. It is tempting to leave the drying compress in place and to wet it again by pouring solution onto the cloth. Although evaporative cooling will continue, irritation may occur from the accumulation of scale, crust, serum, and the increased concentration of aluminum sulfate and calcium acetate, the active ingredients in Burrow's powder.

Oral corticosteroids. Oral corticosteroids such as prednisone are useful for controlling intense or widespread inflammation and may be used in addition to wet dressings. Prednisone controls most cases of poison ivy when it is taken in 20-mg doses twice a day for 7 to 14 days (for adults); however, to treat intense or generalized inflammation, prednisone may be started at 30 mg or more twice a day and maintained at that level for 3 to 5 days. Sometimes 21 days of treatment are required for adequate control. The dosage should not be tapered for these relatively short courses because lower dosages may not give the desired antiinflammatory effect. Inflammation may reappear as diffuse erythema and may even be more extensive if the dosage is too low or is tapered too rapidly. Commercially available steroid dose packs taper the dosage and provide treatment for too short a time and so should not be used. Topical corticosteroids are of little use in the acute stage because the cream does not penetrate through the vesicles.

Antihistamines. Antihistamines, such as diphenhydramine (Benadryl) and hydroxyzine (Atarax), do not alter the course of the disease, but they relieve itching and provide enough sedation so patients can sleep. They are given every 4 hours as needed.

Antibiotics. The use of oral antibiotics may greatly hasten resolution of the disease if signs of superficial secondary infection, such as pustules, purulent material, and crusts, are present. Staphylococcus is the usual pathogen, and cultures are not routinely necessary. Deep infection (cellulitis) is rare with acute eczema. Erythromycin, cephalexin, and dicloxacillin are effective; topical antibiotics are much less effective.

Subacute eczematous inflammation

PHYSICAL FINDINGS. Erythema and scale are present in various patterns, usually with indistinct borders (Figures 3-3 and 3-4). The redness may be faint or intense (Figures 3-5 through 3-8). Psoriasis, superficial fungal infections, and eczematous inflammation may have a similar appearance (Figures 3-9 through 3-11). The borders of the plaques of psoriasis and superficial fungal infections are well defined. Psoriatic plaques have a deep, rich red color and silvery white scales.

SYMPTOMS. These vary from no itching to intense itching.

COURSE. Subacute eczematous inflammation may be the initial stage or it may follow acute inflammation. Irritation, allergy, or infection can convert a subacute process into an acute one. Subacute inflammation resolves spontaneously without scarring if all sources of irritation and allergy are withdrawn. Excess drying created from washing or continued use of wet dressings causes cracking and fissures. If excoriation is not controlled, the subacute process can be converted to a chronic one. Diseases that have subacute eczematous inflammation as a characteristic are listed in Box 3-1.

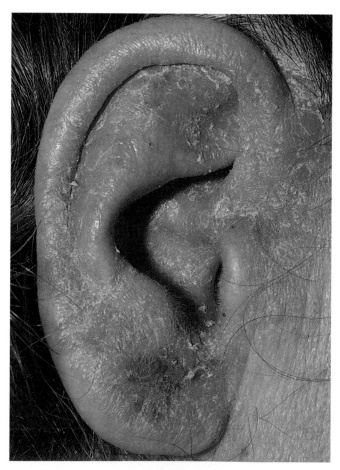

Figure 3-3 Subacute and chronic eczematous inflammation. The skin is dry, red, scaling, and thickened.

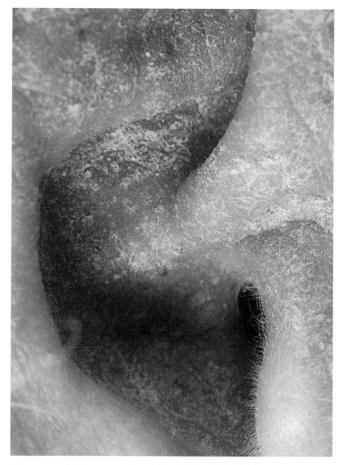

Figure 3-4 Subacute and chronic eczematous inflammation. The ear canal is red, scaling, and thickened from chronic excoriation.

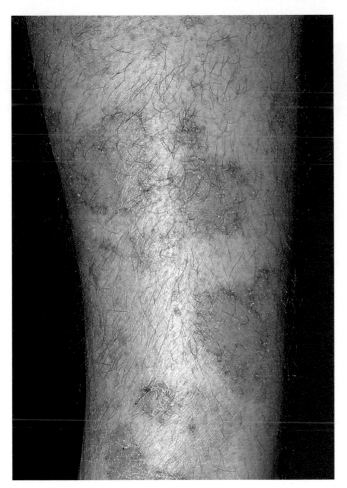

Figure 3-5 Red, scaling, nummular (round) superficial plaques occurred during the winter months from excessive washing.

Box 3-1 Diseases Presenting as Subacute Eczematous Inflammation

Allergic contact dermatitis	Intertrigo
Asteatotic eczema	Irritant contact dermatitis
Atopic dermatitis	Irritant hand eczema
Chapped fissured feet (sweaty sock dermatitis)	Nipple eczema (nursing mothers)
Circumileostomy eczema	Nummular eczema
Diaper dermatitis	Perioral lick eczema
Exposure to chemicals	Statis dermatitis

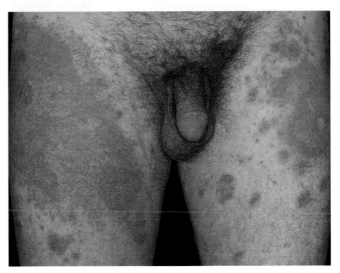

Figure 3-6 Erythema and scaling are present, the surface is dry, and the borders are indistinct.

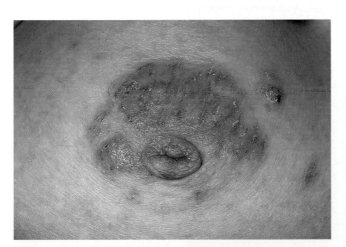

Figure 3-7 The areolae of both breasts are red and scaly. Inflammation of one areola is characteristic of Paget's disease.

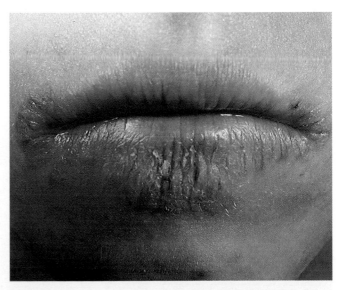

Figure 3-8 Wetting the lip by licking will eventually cause chapping and then eczema.

SUBACUTE ECZEMATOUS INFLAMMATION

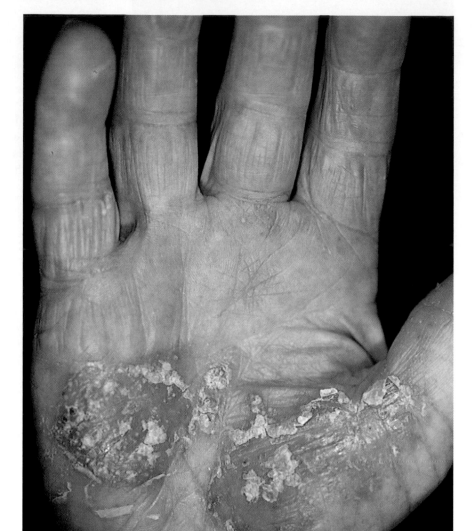

Figure 3-9 Acute vesicular eczema has evolved into subacute eczema with redness and scaling.

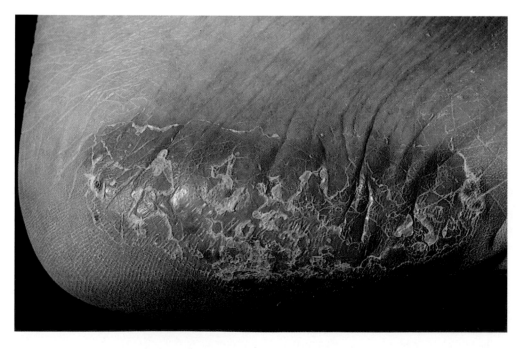

Figure 3-10 Acute and subacute eczematous inflammation. Acute vesicular eczema is evolving into subacute eczema. Vesicles, redness, and scaling are all present in this lesion undergoing transition.

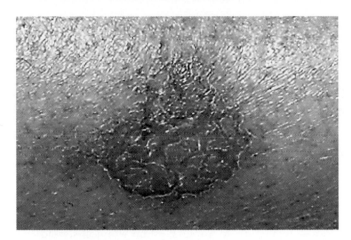

Figure 3-11 Subacute eczematous inflammation. Erythema and scaling in a round or nummular pattern.

TREATMENT. It is important to discontinue wet dressings when acute inflammation evolves into subacute inflammation. Excess drying creates cracking and fissures, which predispose to infection.

Topical corticosteroids. These agents are the treatment of choice (see Chapter 2). Creams may be applied 2 to 4 times a day or with occlusion. Ointments may be applied 2 to 4 times a day for drier lesions. Subacute inflammation requires groups III through V corticosteroids for rapid control. Occlusion with creams hastens resolution, and less expensive, weaker products such as triamcinolone cream 0.1% (Kenalog) give excellent results. *Staphylococcus aureus* colonizes eczematous lesions, but studies show their numbers are significantly reduced following treatment with topical steroids.[1]

Topical macrolide immune suppressants. Tacrolimus ointment (Protopic) and pimecrolimus cream (Elidel) are the first topical macrolide immune suppressants that are not hydrocortisone derivatives. They inhibit the production of inflammatory cytokines in T cells and mast cells and prevent the release of preformed inflammatory mediators from mast cells. Dermal atrophy does not occur. These agents are effective for the treatment of inflammatory skin diseases, such as atopic dermatitis, allergic contact dermatitis, and irritant contact dermatitis. They are approved for use in children 2 years or older. Response to these agents is slower than the response to topical steroids. Topical steroids may be used for several days before the use of these agents to obtain rapid control.

Pimecrolimus (Elidel) cream. Pimecrolimus permeates through skin at a lower rate than tacrolimus, indicating a lower potential for percutaneous absorption. The cream is applied twice a day and may be used on the face. There are no restrictions on duration of use.

Tacrolimus ointment (Protopic). Tacrolimus is effective in the treatment of children (aged 2 years and older) and adults with atopic dermatitis and eczema. The most prominent adverse event is application site burning and erythema. It is available in 0.03% and 0.1% ointment formulations. Some clinicians find the 0.03% concentration to be marginally effective.

Doxepin cream. A topical form of the antidepressant doxepin (doxepin 5% cream; Zonalon) is effective for the relief of pruritus associated with eczema in adults and children aged over 12 years. The two most common adverse effects are stinging at the site of application and drowsiness. The medication can be applied four times a day as needed.

Lubrication. This is a simple but essential part of therapy. Inflamed skin becomes dry and is more susceptible to further irritation and inflammation. Resolved dry areas may easily relapse into subacute eczema if proper lubrication is neglected. Lubricants are best applied a few hours after topical steroids and should be continued for days or weeks after the inflammation has cleared. Frequent application (1 to 4 times a day) should be encouraged. Applying lubricants directly after the skin has been patted dry following a shower seals in moisture. Lotions or creams with or without the hydrating chemicals urea and lactic acid may be used. Bath oils are very useful if used in amounts sufficient to make the skin feel oily when the patient leaves the tub.

Lotions. Curel, DML, Lubriderm, Cetaphil or any of the other lotions listed in the Formulary are useful.

Creams. DML, Moisturel, Neutrogena, Nivea, Eucerin, and Acid Mantle or any of the other creams listed in the Formulary are useful.

Mild soaps. Frequent washing with a drying soap, such as Ivory, delays healing. Infrequent washing with mild or superfatted soaps (e.g., Dove, Cetaphil, Basis—see the Formulary) should be encouraged. It is usually not necessary to use hypoallergenic soaps or to avoid perfumed soaps. Although allergy to perfumes occurs, the incidence is low.

Antibiotics. Eczematous plaques that remain bright red during treatment with topical steroids may be infected. Infected subacute eczema should be treated with appropriate systemic antibiotics, which are usually those active against staphylococci. Systemic antibiotics are more effective than topical antibiotics or antibiotic-steroid combination creams.

Tar. Tar ointments, baths, and soaps were among the few effective therapeutic agents available for the treatment of eczema before the introduction of topical steroids. Topical steroids provide rapid and lasting control of eczema in most cases. Some forms of eczema, such as atopic dermatitis and irritant eczema, tend to recur. Topical steroids become less effective with long-term use. Tar is sometimes an effective alternative in this setting. Tar ointments or creams may be used for long-term control or between short courses of topical steroids.

Chronic eczematous inflammation

ETIOLOGY. Chronic eczematous inflammation may be caused by irritation of subacute inflammation, or it may appear as lichen simplex chronicus.

PHYSICAL FINDINGS. Chronic eczematous inflammation is a clinical-pathologic entity and does not indicate simply any long-lasting stage of eczema. If scratching is not controlled, subacute eczematous inflammation can be modified and converted to chronic eczematous inflammation (Figure 3-12). The inflamed area thickens, and surface skin markings may become more prominent. Thick plaques with deep parallel skin marking ("washboard lesion") are said to be lichenified (Figure 3-13). The border is well defined but not as sharply defined as it is in psoriasis (Figure 3-14). The sites most commonly involved are those areas that are easily reached and associated with habitual scratching (e.g., dorsal feet, lateral forearms, anus, and occipital scalp), areas where eczema tends to be long-lasting (e.g., the lower legs, as in stasis dermatitis), and the crease areas (antecubital and popliteal fossa, wrists, behind the ears, and ankles) in atopic dermatitis (Figures 3-15, 3-16, and 3-17).

SYMPTOMS. There is moderate to intense itching. Scratching sometimes becomes violent, leading to excoriation and digging, and ceases only when pain has replaced the itch. Patients with chronic inflammation scratch while asleep.

COURSE. Scratching and rubbing become habitual and are often done unconsciously. The disease then becomes self-perpetuating. Scratching leads to thickening of the skin, which itches more than before. It is this habitual manipulation that causes the difficulty in eradicating this disease. Some patients enjoy the feeling of relief that comes from scratching and may actually desire the reappearance of their disease after treatment.

TREATMENT. Chronic eczematous inflammation is resistant to treatment and requires potent steroid therapy.

Topical steroids. Groups II through V topical steroids are used with occlusion each night until the inflammation clears—usually in 1 to 3 weeks; group I topical steroids are used without occlusion.

Intralesional injection. Intralesional injection (Kenalog, 10 mg/ml) is a very effective mode of therapy. Lesions that have been present for years may completely resolve after one injection or a short series of injections. The medicine is delivered with a 27- or 30-gauge needle, and the entire plaque is infiltrated until it blanches white. Resistant plaques require additional injections given at 3- to 4-week intervals.

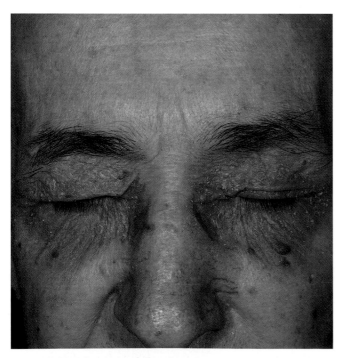

Figure 3-12 Subacute and chronic eczema. Dermatitis of the lids may be allergic, irritant, or atopic in origin. This atopic patient rubs the lids with the back of the hands.

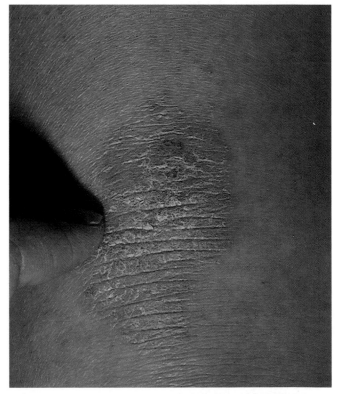

Figure 3-13 Chronic eczematous inflammation. Chronic excoriations thicken the epidermis, which results in accentuated skin lines. Chronic eczema created by picking is called lichen simplex chronicus.

CHRONIC ECZEMATOUS INFLAMMATION

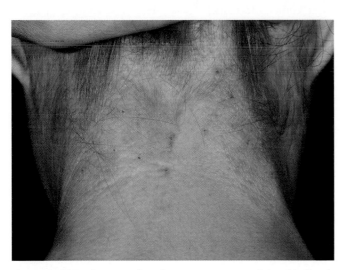

Figure 3-14 Erythema and scaling are present, and the skin lines are accentuated, creating a lichenified or "washboard" lesion.

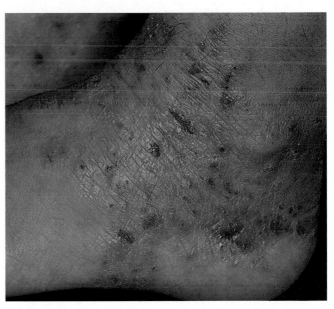

Figure 3-15 Atopic dermatitis. Atopic dermatitis is common in the crease areas. Atopic patients scratch, lichenify the skin, and often create a chronic process.

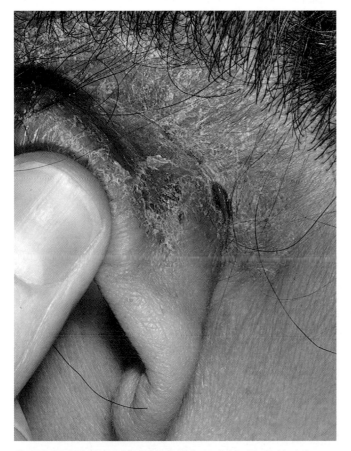

Figure 3-16 Picking and rubbing thickened the skin behind the ear.

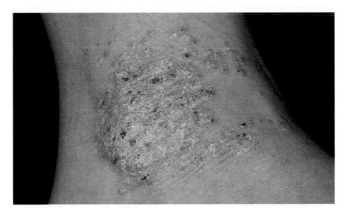

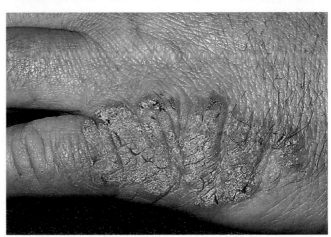

Figure 3-17 A plaque of lichen simplex chronicus created by excoriation is present. Accentuated skin lines and eczematous papules beyond the border help to differentiate this process from psoriasis.

Hand Eczema

Inflammation of the hands is one of the most common problems encountered by the dermatologist. Hand dermatitis causes discomfort and embarrassment and, because of its location, interferes significantly with normal daily activities. Hand dermatitis is common in industrial occupations: it can threaten job security if inflammation cannot be controlled.[2,3] Box 3-2 lists instructions for patients with irritant hand dermatitis.

EPIDEMIOLOGY. A large study provided the following statistics: the prevalence of hand eczema was approximately 5.4% and was twice as common in females as in males. The most common type of hand eczema was irritant contact dermatitis (35%), followed by atopic hand eczema (22%), and allergic contact dermatitis (19%). The most common contact allergies were to nickel, cobalt, fragrance mix, balsam of Peru, and colophony. Of all the occupations studied, cleaners had the highest prevalence at 21.3%. Hand eczema was more common among people reporting occupational exposure. The most harmful exposure was to chemicals, water and detergents, dust, and dry dirt. A change of occupation was reported by 8% and was most common in service workers. Hairdressers had the highest frequency of change. Hand eczema was shown to be a long-lasting disease with a relapsing course; 69% of the patients had consulted a physician, and 21% had been on sick leave at least once because of hand eczema. The mean total sick-leave time was 18.9 weeks; the median was 8 weeks.[4] The most important predictive factors for hand eczema are listed in Box 3-3.

Box 3-2 Irritant Hand Dermatitis Instructions for Patients

1. Wash hands as infrequently as possible. Ideally, soap should be avoided and hands simply washed in lukewarm water.

2. Shampooing must be done with rubber gloves or by someone else.

3. Avoid direct contact with household cleaners and detergents. Wear cotton, plastic, or rubber gloves when doing housework.

4. Do not touch or do anything that causes burning or itching (e.g., wool; wet diapers; peeling potatoes or handling fresh fruits, vegetables, and raw meat).

5. Wear rubber gloves when irritants are encountered. Rubber gloves alone are not sufficient because the lining collects sweat, scales, and debris and can become more irritating than those objects to be avoided. Dermal white cotton gloves should be worn next to the skin under unlined rubber gloves. Several pairs of cotton gloves should be purchased so they can be changed frequently. Try on the rubber gloves over the white cotton gloves at the time of purchase to ensure a comfortable fit.

Box 3-3 Predictive Factors for Hand Eczema

History of childhood eczema (most important predictive factor)

Female sex

Occupational exposure

History of asthma and/or hay fever

Service occupation (cleaners, etc.)

From Meding B, Swanbeck G: *Contact Dermatitis* 23:154, 1990.

Table 3-2 Hand Dermatitis: Differential Diagnosis and Distribution

Location	Redness and scaling	Vesicles	Pustules
Back of hand	Atopic dermatitis	Id reaction	Bacterial infection
	Irritant contact dermatitis	Scabies (web spaces)	Psoriasis
	Lichen simplex chronicus		Scabies (web spaces)
	Nummular eczema		Tinea
	Psoriasis		
	Tinea		
Palmar surface	Fingertip eczema	Allergic contact dermatitis	Bacterial infection
	Hyperkeratotic eczema	Pompholyx (dyshidrosis)	Pompholyx (dyshidrosis)
	Recurrent focal palmar peeling		Psoriasis
	Psoriasis		
	Tinea		

DIAGNOSIS. The diagnosis and management of hand eczema is a challenge. There is almost no association between clinical pattern and etiology. No distribution of eczema is typically allergic, irritant, or endogenous.[5] Not only are there many patterns of eczematous inflammation (Table 3-2), but there are other diseases, such as psoriasis, that may appear eczematous. The original primary lesions and their distribution become modified with time by irritants, excoriation, infection, and treatment. All stages of eczematous inflammation may be encountered in hand eczema (Box 3-4).

Irritant contact dermatitis

Irritant hand dermatitis (housewives' eczema, dishpan hands, detergent hands) is the most common type of hand inflammation. Some people can withstand long periods of repeated exposure to various chemicals and maintain normal skin. At the other end of the spectrum, there are those who develop chapping and eczema from simple hand washing. Patients whose hands are easily irritated may have an atopic diathesis.

PATHOPHYSIOLOGY. The stratum corneum is the protective envelope that prevents exogenous material from entering the skin and prevents body water from escaping. The stratum corneum is composed of dead cells, lipids (from sebum and cellular debris), and water-binding organic chemicals. The stratum corneum of the palms is thicker than that of the dorsa and is more resistant to irritation. The pH of this surface layer is slightly acidic. Environmental factors or elements that change any component of the stratum corneum interfere with its protective function and expose the skin to irritants. Factors such as cold winter air and low humidity promote water loss. Substances such as organic solvents and alkaline soaps extract water-binding chemicals and lipids. Once enough of these protective elements have been extracted, the skin decompensates and becomes eczematous.

CLINICAL PRESENTATION. The degree of inflammation depends on factors such as strength and concentration of the chemical, individual susceptibility, site of contact, and time of year. Allergy, infection, scratching, and stress modify the picture.

STAGES OF INFLAMMATION. Dryness and chapping are the initial changes (Figure 3-18). Very painful cracks and fissures occur, particularly in joint crease areas and around the fingertips. The backs of the hands become red, swollen, and tender. The palmar surface, especially that of the fingers, becomes red and continues to be dry and cracked. A red, smooth, shiny, delicate surface that splits easily with the slightest trauma may develop. These are subacute eczematous changes (Figures 3-19 and 3-20).

Acute eczematous inflammation occurs with further irritation creating vesicles that ooze and crust. Itching intensifies, and excoriation leads to infection (Figures 3-21 and 3-22).

Necrosis and ulceration followed by scarring occur if the irritating chemical is too caustic.

Box 3-4 Various Types of Hand Eczema	
Irritant	Recurrent focal palmar peeling
Atopic	Fingertip
Allergic	Hyperkeratotic
Nummular	Pompholyx (dyshidrosis)
Lichen simplex chronicus	Id reaction

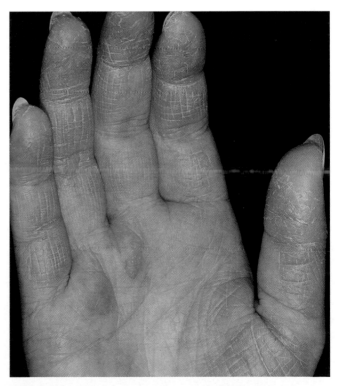

Figure 3-18 Early irritant hand dermatitis with dryness and chapping.

IRRITANT HAND DERMATITIS

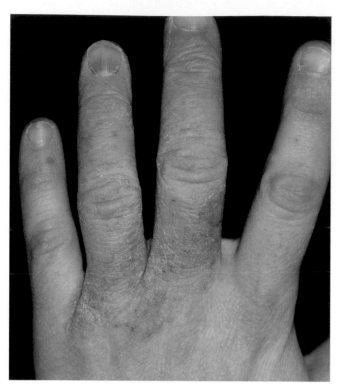

Figure 3-19 Subacute eczematous inflammation appeared on the dry, chapped third and fourth fingers.

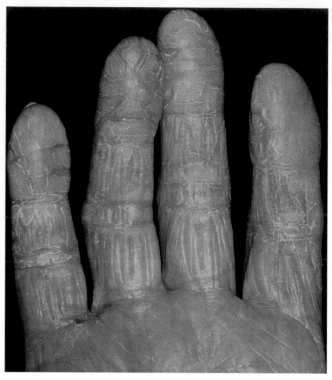

Figure 3-20 Subacute and chronic eczematous inflammation with severe drying and splitting of the fingertips.

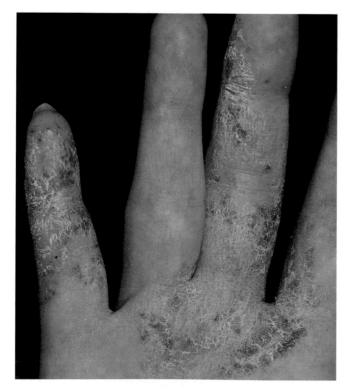

Figure 3-21 Numerous tiny vesicles suddenly appeared on these chronically inflamed fingers.

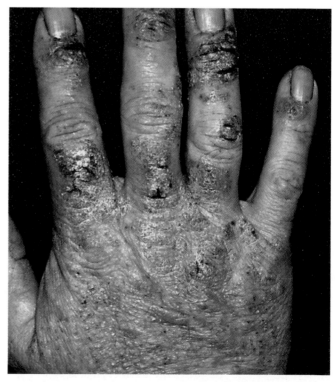

Figure 3-22 Chronic eczematous inflammation. Scratching has thickened the skin. Crusts are signs of infection.

PATIENTS AT RISK. Individuals at risk include mothers with young children (changing diapers), individuals whose jobs require repeated wetting and drying (e.g., surgeons, dentists, dishwashers, bartenders, fishermen), industrial workers whose jobs require contact with chemicals (e.g., cutting oils), and patients with the atopic diathesis.

PREVENTION. One study revealed that hospital staff members who used an emulsion cleanser (e.g., Cetaphil lotion, Duosoft [in Europe]) had significantly less dryness and eczema than those who used a liquid soap.[6] Regular use of emollients prevented irritant dermatitis caused by a detergent.[7]

BARRIER-PROTECTANT CREAMS. Loss of skin barrier function by mechanical or chemical insults may result in water loss and hand eczema. Barrier creams (see Box 3-5) applied at least twice a day on all exposed areas) protect the skin and are formulated to be either water-repellent or oil-repellent. The water-repellent types offer little protection against oils or solvents.

TREATMENT. The inflammation is treated as outlined in the section on stages of eczematous inflammation. Lubrication and avoidance of further irritation helps to prevent recurrence. A program of irritant avoidance should be carefully outlined for each patient (see Box 3-2).

Atopic hand dermatitis

Hand dermatitis may be the most common form of adult atopic dermatitis (see Chapter 5). Hand eczema is significantly more common in people with a history of atopic dermatitis than in others.[8] The following factors predict the occurrence of hand eczema in adults with a history of atopic dermatitis[9]:

- Hand dermatitis before age 15
- Persistent eczema on the body
- Dry or itchy skin in adult life
- Widespread atopic dermatitis in childhood

Many people with atopic dermatitis develop hand eczema independently of exposure to irritants, but such exposure causes additional irritant contact dermatitis.

The backs of the hands, particularly the fingers, are affected (Figure 3-23). The dermatitis begins as a typical irritant reaction with chapping and erythema. Several forms of eczematous dermatitis evolve; erythema, edema, vesiculation, crusting, excoriation, scaling, and lichenification appear and are intensified by scratching.[10] Management for atopic hand eczema is the same as that for irritant hand eczema.

Box 3-5 Barrier Creams—Applied at Least Twice a Day on All Exposed Areas
Water repellent
• North 201
• SBS-44
• Kerodex #71
For oil- or solvent-based materials
• Kerodex #51
• SBS-46
• North 222
• Dermashield (both oil- and water-based materials)
General purpose barrier protective creams
• SBR-Lipocream
• TheraSeal

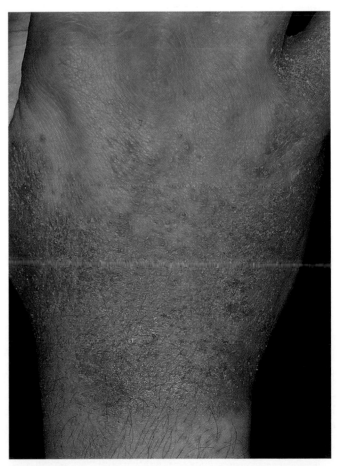

Figure 3-23 Irritant hand dermatitis in a patient with the atopic diathesis. Irritant eczema of the backs of the hands is a common form of adult atopic dermatitis.

Allergic contact dermatitis

Allergic contact dermatitis of the hands is not as common as irritant dermatitis. However, allergy as a possible cause of hand eczema, no matter what the pattern, should always be considered in the differential diagnosis; it may be investigated by patch testing in appropriate cases. The incidence of allergy in hand eczema was demonstrated by patch testing in a study of 220 patients with hand eczema.[11] In 12% of the 220 patients, the diagnosis was established with the aid of a standard screening series now available in a modified form (T.R.U.E. TEST).[12] Another 5% of the cases were diagnosed as a result of testing with additional allergens. The hand eczema in these two groups (17%) changed dramatically after identification and avoidance of the allergens found by patch testing. Table 3-3 lists some possible causes of allergic hand dermatitis.

PHYSICAL FINDINGS. The diagnosis of allergic contact dermatitis is obvious when the area of inflammation corresponds exactly to the area covered by the allergen (e.g., a round patch of eczema under a watch or inflammation in the shape of a sandal strap on the foot). Similar clues may be present with hand eczema, but in many cases allergic and irritant hand eczemas cannot be distinguished by their clinical presentation. Hand inflammation, whatever the source, is increased by further exposure to irritating chemicals, washing, scratching, medication, and infection. Inflammation of the dorsum of the hand is more often irritant or atopic than allergic.

TREATMENT. Allergy may initially appear as acute, subacute, or chronic eczematous inflammation and is managed accordingly.

Table 3-3 Allergic Hand Dermatitis: Some Possible Causes

Allergens	Sources
Nickel	Door knobs, handles on kitchen utensils, scissors, knitting needles, industrial equipment, hairdressing equipment
Potassium dichromate	Cement, leather articles (gloves), industrial machines, oils
Rubber	Gloves, industrial equipment (hoses, belts, cables)
Fragrances	Cosmetics, soaps, lubricants, topical medications
Formaldehyde	Wash-and-wear fabrics, paper, cosmetics, embalming fluid
Lanolin	Topical lubricants and medications, cosmetics

Nummular eczema

Eczema that appears as one or several coin-shaped plaques is called *nummular eczema*. This pattern often occurs on the extremities but may also present as hand eczema. The plaques are usually confined to the backs of the hands (Figure 3-24). The number of lesions may increase, but once they are established they tend to remain the same size. The inflammation is either subacute or chronic and itching is moderate to intense. The cause is unknown. Thick, chronic, scaling plaques of nummular eczema look like psoriasis; treatment for nummular eczema is the same as that for subacute or chronic eczema.

Lichen simplex chronicus

A localized plaque of chronic eczematous inflammation that is created by habitual scratching is called *lichen simplex chronicus* or *localized neurodermatitis*. The back of the wrist is a typical site. The plaque is thick with prominent skin lines (lichenification) and the margins are fairly sharp. Once established, the plaque does not usually increase in area. Lichen simplex chronicus is treated in the same manner as chronic eczematous inflammation.

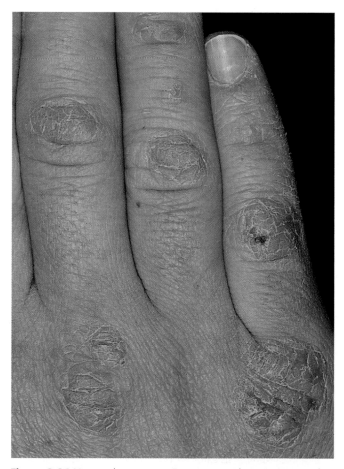

Figure 3-24 Nummular eczema. Eczematous plaques are round (coin-shaped).

Recurrent focal palmar peeling

Keratolysis exfoliativa or recurrent focal palmar peeling is a common, chronic, asymptomatic, noninflammatory, bilateral peeling of the palms of the hands and occasionally soles of the feet; its cause is unknown[13] (Figure 3-25). The eruption is most common during the summer months and is often associated with sweaty palms and soles. Some people experience this phenomenon only once, whereas others have repeated episodes. Scaling starts simultaneously from several points on the palms or soles with 2 or 3 mm of round scales that appears to have originated from a ruptured vesicle; however, these vesicles are never seen. The scaling continues to peel and extend peripherally, forming larger, roughly circular areas that resemble ringworm whereas the central area becomes slightly red and tender. The scaling borders may coalesce. The condition resolves in 1 to 3 weeks and requires no therapy other than lubrication.

Hyperkeratotic eczema

A very thick, chronic form of eczema that occurs on the palms and occasionally the soles is seen almost exclusively in men. One or several plaques of yellow-brown, dense scale increase in thickness and form deep interconnecting cracks over the surface, similar to mud drying in a river bed (Figure 3-26). The dense scale, unlike callus, is moist below the surface and is not easily pared with a blade. Patients discover that the scale is firmly adherent to the epidermis when they attempt to peel off the thick scale and this exposes tender bleeding areas of dermis. Hyperkeratotic eczema may result from allergy or excoriation and irritation, but in most cases the cause is not apparent. The disease is chronic and may last for years. Psoriasis and lichen simplex chronicus must be considered in the differential diagnosis. The disease is treated like chronic eczema; although the plaques respond to group II steroid cream and occlusion, recurrences are frequent. Patch testing is indicated for recurrent disease.

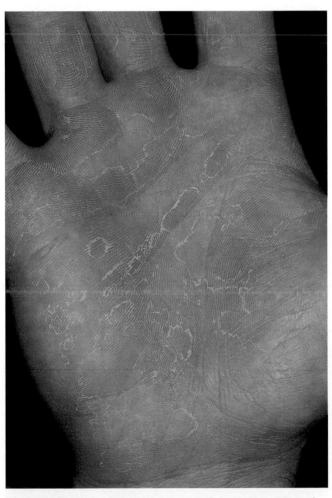

Figure 3-25 Keratolysis exfoliativa. Noninflammatory peeling of the palms that is often associated with sweating. The eruption must be differentiated from tinea of the palms.

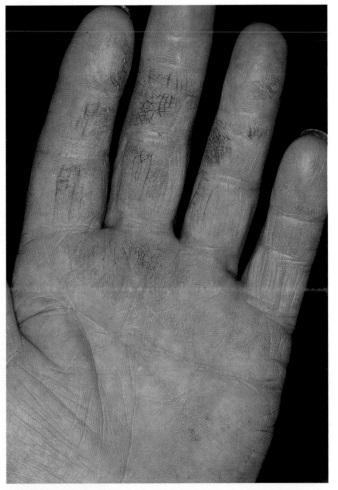

Figure 3-26 Hyperkeratotic eczema. Patches of dense yellow-brown scale occur on the palms. This patient was allergic to a steering wheel.

FINGERTIP ECZEMA

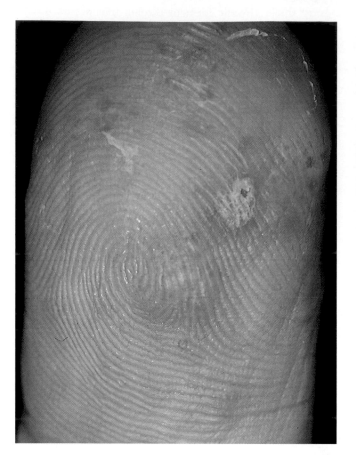
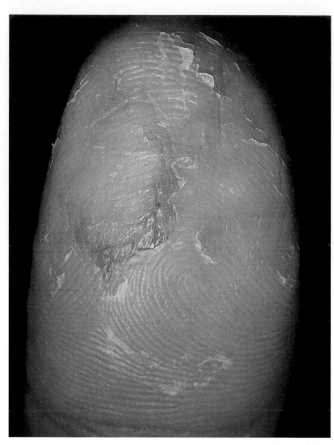

Figure 3-27

A, An early stage. The skin is moist. A vesicle is present. Redness and cracking have occurred in the central area.

B, A more advanced stage. Peeling occurs constantly. The skin lines are lost.

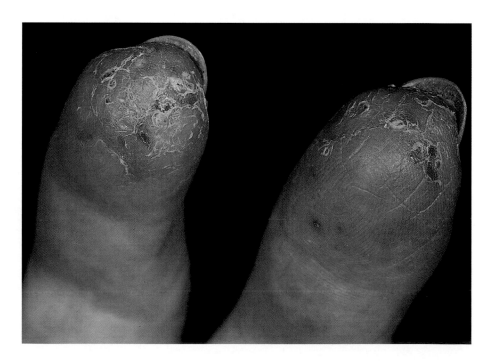

Figure 3-28 Asteatotic eczema. Excessive washing produced this advanced case with cracking and fissures.

Fingertip eczema

A very dry, chronic form of eczema of the palmar surface of the fingertips may be the result of an allergic reaction (e.g., to plant bulbs or resins) or may occur in children and adults as an isolated phenomenon of unknown cause. One finger or several fingers may be involved. Initially the skin may be moist and then may become dry, cracked, and scaly (Figure 3-27). The skin peels from the fingertips distally, exposing a very dry, red, cracked, fissured, tender, or painful surface without skin lines (Figures 3-27, 3-28, and 3-29). The process usually stops shortly before the distal interphalangeal joint is reached (Figures 3-29 and 3-31). Fingertip eczema may last for months or years and is resistant to treatment. Topical steroids with or without occlusion give only temporary relief. Once allergy and psoriasis have been ruled out, fingertip eczema should be managed the same way as subacute and chronic eczema, by avoiding irritants and lubricating frequently. Elidel or Protopic is sometimes effective; tar creams such as Fototar applied twice each day have at times provided relief.

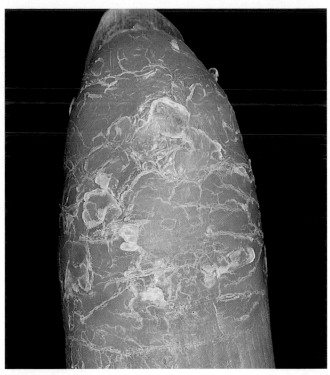

Figure 3-30 Severe chronic inflammation. The skin lines are lost. The dry skin is fragile and cracks easily. Patients are tempted to peel away the dry loose scale.

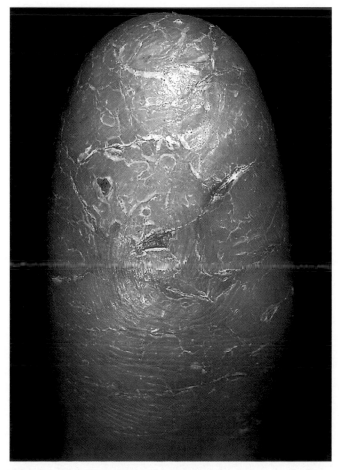

Figure 3-29 Fingertip eczema. Inflammation has been present for months and responded poorly to topical steroids.

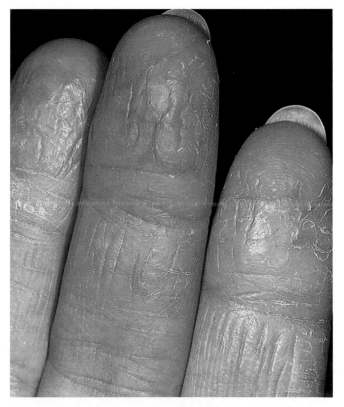

Figure 3-31 The fingers are dry and wrinkled, and the skin is fragile. The skin peels but does not form the thick scale shown in Figures 3-29 and 3-30.

POMPHOLYX (DYSHIDROSIS)

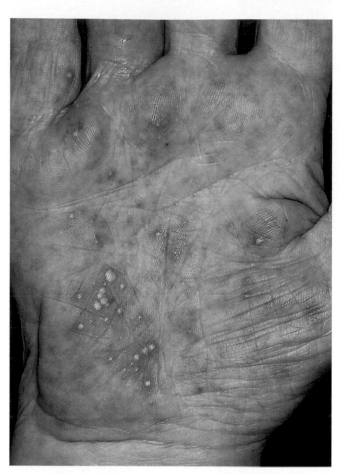

Figure 3-32 Vesicles have evolved into pustules. The eruption has persisted for many weeks.

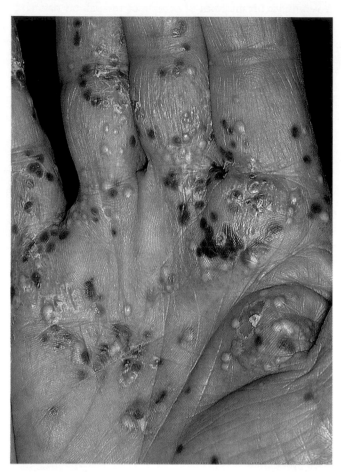

Figure 3-33 Vesicles have become infected. Pustular lesions occurred and then became more numerous.

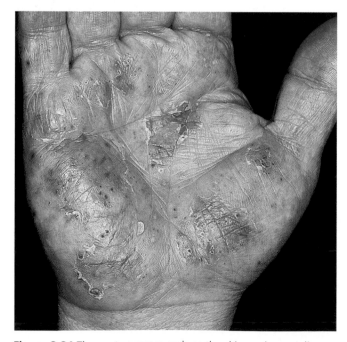

Figure 3-34 The acute process ends as the skin peels, revealing a red, cracked base with brown spots. The brown spots are sites of previous vesiculation.

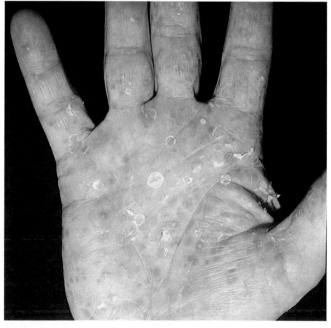

Figure 3-35 A severe form (with large, deep vesicles and blisters) that is indistinguishable from pustular psoriasis of the palms and soles.

Pompholyx

Pompholyx (dyshidrosis) is a distinctive reaction pattern of unknown etiology presenting as symmetric vesicular hand and foot dermatitis (Figure 3-32). Moderate to severe itching precedes the appearance of vesicles on the palms and sides of the fingers (Figure 3-33). The palms may be red and wet with perspiration, hence the name *dyshidrosis*. The vesicles slowly resolve in 3 to 4 weeks and are replaced by 1- to 3-mm rings of scale (Figures 3-34 and 3-35). Chronic eczematous changes with erythema, scaling, and lichenification may follow. Waves of vesiculation may appear indefinitely. Pustular psoriasis of the palms and soles may resemble pompholyx, but the vesicles of psoriasis rapidly become cloudy with purulent fluid, and pain rather than itching is the chief complaint. Pustular psoriasis is chronic and the pustules do not evolve and disappear as rapidly as those of pompholyx. Patients with atopic dermatitis are affected as frequently as others.

The cause of pompholyx is unknown, but there seems to be some relationship to stress. Pompholyx is a disease that disrupts the skin and allows sensitization to contact allergens to occur, but direct contact with the allergen does not seem to be the cause of the disease. Ingestion of allergens such as chromate, neomycin, quinoline, or nickel may cause some cases.[14] Ingestion of nickel, cobalt, and chromium can elicit pompholyx in patients who are patch test negative to these metals.[15,16] The perspiration volume of pompholyx patients was found to be 2.5 times higher than that of age-matched normal control; 20% of patients showed sensitivity to chromate, 16% to cobalt, and 28% to nickel on patch testing. Some patients with positive results who are challenged orally with nickel, cobalt, or chromium show vesicular reactions on their hands. Sensitivity to orally ingested metal compounds in combination with local hyperhidrosis may contribute to the development of vesicular lesions in pompholyx.[17]

TREATMENT. Topical steroids, cold wet compresses, and possibly oral antibiotics are used as the initial treatment, but the response is often disappointing. Short courses of oral steroids are sometimes needed to control acute flares. Resistant cases might respond to PUVA.[18] Patients (64%) who flared after oral challenge to metal salt cleared or markedly improved on diets low in the incriminated metal salt, and 78% of those patients remained clear when the diet was rigorously followed (a suggested diet for nickel-sensitive patients with pompholyx appears on p. 94).[19] Attempts to control pompholyx with elimination diets may be worth a trial in difficult cases.

Patients with severe pompholyx who did not respond to conventional therapy or who had debilitating side effects from corticosteroids were treated with low-dose methotrexate (15 to 22.5 mg per week). This led to significant improvement or clearing, and the need for oral corticosteroid therapy was substantially decreased or eliminated.[20]

Complete remission of severe dyshidrotic eczema was achieved with low-dose external beam megavoltage therapy.[21]

Id reaction

Intense inflammatory processes, such as active stasis dermatitis or acute fungal infections of the feet, can be accompanied by an itchy, dyshidrotic-like vesicular eruption ("id reaction"; Figure 3-36). These eruptions are most common on the sides of the fingers but may be generalized. The eruptions resolve as the inflammation that initiated them resolves. The id reaction may be an allergic reaction to fungi or to some antigen created during the inflammatory process. Almost all dyshidrotic eruptions are incorrectly called id reactions. The diagnosis of an id reaction should not be made unless there is an acute inflammatory process at a distant site and the id reaction disappears shortly after the acute inflammation is controlled.

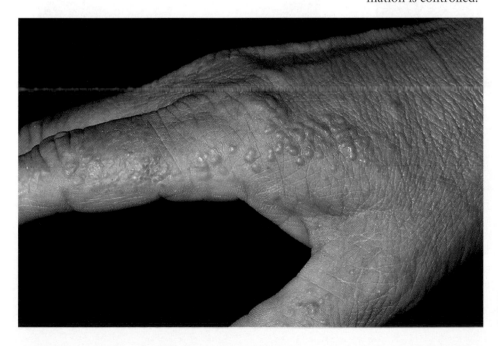

Figure 3-36 Id reaction. An acute vesicular eruption most often seen on the lateral aspects of the fingers

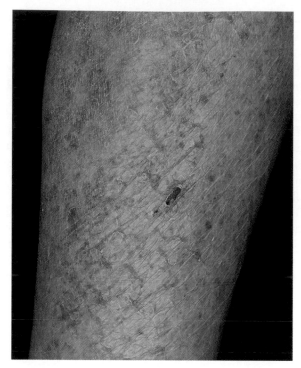

Figure 3-37 Asteatotic eczema (xerosis). The skin is extremely dry, cracked, and scaly. This pattern appears in the winter months when the air is dry.

Eczema: Various Presentations

Asteatotic eczema

Asteatotic eczema (eczema craquele) occurs after excess drying, especially during the winter months and among the elderly. Patients with an atopic diathesis are more likely to develop this distinctive pattern. The eruption can occur on any skin area, but it is most commonly seen on the anterolateral aspects of the lower legs. The lower legs become dry and scaly and show accentuation of the skin lines (xerosis) (Figure 3-37). Red plaques with thin, long, horizontal superficial fissures appear with further drying and scratching (Figure 3-38). Similar patterns of inflammation may appear on the trunk and upper extremities as the winter progresses. A cracked porcelain or "crazy paving" pattern of fissuring develops when short vertical fissures connect with the horizontal fissures. The term *eczema craquele* is appropriately used to describe this pattern. The severest form of this type of eczema shows an accentuation of the above pattern with deep, wide, horizontal fissures that ooze and are often purulent (Figure 3-39). Pain, rather than itching, is the chief complaint with this condition. Scratching or treatment with drying lotions such as calamine aggravates the eczematous inflammation and leads to infection with accumulation of crusts and purulent material.

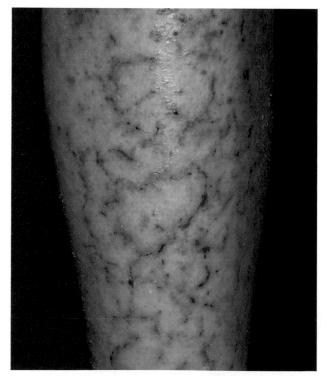

Figure 3-38 Asteatotic eczema (xerosis). Excessive washing of the dry skin shown in Figure 3-37 may result in horizontal, parallel cracks.

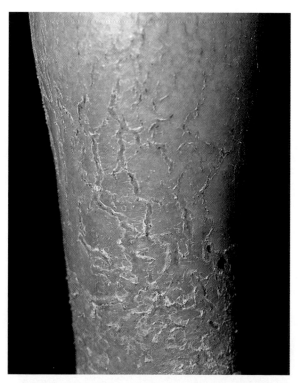

Figure 3-39 Asteatotic eczema (eczema craquele). Excessive drying on the lower legs may eventually become so severe that long, horizontal, superficial fissures appear. The fissures eventually develop a cracked porcelain or "crazy paving" pattern when short vertical fissures connect with the horizontal fissures.

TREATMENT. The initial stages are treated as subacute eczematous inflammation with groups III or IV topical steroid ointments. The severest form may have to be treated as acute eczema. The treatment involves wet compresses and antibiotics to remove crust and suppress infection before group V topical steroids and lubricants are applied. Wet compresses should be used only for a short time (one or two days). Prolonged use of wet compresses results in excessive drying. Lubricating the dry skin during and after topical steroid use is essential. The use of oral steroids should be avoided; the disease flares within 1 or 2 days once they are discontinued.

Nummular eczema

Nummular eczema is a common disease of unknown cause that occurs primarily in the middle-aged and elderly. The typical lesion is a coin-shaped, red plaque that averages 1 to 5 cm in diameter (Figure 3-40). The lesions can itch, and scratching often becomes habitual. In these cases, the term *nummular neurodermatitis* has been used (Figure 3-41). The plaque may become thicker and vesicles appear on the surface; vesicles in ringworm, if present, are at the border. Unlike the thick, silvery scale of psoriasis, this scale is thin and sparse. The erythema in psoriasis is darker. Once the disease is established, lesions may become more numerous, but individual lesions tend to remain in the same area and do not increase in size. The disease is worse in the winter. The back of the hand is the most commonly involved site; usually only one lesion or a few lesions are present (see Figure 3-23). Other frequently involved areas are the extensor aspects of the forearms and lower legs, the flanks, and the hips. Lesions in these other sites tend to be more numerous. An extensive form of the disease can occur suddenly in patients with dry skin that is exposed to an irritating medicine or chemical, or in patients who have an active eczematous process at another site, such as stasis dermatitis on the lower legs. The lesions in these cases are round, faintly erythematous, dry, cracked, superficial, and usually confluent.

The course is variable, but it is usually chronic, with some cases resisting all attempts at treatment. Many cases become inactive after several months. Lesions may reappear at previously involved sites in recurrent cases.

TREATMENT. Treatment depends on the stage of activity; all stages of eczematous inflammation may be present simultaneously. The red vesicular lesions are treated as acute, the red scaling plaques as subacute, and the habitually scratched thick plaques as chronic eczematous inflammation.

ADULT-ONSET RECALCITRANT ECZEMA AND MALIGNANCY. Generalized eczema or erythroderma may be the presenting sign of cutaneous T-cell lymphoma. Intractable pruritus has been associated with Hodgkin's lymphoma. Unexplained eczema of adult onset may be associated with an underlying lymphoproliferative malignancy. Patients may have widespread erythematous plaques that are poorly responsive to therapy. When a readily identifiable cause (e.g., contactants, drugs, or atopy) is not found, a systematic evaluation should be pursued.[22]

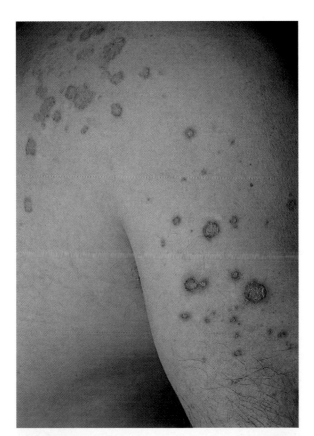

Figure 3-40 Nummular eczema. This form of eczema is of undetermined origin and is not necessarily associated with dry skin or atopy. The round, coin-shaped, eczematous plaques tend to be chronic and resistant to treatment.

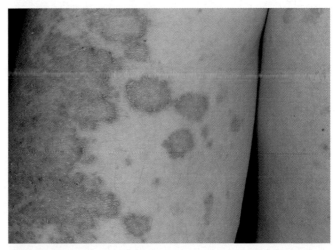

Figure 3-41 Nummular eczema. Round, eczematous plaques formed on the trunk and arms become confluent.

Chapped Fissured Feet

CLINICAL PRESENTATION. Chapped fissured feet (sweaty sock dermatitis, peridigital dermatitis, juvenile plantar dermatosis) are seen initially with scaling, erythema, fissuring, and loss of the epidermal ridge pattern. The tendency to severe chapping declines with age and is gone around the age of puberty. The mean age of onset is 7.3 years; the mean age of remission is 14.3 years.[23] Onset is in early fall when the weather becomes cold and heavy socks and impermeable shoes or boots are worn. An artificial intertrigo is created when moist socks are kept in contact with the soles. The skin in pressure areas, toes, and metatarsal regions becomes dry, brittle, and scaly, and then fissured (Figure 3-42, A). The chapping extends onto the sides of the toes. Eventually, the entire sole may be involved; sometimes the hands are also affected (Figure 3-42, B).

The eruption lasts throughout the winter, clears without treatment in the late spring, and predictably recurs the next fall. Earlier descriptions referred to this entity as *atopic winter feet* in children, but the name has been changed to include patients who do not have atopic dermatitis. Atopic dermatitis of the feet in children occurs on the dorsal toes and usually not on the plantar surface, and it is itchy. The role of atopy is not yet defined.[24] Children with chapped fissured feet complain of soreness and pain. Affected individuals must be predisposed to chapping because their wearing of moist socks and impermeable boots does not differ from that of unaffected children.

DIFFERENTIAL DIAGNOSIS. The differential diagnosis includes psoriasis, tinea pedis, and allergic contact dermatitis. The erythema in psoriasis is darker and the scales shed; the scales in chapped fissured feet are adherent, and removal of the scales causes bleeding. Tinea of the feet in children is rare. Feet with the rare case of familial *Trichophyton rubrum* are pale brown and have a fine scale. Fissuring is minimal, and there is little seasonal variation. Allergic contact dermatitis to shoes usually affects the dorsal aspect and spares the soles, webs, and sides of the feet. The eruption is bright red and scaly rather than pale red and chapped.

TREATMENT. Treatment is less than satisfactory. Topical steroids and lubrication provide some relief. Group II or III topical steroids are applied twice each day or, preferably, with plastic wrap occlusion at bedtime. Elidel cream or Protopic ointment may be effective. Lubricating creams are applied several times each day, especially directly after removing moist socks to seal in moisture. The feet should not be allowed to remain moist inside shoes. Preventive measures include changing into light leather shoes after removing boots at school and changing cotton socks 1 or 2 times each day.

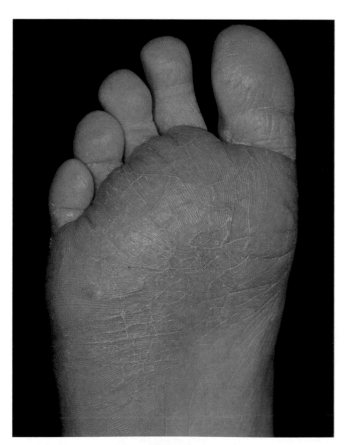

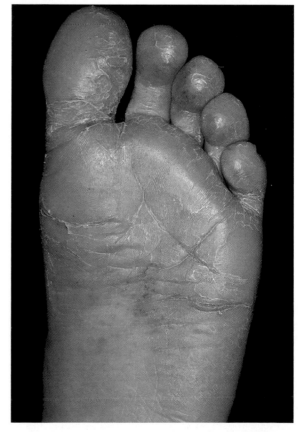

Figure 3-42 Chapped fissured feet. **A,** An early stage with erythema and cracking on pressure areas.

B, An advanced case in which the entire plantar surface is severely dried and fissured.

Self-Inflicted Dermatoses

A number of skin disorders are created or perpetuated by manipulation of the skin surface[25-35] (Table 3-4). Patients may benefit from both dermatologic and psychiatric care. The most common self-inflicted dermatoses are discussed here.

Lichen simplex chronicus

Lichen simplex chronicus (Figures 3-43 through 3-48), or circumscribed neurodermatitis, is an eczematous eruption that is created by habitual scratching of a single localized area. The disease is more common in adults, but may be seen in children. The areas most commonly affected are those that are conveniently reached. These are listed in Box 3-6 in approximate order of frequency. Patients derive great pleasure in the relief that comes with frantically scratching the inflamed site. Loss of this pleasurable sensation or continued subconscious habitual scratching may explain why this eruption frequently recurs.

A typical plaque stays localized and shows little tendency to enlarge with time. Red papules coalesce to form a red, scaly, thick plaque with accentuation of skin lines *(lichenification)*. Lichen simplex chronicus is a chronic eczematous disease, but acute changes may result from sensitization with

Box 3-6 Lichen Simplex Chronicus: Areas Most Commonly Affected Listed in Approximate Order of Frequency

Outer lower portion of lower leg
Scrotum, vulva, anal area, pubis
Wrists and ankles
Upper eyelids
Back (lichen simplex nuchae) and side of neck
Orifice of the ear
Extensor forearms near elbow
Fold behind the ear
Scalp-picker's nodules

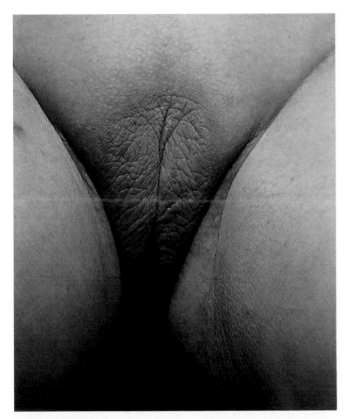

Figure 3-43 Lichen simplex chronicus of the vulva. The skin lines are markedly accentuated from years of rubbing and scratching

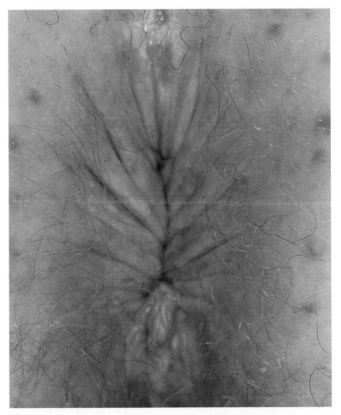

Figure 3-44 Anal excoriations. Scratching has produced focal erosions and thickening of the skin about the anus.

topical medication. Moist scale, serum, crusts, and pustules are signs of infection.

Lichen simplex nuchae occur almost exclusively in women who reach for the back of the neck during stressful situations (see Figure 3-46). The disease may spread beyond the initial well-defined plaque. Diffuse dry or moist scale, crust, and erosions extend into the posterior scalp beyond the neck. Secondary infection is common. Nodules, usually less than 1 cm and scattered randomly in the scalp, occur in patients who frequently pick at the scalp; there may be few nodules or many.

CHRONIC VULVAR ITCHING. Women who have chronic vulvar itching usually have eczema. The degree of itching may not correspond to the appearance of the skin. Scratching begins a cycle that makes the skin rough, red and irritated, producing more itching. Lichen sclerosus, contact dermatits, lichen planus, psoriasis and Paget's disease are other causes of itching. A 2 to 4 week course of a group I topical steroid is usually very effective.

RED SCROTUM SYNDROME. Lichen simplex of the scrotum is a common finding, and thickened skin with accentuated skin markings is typical. Some patients present with persistent redness of the anterior half of the scrotum that may involve the base of the penis. There is persistent itching, burning or pain. The cause is unknown and it is resistant to treatment.[36]

TREATMENT. The patient must first understand that the rash will not clear until even minor scratching and rubbing is stopped. Scratching frequently takes place during sleep, and the affected area may have to be covered. Lichen simplex chronicus is chronic eczema and is treated as outlined in the section on eczematous inflammation. Treatment of the anal area or the fold behind the ear does not require potent topical steroids as do other forms of lichen simplex; rather, these intertriginous areas respond to group V or VI topical steroids. Lichen simplex nuchae, because of its location, is difficult to treat. Dry inflammation that extends into the scalp may be treated with a group II steroid gel such as fluocinonide (Lidex) applied twice each day. Moist, secondarily infected areas respond to oral antibiotics and topical steroid solutions (e.g., Cormax Scalp Solution). A 2- to 3-week course of prednisone (20 mg twice daily) should be considered when an extensively inflamed scalp does not respond rapidly to topical treatment. Nodules caused by picking at the scalp may be very resistant to treatment, requiring monthly intralesional injections with triamcinolone acetonide (Kenalog 10 mg/ml). Botulinum toxin A injected intradermally into lichenified lesions may block acetylcholine release and control pruritus. Pruritus subsided within 3 to 7 days and lesions cleared in 2 to 4 weeks.[37]

Table 3-4 Self-Inflicted and Self-Perpetuated

Dermatologic complaint that is a primary psychiatric symptom	Dermatologic features
Psychogenic parasitosis (Delusions of parasitosis)	Focal erosions and scars Patients convinced they are infested and angry with doctors because "no one believes them"
Factitial dermatitis	Cutaneous lesions are wholly self-inflicted; patient denies their self-inflicted nature Wide range of lesions, blisters, ulcers, burns Bizarre patterns not characteristic of any disease Often a diagnosis of exclusion Adolescents, young adults
Neurotic excoriations and acne excoriée	Possibly initiated by itchy skin disease Repetitive self-excoriation—patient admits self-inflicted nature Linear excoriations in easily reached areas Groups of round or linear scars
Trichotillomania	Compulsive extraction of hair Nonscarring alopecia as a result of self-plucking of hair; patients deny that their alopecia is self-induced in 43% of cases Hairs of various lengths Area not completely devoid of hair
Lichen simplex chronicus	Created and perpetuated by constant scratching and rubbing Very thick oval plaques Usually just one lesion Severe itching Lasts indefinitely Recurs frequently
Prurigo nodularis	0.5-1 cm itchy nodules on arms and legs; lasts for years

Adapted from Gupta AK, Gupta MA: Dermatol 2000; Clin 18(4), and Gupta MD, Gupta AK: J Am Acad Dermatol 1996; 34:1030.
SSRIs, Selective serotonin reuptake inhibitors.

Dermatoses

Possible associated psychiatric disorder	Diagnosis	Treatment
Delusional disorder, somatic type, or monosymptomatic hypochondriacal psychosis; shared psychotic disorder with another person (folie a deux); major depressive disorder with psychotic features; incipient schizophrenia	Most patients are women over 50	Antipsychotics (pimozide [Orap]) Antidepressants may be used for co-morbid depressive disease Anxiolytics and hypnotics may be used in conjunction with antipsychotics in some cases
Personality disorder, cutaneous lesions are an *appeal for help* Posttraumatic stress disorder Rule out sexual and child abuse Depression, psychosis, obsessive-compulsive disorder, malingering, and Munchausen's syndrome	Ratio of female to male patients is 4 to 1 Sudden appearance of lesions "Hollow history"; patient cannot describe how lesion evolved	Empathic, supportive approach None in most cases Antipsychotics and antidepressants may be used in posttraumatic stress disorder
Depression, obsessive-compulsive disorder, perfectionistic traits, presence of significant psychosocial stressor in 33%-98% of patients Body image problems, including eating disorders, in acne excoriée	Exclude systemic causes of itching Patient admits self-inflicted nature	Empathic, supportive approach Antidepressants, especially SSRIs; antianxiety and antipsychotic drugs may be used as adjunctive therapies where indicated
A variant of obsessive-compulsive disorder Many causes Depressive illness Disturbed parent-child relationship Stressful life situation Usually not a primary psychiatric disorder	Many patients are girls between 5 and 12 Patients may deny pulling hair KOH exam rules out tinea Biopsy shows no hair in follicle Hair pluck shows 100% of hairs in anagen	Antidepressants, especially the SSRIs, for some patients. Underlying psychiatric pathology should be diagnosed before psychotropic agents are used Psychotherapy and family therapy
No known psychopathology Triggered by stress	Biopsy shows eczematous inflammation or resembles psoriasis	Topical steroids and plastic occlusion Cordran tape Intralesional steroids
Severe pruritus interferes with life activities and sleep	Biopsy shows very thick epidermis and hyperplasia of nerve fibers	Intralesional steroids Cryotherapy Excision Capsaicin cream Calcipotriol ointment

LICHEN SIMPLEX CHRONICUS

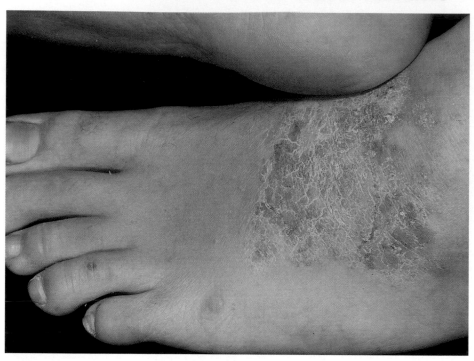

Figure 3-45 This localized plaque of chronic eczematous inflammation was created by rubbing with the opposite heel.

Figure 3-46 Lichen simplex nuchae occurs almost exclusively in women who scratch the back of their neck in stressful situations.

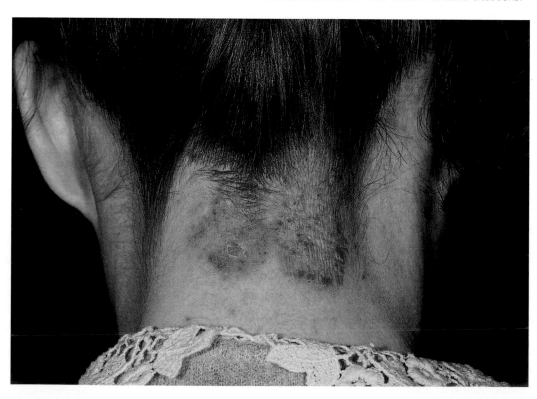

LICHEN SIMPLEX CHRONICUS

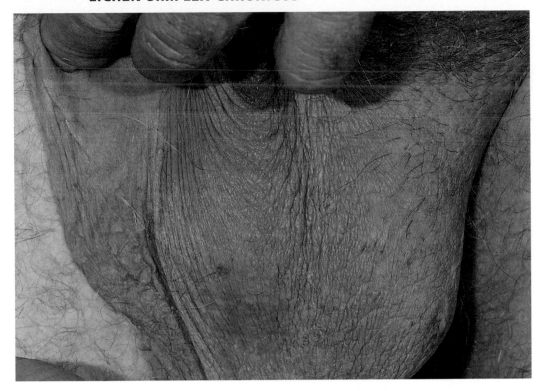

Figure 3-47 Lichen simplex chronicus of the scrotum. The skin is thickened and skin lines are accentuated, unlike the adjacent scrotal skin.

Figure 3-48 Two linear areas are picked and scratched, causing the skin to become very thick. The patient scratches during the day and while asleep.

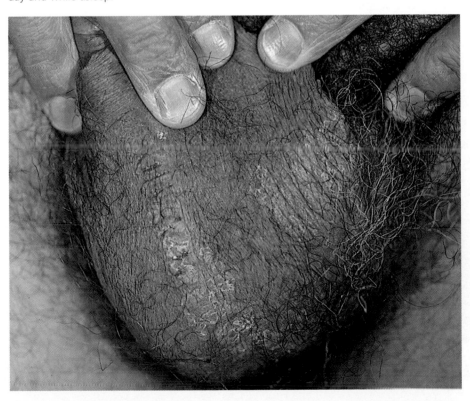

Prurigo nodularis

Prurigo nodularis is an uncommon disease of unknown cause that may be considered a nodular form of lichen simplex chronicus. There is intractable pruritus. It resembles picker's nodules of the scalp except that the few to 20 or more nodules are randomly distributed on the extensor aspects of the arms and legs (Figures 3-49 and 3-50). They are created by repeated scratching. The nodules are red or brown, hard, and dome-shaped with a smooth, crusted, or warty surface; they measure 1 to 2 cm in diameter. Hypertrophy of cutaneous papillary dermal nerves is a relatively constant feature.[38] Complaints of pruritus vary. Some patients claim there is no itching and that scratching is only habitual, whereas others complain that the pruritus is intense.

TREATMENT. Prurigo nodularis is resistant to treatment and lasts for years. As with picker's nodules of the scalp, repeated intralesional steroid injections may be effective. Excision of individual nodules is sometimes helpful. Cryotherapy is sometimes successful. Capsaicin 0.025% (Zostrix cream) and capsaicin 0.075% - HP (Zostrix-HP cream) interferes with the perception of pruritus and pain by depletion of neu-ropeptides in small sensory cutaneous nerves. Application of the cream 4 to 6 times daily for up to 10 months resulted in cessation of burning and pruritus within 12 days. Lesions gradually healed. Pruritus returned within 2 months in some patients who stopped treatment.[39] Calcipotriol ointment applied twice a day to nodules was effective. The use of combination or sequential topical calcipotriol with topical steroids might maximize the benefits and decrease the potential adverse effects of both drugs.[40] Naltrexone (50 mg daily), an orally active opiate antagonist, was found to be effective therapy for pruritic symptoms in many diseases.[41]

Neurotic excoriations

Neurotic excoriations are patient-induced linear excoriations. Patients dig at their skin to relieve itching or to extract imaginary pieces of material that they feel is imbedded in or extruding from the skin. Itching and digging become compulsive rituals. Most patients are aware that they create the lesions. The most consistent psychiatric disorders reported are perfectionistic and compulsive traits; patients manifest repressed aggression and self-destructive behavior.

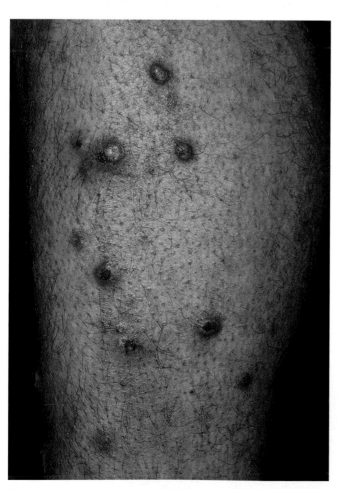

Figure 3-49 Prurigo nodularis. Thick, hard nodules usually present on the extensor surfaces of the forearms and legs from chronic picking.

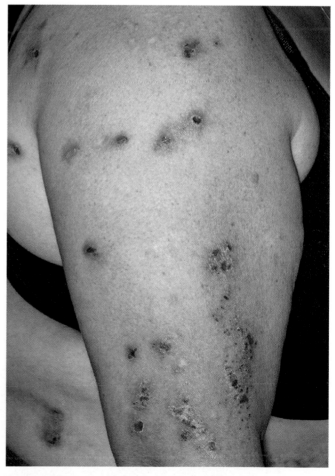

Figure 3-50 Prurigo nodularis. Thick papules and linear excoriations are features of both prurigo nodularis and neurotic excoriations.

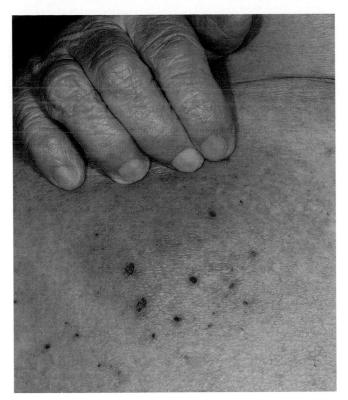

Figure 3-51 Neurotic excoriations. The upper back is one of the most common sites attacked by chronic pickers. Several white, round scars are evidence of past activity.

CLINICAL APPEARANCE. Repetitive scratching and digging produces few to several hundred excoriations; all lesions are of similar size and shape. They tend to be grouped in areas that are easily reached, such as the arms, legs, and upper back (Figures 3-51 through 3-54). Recurrent picking at crusts delays healing. Groups of white scars surrounded by brown hyperpigmentation are typical; their presence alone can indicate past difficulty.

TREATMENT. The use of group I topical steroids applied twice a day or group V topical steroids under plastic wrap occlusion combined with systemic antibiotics produces gratifying results. Frequent lubrication and infrequent washing and with only mild soaps should be encouraged once areas are healed. Patients should try to substitute the ritual of applying lubricants for the ritual of digging. An empathic, supportive approach has been reported to be significantly more effective than insight-oriented psychotherapy, which often exacerbates the symptoms.

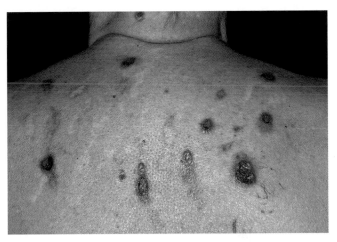

Figure 3-53 Neurotic excoriations. Severe involvement of the upper back. Picking causes shallow erosions and small, round scars. Long, linear scars occur from deep gouging.

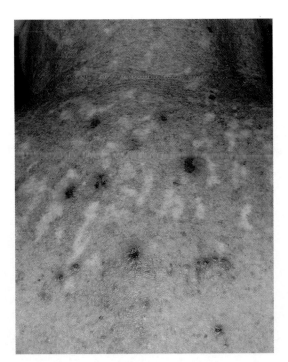

Figure 3-52 Neurotic excoriations. Lesions appear on any area of the trunk and extremities that is easily reached.

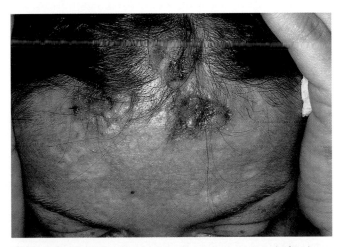

Figure 3-54 Neurotic excoriations. Deep scars occurred after long periods of aggressive picking.

Psychogenic Parasitosis

Patients with psychogenic parasitosis believe they are infested with parasites. They move from one physician to another looking for someone who will believe them. A variety of psychiatric disorders may be associated with this disorder, but suggesting psychiatric referral may offend the patient. A supportive, therapeutic relationship is essential.[42]

THE DELUSION. Patients report seeing and feeling parasites. Involvement of the ears, eyes, and nose is common. They present with the "matchbox" sign, in which small bits of excoriated skin, dried blood, debris or insect parts are brought in matchboxes or other containers as "proof" of infestation. Body fluids thought to contain parasites are brought in jars. Pest control officers may have been hired to rid the house of parasites.

THE SKIN. Excoriations and ulcers and linear scars are common on easily reached areas of the forearms, legs, trunk, and face (Figure 3-55).

CLASSIFICATION. Classify patients (see diagram on the facing page) with psychogenic parasitosis into four groups: anxiety/hypochondriasis, anxiety/hypochondriasis with depression, delusional parasitosis, and delusional parasitosis with depression.[43] Patients suffering from anxiety/hypochondriasis may believe that they are infested by parasites but may also express doubt about their infestation, express fears of "going crazy," and agree that parasites may not be present. Patients with anxiety/hypochondriasis and depression may agree to undergo a psychiatric evaluation. Patients who have a true delusion are convinced that they have a parasitic infestation that none of the doctors can find; these patients may have an underlying major depression.

MANAGEMENT. A majority of patients with short-term illness can be cured with suggestion; the remainder have a true delusion. Patients with symptoms for over 3 months are usually not cured by suggestion alone. Listen and show concern; examine the skin with magnification and prepare scrapings; rule out true infestation. Animal and bird mites and scabies may actually be present. Do not suggest that the diagnosis is obvious on the first visit. The second visit can be lengthy. Collect specimens brought in by the patient and set them aside for later evaluation. Conduct a thorough examination and listen for indicators of depression. After two or more visits patients may suggest that this may be "all in my head." At this point, explain that some patients actually see and feel parasites that are not real. Explain that this is an illness that affects sane people. The clinician may sense that the patient doubts the existence of the infestation (i.e., the belief is shakable). The patient is then offered a benzodiazepine to help with anxiety while waiting for the next visit 2 weeks later; a psychiatric referral is suggested at that 2-week follow-up visit.

Patients whose belief is unshakable are considered to have a delusional disorder. Suggest psychiatric referral. If that is refused, offer a neuroleptic medication such as pimozide (Orap) or haloperidol (Haldol). Intramuscular Haldol is available. Explain that many other patients with similar symptoms have been helped with this treatment and that the medication can be taken as a "therapeutic trial." Psychiatric referral may be more acceptable after a short course of medication.

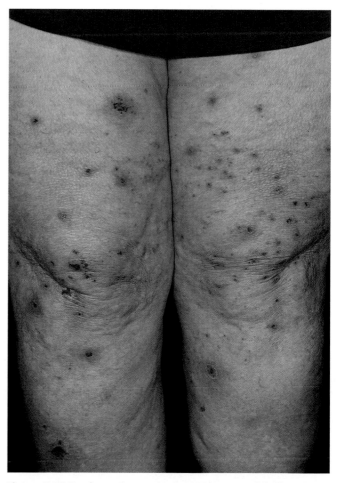

Figure 3-55 Psychogenic parasitosis. Attempts to pick "bugs" out of the skin produce focal erosions on easily accessed areas such as the arms and legs.

TREATMENT FOR PSYCHOGENIC PARASITOSIS

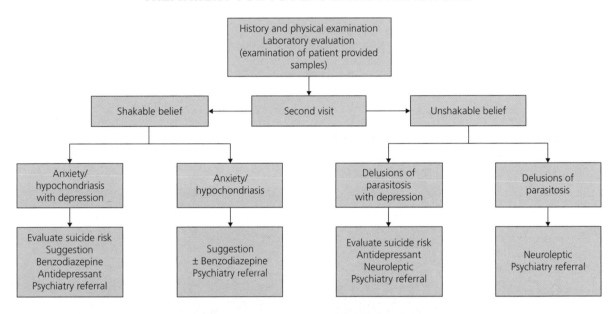

Benzodiazepine: 0.5 mg po tid and 1 mg po qhs; clonazepam 0.5 mg po q am and 1 mg po qhs
Antidepressant: sertraline 50 mg q am; paroxetine 20 mg po q am; fluoxetine 20 mg po q am
Neuroleptic: pimozide 4–6 mg po q am, haloperidol 5 mg–10 mg po bid; depot haloperidol 50 to 100 mg IM q monthly

Adapted from Zanol K, Slaughter J, Hall R: Intl J Dermatol 1998; 37(1):56.

Stasis Dermatitis and Venous Ulceration: Postphlebitic Syndromes

Stasis dermatitis

ETIOLOGY. Stasis dermatitis is an eczematous eruption that occurs on the lower legs in some patients with venous insufficiency. The dermatitis may be acute, subacute, or chronic and recurrent, and it may be accompanied by ulceration. Most patients with venous insufficiency do not develop dermatitis, which suggests that genetic or environmental factors may play a role. The reason for its occurrence is unknown. Some have speculated that it represents an allergic response to an epidermal protein antigen created through increased hydrostatic pressure, whereas others believe that the skin has been compromised and is more susceptible to irritation and trauma.

ALLERGY TO TOPICAL AGENTS. Patients with stasis dermatitis have significantly more positive reactions when patch tested with components of previously used topical agents. Topical medications that contain potential sensitizers such as lanolin, benzocaine, parabens, and neomycin should be avoided by patients with stasis disease. Allergy to corticosteroids in topical medication is also possible.

Types of eczematous inflammation
Subacute inflammation

Subacute inflammation usually begins in the winter months when the legs become dry and scaly. Brown staining of the skin (hemosiderin) may have appeared slowly for months (Figure 3-56). The pigment is iron left after disintegration of red blood cells that leaked out of veins because of increased hydrostatic pressure. Scratching induces first subacute and then chronic eczematous inflammation (Figure 3-57). Attempts at self-treatment with drying lotions (calamine) or potential sensitizers (e.g., neomycin-containing topical medicines) exacerbate and prolong the inflammation.

Acute inflammation

A red, superficial, itchy plaque may suddenly appear on the lower leg. This acute process may be eczematous inflammation, cellulitis, or both. Weeping and crusts appear (Figure 3-57). A vesicular eruption (id reaction) on the palms, trunk, and/or extremities sometimes accompanies this acute inflammation. The inflammation responds to systemic antibiotics, wet compresses, and group III to V topical steroids. Wet compresses should be discontinued before excessive drying occurs. The id reaction resolves spontaneously as the primary site improves.

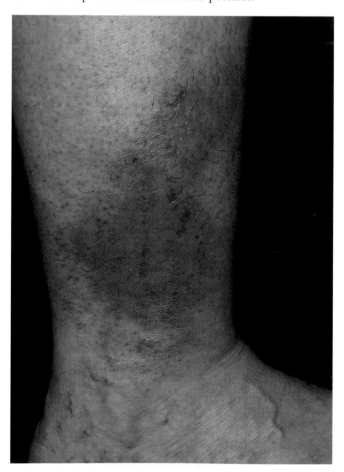

Figure 3-56 Stasis dermatitis in an early stage. Erythema and erosions produced by excoriations are shown.

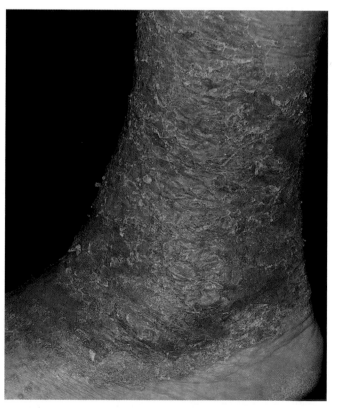

Figure 3-57 Stasis dermatitis (severe inflammation). A red, itchy plaque may suddenly develop acute inflammation and/or cellulitis. Weeping, crusts, and fissuring may be extensive.

Chronic inflammation

Recurrent attacks of inflammation eventually compromise the poorly vascularized area, and the disease becomes chronic and recurrent (Figures 3-58 and 3-59). The typical presentation is a cyanotic red plaque over the medial malleolus. Fibrosis following chronic inflammation leads to permanent skin thickening. The skin surface in these irreversibly changed areas may have a bumpy, cobblestone appearance that results from fibrosis and venous and lymph stasis. The skin remains thickened and diffusely dark brown *(postinflammatory hyperpigmentation)* during quiescent periods.

TREATMENT OF STASIS DERMATITIS

Topical steroids and wet dressings. The early, dry, superficial stage is managed as subacute eczematous inflammation with group II to V topical steroid creams or ointments and lubricating creams or lotions. Oral antibiotics (usually those active against staphylococci, e.g., cephalexin) hasten resolution if cellulitis is present. Moist exudative inflammation and moist ulcers respond to tepid wet compresses of Burrow's solution or just saline or water for 30 to 60 minutes several times a day. Wet dressings suppress inflammation while debriding the ulcer. Adherent crust may be carefully freed with blunt-tipped scissors. Group V topical steroids are applied to eczematous skin at the periphery of the ulcer. Patients must be warned that steroid creams placed on the ulcer stop the healing process. Elevation of the legs encourages healing.

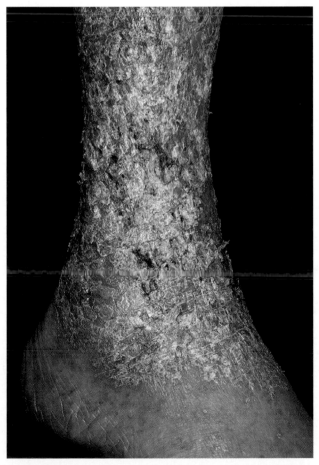

Figure 3-58 Stasis dermatitis. Severe, painful, exudative, weeping, infected eczema with moist crust. Oral antibiotics and cool compresses are initial treatment followed in a few days with group II to V topical steroid creams or ointments.

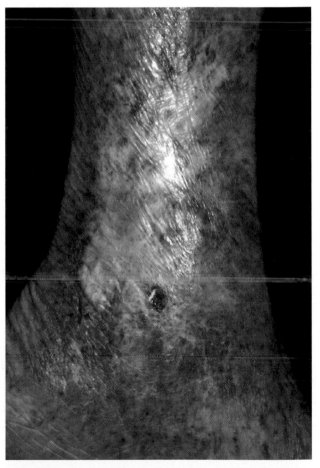

Figure 3-59 Stasis dermatitis. Cycles of inflammation, ulceration, and healing produce scarring. The surrounding chronically inflamed skin is hyperpigmented from deposits of hemosiderin from extravasated erythrocytes.

Venous leg ulcers

The three main types of lower-extremity ulcers are *venous, arterial,* and *neuropathic* (Table 3-5.) Most leg ulcers are venous; foot ulcers are more often caused by arterial insufficiency or neuropathy. Most venous ulcers are located over the medial malleolus and are often larger than other ulcers. Diabetes is a common underlying condition.

DIFFERENTIAL DIAGNOSIS OF LEG ULCERS. Many diseases cause leg ulcers (Table 3-6). Biopsy (basal cell carcinomas, squamous cell carcinomas) and culture (fungal, atypical mycobacterial) chronic ulcers that do not respond to conventional therapy. Vasculitis, pyoderma gangrenosum, rheumatoid arthritis, and systemic lupus erythematosus may be associated with lower-extremity ulcers.

PATHOPHYSIOLOGY OF VENOUS INSUFFICIENCY. The leg has superficial, communicating, and deep veins. The superficial system contains the long (medial) and short (lateral) saphenous veins. Perforator veins connect the superficial veins to the deep venous system. Normally blood flows from the superficial to the deep system. Venous hypertension ("chronic venous insufficiency") occurs if any of the valves dysfunction, a thrombosis blocks the deep system, or there is calf muscle pump failure. Increased pressure causes diffusion of substances, including fibrin, out of capillaries. Fibrotic tissue may predispose the tissue to ulceration.

ETIOLOGY AND LOCATION. Venous insufficiency followed by edema is the fundamental change that predisposes to dermatitis and ulceration. Venous insufficiency occurs when venous return in the deep, perforating, or superficial veins is impaired by vein dilation and valve dysfunction. Deep vein thrombophlebitis, which may have been asymptomatic earlier, is the most frequent precursor of lower leg venous insufficiency. Blood pools in the deep venous system and causes deep venous hypertension and dilation of the perforators that connect the superficial and deep venous systems. Venous hypertension is then transmitted to the superficial venous system. The largest perforators are posterior and superior to the lateral and medial malleoli. These are the same areas where dermatitis and ulceration are most prevalent. Superficial varicosities alone are unlikely to produce venous insufficiency.

Table 3-5 The Three Common Types of Leg Ulcers

	Venous	Arterial	Neuropathic
Ulcer location	Medial malleolus; trauma or infection may localize ulcers laterally or more proximally	Distal, over bony prominences; trauma may localize ulcers proximally	Pressure points on feet (e.g., junction of great toe and plantar surface, metatarsal head, heel)
Ulcer appearance	Shallow, irregular borders; base may be initially fibrinous but later develops granulation tissue	Round or punched-out, well-demarcated border; fibrinous yellow base or true necrotic eschar; bone and tendon exposure may be seen	Callus surrounding the wound and undermined edges are characteristic; blister, hemorrhage, necrosis, and exposure of underlying structures are commonly seen
Physical examination	Varicose veins, leg edema, atrophie blanche, dermatitis, lipodermatosclerosis, pigmentary changes, purpura	Loss of hair, shiny, atrophic skin, dystrophic toenails, cold feet, femoral bruit, absent or decreased pulses, prolonged capillary refilling time	No sensation to monofilament; bone resorption, claw toes, flat foot, Charcot joints
Frequent symptoms	Pain, odor, and copious drainage from the wound; pruritus	Claudication, resting ischemic pain	Foot numbness, burning, paresthesia
Ankle-to-brachial blood pressure ratio (ankle/brachial index [ABI]) measured by Doppler ultrasonography	>0.9	ABI <0.7 suggests arterial disease; calcification of vessels gives falsely high Doppler readings	Normal, unless associated with arterial component
Risk factors	Deep venous thrombosis, significant leg injury, obesity	Diabetes, hypertension, cigarette smoking, hypercholesterolemia	Diabetes, leprosy, frostbite
Complications	Allergic contact dermatitis, cellulitis	Gangrene	Underlying osteomyelitis
Treatment pearl	Compression therapy, leg elevation	Pentoxifylline, vascular surgery assessment if ABI <5	Vigorous surgical debridement, pressure avoidance

From Valencia IC et al: J Am Acad Dermatol, 2001; 44:401.

VENOUS ULCER—CLINICAL FEATURES. Ulceration is almost inevitable once the skin has been thickened and circulation is compromised. Ulceration may occur spontaneously or after the slightest trauma (Figure 3-60). The ulcer may remain small or may enlarge rapidly without any further trauma. A dull, constant pain that improves with leg elevation is present. Pain from ischemic ulcers is more intense and does not improve with elevation.

Ulcers have a sharp or sloping border and are deep or superficial. Removal of crust and debris reveals a moist base with granulation tissue. The base and surrounding skin is often infected. Healing is slow, taking several weeks or months. After healing, it is not uncommon to see ulcers rapidly recur. The ulcers are replaced with ivory-white sclerotic scars. Despite the pain and the inconvenience of treatment, most patients tolerate this disease well and remain ambulatory.

CHANGES IN SURROUNDING SKIN. Edema is a common finding; it is usually pitting and disappears at night with elevation. Chronic edema, trauma, infection, and inflammation lead to subcutaneous tissue fibrosis, giving the skin a firm, nonpitting, "woody" quality. Fat necrosis may follow thrombosis of small veins, and this may be the most important underlying change that predisposes to ulceration. Recurrent ulceration and fat necrosis is associated with loss of subcutaneous tissue and a decrease in lower leg circumference (lipodermatosclerosis). Advanced disease is represented by an "inverted bottle leg," in which the proximal leg swells from chronic venous obstruction and the lower leg shrinks from chronic ulceration and fat necrosis.

Table 3-6 Leg Ulcers: Differential Diagnosis

Venous	Neoplastic
Postphlebitic syndrome	Basal cell carcinoma
Arteriovenous malformation	Cutaneous T-cell lymphoma
	Metastatic tumors
Arterial	Sarcoma (e.g., Kaposi's)
Atherosclerosis	Squamous cell carcinoma
Cholesterol embolism	**Metabolic**
Thromboangiitis obliterans	Diabetes
Lymphatic (lymphedema)	Gout
Neuropathic	**Bacterial infections**
Diabetes	Ecthyma gangrenosum
Spinal cord lesions	Furuncle
Tabes dorsalis	Gram-negative
Vasculitic	Mycobacterial
Atrophie blanche	Septic emboli
Hypersensitivity vasculitis	Syphilis
Lupus erythematosus	**Fungal infection**
Nodular vasculitis	Deep fungal
Polyarteritis nodosa	Trichophytin granuloma
Rheumatoid arthritis	**Infestations**
Scleroderma	Spider bites
Wegener's granulomatosis	Protozoal (leishmania)
Hematologic	**Panniculitis**
Sickle cell anemia	Necrobiosis lipoidica
Thalassemia	Pancreatic fat necrosis
Traumatic	Weber-Christian disease
Burns (thermal, radiation)	**Others**
Cold	Necrobiosis lipoidica
Factitial	Pyoderma gangrenosum
Pressure	Sarcoidosis

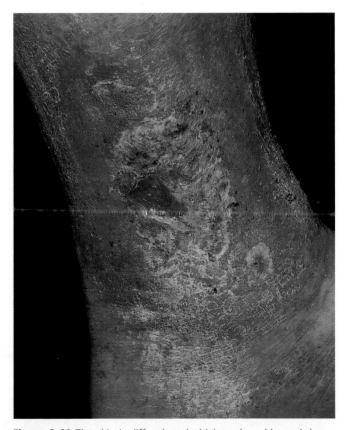

Figure 3-60 The skin is diffusely red, thickened, and bound down by fibrosis. Ulceration occurs with the slightest trauma.

STASIS PAPILLOMATOSIS. Stasis papillomatosis is a condition usually found in chronically congested limbs. Lesions vary from small to large plaques that consist of aggregated brownish or pinkish papules with a smooth or hyperkeratotic surface (Figure 3-61). The lesions most frequently affect the dorsum of the foot, the toes, the extensor aspect of the lower leg, or the area surrounding a venous ulcer. This condition occurs in patients with local lymphatic disturbances; patients with primary lymphedema, chronic venous insufficiency, trauma, and recurrent erysipelas are at greatest risk.[40]

POSTPHLEBITIC SYNDROMES (CLINICAL VARIANTS). Impairment of venous return leads to increased hydrostatic pressure and interstitial fluid accumulation. Six clinical variants (Table 3-7) occur with venous hypertension.

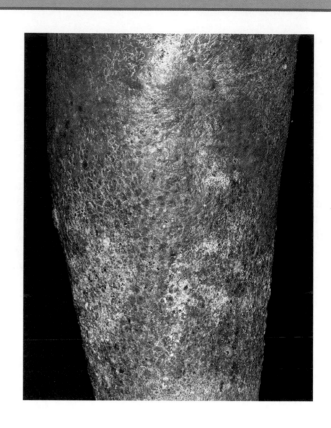

Figure 3-61 Stasis papillomatosis. Chronic inflammation may cause long standing lymphatic obstruction. This sometimes results in the bizarre appearance of numerous dome shaped red, blue papules. These changes are irreversible.

Table 3-7 Venous Ulceration Syndromes (Postphlebitic Syndromes)

Syndrome	Clinical features	Pathophysiology	Management
Dependent edema and ulceration	Pitting edema reversed by elevation Hyperpigmentation	Increased capillary hydrostatic static pressure	Compression bandages Unna's boot Bed rest (short periods) Elevation
Lipodermatosclerosis and ulceration	Induration of skin and subcutaneous tissue Extensive hyperpigmentation Pitting edema Erythema secondary to capillary proliferation	Prolonged high pressure in veins Biopsy shows fibrin deposits around capillaries Fibrin prevents O_2 diffusion to epidermis	Fibrinolytic therapy; stanozol 5 gm twice daily Hyperbaric O_2
Atrophie blanche	White, smooth, flat scars with focal dilated capillaries May be preceded by small painful ulcers	Statis and platelet sludging causes platelet thrombi Dermal capillary occlusion causes infarction of overlying dermis; heals with white scars	Antiplatelet therapy; aspirin Compression therapy makes ulcers worse Elevation promotes venous return
Ankle blow out syndrome	Multiple small, tortuous veins below and behind the malleoli Ulcers usually above and behind medial malleolus in midst of veins Trauma, eczema, bursting of vein causes ulcer	Localized venous valvular incompetence of lower third of leg Exercise makes condition worse	Surgical ligation of localized incompetent veins
Secondary venous varicosity with ulceration	Tortuous saphenous systems	Transmission of hypertension to saphenous system	Compression bandages Hyperbaric O_2
Secondary lymphedema with ulceration	Nonpitting edema	Lymphedema may complicate the lipodermatosclerosis syndrome because of involvement of lymphatic channels by the fibrotic process	Hyperbaric O_2

Modified from Heng MCY: Int J Dermatol 1987; 26:14–21.

Management of venous ulcers

INITIAL EVALUATION AND TREATMENT. Once other causes of lower leg ulcers have been excluded, the area around the ulcer must be prepared for definitive treatment. Ulcers do not heal if edema, infection, or eczematous inflammation are present. The venous system should be investigated. Surgery or sclerotherapy may be needed to control venous reflux.

VARICOSE VEINS. Varicose veins are superficial vessels that are caused by defective venous valves. Perforator vein incompetence may lead to ulceration. Varicose veins cause venous hypertension that leads to edema, cutaneous pigmentation, stasis dermatitis, and ulceration. The goal of therapy is to normalize venous physiology. Deep venous hypertension is managed with compression therapy. Sclerotherapy is used to treat isolated perforator incompetence, even through an ulcer if necessary. Saphenous vein insufficiency is usually managed by surgery.

LABORATORY EVALUATION. Initial evaluation includes CBC, blood glucose, and sedimentation rate. Consider curet or biopsy of the ulcer for bacterial culture. Biopsy the edge of ulcers that do not heal with conventional therapy to rule out basal cell or squamous cell carcinoma. X-ray film deep ulcers to rule out osteomyelitis.

FUNCTION STUDIES. A duplex ultrasound scan confirms the site and extent of venous reflux. Arterial pulses may not be palpable if edema is present. A hand-held Doppler flowmeter is used to measure the ankle-brachial pressure index (ABI); see Table 3-5. This is the ratio of systolic pressure in the ankle to that in the arm when the patient is in the supine position. Patients with a ratio of 0.7 or less usually have moderate to severe arterial disease, and arterial reconstruction may be necessary. In diabetic patients with inelastic vessels, the ankle-brachial pressure index is not helpful; arteriography should be performed.

TREATMENT. Hospital-based wound care clinics are available for treatment. Venous pressure and leg edema can be reduced with bed rest, leg elevation, and compression. Contributing systemic disease, local infection, and inflammation should be treated (see diagram at right). Stop cigarette smoking and excessive alcohol intake. Encourage good nutrition. Multivitamin supplements that contain vitamins C and E and zinc may help.

LEG ELEVATION. Venous hypertension must be reversed. Bed rest and leg elevation are effective. Elevation of the legs above the heart level for 30 minutes, 3 to 4 times per day, allows swelling to subside. Leg elevation at night is accomplished by raising the foot end of the patient's bed on blocks 15 to 20 cm high.

TREATMENT OF VENOUS ULCERS

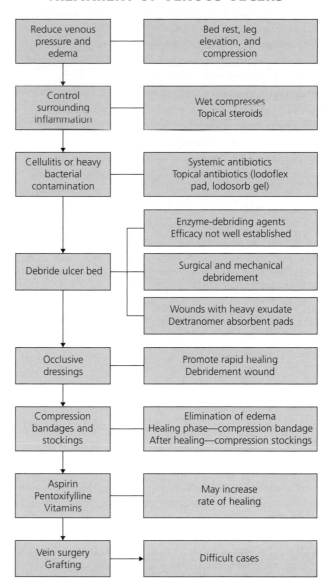

INFLAMMATION SURROUNDING THE ULCER. Tepid saline or silver nitrate (0.5%) wet compresses rapidly control inflammation. Silver nitrate is preferred when infection is present. Fresh compresses (replaced hourly) should be kept in place almost continuously for 24 to 72 hours. Fluids should not be added to dressings that are in place. Group V topical steroids are applied 2 to 4 times each day and may be covered with the compress. Patients with venous ulcers are prone to developing allergic reactions to topical medications in the surrounding compromised skin. Neomycin, paraben preservatives, and lanolin should be avoided. If inflammation persists after appropriate treatment, patch testing should be undertaken.

SYSTEMIC ANTIBIOTICS. Ulcers are typically contaminated with different aerobic and anaerobic bacteria, but routine administration of systemic antibiotics does not increase healing rates. Topical and/or systemic antibiotics may enhance wound healing when heavy bacterial contamination is present. Cellulitis must be treated with systemic antibiotics (see Chapter 9). Stasis dermatitis and cellulitis have a similar appearance and are often confused. Stasis dermatitis may act as a reservoir for infection. Dermatitis is easily treated with short courses of group I to IV topical steroids.

TOPICAL ANTIBIOTICS. Cadexomer-iodine (Iodoflex pad, Iodosorb gel) preparations have antimicrobial properties, debride wounds, and stimulate granulation tissue; other topical antiseptics may be toxic for wounds.

DEBRIDEMENT OF ULCER BED. Once cellulitis and eczematous inflammation have been controlled, the ulcer must be prepared for definitive treatment. Exudate and crust must be removed to expose granulation tissue, the foundation for new epithelium.

Wound debridement. Ulcers should be debrided of necrotic and fibrinous debris. Occlusive dressing, chemical debridement, and surgical and mechanical debridement are three methods that help to remove necrotic tissue and promote granulation tissue.

Occlusive dressings. Many products are available (Table 3-8); the choice is usually determined by the type of wound and the amount of exudate. These dressings should be used with compression for maximum benefit.

Chemical debridement. Enzyme-debriding agents may be considered to remove necrotic tissue. Santyl (collagenase), Panafil (papain), Granulex (trypsin), or Accuzyme is applied one or several times each day. The efficacy of all of these agents is not well established; Elase is ineffective.

Surgical or mechanical debridement. Debridement with sharp surgical instruments must be performed with great care so as not to damage delicate viable tissue. Whirlpool, wound irrigation, wet dressings, and hydrotherapy are all commonly used.

Dextranomer absorbent pads contain Debrisan beads, which are highly absorbent and are useful for wounds with heavy exudate. They should not be used to treat dry wounds or deep narrow wounds or sinuses from which removal may be difficult.

DEFINITIVE TREATMENT
1. Measure the ulcer at each visit.
2. Encourage elevation and periods of exercise and ambulation.
3. Minimize bacteria and necrotic debris.
4. Promote granulation tissue formation.
5. Induce reepithelialization.
6. Reduce edema.
7. Protect from trauma.

Table 3-8 Occlusive Wound Dressings Used for Leg Ulcers

Type (examples)	Advantages	Disadvantages	Indications
Hydrogels (e.g., IntraSite Gel, Nu-gel, Vigilon)	Semitransparent, soothing, do not adhere to wounds, absorbent	Require secondary dressing and frequent dressing changes; expensive	Painful, laser, and partial-thickness wounds; after dermabrasion or chemical peel
Alginates (e.g., AlgiDerm, Kaltostat, Sorbsan)	Absorbent, hemostatic, do not adhere to wounds, fewer dressing changes. Can be used on infected wounds	Require secondary dressing; gel has foul smell. Not to be used on low-exudating wounds/dry necrotic wounds	Highly exudative wounds, partial- or full-thickness wounds; after surgery
Hydrocolloids (e.g., Comfeel, DuoDerm, Restore)	Fibrinolytic, enhance angiogenesis, absorbent, create bacterial and physical barrier	Opaque, gel has foul smell, expensive	Partial- or full-thickness wounds; stage 1-4 pressure ulcers
Foams (e.g., Allevyn, Curafoam, Lyofoam)	Use on fragile skin; highly absorbent; frequency of dressing change depends on level of exudate (1-6 days)	Opaque, require secondary dressing, may adhere to wounds, expensive	Partial-thickness exudative wounds; for pressure relief
Films (e.g., OpSite, Polyskin 11, Tegaderm)	Transparent, create bacterial barrier, adhesive without secondary dressing	May adhere to wounds; can cause fluid collection	Donor sites, superficial burns, partial-thickness wounds with minimal exudate

Adapted from Phillips TJ: Postgrad Med 1999; 105:5.

Occlusive dressings. Occlusive dressings promote rapid healing of leg ulcers. Five types are available that achieve debridement less painfully but more slowly than surgical debridement. Crust formation is suppressed, and epidermis migrates rapidly over the moist granulation tissue. There is no set amount of time that occlusive dressings should stay on a wound; they can be left in place for several days at a time. Dressings should be left in place until fluid begins to leak from around their edges. Early removal of dressings can lead to stripping of delicate new epithelium. Initially, dressings usually need to be changed every other day. Thereafter they may be left in place for many days if excess fluid does not accumulate. Dressings applied over fresh wounds accumulate large amounts of fluid. This can be removed by needle aspiration. Dressings should not be applied to inflamed eczematous skin at the borders of ulcers because this increases bacterial flora. Treatment should be interrupted only if clinical signs of infection appear. Patients remain ambulatory, and relief of pain is significant. Patients should be warned that an unpleasant odor occurs with fluid buildup. The choice of dressing is determined by the type of wound, the amount of exudate, and the cost (see Table 3-8).

COMPRESSION. Compression is the cornerstone of therapy for venous ulcers. Elimination of edema is essential during treatment and after resolution. This is accomplished by applying external compression bandages during the healing phase and graded compression stockings after healing to prevent recurrence. Compression bandages can be applied over occlusive dressing during the healing phase. Some patients may have arterial insufficiency, as well as venous disease. Measure the ankle-brachial pressure index before compression to avoid necrosis or gangrene of the foot.

Compression bandages. Compression therapy and maintenance of a moist wound environment are essential. Compression improves venous hypertension and relieves edema. An external pressure of at least 35 to 40 mm Hg at the ankle is desirable. Many bandage systems are available.

MULTI-LAYER BANDAGES. The new multi-layered bandage systems (e.g., three-layered padding or Dynaflex and four-layered padding or Profore) are expensive but produce the fastest healing rates. They achieve uniform, sustained compression and can be left in place for a week.

GRADED ELASTIC COMPRESSION STOCKINGS. These stockings exert high pressure at the ankle, with pressure decreasing to the thigh. After healing, compression stockings should be worn to prevent ulcer recurrence. These stockings are put on in the morning soon after the patient gets out of bed. Patients with arthritis who have difficulty putting these stockings on may use the zip-up type. The amount of compression can be specified by the physician (see Table 3-9). Patients with chronic venous insufficiency who have had stasis dermatitis or ulceration require a compression of between 35 and 40 mm Hg. Various lengths can be purchased; an

Class	Ankle pressure (mm Hg)	Indications
I	20 to 30	Varicose veins, mild edema, or leg fatigue
II	30 to 40	Moderate leg edema, severe varicosities, and moderate venous insufficiency
III	40 to 50	Severe edema or elephantiasis and severe venous insufficiency with secondary post-thrombotic edema
IV	60	

Table 3-9 Compression Stockings (e.g., Jobst, Juzo, Sigvaris)

Adapted from: Isabel C et al: J Am Acad Dermatol 2001; 44:401.

above-the-knee stocking may give the best results but knee-high stockings are most commonly used. The stockings may be difficult for older patients to put on; also, the stockings must be replaced periodically because they may stretch, thereby losing elasticity. Firmly applied Ace bandages are a less effective but convenient alternative.

There are 4 classes of stockings based on the compression exerted at the ankle.

Nonelastic bandages. Unna's boots (e.g., Domepaste, GELOCAST BANDAGE, UnnaFlex) are gauze bandages impregnated with zinc oxide paste to create a semirigid "boot" when applied. They protect ulcers from the environment and help control edema and are especially helpful in elderly or noncompliant patients because they can be left in place for 7 to 10 days. Because such a bandage does not eliminate existing edema fluid, it should be applied in the morning after edema has drained. However, when ulcers produce a large amount of exudate, the boot should be changed more often. Unna's boots are not applied over synthetic dressings.

Pneumatic compression pumps. Intermittent-compression pumps are considered when a venous ulcer does not respond to treatment with standard compression dressings.

ASPIRIN. Oral enteric-coated aspirin (300 mg) increased the rate of venous ulcer healing.[44]

Pentoxifylline. Pentoxifylline (800 mg tid) accelerated the healing rate of venous ulcers and was more effective than the conventional dose (400 mg tid).[45]

Vitamins. Patients with signs of malnutrition, such as low serum albumin or transferrin concentrations, may benefit from dietary supplementation. Ascorbic acid (1 to 2 gm/day), zinc sulfate (220 mg tid), and vitamin E (200 mg/day) may be used for supplementation. These vitamins are essential for wound healing but should not be prescribed in excessively high dosages.

Grafting. Skin grafts promote healing even if they do not take because they stimulate wound epithelialization. Split-thickness skin grafting is used for large ulcers. Meshed grafts are useful for large ulcers because they allow exudate to escape through the graft interstices. The donor site may be painful and slow to heal, especially in elderly patients. Pinch grafting is a useful for smaller wounds. Multiple small pinches or superficial punch biopsies are taken from a donor site (e.g., thigh) and placed dermal side down on the ulcer bed. The tissue-engineered human skin equivalent, Apligraf, is effective for treating long-standing deep ulcers.

Vein surgery. Ligation or sclerosis of the long and short saphenous systems, with or without communicating vein ligation or sclerosis, is useful only if the deep veins are competent. Superficial vein surgery does not improve the healing rate of venous ulcers.

References

1. Nilsson E, Henning C, Hjorleifsson M-L: Density of the microflora in hand eczema before and after topical treatment with a potent corticosteroid, J Am Acad Dermatol 1986; 15:192.

2. Meding B, Swanbeck G: Occupational hand eczema in an industrial city, Contact Dermatitis 1990; 22:13.

3. Meding B, Swanbeck G: Consequences of having hand eczema, Contact Dermatitis 1990; 23:6.

4. Meding B: Epidemiology of hand eczema in an industrial city, Acta Derm Venereol (Suppl) 1990; 153:1.

5. Cronin E: Clinical patterns of hand eczema in women, Contact Dermatitis 1985; 13:153.

6. Lauharanta J, et al: Prevention of dryness and eczema of the hands of hospital staff by emulsion cleansing instead of washing with soap, J Hosp Infect 1991; 17:207.

7. Hannuksela A, Kinnunen T: Moisturizers prevent irritant dermatitis, Acta Derm Venereol 1992; 72:42.

8. Rystedt I: Atopy, hand eczema, and contact dermatitis: summary of recent large-scale studies, Semin Dermatol 1986; 5:290.

9. Rystedt I: Factors influencing the occurrence of hand eczema in adults with a history of atopic dermatitis in childhood, Contact Dermatitis 1985; 12:185.

10. Rystedt I: Hand eczema in patients with history of atopic manifestations in childhood, Acta Derm Venereol (Stockh) 1985; 65:305.

11. Jordan WP Jr: Allergic contact dermatitis in hand eczema, Arch Dermatol 1974; 110:567.

12. Adams RM: Patch testing: a recapitulation, J Am Acad Dermatol 1981; 5:629.

13. Lee Y et al: Recurrent focal palmar peeling, Australas J Dermatol 1996; 37(3):143.

14. Thelin I, Agrup G: Pompholyx: a one-year series, Acta Derm Venereol (Stockh) 1985; 65:214.

15. Veien NK et al: Oral challenge with metal salts: vesicular patch-test negative reaction, Contact Dermatitis 1983; 9:402.

16. Lodi A et al: Epidemiological, clinical and allergological observations on pompholyx, Contact Dermatitis 1992; 26:17.

17. Yokozeki H et al: The role of metal allergy and local hyperhidrosis in the pathogenesis of pompholyx, J Dermatol 1992;19:964.

18. LeVine MJ, Parrish JA, Fitzpatrick TB: Oral methoxsalen photochemotherapy (PUVA) of dyshidrotic eczema, Acta Derm Venereol (Stockh) 1981; 61:570.

19. Egan C et al: Low-dose oral methotrexate treatment for recalcitrant palmoplantar pompholyx, J Am Acad Dermatol 1999; 40(4):612.

20. Egan CA, et al: Low-dose oral methotrexate treatment for recalcitrant palmoplantar pompholyx, J Am Acad Dermatol 1999; 40:612.

21. Stambaugh M et al: Complete remission of refractory dyshidrotic eczema with the use of radiation therapy, Cutis 2000; 65(4):211.

22. Callen J et al: Adult-onset recalcitrant eczema: a marker of noncutaneous lymphoma or leukemia, J Am Acad Dermatol 2000; 43(2):207.

23. Jones SK et al: Juvenile plantar dermatosis: an 8-year follow-up of 102 patients, Clin Exp Dermatol 1987; 12:5.

24. Ashton RE, Griffiths WAD: Juvenile plantar dermatosis: atopy or footwear? Clin Exp Dermatol 1986; 11:529.

25. Lyell A: Cutaneous artifactual disease, J Am Acad Dermatol 1979; 1:391.

26. Doran AR, Roy A, Wolkowitz OW: Self-destructive dermatoses, Psychiatr Clin North Am 1985; 8:291.

27. Gupta MA, Gupta AK, Haberman HF: The self-inflicted dermatoses: a critical review, Gen Hosp Psychiatry 1987; 9:45.

28. Medansky RS, Handler RM: Dermatopsychosomatics: classification, physiology, and therapeutic approaches, J Am Acad Dermatol 1981; 5:125.

29. Munro A: Delusional parasitosis: a form of monosymptomatic hypochondriacal psychosis, Semin Dermatol 1983; 2:197.

30. Koo JY, Pham CT: Psychodermatology: practical guidelines on pharmacotherapy, Arch Dermatol 1992; 128:381.

31. Van MM: Psychodermatology: an overview, Psychother Psychosom 1992; 58:125.

32. Koblenzer CS: Cutaneous manifestations of psychiatric disease that commonly present to the dermatologist—diagnosis and treatment, Intl J Psychiatry Med 1992; 22:47.

33. Folks DG, Kinney FC: The role of psychological factors in dermatologic conditions, Psychosomatics 1992; 33:45.

34. Moffaert MV: Localization of self-inflicted dermatological lesions: what do they tell the dermatologist? Acta Derm Venereol (Stockh) 1991; 156(suppl):23.

35. Hatch ML et al: Obsessive-compulsive disorder in patients with chronic pruritic conditions: case studies and discussion, J Am Acad Dermatol 1992; 26:549.

36. Fisher B: The red scrotum syndrome, Cutis 1997; 60(3):139.

37. Heckmann M et al: Botulinum toxin type A injection in the treatment of lichen simplex: an open pilot study, J Am Acad Dermatol 2002; 46(4):617.

38. Harris B t al: Demonstration by S-100 protein staining of increased numbers of nerves in the papillary dermis of patients with prurigo nodularis, J Am Acad Dermatol 1992; 26:56.

39. Stander S, Luger T, Metze D: Treatment of prurigo nodularis with topical capsaicin, J Am Acad Dermatol 2001; 44(3):471.

40. Wong S, Goh C: Double-blind, right/left comparison of calcipotriol ointment and betamethasone ointment in the treatment of prurigo nodularis, Arch Dermatol 2000; 136(6): 807.

41. Metze D et al: Efficacy and safety of naltrexone, an oral opiate receptor antagonist, in the treatment of pruritus in internal and dermatological diseases, J Am Acad Dermatol 1999; 41(4):533.

42. Slaughter J et al: Psychogenic parasitosis: a case series and literature review, Psychosomatics 1998; 39(6):491.

43. Zanol K, Slaughter J, Hall R: An approach to the treatment of psychogenic parasitosis, Intl J Dermatol 1998; 37(1):56.

44. Layton A et al: Randomised trial of oral aspirin for chronic venous leg ulcers, Lancet 1994, 334.164.

45. Falanga V et al: Systemic treatment of venous leg ulcers with high doses of pentoxifylline: efficacy in a randomized, placebo-controlled trial, Wound Repair Regen 1999; 7(4):208.

Contact Dermatitis and Patch Testing

❏ **Irritant contact dermatitis**

❏ **Allergic contact dermatitis**
   Systemically induced allergic contact
      dermatitis
   Clinical presentation
   Rhus dermatitis
   Natural rubber latex allergy
   Shoe allergy
   Metal dermatitis
   Cement dermatitis and burns
   Further examples of allergic contact dermatitis
   Patients with leg ulcers
   Cosmetic and fragrance allergy

❏ **Diagnosis of contact dermatitis**
   Patch testing

Contact dermatitis is an eczematous dermatitis caused by exposure to substances in the environment. Those substances act as irritants or allergens and may cause acute, subacute, or chronic eczematous inflammation. To diagnose contact dermatitis one must first recognize that an eruption is eczematous. Contact allergies often have characteristic distribution patterns indicating that the observed eczematous eruption is caused by external rather than internal stimuli. Elimination of the suspected offending agent and appropriate treatment for eczematous inflammation usually serve to manage patients with contact dermatitis effectively. However, in the many cases in which this direct approach fails, patch testing is useful.

It is important to differentiate contact dermatitis resulting from irritation from that caused by allergy. An outline of these differences is listed in Table 4-1.

Table 4-1 Contact Dermatitis: Irritant versus Allergic

	Irritant	Allergic
People at risk	Everyone	Genetically predisposed
Mechanism of response	Nonimmunologic; a physical and chemical alteration of epidermis	Delayed hypersensitivity reaction
Number of exposures	Few to many; depends on individual's ability to maintain an effective epidermal barrier	One or several to cause sensitization
Nature of substance	Organic solvent, soaps	Low molecular weight hapten (e.g., metals, formalin, epoxy)
Concentration of substance required	Usually high	May be very low
Mode of onset	Usually gradual as epidermal barrier becomes compromised	Once sensitized, usually rapid; 12 to 48 hours after exposure
Distribution	Borders usually indistinct	May correspond exactly to contactant (e.g., watch band, elastic waistband)
Investigative procedure	Trial of avoidance	Trial of avoidance, patch testing, or both
Management	Protection and reduced incidence of exposure	Complete avoidance

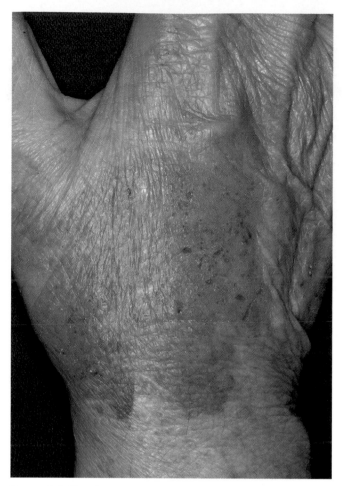

Figure 4-1 Chronic exposure to soap and water has caused subacute eczematous inflammation over the backs of the hands and fingers.

Irritant Contact Dermatitis

Irritation of the skin is the most common cause of contact dermatitis. The epidermis is a thin cellular barrier with an outer layer composed of dead cells in a water-protein-lipid matrix. Any process that damages any component of the barrier compromises its function, and a nonimmunologic eczematous response may result. Repeated use of strong alkaline soap or industrial exposure to organic solvents extracts lipid from the skin. Acids may combine with water in the skin and cause dehydration. When the skin is compromised, exposure to even a weak irritant sustains the inflammation. The intensity of the inflammation is related to the concentration of the irritant and the length of exposure. Mild irritants cause dryness, fissuring, and erythema; a mild eczematous reaction may occur with continuous exposure. Continuous exposure to moisture in areas such as the hand, the diaper area, or the skin around a colostomy may eventually cause eczematous inflammation. Strong chemicals may produce an immediate reaction; Figures 4-1 through 4-4 show examples of irritant dermatitis.

Patients vary in their ability to withstand exposure to irritants. Some people cannot tolerate frequent hand washing whereas others may work daily with harsh cleaning solutions without any difficulty.

Figure 4-2 Long exposure to wet diapers followed by frequent washing has resulted in diffuse erythema and dry, cracked, fissured skin.

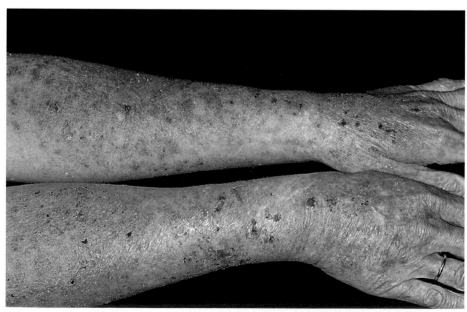

IRRITANT DERMATITIS

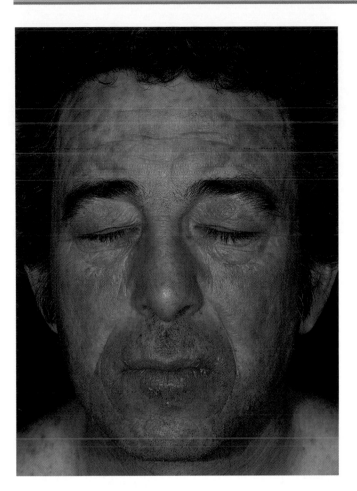

Figure 4-3 Exposure to industrial solvents has resulted in diffuse erythema with dryness and fissuring about the mouth.

Figure 4-4 Repeated cycles of wetting and drying by lip licking resulted in irritant dermatitis.

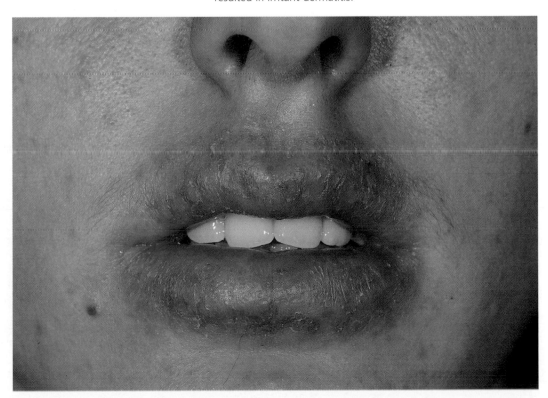

Allergic Contact Dermatitis

Allergic contact dermatitis is an inflammatory reaction that follows absorption of antigen applied to the skin and recruitment of previously sensitized, antigen-specific T lymphocytes into the skin. It affects a limited number of individuals. The antigens are usually low-molecular-weight substances that readily penetrate the stratum corneum. Most contact allergens are weak and require repeated exposure before sensitization occurs. Strong antigens, such as poison ivy, require only two exposures for sensitization.

Interaction between antigen and T lymphocytes is mediated by antigen-presenting epidermal cells (Langerhans' cells) and is divided into two sequential phases: an initial sensitization phase and an elicitation phase. Langerhan's cells are abundant in skin and sparse at mucosal sites.[1]

Allergic contact dermatitis phases

SENSITIZATION PHASE. Antigen is applied to the skin surface, penetrates the epidermal barrier (stratum corneum) and is taken up by Langerhans' cells in the epidermal basal layer. The antigen is "processed" and displayed on the surface of the Langerhans' cell. This cell migrates to the regional lymph nodes and presents the antigen to T lymphocytes. Cytokine-induced proliferation and clonal expansion within the lymph nodes results in T lymphocytes bearing receptors that recognize the specific antigen. These antigen-specific T lymphocytes enter the bloodstream and circulate back to the epidermis.

ELICITATION PHASE. The elicitation phase occurs in sensitized patients with reexposure to the antigen. Langerhans' cells bearing the antigen interact with antigen-specific T lymphocytes that are circulating in the skin. This interaction results in cytokine-induced activation and proliferation of the antigen-specific T lymphocytes and the release of inflammatory mediators. Allergic contact dermatitis develops within 12 to 48 hours of antigen exposure and persists for 3 or 4 weeks.

Cross-sensitization

An allergen, the chemical structure of which is similar to the original sensitizing antigen, may cause inflammation because the immune system is unable to differentiate between the original and the chemically related antigen. For example, the skin of patients who are allergic to balsam of Peru, which is present in numerous topical preparations, may become inflamed when exposed to the chemically related benzoin in tincture of benzoin.

Systemically induced allergic contact dermatitis

Systemic contact dermatitis results from the exposure to an allergen by ingestion, inhalation, injection, or percutaneous penetration in a person previously sensitized to the allergen by cutaneous contact. Patients allergic to poison ivy develop diffuse inflammation following the ingestion of raw cashew nuts (Figure 4-5). Cashew nut oil [2,3] is chemically related to the oleoresin of the poison ivy plant. Persons allergic to balsam of Peru and/or fragrance mix benefit from dietary avoidance of balsams.[4]

Clinical presentation

SHAPE AND LOCATION. The shape and location of the rash are the most important clues to the cause of the allergen (Table 4-2). The pattern of inflammation may correspond exactly to the shape of the offending substance (Figures 4-6, 4-7, and 4-8). The diagnosis is obvious when inflammation is confined specifically to the area under a watchband, shoe, or elastic waistband. Plants (e.g., poison ivy) produce linear lesions.

Unfortunately most allergic reactions do not conform precisely to the areas contacting the allergen. The woman allergic to an ingredient in her facial cosmetic typically presents with a patchy facial eczema, rather than with a diffuse der-

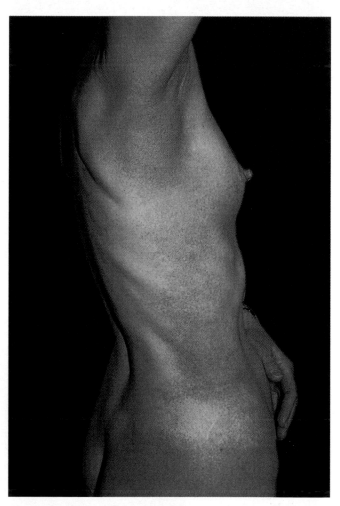

Figure 4-5 Diffuse allergic reaction occurring in a patient allergic to poison ivy who has ingested raw cashew nuts, the oil of which cross-reacts with the oleoresin of poison ivy.

Table 4-2 Contact Dermatitis: Distribution Diagnosis

Location	Material
Scalp and ears	Shampoos, hair dyes, topical medicines, metal earrings, eyeglasses, rubber ear plugs
Face	Cosmetics (preservatives, emulsifiers, fragrances) Acne medications (e.g., benzoyl peroxide), aftershave lotions Respirators, masks, aerosolized mists (machinists), volatile organic substances (e.g., amine hardeners in the plastic industry) Chemicals (hair dyes) applied to the scalp spread to face, ears, and neck—spares the scalp (scalp is resistant) Airborne allergens (poison ivy from burning leaves, ragweed) Photoallergic reactions—spare the upper lip and have a sharp cut-off at the jawline (sunscreen ingredients—oxybenzone, benzophenone No. 3)
Eyelids	Nail polish (transferred by rubbing), cosmetics, contact lens solution, metal eyelash curlers, make-up sponges (rubber) Lower lids (topical medications) Periocular area (goggles)
Upper and lower eyelids	Cause is usually not allergic (atopic dermatitis, seborrheic dermatitis, psoriasis)
Facial and eyelid accentuation	Airborne contact dermatitis (ragweed, volatile organic substances, fragrances, chemicals in smoke) Products applied to the hands and transferred to the face (nail enamels)
Mucosal	Most patients allergic to allergens applied intraorally have cheilitis but not stomatitis. Individual who reacts to nickel, mercury, palladium, or gold in dental amalgams presents with a systemic contact dermatitis with or without a localized stomatitis
Neck	Necklaces (metals, exotic woods), airborne allergens (ragweed), perfumes, aftershave lotion. Cosmetic allergens. Textile dermatitis (dyes, formaldehyde resins in clothing)
Trunk	Textile (sparing of the axillary and undergarment areas) Azo-aniline dyes (color clothing) Urea formaldehyde resins (wrinkle-resistant clothing) NOTE: Para-phenylenediamine (PPD) and formaldehyde are not adequate screens for patch testing for allergy to textile dyes and resins Rubber allergens Elasticized waist bands, spandex bras NOTE: standard rubber patch test allergens may be negative. Patch test with a portion of the elastic band from a garment that has been bleached. Generalized reactions Fragrances, preservatives in moisturizing lotions, topical medication, sunscreens; poison ivy; plants (phototoxic reactions); metal belt buckles Laundry detergents rarely cause allergic contact dermatitis[6]
Scattered, generalized dermatitis	"Systemic contact dermatitis"—an individual who has been sensitized topically to an allergen and is subsequently reexposed systemically (drug/chemical introduced intramuscularly, intravenously, orally, rectally, or vaginally), foods, medical or dental devices that contact mucosal surfaces or that have been implanted surgically into the body. Cinnamic aldehyde and balsam (cosmetics, topical medications, suppositories, dental liquids, and flavorings) or parabens (food preservatives). Contaminants in foodstuffs, such as nickel
Arms	Same as hands; watch and watchband. Photosensitive process (rash ends at mid-upper arm). Soap, moisturizing creams
Fingertips	Hairdressers—glyceryl monothioglycolate in permanent solutions or para-phenylenediamine in hair dyes. Nurses—glutaraldehyde in disinfectants Dental and orthopedic personnel—glue (methylmethacrylate) Many chemicals penetrate standard gloves
Axillae	Deodorant (axillary vault), clothing (axillary folds)
Hands	Soaps and detergents, foods, spices, poison ivy, industrial solvents and oils, cement, metal (pots, rings), topical medications, rubber gloves in surgeons
Genitals	Poison ivy (transferred by hand), rubber condoms, diaphragms, pessaries
Anal region	Hemorrhoid preparations (benzocaine, Nupercaine)
Lower legs, popliteal fossa, and inner thigh	Topical medication (benzocaine, lanolin, neomycin, parabens) Fragrances, preservatives, and vehicles in moisturizers and cosmetics Dyes in pantyhose (especially blue disperse dyes in darker-colored hose and disperse yellow No. 3 in flesh-colored hose) Textiles
Feet	Shoes—paratertiary butylphenol formaldehyde resin (a component of shoe glues), rubber components, and chromate (used to tan leather) Cement spilling into boots

Adapted from Belsito DV: Dermatol Clin 1999; 17:3.

ALLERGIC CONTACT DERMATITIS

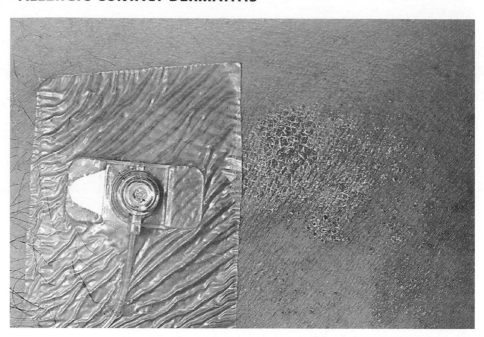

Figure 4-6 Adhesives allergy.

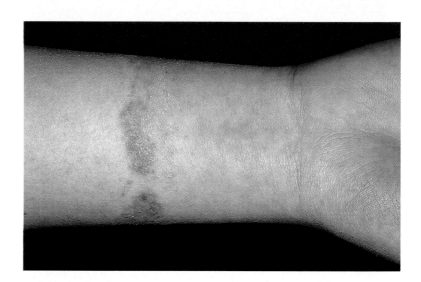

Figure 4-7 Potassium dichromate allergy (leather watch band).

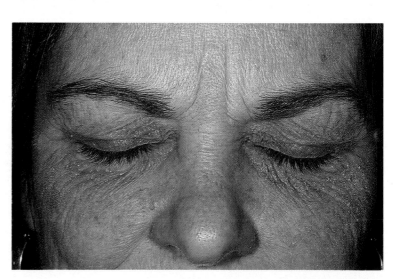

Figure 4-8 Eye cosmetic allergy. Open patch testing with the cosmetic proved the diagnosis. Routine patch testing was positive for fragrance mix.

matitis involving all areas of the face to which the cosmetic was applied. An allergen may be spread to other sites by inadvertent contact. The scalp, palms, and soles are resistant to allergic contact dermatitis and may show only minimal inflammation despite contact with an allergen that produces dermatitis in adjacent area.[5]

Aeroallergens inflame the exposed skin and spare clothed areas. Clothing allergens cause dermatitis of clothed areas. Table 4-2 lists substances that are common causes of inflammation in specific body regions. Table 4-3 lists substances commonly encountered in specific professions.

The failure of an eczematous dermatitis to respond to standard treatments also suggest that the dermatitis is allergic and not irritant.

INTENSITY AND PATTERNS. The intensity of inflammation depends on the degree of sensitivity and the concentration of the antigen. Strong sensitizers such as the oleoresin of poison ivy may produce intense inflammation in low concentrations whereas weak sensitizers may cause only erythema. The appearance also depends on location and duration. Acute inflammation appears as macular erythema, edema, vesicles, or bullae. Chronic inflammation is characterized by lichenification, scaling, or fissures. Contact allergies may have noneczematous patterns that include the cellulitis-like appearance of dermal contact hypersensitivity, lichenoid variants, contact leukoderma, contact purpura, and erythema multiforme.[5]

DIRECT VERSUS AIRBORNE CONTACT. Acute and chronic dermatitis of exposed parts of the body, especially the face, may be caused by chemicals suspended in the air. Sprays, perfumes, chemical dusts, and plant pollen (e.g., ragweed) are possible sources. Inflammation from airborne sensitizers tends to be more diffuse. Photodermatitis can have the same distribution. Airborne material easily collects on the upper eyelids; this area is particularly susceptible. Volatile substances can collect in clothing.

Allergic contact dermatitis in children
Allergic contact dermatitis may account for as many as 20% of all cases of dermatitis in children. Poison ivy, nickel (jewelry), rubber (shoe dermatitis), balsam of Peru (hand and face dermatitis), formaldehyde (cosmetics and shampoos), and neomycin (topical antibiotic ointments) are the common allergens.

MANAGEMENT OF ALLERGIC CONTACT DERMATITIS
1. Minimize products for topical use
2. Use ointments instead of creams (creams contain preservatives and are complex mixtures of chemicals)
3. Botanical extracts may be used in "fragrance-free" products
4. When patch testing, also test to the patient's consumer products
5. Read product labels carefully. Many "dermatologist recommended" products contain sensitizers (e.g., lanolin, fragrance, Quaternium 15, parabens, methylchloroisothiazolinone/mentylisothiazolinone)

Table 4-3 Contact Dermatitis: Occupational Exposure

Occupation	Irritants	Allergens
Beauticians	Wet work (shampoos)	Hair tints, permanent solution, shampoos (formaldehyde)
Construction workers	Fuels, lubricants, cement	Cement (chromium, cobalt), epoxy, glues, paints, solvents, rubber, chrome-tanned leather gloves
Chefs, bartenders, bakers	Moist foods, juices, corn, pineapple juice	Orange and lemon peel (oil of limonene), mango, carrot, parsnips, parsley, celery; spices (e.g., capsicum, cinnamon, cloves, nutmeg, vanilla)
Farmers	Milker's eczema (detergents), tractor lubricants and fuels	Malathion, pyrethrium insecticides, fungicides, rubber, ragweed, marsh elder
Forest products industry	Wet work (wood processing)	Poison ivy and oak, plants growing on bark (e.g., lichens, liverworts)
Medical and surgical personnel	Surgical scrubbing	Rubber gloves, glutaraldehyde (germicides), acrylic monomer in cement (orthopaedic surgeons), penicillin, chlorpromazine, benzalkonium chloride, neomycin
Printing industry	Alcohols, alkalis, grease	Polyfunctional acrylic monomers, epoxy acrylate oligomers, isocyanate compounds (all used in a new ink-drying method)

Rhus dermatitis

In the United States poison ivy, poison oak, and poison sumac produce more cases of allergic contact dermatitis than all other contactants combined. The allergens responsible for poison ivy and poison oak allergic contact dermatitis are contained within the resinous sap material termed *urushiol.* Urushiol is composed of a mixture of catechols. All parts of the plant contain the sap. These plants belong to the *Anacardiaceae* family and the genus *Rhus.* Other plants in that family, such as cashew trees, mango trees, Japanese laquer trees, and ginkgo contain allergens identical or related to those in poison ivy. Thousands of workers on cashew nut farms in India develop hand dermatitis from direct contact with the irritating resinous oil from cashew nut shells. Poison ivy and poison oak are neither ivy nor oak species.

CLINICAL PRESENTATION. *Rhus* dermatitis occurs from contact with the leaf or internal parts of the stem or root and can be acquired from roots or stems in the fall and winter. The clinical presentation varies with the quantity of oleoresin that contacts the skin, the pattern in which contact was made, individual susceptibility, and regional variations in cutaneous reactivity. Small quantities of oleoresin produce only erythema whereas large quantities cause intense vesiculation (Figures 4-9, 4-10, and 4-11).

The highly characteristic linear lesions are created when part of the plant is drawn across the skin or from streaking the oleoresin while scratching. Diffuse or unusual patterns of inflammation occur when the oleoresin is acquired from contaminated animal hair or clothing or from smoke while burning the plant. The eruption may appear as quickly as 8 hours after contact or may be delayed for a week or more. The appearance of new lesions a week after contact may be confusing to the patient, who may attribute new lesions to the spread of the disease by touching active lesions or to contamination with blister fluid. Blister fluid does not contain the oleoresin and, contrary to popular belief, cannot spread the inflammation.

PREVENTION. Washing the skin with any type of soap inactivates and removes all surface oleoresin, thereby preventing further contamination. Washing must be performed immediately after exposure. After 10 minutes, only 50% of urushiol can be removed; after 30 minutes, only 10% can be removed; and after 60 minutes, none can be removed.

BARRIER CREAMS. An organoclay compound, 5% quaternium-18 bentonite lotion ("Ivy-Block") prevents dermatitis in more than 50% of sensitized and exposed patients.

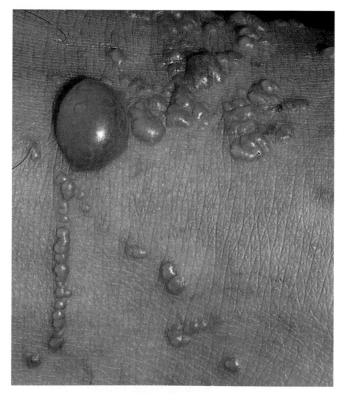

Figure 4-9 Poison ivy. A classic presentation with vesicles and blisters. A line of vesicles (linear lesions) caused by dragging the resin over the surface of the skin with the scratching finger is a highly characteristic sign of plant contact dermatitis.

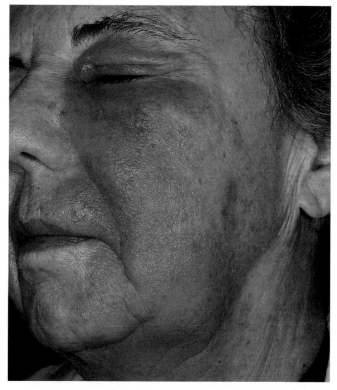

Figure 4-10 Poison ivy dermatitis. Diffuse erythema with vesicles over the entire surface.

TREATMENT OF INFLAMMATION

Wet compresses. Blisters and intense erythema are treated with cold, wet compresses, and they are highly effective during the acute blistering stage. Cold compresses should be used for 15 to 30 minutes several times a day for 1 to 3 days until blistering and severe itching is controlled. Topical steroids do not penetrate through blisters. Short, cool tub baths with or without colloidal oatmeal (Aveeno) are very soothing and help to control widespread acute inflammation. Calamine lotion controls itching but prolonged use causes excessive drying. Hydroxyzine and diphenhydramine control itching and encourage sleep.

Topical steroids. Mild to moderate erythema may respond to topical steroids. Groups I to V creams or gels applied 2 to 4 times a day rapidly suppress erythema and itching.

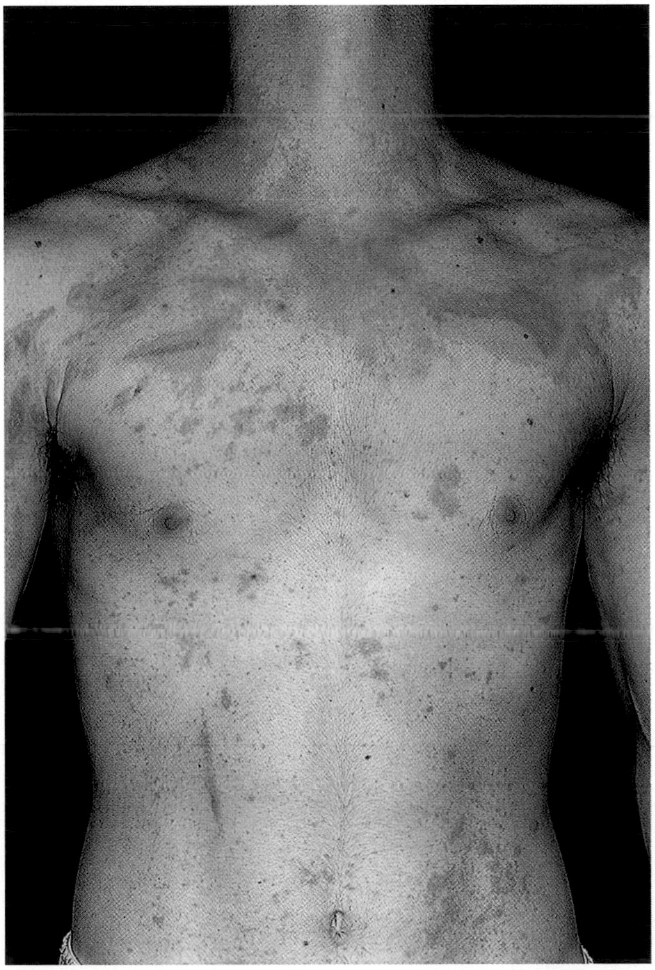

Prednisone. Severe poison ivy is treated with prednisone. A single dose treatment schedule is shown in Box 4-1. Prednisone, administered in a dosage of 20 mg twice each day for at least 7 days, is an alternative schedule for severe, widespread inflammation. Tapering the dosage after this short course is usually not necessary. Patients who may have trouble adhering to a medication schedule may be treated with triamcinolone acetonide (Kenalog, Aristocort; 40 mg suspension) given intramuscularly. Commercially available steroid dose packs (e.g., Medrol Dosepak) should be avoided because they provide an inadequate amount of medicine and may cause recurrence of rash and pruritus after initial partial amelioration of symptoms during the first days of treatment.[7] Patients who do not initially seem to require medication may become much worse 1 or 2 days after an office visit; they should be advised that prednisone is available if their conditions worsen.

DIAGNOSIS. The diagnosis is usually obvious. The intense, often linear, vesicular eruption is highly characteristic. Patch testing is not done because the risk of inducing allergic reactions in individuals who have not yet been sensitized is high.

PROPHYLACTIC TREATMENT. Complete desensitization cannot be accomplished. Poison ivy oleoresin in capsules and injectable syringes for hyposensitization has been removed from the market by the FDA.

Figure 4-11 Poison ivy dermatitis. Acute inflammation over wide areas. The asymmetrical distribution of intense erythema and vesicles suggests the diagnosis of an external insult. Linear lesions are highly characteristic. Inflammation of this intensity usually requires prednisone.

Box 4-1 Prednisone for Severe Poison Ivy Dermatitis (Adults)	
Day	**Dosage mg/day**
	10-mg tablets, taken as a single dose each morning
1-4	60
5-6	50
7-8	40
9-10	30
11-12	20
13-14	10

Natural rubber latex allergy

Allergy to natural rubber latex (NRL) is a national health problem. Groups at highest risk include health care workers, rubber industry workers, and persons who have undergone multiple surgical procedures.[8]

Types of allergies. There are three reactions to NRL products: irritant contact dermatitis, allergic contact dermatitis, and immediate-type hypersensitivity reaction.[9]

IRRITANT CONTACT DERMATITIS. Irritant contact dermatitis is a nonimmune eczematous reaction caused by moisture, heat, and friction under gloves. Reaction severity depends on duration of exposure, degree of skin occlusion, and skin temperature. There is itching, erythema, and scaling followed by thickened crusted plaques. The use of a cotton liner under NRL gloves can help.

ALLERGIC CONTACT DERMATITIS (TYPE IV ALLERGY). Of 100 cases of chronic hand dermatitis in surgeons, dentists, and surgical personnel, 11 patients were allergic to latex rubber surgical gloves.[10] Latex allergy occurs in up to 10% of operating room nurses.[11] Delayed-type hypersensitivity (type IV) T-cell-mediated sensitization to rubber accelerators (e.g., thiurams, carbamates, mercapto compounds) and antioxidants (not latex proteins) in latex gloves causes an allergic contact dermatitis usually limited to the sites of direct contact (e.g., dorsum of the hand) (Figure 4-12). Glove allergy was caused by thiurams in 72% of cases, carbamates in 25% of cases, and mercapto compounds in 3% of cases. Once sensitized, subsequent challenges from the same allergen will cause an eczematous dermatitis (erythema, scaling, vesiculation). Type IV allergy accounts for about 80% of occupationally acquired rubber allergy. The diagnosis is made by patch testing. The standard patch test screening series (see p. 101) contains the chemicals found in latex products. Patch testing with a thin piece of an NRL product (e.g., glove) may be helpful, but not in patients with suspected type I allergy to NRL. Hand dermatitis and atopy are risk factors for NRL allergy. Allergy to other forms of rubber also occurs (Figures 4-13 and 4-14).

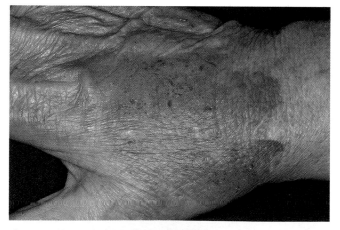

Figure 4-12 Latex glove allergy should be suspected in health care workers who present with eczema on the back of the hands.

TREATMENT. Once the allergen has been identified by patch testing, alternative rubber articles that utilize different rubber manufacturing chemicals can be obtained.[12,19] Patients who have undergone or will require multiple surgical procedures should be offered a latex-safe hospital environment.

Surgeons with rubber sensitivity may use Elastyren hypoallergenic surgical gloves (1-800-ELASTYN). Unlike latex rubber, Elastyren is not vulcanized and therefore contains no metal oxides, sulfur, accelerators, or mercaptobenzothiazole, sensitizers commonly found in rubber products. Allerderm vinyl gloves, for household use, can be used with a cotton liner. Hypoallergenic vinyl gloves for examination are generally available.

IMMEDIATE-TYPE HYPERSENSITIVITY (TYPE I ALLERGY). This IgE-mediated reaction requires previous sensitization. Reexposure to the allergen induces the release of histamine and other mediators. Skin exposure causes contact urticaria. Exposure to latex in the air elicits allergic rhinitis, conjunctivitis, asthma, anaphylaxis, and death. Allergic patients are vulnerable in the hospital setting. Latex allergy can present as IgE-mediated anaphylaxis during surgery, barium enema, or dental work. Intraoperative anaphylaxis and death can occur as a result of mucosal latex absorption at the time of surgery or procedure because of exposure to the surgeon's latex gloves. Mucosal exposure can occur from airborne powder particles, used as dry lubricant on gloves. The powder acts as a carrier for the latex proteins in the air. These particles can be dispersed when removing gloves and cause aerosol contamination, resulting in asthma. Patients with Type I NRL allergy can have a cross-reaction to certain foods. Anaphylactic reactions (to banana, avocado, tomato, or kiwi) or local irritation when working with such foods have been reported.

DIAGNOSIS. Patients with a history of symptoms from rubber exposure can be screened with a RAST test to detect latex-specific IgE. If the RAST is positive, no further testing should be done. If negative (RASTs may have a false-negative rate of >30%), a "use" test utilizing a latex glove in a supervised setting may be performed, first with one finger, then an entire hand. If still negative, a skin-prick test should be done with eluted latex protein in solution. Anaphylactic reactions can occur with use and skin-prick tests, so life support equipment must be available.

TREATMENT. Nonlatex glove alternatives should be provided to health care workers who have type I reactions, and low-allergen, powder-free gloves should be worn by other health care workers at that worksite.

Vinyl gloves may leak and not provide an acceptable barrier for exposure to blood and bodily fluids. Double-gloving with vinyl gloves may provide greater protection during the performance of mucosal examinations (e.g., oral, rectal, vaginal). Thermoplastic elastomer gloves are more expensive but provide a barrier as effective as NRL gloves.

ALLERGIC CONTACT DERMATITIS

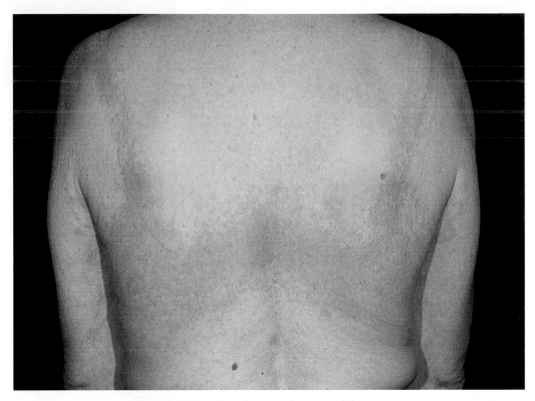

Figure 4-13 Spandex rubber in a bra caused this reaction.

Figure 4-14 Allergy to the rubber band of underwear. Washing clothes with bleach may make the rubber allergenic.

Shoe allergy

All patients with foot dermatitis that does not respond to treatment should be patch tested to exclude shoe allergy. Shoe allergy typically appears as subacute eczematous inflammation with redness and scaling over the dorsa of the feet, particularly the toes (Figures 4-15 and 4-16). The interdigital spaces are spared, in contrast to tinea pedis. Inflammation is usually bilateral, but unilateral involvement does not preclude the diagnosis of allergy. The thick skin of the soles is more resistant to allergens.

DIFFERENTIAL DIAGNOSIS. Fungal infections, psoriasis, and atopic dermatitis are common causes of inflammation of the feet. Shoe allergy should always be considered in the differential diagnosis of inflammation of the feet, particularly in children. Sweaty sock dermatitis, an irritant reaction in children caused by excessive perspiration, presents as diffuse dryness with fissuring on the toes, webs, and soles (see Figure 3-42). These irritated areas may become eczematous and appear as shoe contact dermatitis.

DIAGNOSIS. Patch testing is required to confirm the diagnosis of allergy. The standard patch test series can be used for screening. Special shoe patch testing trays are used by patch testing experts.[13] Pieces of the shoe that cover the inflamed site should also be used for the patch test (Figure 4-17).

1. Cut a 1-inch square piece of material from the shoe and round off the corners.
2. Seperate glued surfaces and patch test with all layers.
3. Moisten each layer with water, apply the samples to the upper outer arm, cover with tape, and proceed as described in the section on patch testing.

Rubber (e.g., mercaptobenzothiazole) is the most common allergen, followed by chromate, p-tertiary-butylphenol-formaldehyde resin, and colophony.[14] Mercaptobenzothiazole is a rubber component of adhesives used to cement shoe uppers, and potassium bichromate is a leather tanning agent. These chemicals are leached out by sweat.

MANAGEMENT. Patients with shoe allergy must control perspiration. Socks should be changed at least once each day. An absorbent powder such as Z-Sorb applied to the feet may be helpful. Aluminum chloride hexahydrate in a 20% solution (Drysol) applied at bedtime is a highly effective antiperspirant. Most vinyl shoes are acceptable substitutes for rubber-sensitive and chrome-sensitive patients. Inflammation of the soles may be prevented by inserting a barrier such as Dr. Scholl's Air Foam Pads or Johnson's Odor-Eaters. Once perspiration is controlled, it may be possible for sensitized patients to wear both leather shoes and shoes that contain rubber cement.

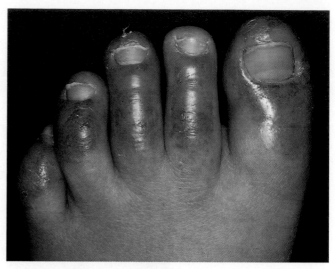

Figure 4-15 Shoe contact dermatitis. The toe webs are spared, in contrast to tinea pedis.

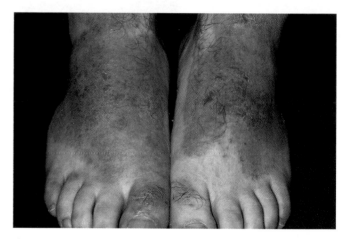

Figure 4-16 Shoe contact dermatitis. Sharply defined plaques formed under a shoe lining impregnated with rubber cement.

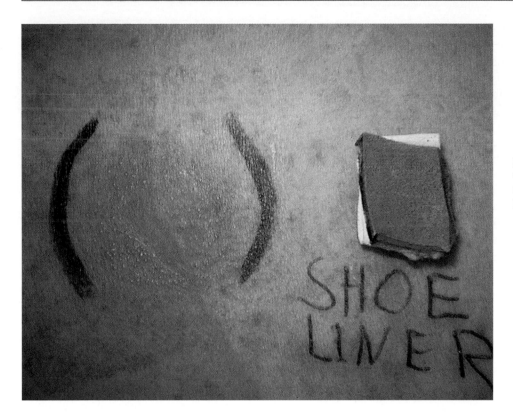

Figure 4-17 Patient in Figure 4-16 was patch tested with a piece of shoe lining. A 2+ positive allergic reaction occurred within 48 hours.

Metal dermatitis
Nickel

Sensitization to nickel is the leading cause of allergic contact dermatitis worldwide. Women are affected much more frequently than men; men are usually sensitized in an industrial setting. The most common symptom of nickel allergy is a history of reacting to jewelry or to other metal contact on the skin. Allergy to other metals found in jewelry (e.g., palladium, gold) may be the cause of jewelry dermatitis. Ear piercing and the wearing of cheap jewelry are the most common causes of nickel sensitization. Previous sites of inflammation are more reactive than normal skin to re-challenge with nickel.[15]

EARRINGS. Ear or body piercing or wearing clip-on earrings brings metal into direct contact with skin, an ideal setting for sensitization to occur (Figure 4-18). Ears should be pierced with stainless steel instruments, and stainless steel or plastic studs should be worn until complete epithelialization takes place. So-called hypoallergenic earrings may sensitize a person to a metal. Some nickel products that contain stainless steel may cause allergic contact dermatitis and others may not. Some gold earrings contain and release nickel. All-plastic earrings with fronts, posts, and backs made of hard nylon are now available.

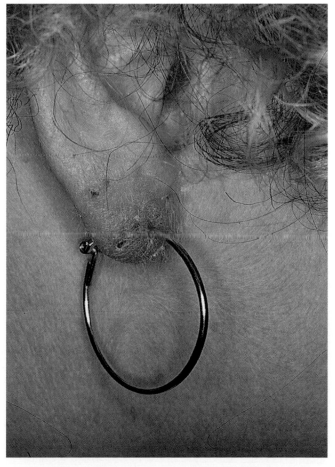

Figure 4-18 Nickel allergy. A classic presentation.

OTHER SOURCES OF NICKEL. Avoidance is the only way to prevent inflammation. Sources of contact are necklaces, metal in clothing, such as jean buttons and zippers, scissors, door handles, watchbands, bracelets, belt buckles (Figure 4-19), keys carried in pockets, hair and eyelash curlers, hooks, buttons, and coined money (common in cashiers).

Nickel-sensitive persons are not at greater risk of developing discomfort in the oral cavity when wearing an intraoral orthodontic appliance.[16] Modern plastic-to-metal joint replacements rarely cause sensitization to composite metals and are safe for nickel-sensitive patients.[17,18] Acrylic bone cement has never been implicated in causing dermatitis, although orthopedic surgeons have become sensitized to the methylmethacrylate monomer used in the cement. Surgical skin clips should not be used in nickel-sensitive patients.[19] Stainless steel pans are not a source of nickel ingestion.

DIMETHYLGLYOXIME SPOT TEST. The dimethylglyoxime spot test for nickel involves adding two solutions to a metal surface. If the solution turns pink, the test is positive. All nickel-sensitive patients should be taught how to use the dimethylglyoxime test (Chemotechnique Nickel Spot test, available from Dormer Laboratories, Inc., Toronto, Ontario, Canada). This enables them to determine which metallic objects they should avoid.

ORAL INGESTION OF NICKEL. Nickel is found in food and water. Some nickel-sensitive patients with periodic vesicular, palmar eczema (pompholyx) may benefit from a low-nickel diet (see Box 4-2).[20-23] Some cases of so-called endogenous pompholyx-like eruptions in nickel-sensitive persons may be the result of exogenous contact with nickel-plated objects.

Oral ingestion of nickel in a person previously sensitized by contact exposure to nickel may elicit an eczematous reaction and the affected sites usually correspond to those involved in prior contact dermatitis.

The term **"baboon syndrome"** or *intertriginous drug eruptions*[24] has been used to describe a symmetric eczematous eruption involving the elbows, axilla, eyelids, and sides of the neck accompanied by bright red ano-genital lesions. The term derives from the skin lesions, which are compared to the red gluteal region of the baboon. An allergic type IV reaction to systemically administered nickel or other allergens probably underlies lesions of this type.

PATCH TESTING. A positive history of allergic contact dermatitis but negative patch test results to nickel does not rule out nickel allergy. There is individual variation in nickel reactivity to patch testing. Some patients have a negative test reaction on one occasion and a positive test reaction at another time.[25] The shorter the time interval between the previous exposure and reexposure, the stronger the reaction.

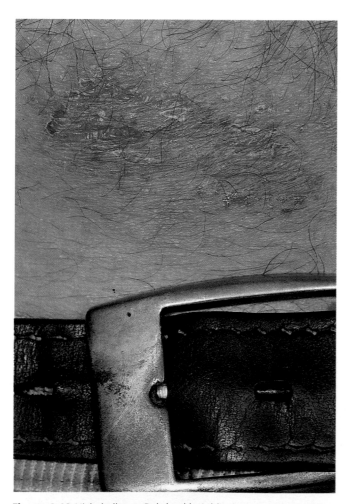

Figure 4-19 Nickel allergy. Belt buckle rubbed against abdomen when the patient bent over.

Box 4-2 Suggested Diet for Nickel-Sensitive Individuals with Pompholyx
Permitted foods: All meats, fish (except herring), poultry, eggs, milk, yogurt, butter, margarine, cheese, one medium-sized potato per day, small amounts of the following: cauliflower, cabbage, carrots, cucumber, lettuce, polished rice, flour (except whole grain), fresh fruits, except pears, marmalade/jam, coffee, wine, beer
Prohibited foods: Canned foods, foods cooked in nickel-plated utensils, herring, oysters, asparagus, beans, mushrooms, onions, corn (maize), spinach, tomatoes, peas, whole grain flour, fresh and cooked pears, rhubarb, tea, cocoa and chocolate, baking powder
Foods preferably should be cooked in aluminum or stainless steel utensils or in utensils that give a negative test for nickel with dimethylgloxime

Mercury dental amalgam

The mercury amalgam that dentists use to fill decayed teeth does not contain nickel. Allergy to mercury is very rare. Patch testing to mercury is unreliable and rarely done.[26,27] Gold alloyed with metal other than mercury is used for mercury-sensitive patients. Gold, however, is also a possible cause of allergic contact dermatitis.[28]

Chromates

Trivalent chromium (insoluble) and hexavalent chromium (soluble) compounds are sensitizers. Trivalent chromium is found in leather gloves and shoes. Hexavalent chromium is found in cement. Chromate is possibly the most common sensitizer for men in industrialized countries. Sources are cement, photographic processes, metal, and dyes. Cement is the most common cause of chromate allergy and it acts both as an irritant and a sensitizer.

Cement dermatitis and burns

Most cement workers experience dryness of the skin when first exposed, but most seem to adapt. Severe deep cutaneous alkali (pH 12) burns may occur on the lower legs of men whose skin is in direct contact with wet cement. Initial symptoms are burning and erythema; ulceration develops after 12 hours.[29] The most severe burns occur when cement spills over the boot top and is held next to the skin[30] (Figures 4-20 and 4-21). Chronic pain and scarring may follow severe burns.[31] Industrial workers sensitized to chromates in cement develop eczematous inflammation on the backs of the hands and forearms. The source of contact frequently is not appreciated until these patients do not respond to both topical and systemic steroids. Once the patient is removed from contact with cement, response to treatment is rapid.

Further examples of allergic contact dermatitis

Allergic contact dermatitis is further illustrated in Figures 4-22 through 4-24.

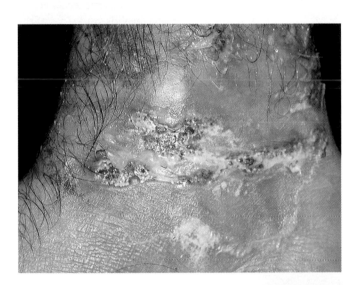

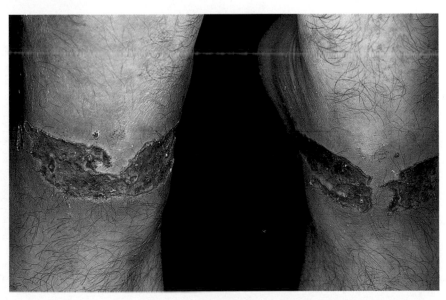

Figure 4-20 Severe irritant dermatitis from contact with wet cement.

Figure 4-21 Deep ulceration occurred after cement poured over the boot tops. This required months of treatment.

ALLERGIC CONTACT DERMATITIS

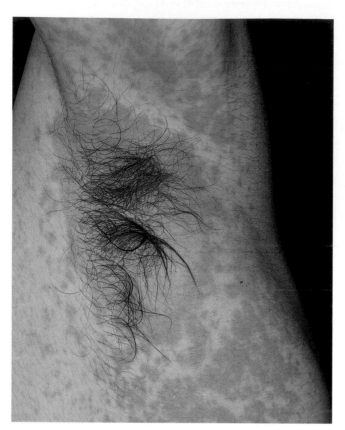

Figure 4-22 Allergic contact dermatitis to a spray deodorant.

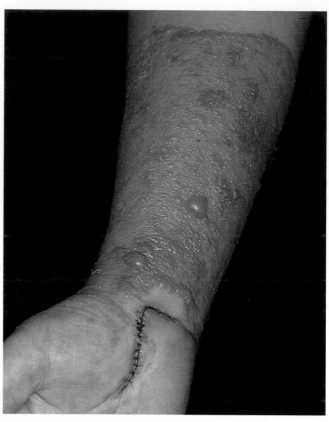

Figure 4-23 Allergic contact dermatitis to benzoin under a cast.

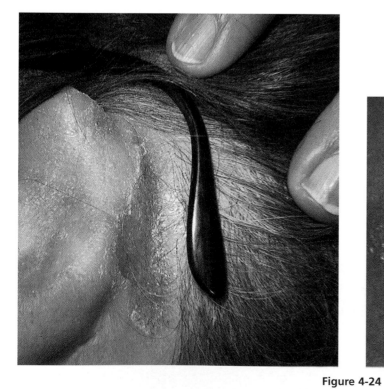

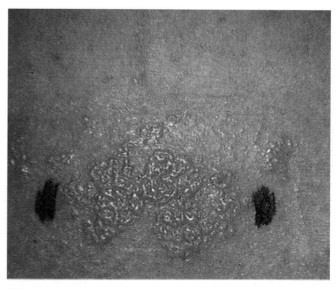

Figure 4-24

A, Allergic contact dermatitis to the plastic in a pair of glasses.

B, Patch testing with the plastic handle applied to the skin under tape for 2 days shows a 3+ positive reaction.

Patients with leg ulcers

Patients with leg ulcers, venous insufficiency, and lower leg edema may have an altered sensitivity to chemicals and are particularly susceptible to contact dermatitis of the lower legs. Topical medicines containing wool alcohols, lanolin, fragrance, parabens, and neomycin and bacitracin should be avoided.

Cosmetic and fragrance allergy

Cosmetics are frequently suspected of causing allergic reactions (Figure 4-25). Preservatives, fragrances, and emulsifiers are implicated. Patch testing can be done with suspected products. The Cosmetic, Toiletry, and Fragrance Association (www.ctfa.org) provides information on product formulation and ingredient characteristics of a wide range of products.

The most common cosmetic allergen is fragrance. Fragrances are ubiquitous and are used in a wide range of products other than cosmetics including perfumes, bath additives, deodorants, and household products. Allergy to the fragrance mix was found in 11.7% of patients who were patch tested by the North American Contact Dermatitis Group. Patch testing with balsam of Peru detects approximately 50% of patients with fragrance allergy. Most often when patients react to fragrance, the source of exposure is a skin or hair product with fragrance. Some so called "fragrance-free" products may contain fragrance chemicals.[32]

BALSAM OF PERU AVOIDANCE DIET. Allergy to fragrance can be associated with systemic contact dermatitis to certain ingested spices and foods and may account for some cases of stomatitis, cheilitis, generalized or resistant palmar dermatitis, and plantar or anogenital dermatitis. Persons allergic to balsam of Peru and/or fragrance mix benefit from dietary avoidance of balsams (see Box 4-3 on foods to avoid if allergic to balsam of Peru or fragrance mix). Patients most likely to benefit from a balsam-restricted diet included those with (1) a chronic dermatitis of at least 1 year's duration, which persists despite avoidance of cutaneous contact with known allergens; (2) a dermatitis that symmetrically involves the hands and/or feet, the anogenital area, and/or the skin folds; and (3) a positive patch test to balsam of Peru and/or fragrance mix. Place these patients on a balsam-restricted diet for at least 4 weeks and, if the dermatitis significantly improves, recommend long-term compliance. Subsequently, one food (e.g., tomatoes) can be reintroduced into the diet every several weeks to ascertain whether this particular substance exacerbated the dermatitis.[33]

TOPICAL GLUCOCORTICOSTEROIDS. The medication used to treat eczema can be the cause. Allergic reactions to glucocorticosteroids may occur, and patch testing is required to prove the diagnosis. Patients can cross-react to multiple steroid preparations (see Chapter 2).

Box 4-3 Balsam of Peru Diet (Foods to Avoid) for Selected Patients with Allergy to Balsam of Peru or Fragrance Mix

- Products that contain citrus fruits* (oranges, lemons, grapefruit, bitter oranges, tangerines, and mandarin oranges), for example, marmalade, juices, and bakery goods
- Flavoring agents such as those found in Danish pastries and other bakery goods, candy, and chewing gum
- Spices* such as cinnamon, cloves, vanilla, curry, allspice, anise, and ginger
- Spicy condiments such as ketchup, chili sauce, barbecue sauce, chutney and the like, and liver paste
- Pickles and pickled vegetables
- Wine, beer, gin, and vermouth
- Perfumed or flavored tea and tobacco, such as mentholated tobacco products
- Chocolate*
- Certain cough medicines and lozenges
- Ice cream
- Cola* and other spiced soft drinks such as Dr Pepper
- Chili*, pizza, Italian and Mexican foods with red sauces
- Tomatoes* and tomato-containing products

*Food items most commonly mentioned as causes of flare-up of dermatitis

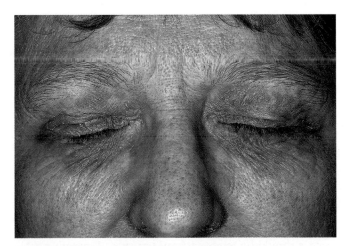

Figure 4-25 This patient bought many different products in an attempt to find something she could tolerate. Fragrance allergy was later proven by patch testing. Fragrance free cosmetics caused no inflammation.

Diagnosis of Contact Dermatitis

Determining the allergens responsible for allergic contact dermatitis requires a medical history, physical examination, and, in some instances, patch testing (see the diagram on p. 99). Historical points of interest are date of onset, relationship to work (i.e., improves during weekends or vacations), and types of products used in skin care. The number of different creams, lotions, cosmetics, and topical medications that patients can accumulate is amazing and persistent questioning may eventually uncover the responsible antigen.

Patch testing should not be attempted until the patient has had time to ponder the questions raised by the physician. In many cases all that is required is to avoid the suspected offending material.

Patch testing

Patch testing is indicated for cases in which inflammation persists despite avoidance of the offending agent and appropriate topical therapy. Patch testing is not useful as a diagnostic test for irritant contact dermatitis because irritant dermatitis is a nonimmunologically mediated inflammatory reaction. Not all positive patch test reactions are relevant to the patient's condition, and it is essential that the relevance of positive reactions be determined.

OPEN PATCH TEST. The suspected allergen is applied to the skin of the upper outer arm and left uncovered. Application is repeated twice daily for 2 days and as described next.

USE TEST. The suspected cream or cosmetic is used on a site distant from the original eruption. Suitable areas for testing are the outer arm or the skin of the antecubital fossa. The material is applied twice daily for at least 7 days. The test is stopped if a reaction occurs.

CLOSED PATCH TEST. The material is applied to the skin and covered with an adhesive bandage. The adhesive bandage is removed in 48 hours for initial interpretation (Figures 4-26, 4-27, and 4-28).

Solid objects such as shoe leather, wood, or rubber materials, or nonirritating material such as skin moisturizers, topical medicines, or cosmetics, are well suited to this technique.

Only bland material should be applied directly to the skin surface. Caustic industrial solvents must be diluted. Patch testing with a high concentration of caustic material may lead to skin necrosis. Petrolatum is generally the most suitable vehicle for dispersion of test materials. The concentration required to elicit a response varies with each chemical, and appropriate concentrations for testing can be found in standard textbooks dealing with contact dermatitis. If intense itching occurs, patches should be removed from test sites. A negative patch test with this direct technique does not rule out the diagnosis of allergy. The concentration of material tested may be too

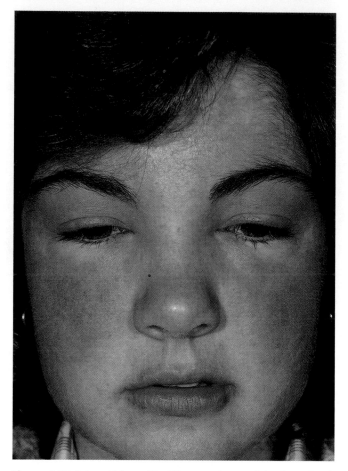

Figure 4-26 A beautician with diffuse erythema of the face. Patch testing showed a positive reaction (Figure 4-27).

weak to elicit a response, or one component of a topical medication (e.g., topical steroids) may suppress the allergic reaction induced by another component of the same cream.

If this technique fails or if the clinical presentation is that of allergic contact dermatitis but a source cannot be uncovered by the history and physical examination, then patch testing with the standard patch test series should be considered.

Patch test allergens

Testing with groups of allergens is generally performed by physicians who frequently see contact dermatitis and have experience with the problems involved in accurately determining the significance of test results. A group of chemicals that have proved to be frequent or important causes of allergic contact dermatitis have been assembled into standard patch test series. The T.R.U.E. TEST is a ready-to-use patch test for the diagnosis of allergic contact dermatitis. It contains

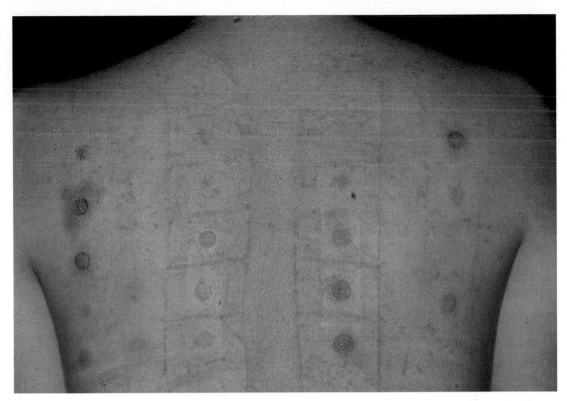

Figure 4-27 The patient in Figure 4-26 was patch tested with several of the preparations used at work. Many positive reactions of varying intensity appeared.

EVALUATION OF ALLERGIC CONTACT DERMAITIS

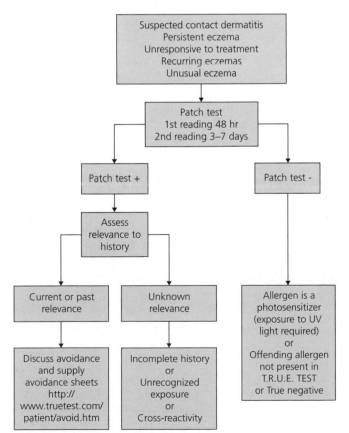

Suspected contact dermatitis
Persistent eczema
Unresponsive to treatment
Recurring eczemas
Unusual eczema

↓

Patch test
1st reading 48 hr
2nd reading 3–7 days

Patch test +

Patch test -

Assess relevance to history

Current or past relevance

Unknown relevance

Allergen is a photosensitizer (exposure to UV light required)
or
Offending allergen not present in T.R.U.E. TEST or True negative

Discuss avoidance and supply avoidance sheets http://www.truetest.com/patient/avoid.htm

Incomplete history
or
Unrecognized exposure
or
Cross-reactivity

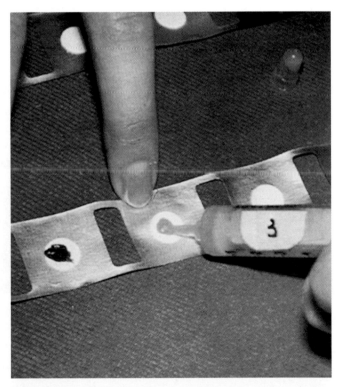

Figure 4-28 Patch testing. Individual allergens are tested on strips obtained from companies that sell individual allergens in syringes.

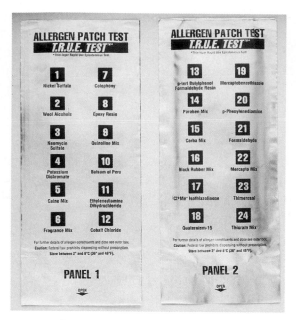

A, The two test panels are packaged in foil.

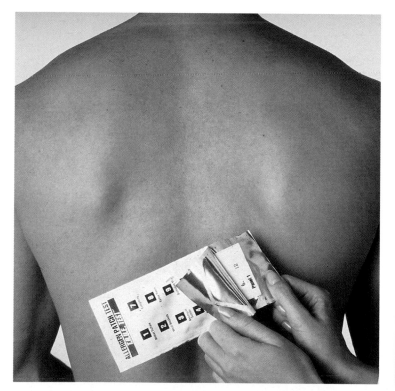

B, Each panel contains 12 allergens fixed to an adhesive tape.

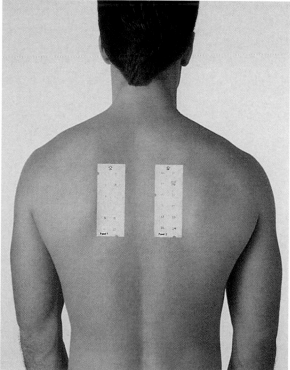

C, The tape is removed and applied to the back.

Figure 4-29

23 allergens and allergen mixes responsible for as much as 80% of allergic contact dermatitis (Table 4-4). Patch testing experts usually use more allergens beyond those available in this standard series. These additional allergens are available from sources outside the United States. Positive reactions to fragrance mix, balsam of Peru, and the rubber additives thiuram and carba mixes may be missed if the T.R.U.E. TEST is used alone.[34] TROLAB Herbal Patch Test Allergens from Europe are distributed in Canada and in many other countries. Search TROLAB on the web for details. They have a very large number of different allergens available. The North American Contact Dermatitis Group Tray contains about 50 antigens.[34]

TECHNIQUE FOR T.R.U.E. TEST. Each of the two T.R.U.E. TEST panels employs 12 standardized allergens or allergen mixes fixed in thin, dehydrated gel layers attached to a waterproof backing. Moisture from the skin after application causes the gels to be rehydrated and to release small amounts of allergen onto the patient's skin. After 48 hours, T.R.U.E. TEST is removed; reactions are then interpreted sometime between 4 and 7 days after application of the patches (Figure 4-29). The second reading is important for elderly patients, who mount an allergic reaction more slowly than younger patients. More than half of the reactions to neomycin are not evident until 96 hours after application of the patch test.

Table 4-4 T.R.U.E. TEST Allergen Patch Test of 23 Allergens (Reference Manual and Allergen Avoidance Sheets are Online at http://www.truetest.com)

Component	Occurrence	Reaction frequency (%)*
1. Nickel sulfate	Jewelry, metal, and metal-plated objects	14.2
2. Wool alcohols	Cosmetics and topical medications	3.3
3. Neomycin sulfate	Topical antibiotics	13.1
4. Potassium dichromate	Cutting oils, antirust paints	2.8
5. Caine mix	Topical anesthetics	2.0
6. Fragrance mix	Fragrances, toiletries, scented household products, flavorings	11.7
7. Colophony	Cosmetics, adhesives, industrial products	2.0
8. Paraben mix	Preservative in topical formulations, industrial preparations	1.7
9. Negative control		
10. Balsam of Peru	Fragrances, flavorings, cosmetics	11.8
11. Ethylenediamine dihydrochloride	Topical medications, eye drops, industrial solvents, anticorrosive agents	2.6
12. Cobalt dichloride	Metal-plated objects, paints, cement, metal	9.0
13. p-tert Butylphenol formaldehyde resin	Waterproof glues, leather, construction materials, paper, fabrics	1.8
14. Epoxy resin	Two-part adhesives, surface coatings, paints	1.9
15. Carba mix	Rubber products, glues for leather, pesticides, vinyl	7.3
16. Black rubber mix	All black rubber products, some hair dye	1.5
17. Cl +Me- Isothiazolinone	Cosmetics and skin care products, topical medications, household cleaning products	2.9
18. Quaternium-15	Preservative in cosmetics and skin care products, household polishes and cleaners, industrial products	9.0
19. Mercaptobenzothiazole	Rubber products, adhesives, industrial products	1.8
20. p-Phenylenediamine (PPD)	Dyed textiles, cosmetics, hair dyes, printing ink, photodeveloper	6.0
21. Formaldehyde	Plastics, synthetic resins, glues, textiles, construction material	9.3
22. Mercapto mix	Rubber products, glues for leather and plastics, industrial products	1.8
23. Thimerosal	Preservative in contact lens solutions, cosmetics, nose and ear drops, injectable drugs	10.9
24. Thiuram mix	Rubber products, adhesives, pesticides, drugs	6.9

North American Contact Dermatitis Group Patch Test Results, 1996-1998 (Arch Dermatol 2000; 136:272-274.)
* These results were obtained with another path testing system used by the North American Patch Test Group.

Figure 4-30 A 1+ positive patch test reaction with erythema.

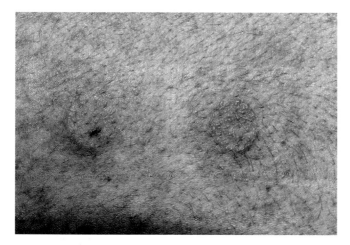

Figure 4-31 A 2+ positive patch test reaction with erythema and vesicles.

Figure 4-32 A 3+ positive patch test reaction with vesicles and bullae.

PATCH TEST READING AND INTERPRETATION. The test reactions are graded at each reading as follows:

+ = Weak (nonvesicular) positive reaction: erythema, infiltration, and possibly papules (Figure 4-30)

++ = Strong (edematous or vesicular) positive reaction (Figure 4-31)

+++ = Extreme (spreading, bullous, ulcerative) positive reaction (Figure 4-32)

− = Negative reaction

IR = Irritant reactions of different types

NT = Not tested

Doubtful reaction (macular erythema only)

Allergic versus irritant test reactions

It is important to determine whether the test response is caused by allergy or by a nonspecific irritant reaction. Strong allergic reactions are vesicular and may spread beyond the test site. Strong irritant reactions exhibit a deep erythema, resembling a burn. There is no morphologic method of distinguishing a weak irritant patch test from a weak allergic test. Commercially prepared antigens are formulated to minimize irritant reactions. Irritant test responses are caused by either hyperirritability of the skin or by the application of an irritating concentration of a test substance. Irritation is avoided by applying tests only on normal skin that has not been washed or cleaned with alcohol.

WHEN NOT TO PERFORM PATCH TESTING. Avoid testing in the presence of an active, flaring dermatitis that covers more than 25% of the body surface area. Under these conditions, the "angry back reaction" with numerous false-positive tests frequently occurs. Defer testing until 1 or 2 weeks following treatments known to interfere with delayed-type hypersensitivity reactions such as systemic corticosteroids, immunosuppressants (cyclophosphamide, azathioprine, etc.), and ultraviolet B or PUVA phototherapy.[5]

STEROIDS AND PATCH TESTING. Corticosteroids such as prednisone in dosages of 15 mg/day or the equivalent may inhibit patch test reactions. If a patient has been treated with systemic corticosteroids, patch testing should be delayed for at least 2 weeks. The prior application of the group V topical steroid triamcinolone acetonide to skin does not strongly influence patch test reactions.[35] If topical corticosteroids are being used on the back, patch testing should be delayed for 3 days. Allergic contact dermatitis to topical corticosteroids is possible (see Chapter 2).

THE EXCITED SKIN SYNDROME (ANGRY BACK). "Eczema creates eczema." The excited skin syndrome is a major cause of false-positive patch test reactions. Single or multiple concomitant positive patch test reactions may produce a state of skin hyperreactivity in which other patch test sites, particularly those with minimal irritation, may become reactive. Patients who have multiple strong test reactions should be retested at a later date with one antigen at a time (Figure

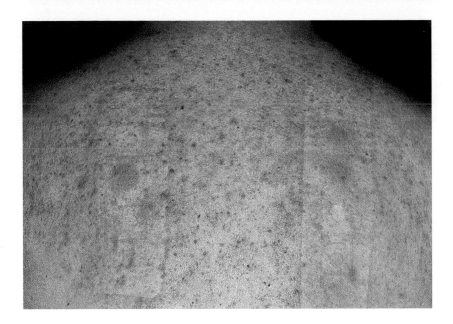

Figure 4-33 The excited skin syndrome. Several tests have become positive, and the severe reactions have stimulated inflammation over the entire back.

4-33). Retesting may show that some of the original tests were false positives. The excited skin syndrome may also be caused by even minimal dermatitis elsewhere.

RELEVANCE OF TEST RESULTS AND MANAGEMENT. A number of possible conclusions may be drawn from the test results:

- The allergen eliciting the positive test is directly responsible for the patient's dermatitis.
- A chemically related or cross-reacting material is responsible for the dermatitis.
- The patient has not recently been in contact with the indicated allergen and, although he or she is allergic to that specific chemical, it is not relevant to the present condition.
- The test is negative but would be positive if a sufficient concentration of the test chemical were used.
- The positive test is an irritant reaction and is irrelevant.

In studies done from 1992 through 1996, fragrance mix, quaternium-15, balsam of Peru, formaldehyde, thiuram mix, nickel sulfate, neomycin, bacitracin, carba mix, and paraphenylenediamine were the 10 leading allergens in clinical importance. Ethylenediamine and benzocaine have markedly decreased in clinical importance. Methylchloroisothiazolinone/methylisothiazolinone has become a leading allergen. A number of important allergens are not included in the T.R.U.E. test, including bacitracin, diazolidinyl urea, glyceryl thioglycate, ethyleneurea melamine-formaldehyde, and imidazolidinyl urea.[36] Consider referral to contact dermatitis experts for further patch testing if T.R.U.E test does not provide relevant information.

Contact allergen alternatives

Review where the allergen is found (including foods), and discuss safe replacements with the patient. Identify potential cross-reacting substances. A list of safe and practical alternatives to common allergens has been published in the Journal of the American Academy of Dermatology.[21] Also visit www.truetest.com.

NEGATIVE TESTS. A number of possibilities exist for a negative test: the eczema may be nonallergic, the responsible chemical may not have been tested, or the result may be a false-negative. Also, a second reading of the test sites after the initial inspection at 48 hours may not have been made. False-negative tests can occur when the concentration of the test allergens is too low to elicit a reaction. Photopatch testing is necessary when the allergen requires photoactivation, as in photoallergic contact dermatitis caused by the sunscreen oxybenzone.

References

1. Weston W, Bruckner A: Allergic contact dermatitis, Pediatr Clin North Am 2000; 47(4): 897.
2. Marks JG Jr et al: Dermatitis from cashew nuts, J Am Acad Dermatol 1984; 10:627.
3. McGovern T: Botanical briefs: the cashew tree—Anacardium occidentale [In Process Citation], Cutis 2001; 68(5):321.
4. Salam T, Fowler J: Balsam-related systemic contact dermatitis, J Am Acad Dermatol 2001; 45(3):377
5. Belsito D: A sherlockian approach to contact dermatitis, Dermatol Clin 1999;17(3): 705.
6. Belsito D, et al: Allergic contact dermatitis to detergents: a multicenter study to assess prevalence, J Am Acad Dermatol 2002; 46(2):200.
7. Moe J: How much steroid for poison ivy? Postgrad Med 1999; 106(4):21.
8. Warshaw E: Latex allergy, J Am Acad Dermatol 1998; 39(1):1; quiz 25.
9. Cohen D, et al: American Academy of Dermatology's position paper on latex allergy, J Am Acad Dermatol 1998; 39(1):98.

10. Fisher AA: Contact dermatitis in surgeons, J Dermatol Surg Oncol 1975; 13:63.

11. Lagier F, et al: Prevalence of latex allergy in operating room nurses, J Allergy Clin Immunol 1992; 90:319.

12. Heese A, et al: Allergic and irritant reactions to rubber gloves in medical health services. Spectrum, diagnostic approach, and therapy, J Am Acad Dermatol 1991; 25(5 Pt 1):831.

13. Van CA, et al: Contact allergens in shoe leather among patients with foot eczema [In Process Citation], Contact Dermatitis 2002; 46(3): 145.

14. Freeman S: Shoe dermatitis, Contact Dermatitis 1997; 36(5): 247.

15. Hindsen M, Bruze M: The significance of previous contact dermatitis for elicitation of contact allergy to nickel, Acta Derm Venereol 1998; 78(5):367.

16. Staerkjaer L, Menne T: Nickel allergy and orthodontic treatment. Eur J Orthod 1990; 12:284.

17. Fisher AA: The safety of artificial hip replacement in nickel-sensitive patients, Cutis 1986; May:333.

18. Gawkrodger DJ: Nickel sensitivity and the implantation of orthopaedic prostheses, Contact Dermatitis 1993; 28:257.

19. Oakley AMM, Ive FA, Carr MM: Skin clips are contraindicated when there is nickel allergy, J R Soc Med 1987; 80:290.

20. Nielsen GD, et al: Nickel-sensitive patients with vesicular hand eczema: oral challenge with a diet naturally high in nickel, Br J Dermatol 1990; 122:299.

21. Adams RM, Fisher AA: Contact allergen alternatives: 1986, J Am Acad Dermatol 1986; 14:951.

22. Veien NK, et al: Low nickel diet: an open, prospective trial, J Am Acad Dermatol 1993; 29:1002.

23. Moller H: Yes, systemic nickel is probably important, J Am Acad Dermatol 1993; 28:511.

24. Le CC, et al: An unusual case of mercurial baboon syndrome, Contact Dermatitis 1996; 35(2):112.

25. Hindsen M, Bruze M, Christensen O: Individual variation in nickel patch test reactivity, Am J Contact Dermat 1999; 10(2):62.

26. Fisher AA: The misuse of the patch test to determine "hypersensitivity" to mercury amalgam dental fillings, Cutis 1985; 35:112.

27. Mackert JR, Jr: Hypersensitivity to mercury from dental amalgams, J Am Acad Dermatol 1985; 12:877.

28. Laeijendecker R, J Van T: Oral manifestations of gold allergy, J Am Acad Dermatol 1994; 30:205.

29. Robinson SM, Tachakra SS: Skin ulceration due to cement, Arch Emerg Med 1992; 9:326.

30. Peters WJ: Alkali burns from wet cement, Can Med Assoc J 1984; 130:902.

31. Lane PR, Hogan DJ: Chronic pain and scarring from cement burns, Arch Dermatol 1985; 121:368.

32. Scheinman P: The foul side of fragrance-free products, J Am Acad Dermatol 2000; 42(6):1087.

33. Belsito D: Surviving on a balsam-restricted diet: cruel and unusual punishment or medically necessary therapy? J Am Acad Dermatol 2001; 45(3):470.

34. Marks J, et al: North American Contact Dermatitis Group patch-test results, 1996-1998, Arch Dermatol 2000; 136(2):272.

35. Dahl MV, Jordan, WP, Jr: Topical steroids and patch tests, Arch Dermatol 1983; 119:3.

36. Maouad M, et al: Significance-prevalence index number: a reinterpretation and enhancement of data from the North American contact dermatitis group, J Am Acad Dermatol 1999; 41(4):573.

Atopic Dermatitis

❑ **Pathogenesis and immunology**

❑ **Clinical aspects**
Infant phase (birth to 2 years)
Childhood phase (2 to 12 years)
Adult phase (12 years to adult)

❑ **Associated features**
Dry skin and xerosis
Ichthyosis vulgaris
Keratosis pilaris
Hyperlinear palmar creases
Pityriasis alba
Atopic pleats
Cataracts and keratoconus

❑ **Triggering factors**
Temperature change and sweating
Decreased humidity
Excessive washing
Contact with irritating substances
Contact allergy
Aeroallergens
Microbic agents
Food
Emotional stress

❑ **Treatment**
Dry skin
Inflammation and infection
Infants
Children and adults
Tar
Hospitalization for severely resistant cases
Lubrication
Sedation and antihistamines
Phototherapy
Diet restriction and breast-feeding

The term *atopy* was introduced years ago to designate a group of patients who had a personal or family history of one or more of the following diseases: hay fever, asthma, very dry skin, and eczema.

Atopic dermatitis (AD) is a chronic, pruritic eczematous disease that nearly always begins in childhood and follows a remitting/flaring course that may continue throughout life. It develops as a result of a complex interrelationship of environmental, immunologic, genetic, and pharmacologic factors. It may be exacerbated by infection, psychologic stress, seasonal/climate changes, irritants, and allergens. The disease often moderates with age, but patients carry a life-long skin sensitivity to irritants, and this atopy predisposes them to occupational skin disease.[1]

The disease characteristics vary with age. Infants have facial and patchy or generalized body eczema. Adolescents and adults have eczema in flexural areas and on the hands. The pattern of inheritance is unknown, but available data suggest that it is polygenic.

DIAGNOSTIC CRITERIA. There are no specific cutaneous signs, no known distinctive histologic features, and no characteristic laboratory findings for atopic dermatitis. There are a variety of characteristics that indicate that the patient has atopic dermatitis (see Box 5-1). The diagnosis is made when the patient has three or more of the major features and three or more of the minor features. Each patient is different, with a unique combination of major and minor features.

PREVALENCE. The prevalence in children is 7% to 17.2%.[2] The prevalence of AD in schoolchildren has increased greatly since the early 1960s.

Genetic factors cannot explain the rapid change in prevalence. Changes in environmental factors and lifestyle, as well as increased recognition of the disease by doctors and families, are contributory factors. Some events in childhood may be of importance (e.g., early infections, early allergen exposure, and early diet).

COURSE AND PROGNOSIS. Factors associated with a low frequency of healing and increased severity of persistent or recurring dermatitis are listed in order of relative importance in Box 5-2.[3] More than 50% of young children with generalized AD develop asthma and allergic rhinitis by the age of 13. Dermatitis improves in most children.[4]

Seventy percent of atopic patients have a family history of one or more of the major atopic characteristics: asthma, hay fever, or eczematous dermatitis.

Box 5-1 Criteria for Diagnoses of Atopic Dermatitis

Major Features (Must Have Three or More)

Pruritus

Typical morphology and distribution

Flexural lichenification in adults

Facial and extensor involvement in infants and children

Dermatitis—chronically or chronically relapsing

Personal or family history or atopy—asthma, allergic rhinitis, atopic dermatitis

Minor Features (Must Have Three or More)

Cataracts (anterior-subcapsular)

Cheilitis

Conjunctivitis—recurrent

Eczema—perifollicular accentuation

Facial pallor/facial erythema

Food intolerance

Hand dermatitis—nonallergic, irritant

Ichthyosis

IgE—elevated

Immediate (Type 1) skin test reactivity

Infections (cutaneous)—*Staphylococcus aureus,* herpes simplex

Infraorbital fold (Dennie-Morgan lines)

Itching when sweating

Keratoconus

Keratosis pilaris

Nipple dermatitis

Orbital darkening

Palmar hyperlinearity

Pityriasis alba

White dermographism

Wool intolerance

Xerosis

Data from Roth HL: Int J Dermatol 1987; 26:139; Hanifin JM, Rajka G: Acta Derm Venereol (Stockh) 1980; 92(suppl):44; and Hanifin JM, Lobitz WC Jr: Arch Dermatol 1977; 113:663.

Box 5-2 Atopic Dermatitis: Unfavorable Prognostic Factors*

Persistent dry or itchy skin in adult life

Widespread dermatitis in childhood

Associated allergic rhinitis

Family history of atopic dermatitis

Associated bronchial asthma

Early age at onset

Female sex

Data from Rystedt I: Acta Derm Venereol (Stockh) 1985; 65:206.
*In order of relative importance.

Pathogenesis and Immunology

ELEVATED IgE AND THE INFLAMMATORY RESPONSE. The role of IgE in AD is unknown. IgE is increased in the serum of many patients with AD, but 20% of AD patients have normal serum IgE and no allergen reactivity. The levels of IgE do not necessarily correlate with the activity of the disease; therefore elevated serum IgE levels can only be considered supporting evidence for the disease.[5] Total IgE is significantly higher in children with coexistent atopic respiratory disease in all age groups. Most persons with AD have a personal or family history of allergic rhinitis or asthma and increased serum IgE antibodies against airborne or ingested protein antigens. AD usually diminishes during the spring hay fever season, when aeroallergens are at maximum concentrations.

BLOOD EOSINOPHILIA. Eosinophils may be major effector cells in AD. Blood eosinophil counts roughly correlated with disease severity, although many patients with severe disease show normal peripheral blood eosinophil counts. Patients with normal eosinophil counts mainly are those with atopic dermatitis alone; patients with severe atopic dermatitis and concomitant respiratory allergies commonly have increased peripheral blood eosinophils. There is no accumulation of tissue eosinophils; however, degranulation of eosinophils in the dermis releases major basic protein that may induce histamine release from basophils and mast cells and stimulate itching, irritation, and lichenification.[6]

REDUCED CELL-MEDIATED IMMUNITY. Several facts suggest that AD patients have disordered cell-mediated immunity. Patients may develop severe diffuse cutaneous infection with the herpes simplex virus (eczema herpeticum) whether or not their dermatitis is active. Mothers with active herpes labialis should avoid direct contact of their active lesion with their children's skin, as in kissing, especially if the child has dermatitis. The incidence of contact allergy (e.g., reduced sensitivity to poison ivy) may be lower than normal in atopic patients;[7] however, some studies show equal rates of sensitization.[8,9] Humoral immunity seems to be normal.

MISCONCEPTIONS. There are two common misconceptions about AD. The first is that it is an emotional disorder. It is true that patients with inflammation that lasts for months or years seem to be irritable, but this is a normal response to a frustrating disease. The second misconception is that atopic skin disease is precipitated by an allergic reaction. Atopic individuals frequently have respiratory allergies and, when skin tested, are informed that they are allergic to "everything." Atopic patients may react with a wheal when challenged with a needle during skin testing, but this is a characteristic of atopic skin and is not necessarily a manifestation of allergy. All evidence to date shows that most cases of AD are precipitated by environmental stress on genetically compromised skin and not by interaction with allergens.

AEROALLERGENS. Aeroallergens may play an important role in causing eczematous lesions. Patch testing rates of reactions are: house dust (70%), mites (70%), cockroaches (63%), mold mix (50%), and grass mix (43%). Patients with AD frequently show positive scratch and intradermal reactions to a number of antigens; avoidance of these antigens rarely improves the dermatitis.

Clinical Aspects

MAJOR AND MINOR DIAGNOSTIC FEATURES. Box 5-1 on the criteria for diagnosing AD lists the major and minor[10] diagnostic features for atopic dermatitis and atopy. Each patient has his or her own unique set of features, and there is no precise clinical or laboratory marker for this genetic disease.[11]

ITCHING, THE PRIMARY LESION. "It is not the eruption that is itchy but the itchiness that is eruptive." Atopic dermatitis starts with itching. Abnormally dry skin and a lowered threshold for itching are important features of AD. It is the scratching that creates most of the characteristic patterns of the disease. Most patients with AD make a determined effort to control their scratching, but during sleep conscious control is lost; under warm covers the patient scratches and a rash appears. The itch-scratch cycle is established, and conscious effort is no longer sufficient to control scratching. The act of scratching becomes habitual, and the disease progresses. Atopic skin is associated with a lowered threshold of responsiveness to irritants.

PATTERNS OF INFLAMMATION. Several patterns and types of lesions may be produced by exposure to external stimuli or may be precipitated by scratching. Acute inflammation begins with erythematous papules and erythema. These are associated with excoriations, erosions, and serous exudate. Subacute dermatitis is associated with erythematous, excoriated, scaling papules. Chronic dermatitis is the result of scratching over an extended period. There are thickened skin, accentuated skin markings (lichenification), and fibrotic papules. Inflammation resolves slowly, leaving the skin in a dry, scaly, compromised condition called *xerosis*. There is no single primary lesion in AD. All three types of reactions can coexist in the same individual. These types of lesions are papules (Figure 5-1), eczematous dermatitis with redness and scaling (Figure 5-2), and lichenification (Figure 5-3). Lichenification represents a thickening of the epidermis. It is a highly characteristic lesion, with the normal skin lines accentuated to resemble a washboard. These responses are altered by excoriation and infection.

Although the cutaneous manifestations of the atopic diathesis are varied, they have characteristic age-determined patterns. Knowledge of these patterns is useful; many patients, however, have a nonclassic pattern. AD may terminate after an indefinite period or may progress from infancy to adulthood with little or no relief; 58% of infants with AD were found to have persistent inflammation 15 to 17 years later.[12] AD is arbitrarily divided into three phases.

ATOPIC DERMATITIS—PATTERNS OF INFLAMMATION

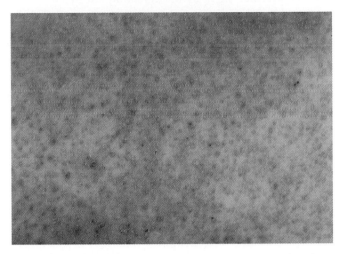

Figure 5-1 Papular lesions are common in the antecubital and popliteal fossae. Papules become confluent and form plaques.

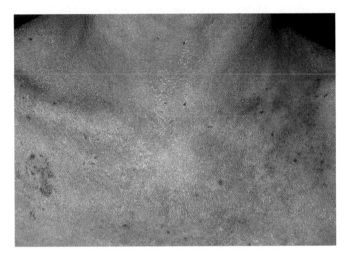

Figure 5-2 Eczematous dermatitis with diffuse erythema and scaling on the neck and chest.

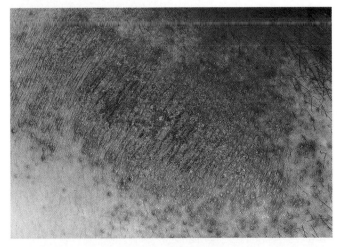

Figure 5-3 Lichenification with accentuation of normal skin lines. This lichenified plaque is surrounded by papules.

Infant phase (birth to 2 years)

Infants are rarely born with atopic eczema, but they typically develop the first signs of inflammation during the third month of life. The most common occurrence is that of a baby who during the winter months develops dry, red, scaling areas confined to the cheeks, but sparing the perioral and paranasal areas (Figures 5-4 and 5-5). This is the same area that becomes flushed with exposure to cold. The chin is often involved and initially may be more inflamed than the cheeks because of the irritation of drooling and subsequent repeated washing. Inflammation may spread to involve the paranasal and perioral area as the winter progresses (Figure 5-6). Habitual lip licking by an atopic child results in oozing, crusting, and scaling on the lips and perioral skin (Figure 5-7).

Many infants do not excoriate during these early stages, and the rash remains localized and chronic. Repeated scratching or washing creates red, scaling, oozing plaques on the cheeks, a classic presentation of infantile eczema. At this stage the infant is uncomfortable and becomes restless and agitated during sleep.

A small but significant number of infants have a generalized eruption consisting of papules, redness, scaling, and areas of lichenification. The scalp may be involved, and differentiation from seborrheic dermatitis is sometimes difficult

(Figure 5-8). The diaper area is often spared (Figure 5-9). Lichenification may occur in the fossae and crease areas, or it may be confined to a favorite, easily reached spot, such as directly below the diaper, the back of the hand, or the extensor forearm (Figures 5-9 through 5-11). Prolonged AD with increasing discomfort disturbs sleep, and both the parents and the child are distraught.

For years, foods have been suspected as etiologic factors.[13] Food testing and breast-feeding are discussed at the end of this chapter. The course of the disease may be influenced by events such as teething, respiratory infections, and adverse emotional stimuli. The disease is chronic, with periods of exacerbation and remission, and resolves in approximately 50% of infants by 18 months; other cases progress to the childhood phase, and a different pattern evolves.

GROWTH IN ATOPIC ECZEMA. Height is significantly correlated with the surface area of skin affected by eczema. The growth of children with eczema affecting less than 50% of the skin surface area appears to be normal, and impaired growth is confined to those with more extensive disease. Treatment with topical steroids has only marginal additional effect on impaired growth.[14]

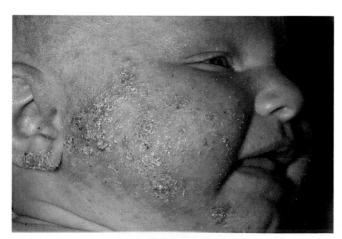

Figure 5-4 Red scaling plaques confined to the cheeks are one of the first signs of atopic dermatitis in an infant.

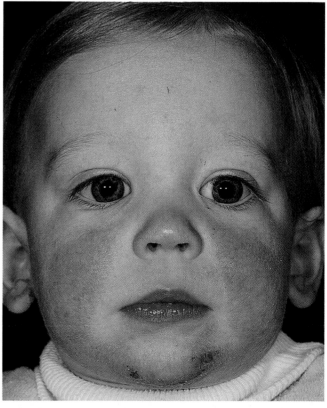

Figure 5-5 Atopic dermatitis. A common appearance in children with erythema and scaling confined to the cheeks and sparing the perioral and paranasal area.

ATOPIC DERMATITIS

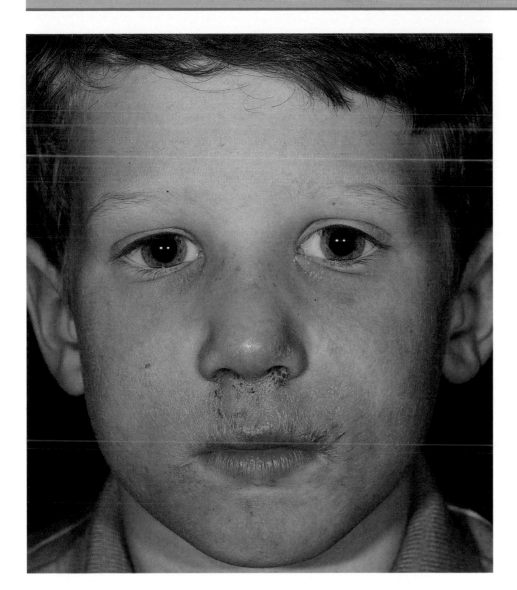

Figure 5-6 Atopic dermatitis. Progression of inflammation to involve the perioral and paranasal areas.

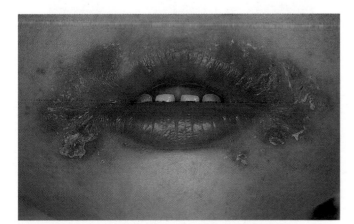

Figure 5-7 Habitual lip licking in an atopic child produces erythema and scaling that may eventually lead to secondary infection.

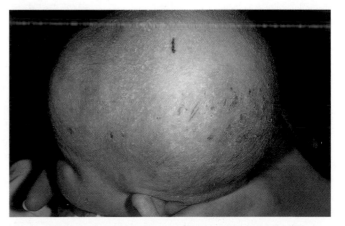

Figure 5-8 Diffuse superficial erythema and scale of the scalp respond rapidly to group VI topical steroids. Hydrocortisone 1% may not be strong enough to control the inflammation.

ATOPIC DERMATITIS

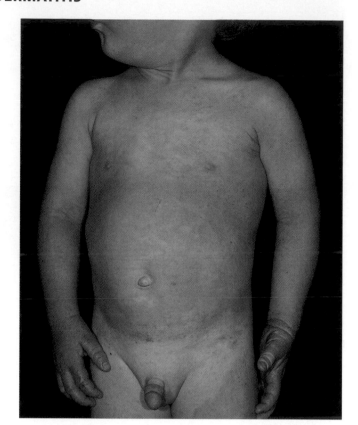

Figure 5-9 Generalized infantile atopic dermatitis sparing the diaper area, which is protected from scratching.

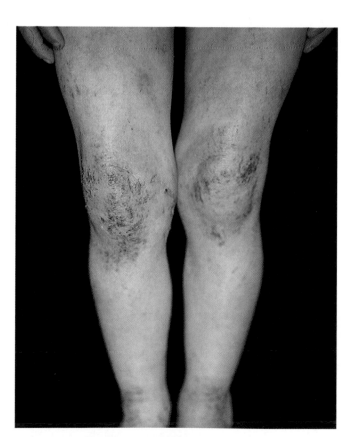

Figure 5-10 Inflammation in the flexural areas is the most common presentation of atopic dermatitis in children.

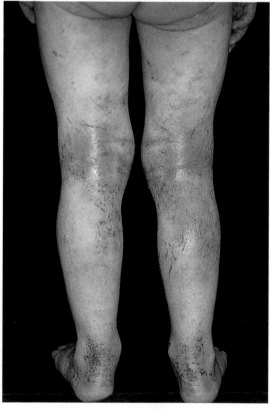

Figure 5-11 Rubbing and scratching the inflamed flexural areas causes thickened (lichenified) skin. These lesions form fissures and are infected with *Staphylococcus aureus*.

Childhood phase (2 to 12 years)

The most common and characteristic appearance of AD is inflammation in flexural areas (i.e., the antecubital fossae, neck, wrists, and ankles [Figures 5-12 through 5-15]). These areas of repeated flexion and extension perspire with exertion. The act of perspiring stimulates burning and intense itching and initiates the itch-scratch cycle. Tight clothing that traps heat about the neck or extremities further aggravates the problem. Inflammation typically begins in one of the fossae or about the neck. The rash may remain localized to one or two areas or progress to involve the neck, antecubital and popliteal fossae, wrists, and ankles. The eruption begins with papules that rapidly coalesce into plaques, which become lichenified when scratched. The plaques may be pale and mildly inflamed with little tendency to change (see Figure 5-13); if they have been vigorously scratched, they may be bright red and scaling with erosions. The border may be sharp and well defined, as it is in psoriasis (Figure 5-15), or poorly defined with papules extraneous to the lichenified areas. A few patients do not develop lichenification even with repeated scratching. The exudative lesions typical of the infant phase are not as common. Most patients with chronic lesions tolerate their disease and sleep well.

Figure 5-12 Atopic dermatitis. Classic appearance of confluent papules forming plaques in the antecubital fossae.

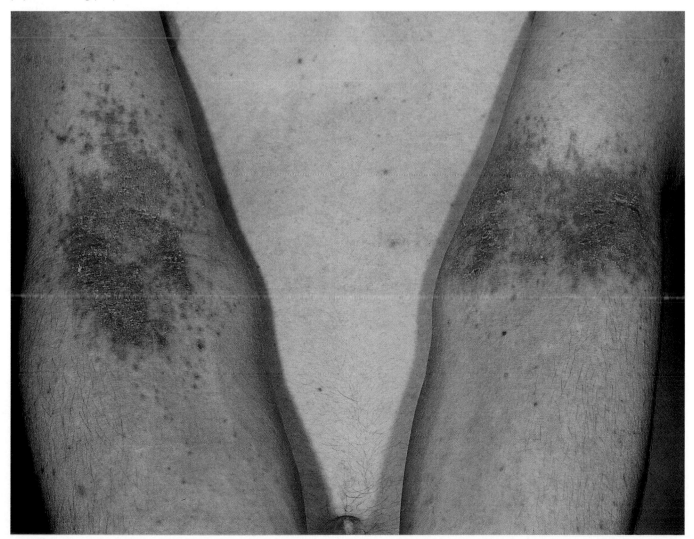

ATOPIC DERMATITIS

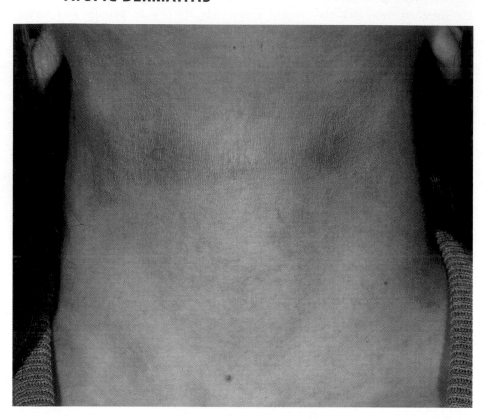

Figure 5-13 Atopic dermatitis. Classic appearance of erythema and diffuse scaling about the neck.

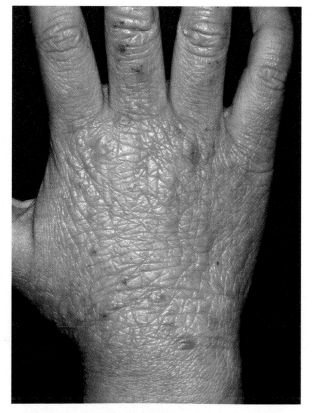

Figure 5-14 Atopic dermatitis. A chronically inflamed lichenified plaque on the wrist and back of hand.

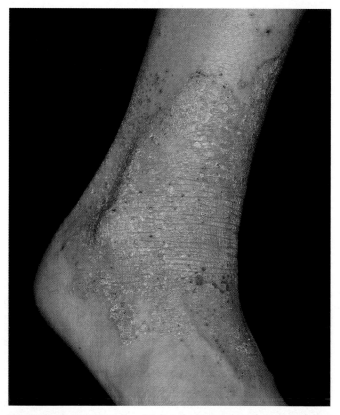

Figure 5-15 Sharply defined lichenified plaque with a silvery scale showing some of the features of psoriasis. Erosions are present.

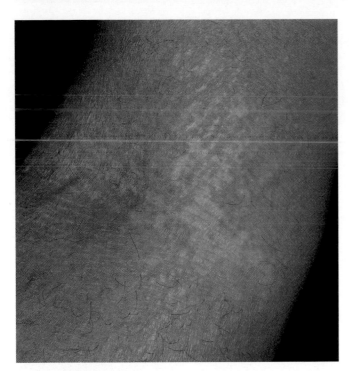

Figure 5-16 Hypopigmentation in the antecubital fossae caused by destruction of melanocytes by chronic scratching.

Constant scratching may lead to destruction of melanocytes, resulting in areas of hypopigmentation that become more obvious when the inflammation subsides. These hypopigmented areas fade with time (Figure 5-16). Additional exacerbating factors such as heat, cold, dry air, or emotional stress may lead to extension of inflammation beyond the confines of the crease areas (Figures 5-17 and 5-18). The inflammation becomes incapacitating. Normal duration of sleep cannot be maintained, and school, work, or job performance deteriorates; these people are miserable. They discover that standing in a hot shower gives considerable temporary relief, but further progression is inevitable with the drying effect produced by repeated wetting and drying. In the more advanced cases, hospitalization is required. Most patients with this pattern of inflammation are in remission by age 30, but in a few patients the disease becomes chronic or improves only to relapse during a change of season or at some other period of transition. Then dermatitis becomes a lifelong ordeal.

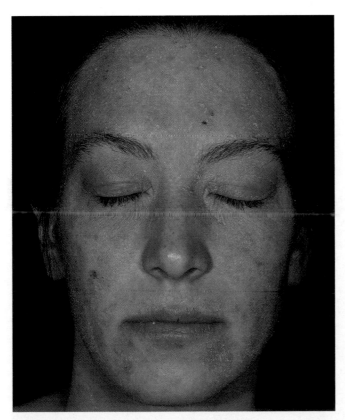

Figure 5-17 Generalized atopic dermatitis. Diffuse erythema and scaling are present.

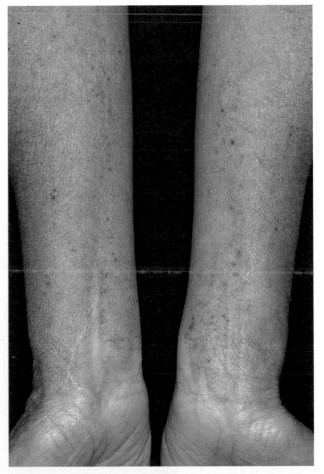

Figure 5-18 The dermatitis has generalized to involve the entire body. Secondary skin infection with *Staphylococcus aureus* is almost always present with this degree of inflammation.

Adult phase (12 years to adult)

The adult phase of AD begins near the onset of puberty. The reason for the resurgence of inflammation at this time is not understood, but it may be related to hormonal changes or to the stress of early adolescence. Adults may have no history of dermatitis in earlier years, but this is unusual. As in the childhood phase, localized inflammation with lichenification is the most common pattern. One area or several areas may be involved, and there are several characteristic patterns.

INFLAMMATION IN FLEXURAL AREAS. This pattern is commonly seen and is identical to childhood flexural inflammation.

HAND DERMATITIS. Hand dermatitis may be the most common expression of the atopic diathesis in the adult. (See the section on hand dermatitis in Chapter 3.) Adults are exposed to a variety of irritating chemicals in the home and at work, and they wash more frequently than do children. Irritation causes redness and scaling on the dorsal aspect of the hand or about the fingers. Itching develops, and the inevitable scratching results in lichenification or oozing and crusting. A few or all of the fingertip pads may be involved. They may be dry and chronically peeling or red and fissured. The eruption may be painful, chronic, and resistant to treatment. Psoriasis may have an identical presentation.

INFLAMMATION AROUND EYES. The lids are thin, frequently exposed to irritants, and easily traumatized by scratching. Many adults with AD have inflammation localized to the upper lids (Figure 5-19). They may claim to be allergic to something, but elimination of suspected allergens may not solve the problem. Habitual rubbing of the inflamed lids with the back of the hand is typical. If an attempt to control inflammation fails, then patch testing should be considered to eliminate allergic contact dermatitis.

LICHENIFICATION OF THE ANOGENITAL AREA. Lichenification of the anogenital area is probably more common in patients with AD than in others. Intertriginous areas that are warm and moist can become irritated and itch. Lichenification of the vulva (see Figure 3-43), scrotum (see Figure 3-48), and rectum (see Figure 3-44) may develop with habitual scratching. These areas are resistant to treatment, and inflammation may last for years. The patient may delay visiting a physician because of modesty, and the untreated lichenified plaques become very thick. Emotional factors should also be considered with this isolated phenomenon.

Figure 5-19 Atopic dermatitis of the upper eyelids, an area that is often rubbed with the back of the hand.

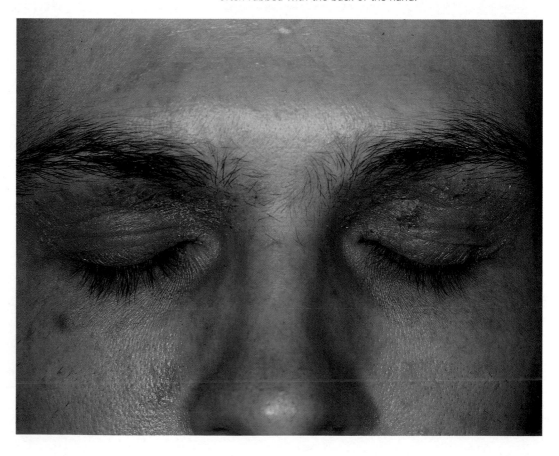

Associated Features

Dry skin and xerosis

Dry skin is an important feature of the atopic state. It is commonly assumed that patients with AD have inherited dry skin. The dryness may, however, reflect mild eczematous changes, concomitant ichthyosis, or a complex of both of these changes.[15]

Dry skin may appear at any age, and it is not unusual for infants to have dry scaling skin on the lower legs. Dry skin is sensitive, easily irritated by external stimuli, and, more importantly, itchy. It is the itching that provides the basis for the development of the various patterns of AD. Scratched itchy skin develops eczema; in other words, it is the itch that rashes.

Dry skin is most often located on the extensor surfaces of the legs and arms, but in susceptible individuals it may involve the entire cutaneous surface. Dryness is worse in the winter when humidity is low. Water is lost from the outermost layer of the skin. The skin becomes drier as the winter continues, and scaling skin becomes cracked and fissured. Dry areas that are repeatedly washed reach a point at which the epidermal barrier can no longer maintain its integrity; erythema and eczema occur. Frequent washing and drying may produce redness with horizontal linear splits, particularly on the lower legs of the elderly, giving a cracked or crazed porcelain appearance (see Chapter 3, Figures 3-37, 3-38, and 3-39). Avoid frequent washing. Use mild soaps (e.g, Dove, Cetaphil Bar) and routinely apply moisturizing creams or lotions. Moisturizers are effectively bound in the skin if they are applied shortly after patting the skin dry following bathing.

Ichthyosis vulgaris

Ichthyosis is a disorder of keratinization characterized by the development of dry, rectangular scales. There are many forms of ichthyosis. Dominant ichthyosis vulgaris may occur as a distinct entity, or it may be found in patients with AD. Atopic patients with ichthyosis vulgaris often have keratosis pilaris and hyperlinear, exaggerated palm creases. Infants may show only dry, scaling skin during the winter, but, with age, the changes become more extensive, and small, fine, white, translucent scales appear on the extensor aspects of the arms and legs (Figure 5-20). These scales are smaller and lighter in color than the large, brown polygonal scales of sex-linked ichthyosis vulgaris, which occurs exclusively in males (Figure 5-21). The scaling of the dominant form does not encroach on the axillae and fossae, as is seen in the sex-linked type. Scaling rarely involves the entire cutaneous surface. The condition tends to improve with age. Application of 12% ammonium lactate lotion or cream (Lac-Hydrin, AmLactin) or Carmol 20 or 40 cream (urea) is very effective.

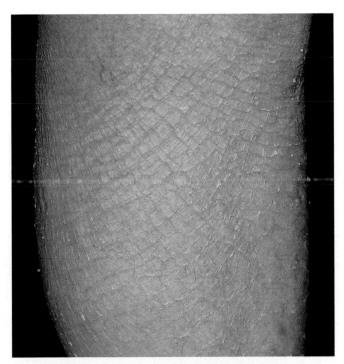

Figure 5-20 Dominant ichthyosis vulgaris. White, translucent, quadrangular scales on the extensor aspects of the arms and legs. This form is significantly associated with atopy.

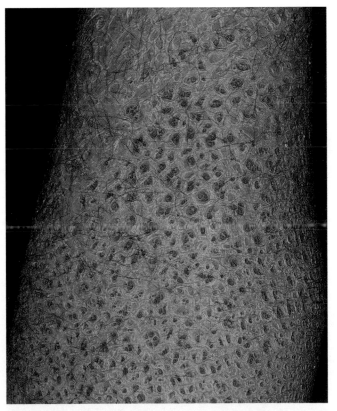

Figure 5-21 Sex-linked ichthyosis vulgaris. Large, brown, quadrangular scales that may encroach on the antecubital and popliteal fossae. Compare this presentation with Figure 5-20. There is no association with atopy.

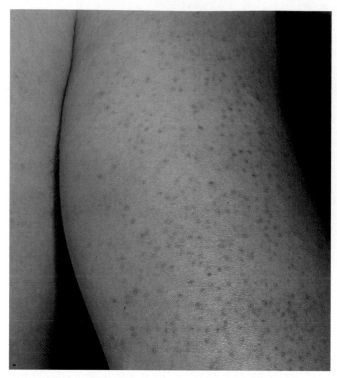

Figure 5-22 Keratosis pilaris. Small, rough, follicular papules or pustules occur most often on the posterolateral aspects of the upper arms and anterior thighs.

Keratosis pilaris

Keratosis pilaris is very common and seems to occur more often and more extensively in patients with AD. Small (1 to 2 mm), rough, follicular papules or pustules may appear at any age and are common in young children (Figure 5-22). The incidence peaks during adolescence, and the problem tends to improve thereafter. Adolescents and adults are disturbed by the appearance.

The posterolateral aspects of the upper arms (Figures 5-22 and 5-23) and anterior thighs are frequently involved, but any area, with the exception of the palms and soles, may be involved. Lesions on the face may be confused with acne, but the uniform small size and association with dry skin and chapping differentiate keratosis pilaris from pustular acne (Figure 5-24). The eruption may be generalized, resembling heat rash or miliaria. Most cases are asymptomatic, but the lesions may be red, inflammatory, and pustular and resemble bacterial folliculitis, particularly on the thighs (Figure 5-25). In the adult generalized form, a red halo appears at the periphery of the keratotic papule. This unusual diffuse pattern in adults persists indefinitely (Figure 5-26). Systemic steroid therapy may greatly accentuate both the lesion and the distribution by creation of numerous follicular pustules.

Treatment with topical retinoids (Retin-A cream or Tazorac cream) may induce improvement, but the irritation is usually unacceptable. Short courses of group II to V topical steroids reduce the unsightly redness and can be offered when temporary relief is desired before an important event. Application of 12% ammonium lactate or lotion (Lac-Hydrin, AmLactin) or Vanamide cream (urea) is probably the most practical and effective way of reducing the roughness; abrasive washing techniques cause further drying.

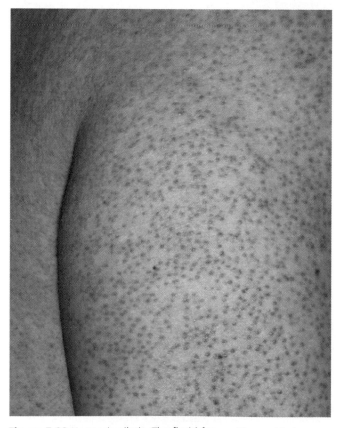

Figure 5-23 Keratosis pilaris. The florid form with a red halo surrounding the follicle can persist in adults.

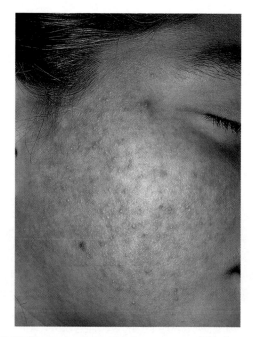

Figure 5-24 Keratosis pilaris. This is common on the face of children and is frequently confused with acne.

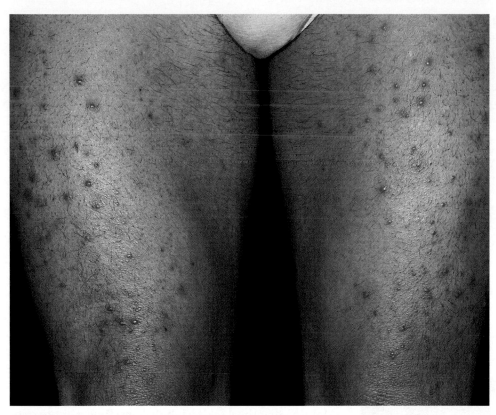

Figure 5-25 Keratosis pilaris. Infected lesions in a uniform distribution. Typical bacterial folliculitis has a haphazard distribution.

Figure 5-26 Keratosis pilaris. Diffuse involvement of the buttock is occasionally seen in adults. This type lasts indefinitely.

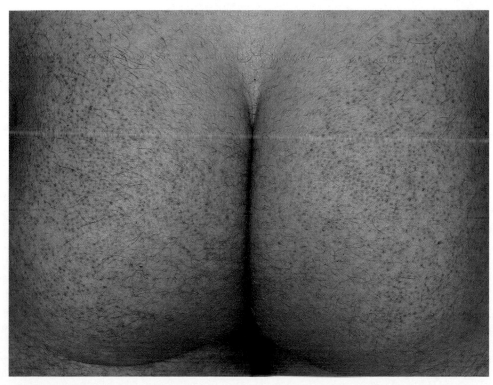

Hyperlinear palmar creases

Atopic patients are frequently found to have an accentuation of the major skin creases of the palms (Figure 5-27). This accentuation may be present in infancy and become more prominent as age and severity of skin inflammation increase. The changes might be initiated by rubbing or scratching. Patients with accentuated skin creases seem to have more extensive inflammation on the body and experience a longer course of disease. Occasionally patients without AD have palm crease accentuation. Moisturizers soften the skin but do not improve crease accentuation.

Pityriasis alba

Pityriasis alba is a common disorder that is characterized by an asymptomatic, hypopigmented, slightly elevated, fine, scaling plaque with indistinct borders. The condition, which affects the face (Figures 5-28 and 5-29), lateral upper arms (Figure 5-30), and thighs (Figure 5-31), appears in young children and usually disappears by early adulthood. The white, round-to-oval areas vary in size, but generally average 2 to 4 cm in diameter (Figure 5-30). Lesions become obvious in the summer months when the areas do not tan.

The loss of pigment is not permanent, as it is in vitiligo. Vitiligo and the fungal infection tinea versicolor both appear to be white, but the margin between normal and hypopigmented skin in vitiligo is distinct. Tinea versicolor is rarely located on the face, and the hypopigmented areas are more numerous and often confluent. A potassium hydroxide examination quickly settles the question. The hypopigmentation usually fades with time. No treatment other than lubrication should be attempted unless the patches become eczematous. Extensive pityriasis alba may respond to a short course of PUVA.[16]

Atopic pleats

The appearance of an extra line on the lower eyelid (Dennie-Morgan infraorbital fold) has been considered a distinguishing feature of patients with AD.[17] The line may simply be caused by constant rubbing of the eyes.[18] This extra line may also appear in people who do not have AD, and it is an unreliable sign of the atopic state.

Cataracts and keratoconus

Analysis of a large group of atopic patients showed that the incidence of cataracts was approximately 10%.[19] The reason for their development is not understood. Most are asymptomatic and can only be detected by slit-lamp examination. Two types have been reported: the complicated type, which begins at the posterior pole in the immediate subcapsular region; and the anterior plaque or shieldlike opacity, which lies subcapsularly and in the pupillary zone.[20] The anterior plaque type is the most frequently described. Posterior subcapsular cataracts are a well-established complication of systemic steroid therapy. Data suggest that there is no safe dosage of corticosteroids and that individual susceptibility may determine the threshold for development of cataracts.[21] It may be that atopic patients have a lower threshold or a greater tendency to develop cataracts, particularly when challenged with systemic steroids. This fact must be considered for the unusual atopic patient who requires systemic steroids for short-term control. Keratoconus (elongation and protrusion of the corneal surface) has been believed to be more common in the atopic state, but the incidence is low, and it does not appear to be associated with cataracts.

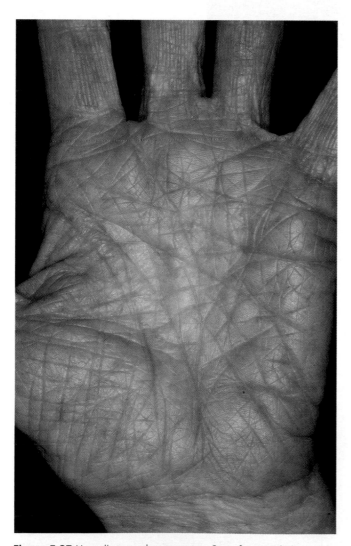

Figure 5-27 Hyperlinear palmar creases. Seen frequently in patients with severe atopic dermatitis.

PITYRIASIS ALBA

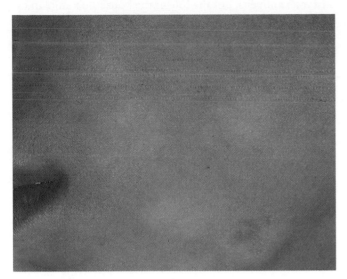

Figure 5-28 Hypopigmented round spots are a common occurrence on the faces of atopic children.

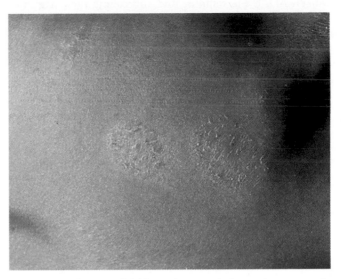

Figure 5-29 The superficial hypopigmented plaques become scaly and inflamed as the dry winter months progress.

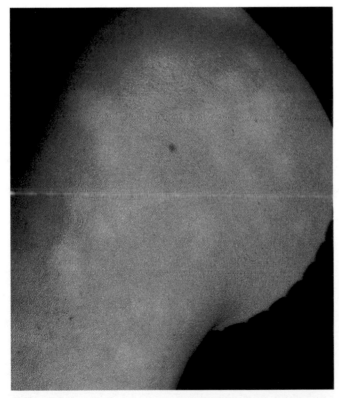

Figure 5-30 Irregular hypopigmented areas are frequently seen in atopic patients and are not to be confused with tinea versicolor or vitiligo.

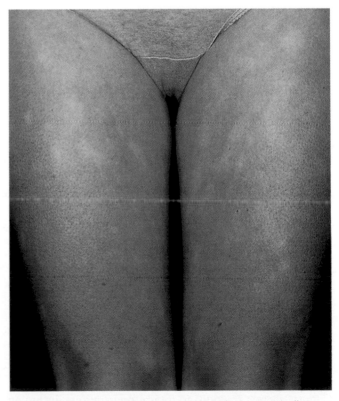

Figure 5-31 Lesions present here are more than are typically seen.

Triggering Factors

Factors that promote dryness or increase the desire to scratch worsen AD. Understanding and controlling these aggravating factors are essential to the successful management of AD.[22] A complete patient history is required because there is no standardized test scheme, like that for rhinitis or asthma, to identify specific triggering factors of AD.

Temperature change and sweating

Atopic patients do not tolerate sudden changes in temperature. Sweating induces itching, particularly in the antecubital and popliteal fossae, to a greater extent in atopic patients than in other individuals. Lying under warm blankets, entering a warm room, and experiencing physical stress all intensify the desire to scratch. A sudden lowering of temperature, such as leaving a warm shower, promotes itching. Patients should be discouraged from wearing clothing that tends to trap heat.

Decreased humidity

The beginning of fall heralds the onset of a difficult period for atopic patients. Cold air cannot support much humidity. The moisture-containing outer layer of the skin reaches equilibrium with the atmosphere and consequently holds less moisture. Dry skin is less supple, more fragile, and more easily irritated. Pruritus is established, the rash appears, and the long winter months in the northern states may be a difficult period to endure. Commercially available humidifiers can offer some relief by increasing the humidity in the house to above 50%.

Excessive washing

Repeated washing and drying removes water-binding lipids from the first layer of the skin. Daily baths may be tolerated in the summer months but lead to excessive dryness in the fall and winter.

Contact with irritating substances

Wool, household and industrial chemicals, cosmetics, and some soaps and detergents promote irritation and inflammation in the atopic patient. Cigarette smoke may provoke eczematous lesions on the eyelids. The inflammation is frequently interpreted as an allergic reaction by patients, who claim that they are allergic to almost everything they touch. The complaints reflect an intolerance of irritation. Atopic patients do develop allergic contact dermatitis, but the incidence is lower than normal.

Contact allergy

Contact allergic reactions to topical preparations, including corticosteroids, should be considered in patients who do not respond to therapy. Patch testing (see Chapter 4) may help to identify the offending agent.

Aeroallergens

The house-dust mite is the most important aeroallergen. Many patients with AD have anti-IgE antibodies to house-dust mite antigens, but the role of the house-dust mite in exacerbations of AD is controversial. Inhalation of house-dust antigen and allergen penetration through the skin may occur. Other aeroallergens such as pollens and allergens from pets, molds, or human dander may contribute to atopic dermatitis. Measures for allergen elimination should be undertaken. Hyposensitization may be effective, but there is little experience with this treatment.

Microbic agents

STAPHYLOCOCCUS AUREUS. S. aureus is the predominant skin microorganism in AD lesions. It is significantly increased in nonaffected skin. Normally S. aureus represents less than 5% of the total skin microflora in persons without atopic dermatitis. Antibiotics given systemically or topically may dramatically improve atopic dermatitis.

Food

Certain foods can provoke exacerbations of AD. Many patients who react to food are not aware of their hypersensitivity. Foods can provoke allergic and nonallergic reactions. The most common offenders are eggs, peanuts, milk, fish, soy, and wheat. Urticaria, an exacerbation of eczema, gastrointestinal or respiratory tract symptoms, or anaphylactic reactions may be signs of a food-induced reaction. Preservatives, colorants, and other low-molecular weight substances in foods may be offenders, but there are no tests for these substances.

Emotional stress

Stressful situations can have a profound effect on the course of AD. A stable course can quickly degenerate, and localized inflammation may become extensive almost overnight. Patients are well aware of this phenomenon and, regrettably, believe that they are responsible for their disease. This notion may be reinforced by relatives and friends who assure them that their disease "is caused by your nerves." Explaining that AD is an inherited disease that is made worse, rather than caused, by emotional stress is reassuring.

Treatment

Treatment goals consist of attempting to eliminate inflammation and infection (Box 5-3), preserving and restoring the stratum corneum barrier by using emollients, using antipruritic agents to reduce the self-inflicted damage to the involved skin, and controlling exacerbating factors (Box 5-4). Most patients can be brought under adequate control in less than 3 weeks. The following are possible reasons for failure to respond: poor patient compliance, allergic contact dermatitis to a topical medicine, the simultaneous occurrence of asthma or hay fever, inadequate sedation, and continued emotional stress.

Box 5-3 Treating Atopic Dermatitis

Topical Therapy

Topical steroids should be used to treat dermatitis until the skin clears, then steroid application should be discontinued. They are also used when pimecrolimus or tacrolimus fails to adequately control inflammation

    Group V creams or ointments for red, scaling skin

    Group I or II creams or ointments for lichenified skin

Parenteral steroids may be used for extensive flares

Prednisone

Topical nonsteroidal antiinflammatory agents may be used without interruption and do not cause atrophy. They are used as initial therapy or following treatment with topical steroids

Pimecrolimus (Elidel)

Tacrolimus (Protopic)

Tar

    Creams (e.g., Fototar)

    Bath oil (e.g., Balnetar)

Moisturizers should be applied after showers and after hand washing

Lipid-free lotion cleansers (e.g., Cetaphil)

Antibiotics

Antibiotics may be prescribed to suppress *Staphylococcus aureus;* they may be administered on a short- or long-term basis.

    Cephalexin (Keflex) 250 mg four times daily

    Cefadroxil (Duricef) 500 mg twice daily

    Dicloxacillin 250 mg four times daily

Antihistamines

Antihistamines control pruritus and induce sedation and sleep

    Hydroxyzine

    Doxepin HCl cream 5% (Zonalon)

Treating severe cases

Corticosteroids

    Oral prednisone

    Intramuscular triamcinolone

Cyclosporin

Mycophenate mofetil

Azathioprine

Hospitalization

    Home hospitalization (see the box on p. 125)

    Topical steroids and rest

    Goeckerman regimen (tar plus UVB)

Light therapy

Combined UVA-UVB

UVA

UVB

UVA1

Narrow-band 311-nm UVB

PUVA

Box 5-4 Controlling Atopic Dermatitis

Protect Skin From the Following Agents

Moisture

Avoid frequent hand washing

Avoid frequent bathing

Avoid lengthy bathing

Use tepid water for baths

Avoid abrasive washcloths

Foods

Avoid prolonged contact (clean food around baby's mouth)

Rough clothing

Avoid wool

Use 100% cotton

Irritants and allergens

Use soaps only in axilla, groin, feet

Avoid perfumes or makeup that burns or itches

Avoid fabric softeners

Scratching

Do not scratch

Pat, firmly press, or grasp the skin

Apply soothing lubricants

Control Environment

Temperature

Maintain cool, stable temperatures

Do not overdress

Limit number of bed blankets

Avoid sweating

Humidity

Humidify the house in winter

Airborne allergens and dust

Do not have rugs in bedrooms

Vacuum drapes and blankets

Use plastic mattress covers

Wet-mop floors

Avoid aerosols

Ventilate cooking odors

Avoid cigarettes

Use artificial plants

Avoid ragweed pollen contact

Minimize animal dander—no cats, dogs, rodents, or birds

Change geographic location

Sudden improvement may occur

Control emotional stress

Pleasant work environment

Learn relaxation techniques

Control diet

Diet control is a controversial treatment method (see text for treatment)

Dry skin

Controlling dry skin is essential in treating AD. Explain to patients that bathing dries the skin through the evaporation of water.

However, bathing also hydrates the skin, when moisturizer is applied immediately after bathing before the water has a chance to evaporate (within 3 minutes), thus retaining the hydration and keeping the skin soft and flexible. Pat the skin dry before moisturizer application. Daily bathing is possible if the 3-minute moisturizing rule is followed. Use of unscented moisturizers, such as an ointment like petrolatum or a cream, is ideal, whereas lotions are less effective emollients.[23]

Inflammation and infection

Inflammation is treated with topical steroids and the new topical nonsteroidal antiinflammatory agents (pimecrolimus and tacrolimus). The combined optimum use of these agents has not been defined. Some clinicians use topical steroids for rapid control and then switch to pimecrolimus or tacrolimus to complete treatment. Low-grade flare-ups are treated in a similar manner. This combination therapy minimizes the side effects of steroids by reducing their frequency of use. Co-administration of topical steroids and tacrolimus may be of benefit for minimizing the initial local irritation associated with tacrolimus.

TOPICAL STEROIDS AND ANTIBIOTICS. Topical steroids control inflammation. If the crusting or pustulation typically seen with *Staphylococcus aureus* infections is present, antibiotics should be prescribed. Oral antibiotics (e.g., cephalexin, cefadroxil) are more effective than topical antibiotics for controlling infection.

HOW TO USE TOPICAL STEROIDS. Topical steroids are very safe and effective medications when used properly. Hydrocortisone and other low-potency topical steroids (groups VI, VII) provide little relief; inflammation persists, therapy becomes prolonged, and patients and parents become discouraged. Use mid-strength to high-strength (adults) topical steroids as initial treatment. Atopic dermatitis will be rapidly controlled in days. Limit treatment to 2 weeks. Ointment-based medications are preferred for dry skin. Moisturizers may also be used. Introduce patients to pimecrolimus cream (Elidel) or tacrolimus ointment (Protopic). Explain that these drugs are also very safe and do not have the side effects associated with long-term use of topical steroids (atrophy, striae, etc.). Patients will learn what combination of medications and bases works best for them and will feel confident that they can control fluctuations in their disease.

SAFETY IN CHILDREN. The group V topical steroid fluticasone propionate cream 0.05% (Cutivate) appears to be safe for the treatment of severe eczema for up to 4 weeks in children 3 months of age and older. Children between 3 months and 6 years with moderate to severe AD (> or =35% body surface area; mean body surface area treated, 64%) were treated with fluticasone propionate cream, 0.05% twice daily for 3 to 4 weeks. Mean cortisol levels were similar at baseline and at the end of treatment.[24]

MAINTAINING CONTROL. Short weekly bursts of topical corticosteroids may play a role in keeping an adult's AD under control. Weekly applications of fluticasone ointment (Cutivate), applied once daily for 2 consecutive days each week to known healed and any newly occurring dermatitis sites maintained the improvements achieved after the initial treatment phase and delayed relapse.[25]

TOPICAL NONSTEROIDAL ANTIINFLAMMATORY AGENTS. Pimecrolimus (Elidel) and tacrolimus (Protopic) are new immunosuppressant topical medications that inhibit a calcium-activated phosphatase called *calcineurin*. The mechanism of action is closely related to that of cyclosporine. They are the first topical immune suppressants that are not hydrocortisone derivatives. They block: the early phase of T-cell activation, degranulation of mast cells and multiple cytokines required to activate cellular immunity. They potently block Langerhans' cells' function and do not cause dermal atrophy.

Pimecrolimus cream 1% (Elidel)

INDICATIONS. Pimecrolimus cream 1% is indicated for short-term and intermittent long-term therapy in the treatment of mild to moderate atopic dermatitis in non-immunocompromised patients 2 years of age and older.

DOSAGE AND ADMINISTRATION. Apply a thin layer to the affected skin twice daily. Pimecrolimus may be used on all skin surfaces, including the head, neck, and intertriginous areas. Pimecrolimus should be used twice daily for as long as signs and symptoms persist. Treatment should be discontinued if resolution of disease occurs. Pimecrolimus cream should not be used with occlusive dressings.

ABSORPTION. Systemic absorption of pimecrolimus is very low.

ADVERSE EFFECTS. Burning does not occur. Patients should avoid excessive exposure to natural or artificial sunlight (tanning beds or UVA/B treatment) while using tacrolimus because of a possible enhancement of ultraviolet carcinogenicity.

Tacrolimus (Protopic)

INDICATIONS. Tacrolimus ointment is indicated for short-term and intermittent long-term therapy of patients with moderate to severe AD.

DOSAGE AND ADMINISTRATION. Two concentrations of tacrolimus (0.03% and 0.1%) are available. In children (2 to 15 years), 0.03% is the only concentration approved by the

Food and Drug Administration. The 0.1% ointment is more effective than 0.03% ointment, does not have a worse side effect profile, is not much more expensive, and has been demonstrated to be safe in children, so it seems reasonable to prescribe the 0.1% ointment. Before starting treatment with tacrolimus, infections at treatment sites should be cleared. Apply a thin layer of ointment to the affected skin areas twice daily. Treatment is continued for 1 week after clearing.[26,27]

EFFICACY OF TACROLIMUS VERSUS GLUCOCORTICOIDS. Tacrolimus ointment has efficacy similar to a mid-potency steroid such as betamethasone valerate (0.12%) ointment.

TREATING THE FACE. Tacrolimus is safe for treating facial dermatoses because of the lack of atrophy and improved safety for the eye. There was no evidence of increased intraocular pressure when applied to the eyelids.

SAFETY IN CHILDREN. Tacrolimus ointment 0.1% can be used daily for periods of up to 1 year without increasing the risk of infection[28] or other nonapplication-site adverse events and without loss of effectiveness, in the treatment of moderate to severe AD in children 2 to 15 years of age.[27]

ABSORPTION. Systemic absorption is minimal even when large areas of skin are treated; blood levels are either undetectable or subtherapeutic. Patients applying large amounts of tacrolimus on severely affected skin may attain significant serum levels of the drug, at least transiently.

ADVERSE EFFECTS. Burning (mild to moderate) at the site of application is the most frequent adverse event, occurring in 31% to 61% of those treated. Burning lasts between 2 minutes and 3 hours and tends to decrease after the first few days of treatment. Tacrolimus ointment is not phototoxic, photosensitizing, or photoallergenic. Patients should avoid excessive exposure to natural or artificial sunlight (tanning beds or UVA/B treatment) while using tacrolimus because of a possible enhancement of ultraviolet carcinogenicity.

Infants
LOCALIZED INFLAMMATION. Topical steroids provide rapid control. Infants with dry, red, scaling plaques on the cheeks respond to group V or VI topical steroids applied twice a day for 7 to 14 days. Elidel cream or Protopic ointment may be used for long-term stability and control. Flares are treated with topical steroids. Parents are instructed to decrease the frequency of washing and start lubrication with a bland lubricant during the initial phase of the treatment period and to continue lubrication long after topical steroids have been discontinued. Antistaphylococcal antibiotics are required only if there is moderate serum and crusting. Cracking about the lips is controlled in a similar fashion, but heavy lubricants (such as petroleum jelly, Aquaphor ointment or Eucerin) are used after the inflammation has cleared.

GENERALIZED INFLAMMATION. Infants with more generalized inflammation require treatment with a group V to VI topical steroid cream or ointment applied two to three times a day for 10 to 21 days. Secondary infection often accompanies generalized inflammation, and a 3- to 7-day course of an antistaphylococcal antibiotic, such as cephalexin suspension, (Keflex) is helpful. Start oral antibiotics 2 days before initiating topical steroid treatment. Sedation with hydroxyzine (10 mg/5 ml) is useful during the initial treatment period. The bedtime dose gives the child a good night's sleep and seems to suppress the unconscious scratching that occurs during disturbed sleep. The parents are grateful; at last they are not up all night with a scratching, crying child.

Potent topical or systemic steroids are potentially hazardous and may be associated with relapse after therapy has been discontinued. Avoidance of certain foods, pets, and house-dust mites is an option; the major drawbacks are the lack of tests to identify triggers or predict response.[29]

Children and adults
LICHENIFIED PLAQUES. Lichenified plaques in older children and adults respond to groups II through V topical steroids used with occlusive dressings (Figure 5-32). Occlusive therapy for 10 to 14 days is preferred if the plaques are resistant to treatment or are very thick. Occlusion may be used as soon as infection has been controlled. Adults may be treated with group I topical steroids for 1 to 4 weeks.

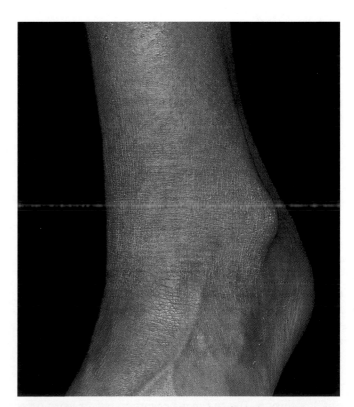

Figure 5-32 Response to treatment. Lichenified plaque shown in Figure 5-15 after 7 days of a group IV topical steroid under occlusive dressing.

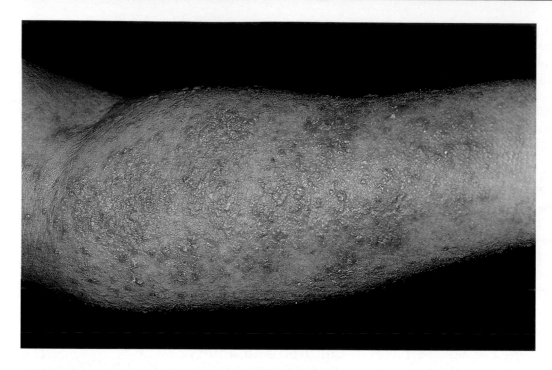

Figure 5-33 Severe generalized atopic dermatitis of this intensity requires prednisone and wet compresses for initial control.

Table 5-1 Prednisone for Atopic Dermatitis (Adults)	
Day	**Dosage mg/day**
	10-mg tablets, taken as a single dose each morning
1-4	60
5-6	50
7-8	40
9-10	30
11-12	20
13-14	10

DIFFUSE INFLAMMATION. Diffuse inflammation involving the face, trunk, and extremities is treated with group V topical steroids applied two to four times a day. Elidel cream or Protopic ointment can be used as initial treatment for mild to moderate inflammation and for maintenance. A 3- to 7-day course of systemic antistaphylococcal antibiotics is almost invariably required. Start oral antibiotics 2 days before initiating topical steroid treatment. Exudative areas (Figure 5-33) with serum and crust are treated with a Burrow's solution compress for 20 minutes three times a day for 2 to 3 days. Dryness and cracking with fissures occur if compressing is prolonged. Resistant cases may be treated with group V topical steroids applied before and after vinyl suit ("psoriasis suit") occlusion. The suit may be worn to bed or worn for 2 hours twice a day. All signs of infection, such as serum and crust, should be clear before initiating occlusive therapy.

SYSTEMIC STEROIDS. Severe AD may be treated with prednisone. A single-dose treatment schedule is shown in Table 5-1. Prednisone, administered in a dosage of 20 mg twice each day for at least 7 days is an alternative schedule for severe, widespread inflammation; later, taper the dosage over the next 2 or 3 weeks. Patients who may have trouble adhering to a medication schedule may be treated with triamcinolone acetonide (Kenalog, Aristocort; 40 mg suspension) given intramuscularly. Commercially available steroid dose packs (e.g., Medrol Dosepak) should be avoided; they provide an inadequate amount of medicine and result in a recurrence of rash and pruritus after initial partial amelioration of symptoms during the first days of treatment.

Oral and intramuscular steroid therapy has a number of disadvantages. The relapse rate is high, with inflammation returning shortly after the medication is discontinued. Enthusiasm for topical therapy diminishes once the patient has experienced the rapid clearing produced by systemic therapy, prompting some patients to request systemic therapy again; this request should be denied. The association of atopic cataracts with systemic steroid therapy has been discussed.

Tar

Tar ointments were the mainstay of therapy before topical steroids were introduced. They were effective and had few side effects but did not work quickly. Tar in a lubricating base such as T-Derm or Fototar applied twice daily is an effective alternative to topical steroids. Intensely inflamed areas should first be controlled with topical steroids. Tar ointments can then be used to complete therapy. Tar can be used as an initial therapy for chronic, superficial plaques.

Hospitalization for severely resistant cases

Some patients with severe, generalized inflammation do not respond to or flare soon after a reasonable trial of topical therapy. These patients are candidates for hospitalization. A short stay in the hospital can rapidly help to control a condition that has had a prolonged, unstable course. A program for "home hospitalization" is outlined in Box 5-5.

Box 5-5 Atopic Dermatitis—Home Hospitalization (Short-Term Intensive Treatment)

Designate family member or friend as nurse.

All treatment is administered by nurse.

Write orders for home nurse.

Treatment starts Friday night and ends Monday morning.

Orders

1. Complete bed rest with bathroom privileges
2. Semi-darkened room
3. No visitors other than nurse
4. Cotton bedclothes; dust-free and animal-free room
5. Temperature 68° to 70° F
6. Humidity 70%
7. Bland diet—no alcohol, spices, or caffeine

Topical therapy

1. Tepid tub bath with bath oil (e.g., Keri Bath Oil), 20 minutes twice a day
2. Emollient bland cream applied to moist body after pat dry immediately on emergence from tub
3. Body lesions covered with group V steroid cream or ointment twice daily
4. Face lesions covered with group V steroid cream or ointment twice daily
5. Scalp inflammation treated with daily shampoo followed by topical steroid lotion in oil (e.g., Dermasmoothe F/S)

Systemic therapy

1. Antibiotics: e.g., cefadroxil 500 mg twice daily or dicloxacillin 250 mg four times daily
2. Sedating antihistamines: hydroxyzine 10 to 25 mg four times daily; doxepin 10 to 25 mg four times daily; or others
3. Phenothiazines for agitated patients: chlorpromazine 25 mg four times daily
4. May give a short-acting injectable steroid before hospitalization (e.g., dexamethasone 8 mg IM or betamethasone 6 mg IM)

Modified from Roth HL: Intl J Dermatol 1987; 26:139-149.

Lubrication

Restoring moisture to the skin increases the rate of healing and establishes a durable barrier against further drying and irritation. A variety of lotions and creams are available, and most are adequate for rehydration. Petroleum jelly (Vaseline) is especially effective. Some products contain urea (e.g., Nutraplus, Carmol 10, 20, 40); others contain lactic acid (e.g., Lac-Hydrin, AmLactin, LactiCare). Urea and lactic acid have special hydrating qualities and may be more effective than other moisturizers. Their use should be encouraged, particularly during the winter months. Patients should be cautioned that lotions may sting shortly after application. This may be a property of the base or of a specific ingredient such as lactic acid. If itching or stinging continues with each application, another product should be selected. If inflammation occurs after use of a lubricant, allergic contact dermatitis to a preservative or a perfume should be considered.

Lubricants are most effective when applied after a bath. The patient should gently pat the skin dry with a towel and immediately apply the lubricant to seal in the moisture. Bath oils (e.g., Keri Bath Oil) are an effective method of lubrication, but they can make the tub slippery and dangerous for older patients. In order to be effective, a sufficient amount of oil must be used to create an oily feeling on the skin when leaving the tub. Septic systems may be adversely affected by prolonged use of bath oils. A mild bar soap should be used infrequently. Cetaphil, Dove, Keri, Purpose, Oilatum, and Basis are adequate; Ivory soap is very drying and should be avoided.

Sedation and antihistamines

ORAL ANTIHISTAMINES. Antihistamines generally have offered only marginal therapeutic benefit. Sedating antihistamines may be useful in relieving pruritus at night by helping patients to sleep. The common practice of prescribing antihistamines is based on individual experiences of patients and physicians. There is no objective evidence to support the effectiveness of sedating or nonsedating antihistamines in treating AD or relieving pruritus.[30] Nonsedating agents may be useful for patients with allergic rhinitis, allergic conjunctivitis, allergen-induced asthma, and chronic urticaria; nonsedating antihistamines are very expensive.

TOPICAL ANTIHISTAMINES. Doxepin HCl cream (Zonalon cream) is an antipruritic cream. The mechanism of action is unknown. Doxepin has potent H_1-receptor and H_2-receptor blocking actions. Zonalon cream is indicated for the short-term (up to 8 days) management of moderate pruritus in adults with AD and lichen simplex chronicus.[31] Drowsiness occurs in more than 20% of patients, especially patients receiving treatment to greater than 10% of their body surface area. The most common local adverse effect is burning and/or stinging. A thin film of cream is applied four times each day with intervals of at least 3 hours between applications.

Phototherapy

Phototherapy is effective for mild or moderate AD. Combined UVA-UVB and UVA or UVB has been shown in the past to be effective. The dosage is considerably lower than that for UVB-treated psoriasis patients.[32] UVA1 irradiation (ranging from 340 to 400 nm) therapy is superior to conventional UVA-UVB phototherapy in patients with severe AD. The optimal dose regarding therapeutic efficacy and possible side effects is still to be determined. A correlation between UVA irradiation and photoaging, skin carcinogenesis, or melanoma induction may exist. Medium dose regimens (50 gm/cm²) have been found to be effective.[33] Programs to avoid rapid relapses are being investigated. Low-dose UVA1 or narrow-band 311-nm UVB twice weekly for 4 weeks and once weekly for another 4 weeks appears to prevent relapse. Narrow-band UVB (311 nm) as monotherapy is also effective for moderate to severe atopic eczema.[34] Photochemotherapy with methoxsalen plus UVA (PUVA) is effective but many clinicians have abandoned its use for AD because of its risk of long-term carcinogenicity.

ORAL IMMUNOSUPPRESSIVE AGENTS. A few patients remain severely affected by AD despite treatment with systemic steroids and phototherapy. Oral immunosuppressive agents may be considered for these few treatment-resistant cases.

CYCLOSPORINE. Cyclosporine A (CsA) is an effective and well-tolerated treatment for severe refractory AD in children and adults. CsA can be prescribed on a short-term basis, both in adults and children. Long-term treatment, up to 1 year, should be considered only in exceptional cases that cannot be controlled by short-time therapy. By starting at a low dose, the therapeutic safety should be further increased. Hence, in severe pediatric AD, CsA microemulsion, when started at a low dose (2.5 mg/kg/day), improves clinical measures of disease.[35] Body-weight–independent dosing with cyclosporine is feasible for short-term treatment. Although the starting dose of 300 mg/day is more effective than 150 mg/day, the 150-mg dose would be preferable for the initiation of therapy because of its excellent renal tolerability.[36] The disease may relapse despite continued treatment or may recur soon after cyclosporine is discontinued. Maintenance therapy may be hampered by side effects in the same way as therapy is hampered by side effects in the treatment of psoriasis. Serum IgE levels and prick test responses are unchanged by cyclosporine.

MYCOPHENOLATE MOFETIL. Mycophenolate mofetil is a highly effective drug for treating moderate-severe AD, with no serious adverse effects. In an open-label pilot study patients were successfully treated with mycophenolate mofetil, 1 gm, given orally twice daily for 4 weeks. At week 5, the dosage was reduced to 500 mg twice daily and stopped at 8 weeks.[37]

AZATHIOPRINE. Limited open studies suggest that azathioprine may be effective. Azathioprine myelotoxicity and drug efficacy are now known to be related to the activity of a key enzyme in azathioprine metabolism, thiopurinemethyltransferase (TPMT). Obtain pretreatment determinations of TPMT. Low levels of TPMT (1 in 300 people) are associated with toxicity (leukopenia, thrombocytopenia).[38] Very high levels are associated with nonresponses. The starting dose is 100-150 mg/day and the maintenance dose is 50-100 mg/day.

CONTROLLING AEROALLERGENS. Atopic dermatitis can be elicited by external contact with an aeroallergen. Eczematous skin lesions are found predominantly in the air-exposed areas of the neck, face, and scalp. IgE-mediated sensitization of questionable clinical relevance is routinely demonstrated in patients with atopic eczema by skin prick test or radioallergosorbent test (RAST). A new test, the atopic patch test, which is not in general use, may be the most specific and relevant.[39] The atopic patch test has a higher specificity with regard to clinical relevance of an allergen compared with skin prick test and RAST.[40] In a large trial, house-dust mite was the most common positive allergen, followed by grass pollen and cat epithelium. Most of the patients were positive only to one allergen, rarely to two or three. A regimen aimed at reducing the presence of house-dust mites can produce clinical improvement in patients with AD who show contact hypersensitivity to mite antigens on skin testing. Reduction of mites with a thorough housecleaning and by covering mattresses may result in dramatic improvement. These home-sanitation programs, which involve cleaning different surfaces, are often recommended by allergists to rhinitis and asthma patients to control aeroallergens such as mites and molds. Allergy Control Products, Inc. (www.allergycontrol.com) offers a full line of supplies to reduce allergen exposure.

Diet restriction and breast-feeding

PREVALENCE OF AD AND FREQUENCY OF FOOD ALLERGY. The prevalence of AD is about 10% to 15% of children.[2] Food hypersensitivity affects about 10% to 40% of children with AD.

FOODS. Food hypersensitivity is usually limited to one or two antigens and may be lost after several years. Five foods account for 90% of the positive oral challenges seen in children; in order of frequency they are: eggs, peanuts, milk, soy, and wheat.

A summary of the role of foods in AD is found in Box 5-6.

A child (especially younger than 7 years) with AD who is unresponsive to routine therapy may have a greater than 50% chance of having food hypersensitivity.[41] A small percentage of children and adults with AD have positive responses to food-challenge tests, resulting in eczematous flares. Significant clinical improvement occurs within 1 or 2 months when an appropriately designed restricted diet is followed. Clinical reactions to food range from mild skin symptoms to life-threatening anaphylactic reactions.

IMMEDIATE-TYPE REACTIONS. Immediate-type clinical reactions to food can easily be identified by history and are associated with a positive skin prick test and specific IgE in serum. Symptoms usually occur within 2 hours of ingesting the food antigen (early-phase reaction). They consist of pruritus, erythema, and edema. A recurrence of pruritus may occur 6 to 8 hours later. This late-phase reaction does not occur in the absence of early-phase reaction. Urticarial lesions are rarely seen. Many patients complain of nausea, abdominal pain, emesis, or diarrhea. Respiratory symptoms, including stridor, wheezing, nasal congestion, and sneezing, may develop. Anaphylactic reactions are uncommon but possible during food testing.

LATE-PHASE REACTIONS. The evaluation of food allergy in the absence of immediate clinical reactions presents diagnostic difficulties in children with AD. Late-phase clinical reactions are associated with a positive atopy patch test but not all clinicians perform this test.[42]

SKIN TEST AND IGE. The most reliable and practical way of diagnosing food allergy has not been determined. The history is of marginal value. In the very young child, either the skin prick tests or circulating specific IgE (as measured by RAST/CAP methods) may be useful as screening tests of IgE-mediated food hypersensitivity. In general, skin prick tests and circulating specific IgE antibody correlate well. False-negative IgE findings are uncommon. False-positive findings are common, particularly in the older child.

PROVOCATION TESTS. Challenge tests are performed to determine the clinical significance of the positive laboratory tests. The double-blind, placebo-controlled food challenge is recognized as the "gold standard" for food allergy, but this test is not practical for most cases. The test is performed in the hospital with emergency equipment available. An open trial is less accurate but more practical. Patients are given a period of antigen avoidance. Foods that produce positive skin prick tests should be eliminated from the patient's diet for 1 to 2 weeks before the oral food challenge.

RESTRICTED DIETS IN ATOPIC DERMATITIS. If food allergy is thought to be a possibility, a limited trial of an exclusion diet can be recommended, after dietary assessment and advice by a pediatric dietician. Food hypersensitivity may be a factor in the activity of AD in very young children, and dietary treatment is of value in these patients. More than 90% of reactions in young children are caused by only five foods: eggs, milk, peanuts, soy, and wheat.

EXCLUSION DIETS IN INFANTS. A relationship between the diversity of diet during the first 4 months (delayed introduction of solid foods) and the development of AD occurs. Itch lessens, and the eczema can improve significantly. The diet must be properly supervised by a pediatric dietitian to ensure that it is free of the allergen(s) while also being nutritionally adequate. Eczema develops in fewer children who receive a casein hydrolysate as compared with those receiving soy or cow's milk formula.

PROGNOSIS. Food allergy does not last indefinitely. A gradual reintroduction of the offending foods should be carefully considered after the child is past the third birthday. Milk and soy allergies usually disappear with aging; egg and fish allergies tend to remain.

Box 5-6 Atopic Dermatitis and Food Allergy

- The history is not a good method of screening for food allergy.
- The most reliable and practical way of diagnosing food allergy has not been determined.

Testing

- Skin prick test
- Determination of specific IgE antibodies
  Sera is analyzed for total IgE and specific IgE antibody titers, e.g., to cow's milk, hen's egg, wheat, and soy. False-negative IgE findings are uncommon. False-positive findings are common, particularly in the older child.

Exclusion diets

- A limited trial of an exclusion diet can be recommended for foods that produce positive skin prick tests or are thought to be a possible cause.
- More than 90% of reactions in young children are caused by only five foods: eggs, milk, peanuts, soy, and wheat.

Maternal diets

- Restricted diets are usually not recommended during pregnancy.
- Nut avoidance during pregnancy and lactation may be of benefit.
- Restricted maternal diet may be necessary in the breast-fed, food-allergic infant if the mother wishes to continue breast-feeding.

Breast-feeding and weaning

1. Exclusive breast-feeding during the first 3 months of life is protective for atopy and atopic dermatitis during childhood in children with a family history of atopy.[43]
2. Food antigens have been identified in breast milk. Infants of mothers who avoid egg whites, cow's milk, fish, peanuts, and soy products during lactation developed less eczema.
3. Prolonged breast-feeding should be encouraged in atopic families.
4. The introduction of solids during the first 4 months should be avoided.

Older children and adults

- Food hypersensivity is rarely a factor.
- Exclusion diets are only rarely helpful.
- Nut and fish allergies are likely to be lifelong.
- Screening tests for IgE of older children (~ >6 years) are not very helpful because false-positive reactions are very common and only rarely indicate food hypersensitivity.

References

1. Hanifin J, Chan S: Biochemical and immunologic mechanisms in atopic dermatitis: new targets for emerging therapies, J Am Acad Dermatol 1999; 41(1):72.

2. Laughter D, et al: The prevalence of atopic dermatitis in Oregon schoolchildren, J Am Acad Dermatol 2000; 43(4):649.

3. Rystedt I: Prognostic factors in atopic dermatitis, Acta Derm Venereol (Stockh) 1985; 65:206.

4. Linna O, et al: Ten-year prognosis for generalized infantile eczema, Acta Paediatr Scand 1992; 81:1013.

5. Fisher D: IgE level and the validation of the diagnostic criteria for atopic dermatitis, Arch Dermatol 1999; 135(12):1550.

6. Leiferman K: A role for eosinophils in atopic dermatitis, J Am Acad Dermatol 2001; 45(1 suppl):S21.

7. de G AC: The frequency of contact allergy in atopic patients with dermatitis, Contact Dermatitis 1990; 22:273.

8. Sutthipisal N, et al: Sensitization in atopic and non-atopic hairdressers with hand eczema, Contact Dermatitis 1993; 29:206.

9. Cronin E, McFadden JP: Patients with atopic eczema do become sensitized to contact allergens, Contact Dermatitis 1993; 28:225.

10. Bohme M, et al: Hanifin's and Rajka's minor criteria for atopic dermatitis: which do 2-year-olds exhibit? J Am Acad Dermatol 2000; 43(5:1):785.

11. Hanifin J: Diagnostic criteria for atopic dermatitis: consider the context, Arch Dermatol 1999; 135(12):1551.

12. Musgrove K, Morgan JK: Infantile eczema, Br J Dermatol 1976; 95:365.

13. Sampson HH, Jolie PL: Increased plasma histamine concentrations after food challenges in children with atopic dermatitis, N Engl J Med 1984; 311:372.

14. Massarano AA, et al: Growth in atopic eczema, Arch Dis Child 1993; 68:677.

15. Uehara M, Miyauchi H: The morphologic characteristics of dry skin in atopic dermatitis, Arch Dermatol 1984; 120:1186.

16. Zaynoun S, Jaber LAA, Kurban AK: Oral methoxsalen photochemotherapy of extensive pityriasis alba, J Am Acad Dermatol 1986; 15:61.

17. Meenan FOC: The significance of Morgan's fold in children with atopic dermatitis, Acta Derm Venereol (Stockh) 1980; 92 (suppl): 42.

18. Uehara M: Infraorbital fold in atopic dermatitis, Arch Dermatol 1981; 117:627.

19. Roth HL, Kierland RR: The natural history of atopic dermatitis, Arch Dermatol 1964; 89:209.

20. Brandonisio T, Bachman J, Sears J: Atopic dermatitis: a case report and current clinical review of systemic and ocular manifestations, Optometry 2001; 72(2):94.

21. Skalka HW, Prachal JT: Effects of corticosteroids on cataract formation, Arch Opthalmol 1980; 98:1773.

22. Morren M-A, et al: Atopic dermatitis: triggering factors, J Am Acad Dermatol 1994; 31:467.

23. Tofte S, Hanifin J: Current management and therapy of atopic dermatitis, J Am Acad Dermatol 2001; 44(1):S13.

24. Friedlander S, Hebert A, Allen D: Safety of fluticasone propionate cream 0.05% for the treatment of severe and extensive atopic dermatitis in children as young as 3 months, J Am Acad Dermatol 2002; 46(3):387.

25. Van DMJ, et al: The management of moderate to severe atopic dermatitis in adults with topical fluticasone propionate: the Netherlands Adult Atopic Dermatitis Study Group, Br J Dermatol 1999; 140(6):1114.

26. Hanifin J, et al: Tacrolimus ointment for the treatment of atopic dermatitis in adult patients: part I—efficacy, J Am Acad Dermatol 2001; 44(1 suppl):S28.

27. Kang S, et al: Long-term safety and efficacy of tacrolimus ointment for the treatment of atopic dermatitis in children, J Am Acad Dermatol 2001; 44(1 suppl):S58.

28. Fleicher AB, et al: Tacrolimus ointment for the treatment of atopic dermatitis is not associated with an increase in cutaneous infections, J Am Acad Dermatol 2002; 47:562.

29. David TJ: Recent developments in the treatment of childhood atopic eczema, J R Coll Physicians Lond 1991; 25:95.

30. Klein P, Clark R: An evidence-based review of the efficacy of antihistamines in relieving pruritus in atopic dermatitis, Arch Dermatol 1999; 135(12):1522.

31. Drake L, et al: Pharmacokinetics of doxepin in subjects with pruritic atopic dermatitis, J Am Acad Dermatol 1999; 41(2:1):209.

32. Jekler J: Phototherapy of atopic dermatitis with ultraviolet radiation, Acta Derm Venereol 1992; 171 (Suppl): 1.

33. von KG, et al: Medium-dose UVA1 cold-light phototherapy in the treatment of severe atopic dermatitis, J Am Acad Dermatol 1999; 41(6):931.

34. Reynolds N, et al: Narrow-band ultraviolet B and broad-band ultraviolet A phototherapy in adult atopic eczema: a randomised controlled trial, Lancet 2001; 357(9273):2012.

35. Bunikowski R, et al: Low-dose cyclosporin A microemulsion in children with severe atopic dermatitis: clinical and immunological effects, Pediatr Allergy Immunol 2001; 12(4):216.

36. Czech W, et al: A body-weight-independent dosing regimen of cyclosporine microemulsion is effective in severe atopic dermatitis and improves the quality of life, J Am Acad Dermatol 2000, 42(4):653.

37. Grundmann-Kollmann M, et al: Mycophenolate mofetil is effective in the treatment of atopic dermatitis, Arch Dermatol 2001; 137(7):870.

38. Meggitt S, Reynolds N: Azathioprine for atopic dermatitis, Clin Exp Dermatol 2001; 26(5):369.

39. Ring J, Darsow U, Behrendt H: Role of aeroallergens in atopic eczema: proof of concept with the atopy patch test, J Am Acad Dermatol 2001; 45(1):S49.

40. Darsow U, Vieluf D, Ring J: Evaluating the relevance of aeroallergen sensitization in atopic eczema with the atopy patch test: a randomized, double-blind multicenter study: Atopy Patch Test Study Group, J Am Acad Dermatol 1999; 40(2:1):187.

41. Lever R: The role of food in etopic eczema, J Am Acad Dermatol 2001; 45 (1 suppl):S57.

42. Niggemann B, Reibel S, Wahn U: The atopy patch test (APT)—a useful tool for the diagnosis of food allergy in children with atopic dermatitis, Allergy 2000; 55(3):281.

43. Gdalevich M, et al: Breast-feeding and the onset of atopic dermatitis in childhood: a systematic review and meta-analysis of prospective studies, J Am Acad Dermatol 2001; 45(4):520.

❏ **Clinical aspects**

❏ **Pathophysiology**

❏ **Initial evaluation of all patients with urticaria**

❏ **Acute urticaria**

❏ **Chronic urticaria**

❏ **Treatment of urticaria**
  Antihistamines
  Epinephrine
  Oral corticosteroids
  Immunotherapy

❏ **Physical urticarias**
  Dermographism
  Pressure urticaria
  Cholinergic urticaria
  Exercise-induced anaphylaxis
  Cold urticaria
  Solar urticaria
  Heat, water, and vibration urticarias
  Aquagenic pruritus

❏ **Angioedema**
  Acquired forms of angioedema
  Hereditary angioedema

❏ **Contact urticaria syndrome**

❏ **Pruritic urticarial papules and plaques of pregnancy**

❏ **Urticarial vasculitis**

❏ **Serum sickness**

❏ **Mastocytosis**

Urticaria, also referred to as *hives* or *wheals*, is a common and distinctive reaction pattern. Hives may occur at any age; up to 20% of the population will have at least one episode. Hives may be more common in atopic patients. Urticaria is classified as *acute* or *chronic*. The majority of cases are acute, lasting from hours to a few weeks. Angioedema frequently occurs with acute urticaria, which is more common in children and young adults. Chronic urticaria (arbitrarily defined as episodes of urticaria lasting more than 6 weeks) is more common in middle-aged women.

Because most individuals can diagnose urticaria and realize that it is a self-limited condition, they do not seek medical attention.

The cause of acute urticaria is determined in many cases, but the cause of chronic urticaria is determined in only 5% to 20% of cases. Patients with chronic urticaria present a frustrating problem in diagnosis and management. History taking is crucial but tedious, and treatment is usually supportive rather than curative.

These patients are often subjected to detailed and expensive medical evaluations that usually prove unrewarding. Studies demonstrate the value of a complete history and physical examination followed by the judicious use of laboratory studies in evaluating the results of the history and physical examination.[1]

Clinical Aspects

DEFINITION. A hive or wheal is a circumscribed, erythematous or white, nonpitting, edematous, usually pruritic plaque that changes in size and shape by peripheral extension or regression during the few hours or days that the individual lesion exists. The edematous, central area (wheal) can be pale in comparison to the erythematous surrounding area (flare).

The evolution of urticaria is a dynamic process. New lesions evolve as old ones resolve. Hives result from localized capillary vasodilation, followed by transudation of protein-rich fluid into the surrounding tissue; they resolve when the fluid is slowly reabsorbed. The edema in urticaria is found in the superficial dermis. Lesions of angioedema are less well demarcated. The edema in angioedema is found in the deep dermis or subcutaneous/submucosal locations. The differential diagnosis of hives is found in Box 6-1.

CLINICAL PRESENTATION. Lesions vary in size from the 2- to 4-mm edematous papules of cholinergic urticaria to giant hives, a single lesion of which may cover an extremity. They may be round or oval; when confluent, they become polycyclic (Figures 6-1 to 6-3). A portion of the border either may not form or may be reabsorbed, giving the appearance of incomplete rings (see Figure 6-2). Hives may be uniformly red or white, or the edematous border may be red and the remainder of the surface white. This variation in color is usually present in superficial hives; thicker plaques have a uniform color (Figures 6-1 to 6-5).

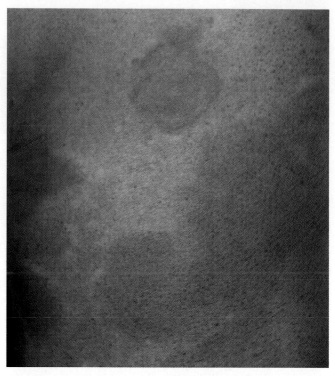

Figure 6-1 Hives. The most characteristic presentation is uniformly red edematous plaques surrounded by a faint white halo. These superficial lesions occur from transudation of fluid into the dermis.

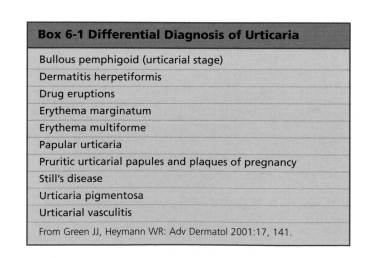

Box 6-1 Differential Diagnosis of Urticaria
Bullous pemphigoid (urticarial stage)
Dermatitis herpetiformis
Drug eruptions
Erythema marginatum
Erythema multiforme
Papular urticaria
Pruritic urticarial papules and plaques of pregnancy
Still's disease
Urticaria pigmentosa
Urticarial vasculitis
From Green JJ, Heymann WR: Adv Dermatol 2001:17, 141.

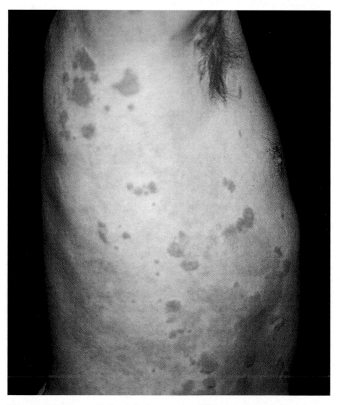

Figure 6-2 Hives. Urticarial plaques in different stages of formation.

HIVES

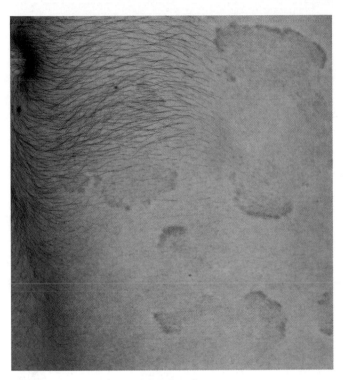

Figure 6-3 Polycyclic pattern.

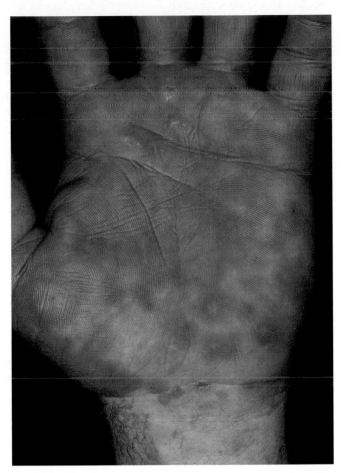

Figure 6-4 The entire palm is affected and is greatly swollen. The lesions resemble those of erythema.

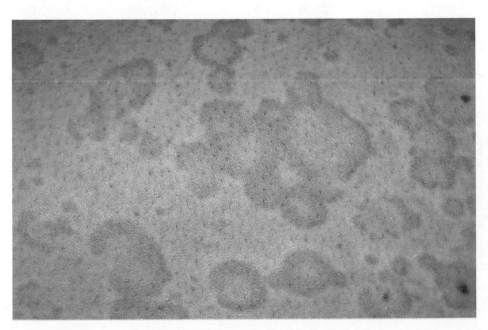

Figure 6-5 Superficial hives vary in color.

Hives may be surrounded by a clear or red halo. Thicker plaques that result from massive transudation of fluid into the dermis and subcutaneous tissue are referred to as *angioedema*. These thick, firm plaques, like typical hives, may occur on any skin surface, but typically involve the lips, larynx (causing hoarseness or a sore throat), and mucosa of the gastrointestinal (GI) tract (causing abdominal pain) (Figures 6-6 and 6-7). Bullae or purpura may appear in areas of intense swelling. Purpura and scaling may result as the lesions of urticarial vasculitis clear. Hives usually have a haphazard distribution, but those elicited by physical stimuli have characteristic features and distribution.

SYMPTOMS. Hives itch. The intensity varies, and some patients with a widespread eruption may experience little itching. Pruritus is milder in deep hives (angioedema) because the edema occurs in areas where there are fewer sensory nerve endings than there are near the surface of the skin.

CLINICAL CLASSIFICATION OF URTICARIA/ANGIOEDEMA. The clinical classification of urticaria and angioedema is found in Box 6-2. Urticaria can be provoked by immunologic and non-immunologic mechanisms, as well as physical stimuli, skin contact, or small vessel vasculitis. Physical and ordinary urticaria may coexist. Angioedema occurs with or without urticaria. Angioedema without urticaria may indicate a C1-esterase inhibitor deficiency. The duration of hives is also an important diagnostic feature (Box 6-3).

Box 6-2 Clinical Classification of Urticaria/Angioedema
Ordinary urticaria (recurrent or episodic urticaria not in the categories below)
Physical urticaria (defined by the triggering stimulus)
Adrenergic urticaria
Aquagenic urticaria
Cholinergic urticaria
Cold urticaria
Delayed pressure urticaria
Dermographism
Exercise-induced anaphylaxis
Localized heat urticaria
Solar urticaria
Vibratory angioedema
Contact urticaria (induced by biologic or chemical skin contact)
Urticarial vasculitis (defined by vasculitis as shown by skin biopsy specimen)
Angioedema (without wheals)

From Brattan CEH: J Am Acad Dermatol 2002, 46:645.

Box 6-3 Duration of Hives	
Type of Urticaria	**Duration**
Ordinary and delayed pressure	4-36 hours
Physical (except delayed pressure)	30 min-2 hours
Contact (may have a delayed phase)	1-2 hours
Urticarial vasculitis	1-7 days

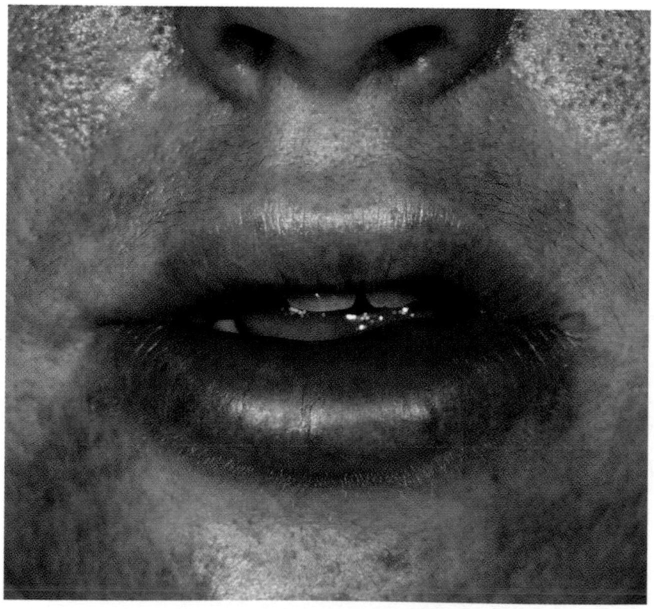

Figure 6-6 Angioedema is a deeper, larger hive than those shown in Figures 6-1 through 6-3. It is caused by transudation of fluid into the dermis and subcutaneous tissue. The lip is a common site.

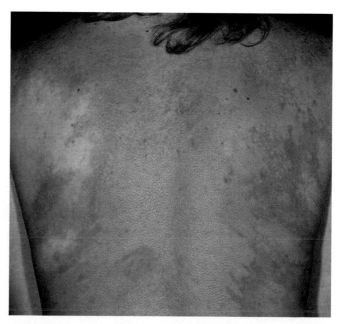

Figure 6-7 Angioedema. Massive swelling of the entire central area of the back.

Pathophysiology

Histamine

Histamine is the most important mediator of urticaria. Histamine is produced and stored in mast cells. There are several mechanisms for histamine release via mast cell surface receptors. A variety of immunologic, nonimmunologic, physical, and chemical stimuli may be responsible for the degranulation of mast cell granules and the release of histamine into the surrounding tissue and circulation. About one third of patients with chronic urticaria have circulating functional histamine-releasing IgG autoantibodies that bind to the high-affinity IgE receptor (Fc epsilon RI). Release of mast cell mediators can cause inflammation and accumulation and activation of other cells, including eosinophils, neutrophils, and possibly basophils. Histamine causes endothelial cell contraction, which allows vascular fluid to leak between the cells through the vessel wall, contributing to tissue edema and wheal formation.

When injected into skin, histamine produces the "triple response" of Lewis, the features of which are local erythema (vasodilation), the flare characterized by erythema beyond the border of the local erythema, and a wheal produced from leakage of fluid from the postcapillary venule. Histamine induces vascular changes by a number of mechanisms (Figure 6-8). Blood vessels contain two (and possibly more) receptors for histamine. The two most studied are designated H_1 and H_2.

H_1 RECEPTORS. H_1 receptors, when stimulated by histamine, cause an axon reflex, vasodilation, and pruritus. Acting through H_1 receptors, histamine causes smooth-muscle contraction in the respiratory and gastrointestinal tracts and pruritus and sneezing by sensory-nerve stimulation. They are blocked by the vast majority of clinically available antihistamines called H_1 antagonists (e.g., chlorpheniramine), which occupy the receptor site and prevent attachment of histamine.

H_2 RECEPTORS. When H_2 receptors are stimulated, vasodilation occurs. H_2 receptors are also present on the mast cell membrane surface and, when stimulated, further inhibit the production of histamine. Activation of H_2 receptors alone increases gastric acid secretion. Cimetidine (Tagamet), ranitidine (Zantac), and famotidine (Pepcid) are H_2 blocking agents (antihistamines). H_2 receptors are present at other sites. Activation of both H_1 and H_2 receptors causes hypotension, tachycardia, flushing, and headache. The H_2 blocking agents are used most often to suppress gastric acid secretion. They are used occasionally, usually in combination with an H_1 blocking agent, to treat urticaria.

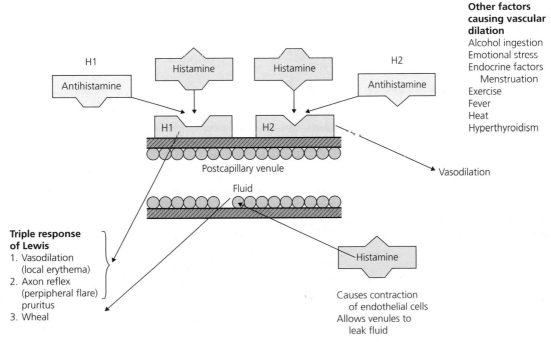

Figure 6-8 Physiology of histamine release.

Box 6-4 Etiologic Classification of Urticaria

Foods

Fish, shellfish, nuts, eggs, chocolate, strawberries, tomatoes, pork, cow's milk, cheese, wheat, yeast

Food additives

Salicylates, dyes such as tartrazine, benzoates, penicillin Aspartame (NutraSweet) probably does not cause hives* Sulfites

Drugs

Penicillin, aspirin, sulfonamides, and drugs that cause a non-immunologic release of histamine (e.g., morphine, codeine, polymyxin, dextran, curare, quinine)

Infections

Chronic bacterial infections (e.g., sinus, dental, chest, gallbladder, urinary tract), *Campylobacter enteritis,* fungal infections (dermatophytosis, candidiasis), viral infections (hepatitis B prodromal reaction, infectious mononucleosis, coxsackie), protozoal and helminth infections (intestinal worms, malaria)

Inhalants

Pollens, mold spores, animal dander, house dust, aerosols, volatile chemicals

Internal disease

Serum sickness, systemic lupus erythematosus, hyperthyroidism, autoimmune thyroid disease, carcinomas, lymphomas, juvenile rheumatoid arthritis (Still's disease), leukocytoclastic vasculitis, polycythemia vera (acne urticaria–urticarial papule surmounted by a vesicle), rheumatic fever, some blood transfusion reactions

Physical stimuli (physical urticarias)

Dermographism, pressure urticaria, cholinergic urticaria, exercise-induced anaphylactic syndrome, solar urticaria, cold urticaria, heat, vibratory, water (aquagenic)

Nonimmunologic contact urticaria

Plants (nettles), animals (caterpillars, jellyfish), medications (cinnamic aldehyde, compound 48/80, dimethyl sulfoxide)

Immunologic or uncertain mechanism contact urticaria

Ammonium persulfate used in hair bleaches, chemicals, foods, textiles, wood, saliva, cosmetics, perfumes, bacitracin

Skin diseases

Urticaria pigmentosa (mastocytosis), dermatitis herpetiformis, pemphigoid, amyloidosis

Hormones

Pregnancy, premenstrual flare-ups (progesterone)

Genetic, autosomal dominant (all rare)

Hereditary angioedema, cholinergic urticaria with progressive nerve deafness, amyloidosis of the kidney, familial cold urticaria, vibratory urticaria

*Geha, R, Buckley CE, et al: J Allergy Clin Immunol 1993; 92:513.

Initial Evaluation of All Patients With Urticaria

1. Determine by skin examination that the patient actually has urticaria and not bites.
2. Rule out the presence of physical urticaria to avoid an unnecessarily lengthy evaluation. Stroking the arm with the wood end of a cotton-tipped applicator will test for dermographism.
3. Determine whether hives are acute or chronic. The difference in duration has been arbitrarily set at 6 weeks. Acute urticaria involves episodes of urticaria that last less than 6 weeks. Chronic urticaria consists of recurrent episodes of widespread urticaria present for longer than 6 weeks.
4. Review the known causes of urticaria listed in Box 6-4 (Etiologic Classification of Urticaria). Knowledge of the etiologic factors helps to direct the history and physical examination.

Acute Urticaria

If the urticaria has been present for less than 6 weeks, it is considered acute (Figure 6-9). The evaluation and management of acute urticaria are outlined in Box 6-5. A history and physical examination should be performed, and laboratory studies are selected to investigate abnormalities.[2] Histamine release that is induced by allergens (e.g., drugs, foods, or pollens) and mediated by IgE is a common cause of acute urticaria, and particular attention should be paid to these factors during the initial evaluation. There are no routine laboratory studies for the evaluation of acute urticaria. Once all possible causes are eliminated, the patient is treated with antihistamines to suppress the hives and stop the itching. Because urticaria clears spontaneously in most patients, an extensive workup is not advised during the early weeks of an urticarial eruption.[3,4]

CHILDREN WITH HIVES. Food origin is important in the etiology of infantile urticaria. In one series it accounted for 62% of patients, more often than drug etiology (22%), physical urticaria (8%), and contact urticaria (8%).[5]

Etiology of acute urticaria

Acute urticaria is IgE-mediated, complement-mediated, or nonimmune-mediated.

IgE-MEDIATED REACTIONS. Type I hypersensitivity reactions are probably responsible for most cases of acute urticaria. Circulating antigens such as foods, drugs, or inhalants interact with cell membrane–bound IgE to release histamine. Food allergies are present in 8% of children less than 3 years of age and in 2% of adults.[6] Food allergies are the most common cause of anaphylaxis. Yellow jackets are the most common cause of insect sting induced urticaria/anaphylaxis in the United States. Latex-induced urticaria is an IgE-mediated reaction.[7]

COMPLEMENT-MEDIATED, OR IMMUNE-COMPLEX MEDIATED, ACUTE URTICARIA. Complement-mediated acute urticaria can be precipitated by administration of whole blood, plasma, immunoglobulins, drugs, and insect stings. Type III hypersensitivity reactions (Arthus reactions) occur with deposition of insoluble immune complexes in vessel walls. The complexes are composed of IgG or IgM with an antigen such as a drug. Urticaria occurs when the trapped complexes activate complement to cleave the anaphylotoxins C5a and C3a from C5 and C3. C5a and C3a are potent releasers of histamine from mast cells. Serum sickness (fevers, urticaria, lymphadenopathy, arthralgias, and myalgias), urticarial vasculitis, and systemic lupus erythematosus are diseases in which hives may occur as a result of immune complex deposition.

NONIMMUNOLOGIC RELEASE OF HISTAMINE. Pharmacologic mediators such as acetylcholine, opiates, polymyxin B, and strawberries react directly with cell membrane–bound mediators to release histamine. Aspirin/NSAIDs cause a nonimmunologic release of histamine. Patients with aspirin/NSAID sensitivity may have a history of allergic rhinitis or asthma. Urticaria may be caused by histamine-containing foods. Fish of the *Scombroidea* family (tuna, mackerel, bonita) accumulate histamine during spoilage. The mechanism of radiocontrast-related urticaria/anaphylaxis is unknown. The incidence varies from 3.1% with newer, lower osmolar agents to 12.7% with older, higher osmolar agents.[8] Atopy is a risk factor for urticaria developing after radiocontrast exposure. The physical urticarias may be induced by both direct stimulation of cell membrane receptors and immunologic mechanisms.

Box 6-5 Acute Urticaria—Evaluation and Management

History and physical examination

1. Ask the patient if he or she knows what causes the hives. In many instances, the patient will have determined the cause.
2. Take a history. See Box 6-4 (**Etiologic Classification Of Urticaria**) for specific etiologies. Drugs are common causes in adults. Viral respiratory infections and streptococcal infections are common causes in children.
3. Perform a physical examination.
4. Stroke the arm to test for dermagraphism.

If the etiology is not determined by history, physical examination, and stroking the arm, order laboratory tests.

Laboratory tests

1. CBC with differential, erythrocyte sedimentation rate (ESR), liver function studies (LFTs), and urinalysis.
2. The history and physical examination may provide evidence that warrants additional tests. Consider: testing for hepatitis A, B, C; infectious mononucleosis; thyroid function tests; thyroid antibodies; and anti-nuclear antibodies (ANA).

Consider allergen testing

1. Skin tests: foods, drugs, aeroallergens, insect venom, natural rubber. Except for penicillin, antibiotics have a high false-positive rate with skin prick testing.
2. Radioallergosorbent tests (RAST) for penicillin, succinylcholine, natural rubber latex.
3. Food testing. Food diaries and elimination diets.
4. Oral challenge testing for food and food additives.

Management

1. Avoid specific allergens.
2. Treat with oral H_1 antagonists.
3. Add H_2 antagonists for resistant cases.[9]
4. Anaphylaxis—subcutaneous epinephrine with or without parenteral H_1 and H_2 antihistamines (e.g., 50 mg of diphenhydramine and 50 mg of ranitidine).[10] Systemic corticosteroids are sometimes useful.
5. Intravenous contrast media reactions—pretreat with H^1 antagonists and corticosteroids.
6. Latex allergic patients—prophylactic administration of corticosteroids prior to surgery.[7]
7. Insect venom reaction—desensitization, preloaded syringes of epinephrine.

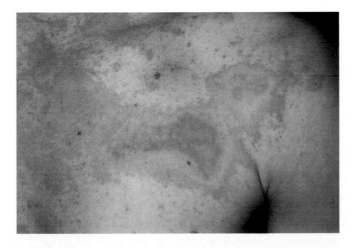

Figure 6-9 Acute urticaria. Wheals vary from a few millimeters to large, continuous plaques that may cover a large area. The plaques have smooth surfaces with curved or polycyclic borders. The degree of erythema varies. Central clearing occurs in expanding lesions.

Chronic Urticaria

Patients who have a history of hives lasting for 6 or more weeks are classified as having chronic urticaria (CU). The etiology is often unclear. The morphology is similar to that of acute urticaria (Figure 6-10). CU is more common in middle-aged women and is infrequent in children. Individual lesions remain for less than 24 hours, and any skin surface can be affected. Itching is worse at night. Respiratory and gastrointestinal complaints are rare. Angioedema occurs in 50% of cases. Angioedema with chronic urticaria differs from hereditary angioedema in that it rarely affects the larynx. CU patients may experience physical urticaria. Symptoms continue for weeks, months, or years. Pressure urticaria, chronic urticaria, and angioedema frequently occur in the same patient. In one study, delayed pressure urticaria was present in 37% of patients with chronic urticaria.[10] Aspirin/NSAIDs, penicillin, angiotensin-converting enzyme (ACE) inhibitors, opiates, alcohol, febrile illnesses, and stress exacerbate urticaria.

Pathogenesis

Urticaria is induced by histamine released from mast cells and basophils. Acute urticaria occurs when mast cells are activated by allergens through cross-linking of cell-surface–bound IgE. The mechanism for histamine release in some patients with chronic urticaria is different.

About one third of patients with chronic urticaria have circulating functional histamine-releasing IgG autoantibodies that bind to the high-affinity IgE receptor (Fc epsilon RIa) or, less commonly, to IgE that resides on the surface of mast cells and basophils.[11,12]

Autoantibody-induced cross-linking of these IgE receptors may be an important mechanism in the pathogenesis of chronic urticaria.[13]

Chronic urticaria has been associated with antithyroid autoantibodies. Most cases of chronic urticaria may ultimately be considered an autoimmune disease rather than an allergic disease.[14]

The evaluation and management of chronic urticaria is outlined in Box 6-6 and in the diagram below.

The patient must understand that the course of this disease is unpredictable; it may last for months or years. During the evaluation, the patient should be assured that antihistamines will decrease discomfort. The patient should also be told that although the evaluation may be lengthy and is often unrewarding, in most cases the disease ends spontaneously. Patients who understand the nature of this disease do not become discouraged so easily, nor are they as apt to go from physician to physician seeking a cure.

There are many studies in the literature on chronic urticaria.[17,18] Most demonstrate that if the cause is not found after investigation of abnormalities elicited during the history and physical examination, there is little chance that it will be determined. It is tempting to order laboratory tests such as antinuclear antibody (ANA) levels and stool examinations for ova and parasites in an effort to be thorough, but results of studies do not support this approach. There are certain tests and procedures that might be considered when the initial evaluation has proved unrewarding.

Box 6-6 Chronic Urticaria—Evaluation and Management

1. CU is a diagnosis of exclusion

Determine that lesions are hives and not insect bites (see Table 6-1 for differential diagnosis). Individual bite lesion lasts longer than 24 hours. Hives last less than 24 hours. Most urticarial plaques are larger than 2 cm. Stroke the patient's arm to rule out dermographism.

2. Take a history

Exact time of onset
Medication
Food and drink

Duration
Acute—days to a few weeks
Chronic—more than 6 weeks

Time of appearance
Time of day
Time of year
  Constant—food, internal disease
  Seasonal—inhalant allergy

Environment
Exposure to pollens, chemicals
  Home—clear while at work or on vacation
  Work—contact or inhalation of chemicals

Appearance after physical stimuli (physical urticaria)

Scratching, pressure, exercise, sun exposure, cold

Associated with arthralgia and fever
Juvenile rheumatoid arthritis, rheumatic fever, serum sickness, systemic lupus erythematosus, urticarial vasculitis, viral hepatitis

Duration of individual lesion
Less than 1 hour—physical urticarias, typical hives
Less than 24 hours—typical hives
More than 25 hours—urticarial vasculitis; scaling and purpura as lesions resolve

3. Physical examination

Stroke the arm to test for dermagraphism, and rule out other types of physical urticaria.

Size
  Papular—cholinergic urticaria, bites
  Plaque—most cases
Thickness
  Superficial—most cases
  Deep—angioedema

Distribution
Generalized—ingestants, inhalants, internal disease
Localized—physical urticarias, contact urticaria

Sources of infection
  Sinus and gum infections
  Cystitis, vaginitis, prostatitis

Dental examination by dentist
  Fix carious teeth
  Treat periodontal disease

Internal disease, thyroid examination, gallbladder symptoms

If the etiology is not determined by history, physical examination, and stroking the arm, then consider ordering laboratory tests.

Laboratory tests

1. Initial screening tests are CBC with differential, erythrocyte sedimentation rate (ESR), liver function studies (LFTs), urinalysis, and studies to confirm findings of history and physical examination.

2. Screening thyroid function tests and tests for thyroid autoimmunity (thyroid microsomal and thyroglobulin antibodies), especially in women, or in those patients with a family history of thyroid disease or other autoimmune diseases.

3. Eosinophilia suggests drug, food, or parasitic causes.

4. Leukocytosis suggests chronic infection.

5. ANA, ESR for patients with connective tissue disease symptoms.

6. Sinus radiographs have been advocated.[2]

7. Oral challenge testing for food additives.

8. Food testing. Food diaries and elimination diets.

9. Lesion biopsy for hives lasting longer than 36 hours (R/O urticarial vasculitis), fever, arthralgias, elevated ESR, petechia.

10. C4 only for patients with angioedema (not for patients with hives).

Management (see also Box 6-8)

1. Second-generation H$_1$ antihistamines: cetirizine (Zyrtec), loratadine (Claritin), fexofenadine (Allegra). Higher doses than suggested by the manufacturers may be required (e.g., 20- to 40-mg of cetirizine each day instead of 10 mg). Sedative side effects increase with higher dosages.

2. Add H$_2$ antagonists if H$_1$ agents do not provide effective control.

3. Hydroxyzine or doxepin are more sedating and can be added at nighttime. Doxepin can interact with other drugs that are metabolized by the cytochrome p450 system (ketoconazole, itraconazole, erythromycin, clarithromycin, etc.).

4. Systemic steroids (short courses) may be used to provide temporary relief.

5. Stop vitamins, laxatives, antacids, toothpaste, cigarettes, cosmetics and all toiletries, chewing gum, household cleaning solutions, aerosols.

6. Stop fruits, tomatoes, nuts, eggs, shellfish, chocolate, alcohol, milk, cheese, bread, diet drinks, junk food.

7. Consider a highly restricted diet such as lamb, rice, and salt (rarely effective).

8. Consider empiric treatment with antibiotics.

9. Leukotriene receptor antagonists—zafirlukast (Accolate 10 mg, 20 mg) and montelukast (Singulair 10 mg/day) may be effective, especially in combination with antihistamines. Leukotriene receptor antagonists may prevent the severe urticaria/angioedema exacerbations that follow the use of NSAIDs in some patients with chronic urticaria.[15]

10. Cyclosporine—patients with severe unremitting chronic urticaria that responded poorly to antihistamines responded to cyclosporine 4 mg/kg daily in combination with cetirizine 20 mg daily.[16]

RULE OUT PHYSICAL URTICARIAS. Unrecognized physical urticarias (see p. 142) may account for approximately 10% of all cases of chronic urticaria. In one large study physical urticarias were present in 71% of patients with chronic urticaria: 22% had immediate dermographism, 37% had delayed pressure urticaria, 11% had cholinergic urticaria, and 2% had cold urticaria.[10]

The presence of physical urticaria should be ruled out by history and appropriate tests (see Table 6-1) before a lengthy evaluation and treatment program is undertaken. Dermographism is the most common type of physical urticaria; it begins suddenly following drug therapy or a viral illness, lasts for months or years, and clears spontaneously. Wheals that appear after the patient's arm is stroked prove the diagnosis.

THYROID AUTOIMMUNE DISEASE. There is a significant association between chronic urticaria and autoimmune thyroid disease (Hashimoto's thyroiditis, Graves' disease, toxic multinodular goiter).[19,20] Thyroid autoimmunity was found in 12% of 140 consecutively seen patients with chronic urticaria in one series; 88% were women.[21] Most patients with thyroid autoimmunity are asymptomatic and have thyroid function that is normal or only slightly abnormal. Guidelines for evaluation and treatment of thyroid related urticaria are presented in Box 6-7.

CHANGE OF ENVIRONMENT. Because the environment consists of numerous antigens, patients should consider a trial period of 1 or 2 weeks of separation from home and work, preferably with a geographic change.

HIGHLY RESTRICTED DIET. A highly restricted diet may be attempted. Patients are fed lamb, rice, sugar, salt, and water for 5 days. The occurrence of new hives after 3 days suggests that foods have no role. If hives disappear, a new food is reintroduced every other day until hives appear.

TREATMENT OF OCCULT INFECTIONS. Patients occasionally respond to antibiotics even in the absence of clinical infection.[23]

SKIN BIOPSY. Urticarial reactions display a wide spectrum of changes, ranging from a mild, mixed dermal inflammatory response to true vasculitis. Patients with hives that are characteristic of urticarial vasculitis should have a biopsy taken of the urticarial plaque. These hives burn rather than itch and last longer than 24 hours.

Dermal edema and dilated lymphatic and vascular capillaries occur. Increased numbers of neutrophils and eosinophils occur in patients with acute urticaria and in those with delayed pressure urticaria. Mast cell numbers are higher in the dermis of lesional and uninvolved skin of all patients with urticaria. Mononuclear infiltrates are more pronounced in cold urticaria and chronic urticaria.[24]

Box 6-7 Guidelines of Evaluation and Treatment of Thyroid Related Chronic Urticaria[22]

1. Screen for thyroid autoimmunity by testing for thyroid microsomal and thyroglobulin antibodies, especially in women (female/male ratio was 7:1), or in those patients with a family history of thyroid disease or other autoimmune disorders.

2. The administration of thyroid hormone may alleviate chronic urticaria and/or angioedema in selected patients.
   If patients with documented thyroid autoimmunity have been unresponsive to standard therapy for chronic urticaria and/or angioedema, consider the use of levothyroxine if the patients are hypothyroid or euthyroid. An appropriate initial dose is 1.7 µg/kg per day.

3. The level of thyroid-stimulating hormone should be monitored by weeks 4 to 6 after the initiation of therapy, being kept in the low normal range, to ensure that the patient is not becoming hyperthyroid.

4. If there has been no response of the chronic urticaria and/or angioedema by week 8 of administration, levothyroxine should be discontinued.

5. After being in remission for at least 1 to 2 months, levothyroxine should be discontinued. Should the chronic urticaria and/or angioedema recur, the hormone may be readministered, with an expectation that most patients will again be responsive to treatment.

Heymann, WR: J Am Acad Dermatol 1999; 40 (2Pt1):229.

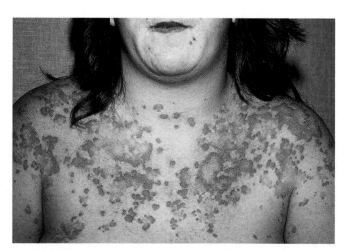

Figure 6-10 Chronic urticaria. Wheals may have the same configuration and intensity as acute urticaria. This patient has red plaques with sharply defined round, oval and annular borders. The central clearing is highly characteristic of urticaria.

Treatment of Urticaria

Box 6-8 below lists the medications used to treat urticaria.

Approach to treatment

Nonsedating H₁ antihistamines (e.g., Allegra 180 mg qd) are the first choice for treatment. Older sedating H₁ antihistamines are more effective and so should be used to treat severe urticaria (e.g., 100 to 200 mg of hydroxyzine or diphenhydramine per day). For patients with severe angioedema (involving swelling of the face, tongue, and pharynx), diphenhydramine is particularly effective.

Patients become accustomed to the sedating effects after about a week, but their performance on driving tests remains impaired. H₂-receptor antagonists have very few side effects

Box 6-8 Medications for Urticaria				
Drug	Initial dose (adult)	Maximal dose* (adult)	Liquid formulation	Tablet formulation
H1-receptor antagonists				
Nonsedating*				
Fexofenadine (Allegra)	180 mg qd	180 mg bid	—	30 mg, 60 mg, 180 mg
Desloratadine (Clarinex)	5 mg	10 mg		5 mg
Loratadine (Claritin)	10 mg qd	20 mg bid	5 mg/5ml	10 mg
Cetirizine (Zyrtec)	10 mg qd	10 mg bid	5 mg/5ml	5 mg, 10 mg
Sedating				
Hydroxyzine (Atarax)	10 mg qid	50 mg qid	10 mg/5 ml susp. 25 mg/5ml	10mg, 25 mg, 50 mg, 100 mg
Diphenhydramine (Benadryl)	25 mg bid	50 mg qid	Elixir 12.5 mg/5ml syrup 6.25 mg/5 ml	25, 50 mg 12.5 chew tab
Cyproheptadine (Periactin)	4 mg qid	8 mg qid	2 mg/5ml	8 mg
H2-receptor antagonists				
Cimetidine (Tagamet)	400 mg bid	800 mg bid	300 mg/5cc	200mg, 300mg, 400 mg, 800 mg
Ranitidine (Zantac)	150 mg bid	300 mg bid	75 mg/5cc	150 mg, 300 mg
Famotidine (Pepcid)	20 mg bid	40 mg bid	40 mg/5cc	20 mg, 40 mg
H1- and H2- receptor antagonists				
Doxepin (Sinequan)	10 mg qid	50 mg qid	10 mg/ml	10 mg, 25 mg, 50 mg, 75 mg, 100 mg, 150 mg
Corticosteroids				
Prednisone	20 mg qod with gradual tapering	Many other dose schedules	5 mg/5 ml	2.5 mg, 5 mg, 10 mg, 20 mg, 50 mg
Methylprednisolone (Medrol)	16 mg qod with gradual tapering	Many other dose schedules	—	2 mg, 4 mg, 8 mg, 16 mg, 24 mg, 32 mg
Leukotriene antagonists		—	—	
Zafirlukast (Accolate)	20 mg bid	—	—	10 mg, 20 mg
Montelukast (Singulair)	10 mg qd	—	—	4 mg chewable, 5 mg chewable, 10 mg
Epinephrine	Injection			
• Ana-Guard (1:1,000)	0.3 mL/dose SC			
• EpiPen (1:1,000)	0.3 mg/dose			
• EpiPen Jr (1:2,000)	Children <12 yr: 0.15 mg/dose			
Immunotherapy				
Cyclosporine	2-3 mg /kg daily	4-6 mg /kg daily	100 mg/ml	25 mg, 50 mg, 100 mg
Methotrexate	2.5 mg PO bid for 3 days of the week	5 mg PO bid for 3 days of the week	25 mg/ml	2.5 mg

*Higher dosages than recommended by the manufacturer may be required for maximum therapeutic effect.

and may be useful as adjunctive therapy. Leukotriene antagonists are considered safe and are worth trying, but severe disease may require prednisone; many regimens have been suggested.

One approach is to start prednisone at 15 to 20 mg as a single morning dose every other day and gradually taper to 2.5 to 5.0 mg every 3 weeks, depending on the patient's response, and discontinue after 4 to 5 months.[25] Side effects are minimized with the use of dietary discretion and exercise. Some patients require a combination of all of these medications.

Patients who have no response to any of these approaches may respond to immunotherapy with 200 to 300 mg of cyclosporine per day or methotrexate.[25]

Antihistamines

For the majority of patients, acute and chronic urticaria may be controlled with antihistamines.

MECHANISM OF ACTION. Antihistamines control urticaria by inhibiting vasodilation and vessel fluid loss. Antihistamines do not block the release of histamine. If histamine has been released before an antihistamine is taken, the receptor sites will be occupied and the antihistamine will have no effect.

INITIATION OF TREATMENT. Antihistamines are the preferred initial treatment for urticaria and angioedema. Cetirizine, loratadine, or fexofenadine are first-line agents and are given once daily. Higher doses than suggested by the manufacturers may be required; see the box on medications for urticaria. Patients with daytime and nighttime symptoms can be treated with combination therapy. These patients can be treated with a low-sedating antihistamine in the morning (e.g., loratadine 10 mg or fexofenadine 180 mg, or cetirizine 10 to 20 mg) and a sedating antihistamine (e.g., hydrolyzing 25 mg) in the evening. Cetirizine can be mildly sedating. Doxepin is an alternative bedtime medication especially for anxious or depressed patients. The initial dose is 10 to 25 mg. Gradually increase the dose up to 75 mg for optimal control. Some patients with chronic urticaria respond when an H_2 receptor antagonist such as cimetidine is added to conventional antihistamines. This may be worth trying in refractory cases.

SIDE EFFECTS. Antihistamines are structurally similar to atropine; therefore they produce atropine-like peripheral and central anticholinergic effects such as dry mouth, blurred vision, constipation, and dizziness. First-generation antihistamines (H_1-receptor antagonists) such as chlorpheniramine, hydroxyzine, and diphenhydramine cross the blood-brain barrier and produce sedation. There is marked individual variation in response and side effects. Antihistamines may produce stimulation in children, especially in those ages 6 through 12.

LONG-TERM ADMINISTRATION. Prolonged use of H_1 antagonists does not lead to autoinduction of hepatic metabolism. The efficacy of H_1-receptor blockade does not decrease with prolonged use. Tolerance of adverse central nervous system effects may or may not develop.

H_1 AND H_2 ANTIHISTAMINES. The majority of available antihistamines are H_1 antagonists (i.e., they compete for the H_1 receptor sites). Cimetidine, ranitidine, and famotidine are H_2 antagonists that are used primarily for the treatment of gastric hyperacidity. Approximately 85% of histamine receptors in the skin are the H_1 subtype, and 15% are H_2 receptors. The addition of an H_2-receptor antagonist to an H_1-receptor antagonist augments the inhibition of a histamine-induced wheal-and-flare reaction once H_1-receptor blockade has been maximized. It would seem that the combination of H_1 and H_2 antihistamines would provide optimum effects. The results of studies are conflicting but generally show that the combination is not much more effective than an H_1 blocking agent used alone.

FIRST-GENERATION (SEDATING) H_1 ANTIHISTAMINES. The first-generation H_1 antihistamines are divided into five classes (see Box 6-8). They are lipophilic, cross the blood-brain barrier and cause sedation, weight gain, and atropine-like complications including dry mouth, blurred vision, constipation, and dysuria. Metabolism occurs via the hepatic cytochrome P-450 (CYP) system. In patients with liver disease, or in patients who are taking CY-P 3A4 inhibitors such as erythromycin or ketoconazole, the plasma half-life may be prolonged. The H_1 antagonists suppress the wheal caused by histamine. Antihistamines given during or after the onset of a hive are less effective. They prevent wheals rather than treat them.

SECOND-GENERATION (LOW-SEDATING) H_1 ANTIHISTAMINES. The second-generation antihistamines are not lipophilic and do not readily cross the blood-brain barrier. They cause little sedation and little or no atropine-like activity.

FEXOFENADINE (ALLEGRA). Fexofenadine in a single dose of 180 mg daily or 60 mg twice daily is the recommended dosage for treating urticaria. Dosage adjustment is not necessary in the elderly or in patients with mild renal or hepatic impairment. Fexofenadine may offer the best combination of effectiveness and safety of all of the low-sedating antihistamines. A dose that is higher than recommended may be required.

CETIRIZINE (ZYRTEC). Cetirizine is a metabolite of the first-generation H_1 antihistamine hydroxyzine. Some patients notice drowsiness after a 10-mg dose. The adult dose is 10 mg daily. A reduced dosage (5 mg daily) is recommended in patients with chronic renal or hepatic impairment. No drug interactions are reported, and there is no cardiotoxicity. A dose higher than recommended may be required.

LORATADINE (CLARITIN). Loratadine is long-acting. A 10-mg dose suppresses whealing for up to 12 hours; suppression lasts longer after a larger dosage. A reduced dosage may be required in patients with chronic liver or renal disease. There are no significant adverse drug interactions. A special form of the medication, Reditabs (10 mg), rapidly disintegrates in the mouth. A dose higher than recommended may be required.

DESLORATADINE (CLARINEX). Desloratadine is an active metabolite of loratadine. A 5-mg dose each day is effective. There is no evidence that it offers any advantage over loratadine.

TRICYCLIC ANTIHISTAMINES (DOXEPIN). Tricyclic antidepressants are potent blockers of histamine H_1 and H_2 receptors. The most potent is doxepin. When taken in dosages between 10 and 25 mg three times a day, doxepin is effective for the treatment of chronic idiopathic urticaria. Few side effects occur at this low dosage. Higher dosages may be tolerated if taken in the evening. Doxepin is a good alternative for patients with chronic urticaria who are not controlled with conventional antihistamines[26,27] and for patients who suffer anxiety and depression associated with chronic urticaria. Lethargy is commonly observed but diminishes with continued use. Dry mouth and constipation are also commonly observed. Doxepin can interact with other drugs that are metabolized by the cytochrome p450 system (e.g., ketoconazole, itraconazole, erythromycin, clarithromycin).

Epinephrine

Severe urticaria or angioedema requires epinephrine. Epinephrine solutions have a rapid onset of effect but a short duration of action. The dosage for adults is a 1:1000 solution (0.2 to 1.0 ml) given either subcutaneously or intramuscularly; the initial dose is usually 0.3 ml. The epinephrine suspensions provide both a prompt and prolonged effect (up to 8 hours). For adults, 0.1 to 0.3 ml of the 1:200 suspension is given subcutaneously.

Oral corticosteroids

Many patients with chronic urticaria and angioedema will have little response to even a combination of H_1- and H_2-receptor blockers. Oral corticosteroids should be considered for these refractory cases.[28] Prednisone 40 mg per day given in a single morning dose or 20 mg bid is effective in most cases. Another approach is to prescribe thirty 20-mg tablets. The patient receives 5 days each of 60 mg, 40 mg, and 20 mg, and the medication is taken once each morning. Others will respond to prednisone 20 mg qod with a gradual taper.

Immunotherapy

Histamine release from mast cells in some patients with chronic urticaria is the result of an autoimmune disease, mediated by autoantibodies to the alpha-subunit of the high-affinity IgE receptor on mast cells and basophils. Removal of these autoantibodies by plasmapheresis, or treatment with intravenous immunoglobulins[29] may cause clinical remission. Cyclosporine A is effective in some patients probably because of a mast cell "stabilizing" effect, leading to reduced release of histamine and other mediators.

CYCLOSPORINE. Cyclosporine might be an effective alternative in some chronic urticaria patients unresponsive to conventional treatments.[16,30] This provides further evidence for a role of histamine-releasing autoantibodies in the pathogenesis of this chronic urticaria. Patients with severe unremitting disease who respond poorly to antihistamines may respond to 4 mg/kg daily of cyclosporine for 4 weeks. Patients requiring initially high doses of glucocorticosteroids and with a long clinical history are less amenable to cyclosporine treatment.[31]

METHOTREXATE. Methotrexate may be considered in resistant cases of urticaria.[32] All symptoms and signs resolved after two weekly cycles of methotrexate (2.5 mg orally twice a day for 3 days of the week).[33]

TOPICAL MEASURES. Itching is controlled with tepid showering, tepid oatmeal baths (Aveeno), cooling lotions that contain menthol (Sarna lotion) and topical pramoxine lotions (Itch-X). Avoid factors that enhance pruritus (e.g., aspirin, drinking alcohol, wearing of tight elasticized apparel, or coarse woolen fabrics).

Physical Urticarias

Physical urticarias are induced by physical and external stimuli, and they typically affect young adults. More than one type of physical urticaria can occur in an individual. Provocative testing confirms the diagnosis. During the initial examination, the physician should determine whether the hives are elicited by physical stimuli (Table 6-1). Patients with these distinctive hives may be spared a detailed laboratory evaluation; they simply require an explanation of their condition and its treatment. Unrecognized physical urticarias may account for approximately 20% of all cases of chronic urticaria. A major distinguishing feature of the physical urticarias is that attacks are brief, lasting only 30 to 60 minutes. In typical urticaria, individual lesions last from hours to a few days. The one exception among physical urticarias is pressure urticaria, in which swelling may last for several hours.

Dermographism

Also known as "skin writing," dermographism is the most common physical urticaria, occurring to some degree in approximately 5% of the population. Scratching, toweling, or other activities that produce minor skin trauma induce itching and wheals. The onset is usually sudden; young patients are affected most commonly. The tendency to be dermographic lasts for weeks to months or years. The condition runs on average a course of 2 to 3 years before resolving spontaneously. It may be preceded by a viral infection, antibiotic therapy (especially penicillin), or emotional upset, but in most cases the cause is unknown.[34] Mucosal involvement and angioedema do not occur. There are no recognized systemic associations (such as atopy or autoimmunity).

The degree of urticarial response varies. A patient will be highly reactive for months and then appear to be in remission, only to have symptoms recur (Figures 6-11 and 6-12).

Table 6-1 Comparison of the Physical Urticarias

Urticaria	Relative frequency	Precipitant	Time of onset	Duration	Local symptoms
Symptomatic dermographism	Most frequent	Stroking skin	Minutes	2-3 hr	Irregular, pruritic wheals
Delayed dermographism	Rare	Stroking skin	30 min-8 hr	≤48 hr	Burning; deep swelling
Pressure urticaria	Frequent	Pressure	3-12 hr	8-24 hr	Diffuse, tender swelling
Solar urticaria	Frequent	Various wavelengths of light	2-5 min	15 min-3 hr	Pruritic wheals
Familial cold urticaria	Rare	Change in skin temperature from cold air	30 min-3 hr	≤48 hr	Burning wheals
Essential acquired cold urticaria	Frequent	Cold contact	2-5 min	1-2 hr	Pruritic wheals
Heat urticaria	Rare	Heat contact	2-5 min (rarely delayed)	1 hr	Pruritic wheals
Cholinergic urticaria	Very frequent	General overheating of body	2-20 min	30 min-1 hr	Papular pruritic wheals
Aquagenic urticaria	Rare	Water contact	Several min-30 min	30-45 min	Papular, pruritic wheals
Vibratory angioedema	Very rare	Vibrating against skin	2-5	1 hr	Angioedema
Exercise-induced anaphylaxis	Rare	Exercise; some cases ingestion of certain foods	During or after exercise	Minutes to hours	Pruritic wheals

From Jorizzo JL, Smith EB: Arch Dermatol 118: 198, 1982; copyright 1982, American Medical Association.

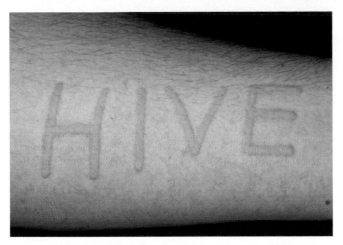

Figure 6-11 Dermographism. The patient complained of itching for the past several months. Occasional swelling was reported.

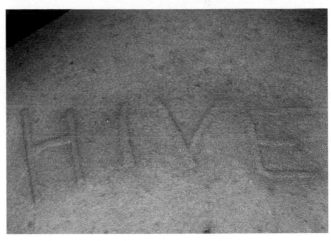

Figure 6-12 Dermographism. Hives occurred every day with the slightest trauma. Nonsedating antihistamines provided control.

Systemic symptoms	Tests	Mechanism	Treatment
None	Scratch skin	Passive transfer; IgE; histamine; possible role of adenosine triphosphate; substance P; possible direct pharmacologic mechanism	Continual hydroxyzine hydrochloride regimen or nonsedating antihistamines; combined H_1 and H_2 blockers
None	Scratch skin; observe early and late	Unknown	Avoidance of precipitants
Flulike symptoms	Apply weight	Unknown	Avoidance of precipitants; if severe, low dosages of corticosteroids given for systemic effect
Wheezing; dizziness; syncope	Phototest	Passive transfer; reverse passive transfer; IgE; possible histamine	Avoidance of precipitants; antihistamines; sunscreens; chloroquine phosphate regimen for short time
Tremor; headache; arthralgia; fever	Expose skin to cold air	Unknown	Avoidance of precipitants
Wheezing; syncope; drowning	Apply ice-filled copper beaker to arm; immerse arm in cold water	Passive transfer; reverse passive transfer IgE (IgM); histamine; vasculitis can be induced	Cyproheptadine hydrochloride regimen; other antihistamines; desensitization; avoidance of precipitants
None	Apply hot water-filled cylinder to arm	Possible histamine; possible complement	Antihistamines; desensitization; avoidance of precipitants
Syncope; diarrhea; vomiting; salivation; headaches	Bathe in hot water; exercise until perspiring; inject methacholine chloride	Passive transfer; possible immunoglobulin; product of sweat gland stimulation; histamine; reduced protease inhibitor	Application of cold water or ice to skin; hydroxyzine regimen; refractory period; anticholinergics
None reported	Apply water compresses to skin	Unknown	Avoidance of precipitants; antihistamines; application of inert oil
None reported	Apply body of vibrating mixer to forearm	Unknown	Avoidance of precipitants
Respiratory distress; hypotension	Exercise testing; immersion tests	Unknown	Antihistamines; ketotifen

Patients complain of linear, itchy wheals from scratching or wheals at the site of friction from clothing. Delayed dermographism, in which the immediate urticarial response is followed in 1 to 6 hours by a wheal that persists for 24 to 48 hours, is rare.

DIAGNOSIS. A tongue blade drawn firmly across the patient's arm or back produces whealing 2 mm or more in width in approximately 1 to 3 minutes (Darier's sign), an exaggerated triple response (Figure 6-13).

1. A red line occurs in 3 to 15 seconds (capillary dilation).
2. Broadening erythema appears (axon reflex flare from arteriolar dilation).
3. A wheal with surrounding erythema replaces the red line (transudation of fluid through dilated capillaries).

As a control, the examining physician can perform this test on his or her own arm at the same time.

Unlike urticaria pigmentosa caused by cutaneous mastocytosis (which also manifests dermographism—Darier's sign), there is no increase in skin mast cell numbers.

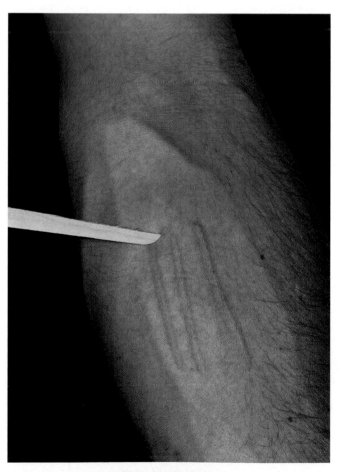

Figure 6-13 Dermographism. A tongue blade drawn firmly across the arm elicits urticaria in susceptible individuals. This simple test should be considered for any patient with acute or chronic urticaria.

TREATMENT. Treatment is not necessary unless the patient is highly sensitive and reacts continually to the slightest trauma. Antihistamines are very effective. Nonsedating H_1 antihistamines or hydroxyzine in relatively low dosages (10 to 25 mg qd to qid) provides adequate relief. Some patients are severely affected and require continuous suppression. Use the lowest dose possible to stop itching. Many patients adapt to a low dose of hydroxyzine and do not feel sedated.

Pressure urticaria

A deep, itchy, burning, or painful swelling occurring 2 to 6 hours after a pressure stimulus and lasting 8 to 72 hours is characteristic of this common form of physical urticaria. The mean age of onset is the early 30s. The disease is chronic, and the mean duration is 9 years (range: 1 to 40 years). Malaise, fatigue, fever, chills, headache, or generalized arthralgia may occur. Many have moderate to severe disease that is disabling, especially for those who perform manual labor.[35] Pressure urticaria, chronic urticaria, and angioedema frequently occur in the same patient. In one study delayed pressure urticaria was present in 37% of patients with chronic urticaria.[10] This explains the frequency of wheals at local pressure sites in patients with chronic urticaria. It also explains the poor response to H_1 antihistamines in some patients because delayed pressure urticaria is generally poorly responsive to this treatment.

The hands, feet, trunk, buttock, lips, and face are commonly affected. Lesions are induced by standing, walking, wearing tight garments, or prolonged sitting on a hard surface.

DIAGNOSIS. Because the swelling occurs hours after the application of pressure, the cause may not be immediately apparent. Repeated deep swelling in the same area is the clue to the diagnosis. Patients with dermographism may have whealing from pressure that occurs immediately, rather than hours later. Tests using weights are used for studies but generally not performed in clinical practice.

TREATMENT. Protect pressure points. Systemic steroids given in short duration tapers are the most effective treatment for severe, disabling delayed pressure urticaria. Dosages of prednisone greater than 30 mg/day may be required. Antihistamines are usually not helpful, but high-dose cetirizine (>30 mg/day) is reported to be effective.[36] Dapsone may be effective.

Cholinergic urticaria

In its milder form, "heat bumps," cholinergic urticaria is the most common of the physical urticarias. It is primarily seen in adolescents and young adults. The overall prevalence is 11.2%; most of the affected persons are older than 20 years. A very small group is severely afflicted. Most persons have mild symptoms that are restricted to fleeting, pinpoint-size wheals. Most affected people do not seek medical attention.[37] Activation of the cholinergic sympathetic innervation of sweat glands is a possible mechanism.

CLINICAL FEATURES. Round, papular wheals 2 to 4 mm in diameter that are surrounded by a slight to extensive red flare are diagnostic of this most distinctive type of hive[38] (Figure 6-14). Typically, the hives occur during or shortly after exercise. However, their onset may be delayed for approximately an hour after stimulation. An attack begins with itching, tingling, burning, warmth, or irritation of the skin. Hives begin within 2 to 20 minutes after the patient experiences a general overheating of the body as a result of exercise, exposure to heat, or emotional stress, and they last for minutes to hours (median: 30 minutes). Cholinergic urticaria may become confluent and resemble typical hives. The incidence of systemic symptoms is very low; however, when they occur, systemic systems include angioedema, hypotension, wheezing, and GI tract complaints.[39]

DIAGNOSIS. The diagnosis is suggested by the history and confirmed by experimentally reproducing the lesions. The most reliable and efficient testing method is to ask the patient to run in place or to use an exercise bicycle for 10 to 15 minutes, and then to observe the patient for 1 hour to detect the typical micropapular hives. Exercise testing should be done in a controlled environment; patients with exercise-induced

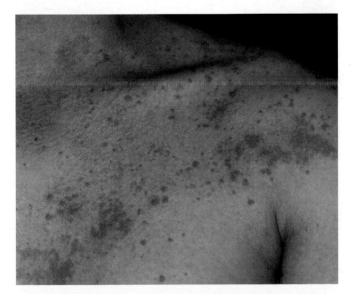

Figure 6-14 Cholinergic urticaria. Round, red, papular wheals that occur in response to exercise, heat, or emotional stress.

anaphylaxis may need emergency treatment. Immersion of half the patient in a bath at 43° C can raise the patient's oral temperature by 1° C to 1.5° C and induce characteristic micropapular hives.[40] The immersion test does not induce hives in patients with exercise-induced anaphylaxis.

TREATMENT. Patients can avoid symptoms by limiting strenuous exercise. Showering with hot water may temporarily deplete histamine stores and induce a 24-hour refractory period. Immediate cooling after sweating, such as a cool shower, can abort attacks. Cetirizine (Zyrtec) at twice its recommended dose of 20 mg is very effective.[41] Hydroxyzine (10 to 50 mg) taken 1 hour before exercise attenuates the eruption, but the side effect of drowsiness is often unacceptable. Oral propranolol may be used with antihistamines. Severely affected unresponsive patients may respond to stanozolol.[42]

Exercise-induced anaphylaxis

Patients develop pruritus, urticaria, respiratory distress, and hypotension after exercise. Symptoms may progress to angioedema, laryngeal edema, bronchospasm, and hypotension, and there is a high frequency of progression to upper airway distress and shock.[43,44] It is associated with different kinds of exercise, although jogging is the most frequently reported. Exercise acts as a physical stimulus that, through an unknown mechanism, provokes mast cell degranulation and elevated serum histamine levels. In contrast to cholinergic urticaria, the lesions are large and are not produced by hot showers, pyrexia, or anxiety. It is differentiated from cholinergic urticaria by a hot-water immersion test (see cholinergic urticaria). Exercise-induced or exercise-accentuated anaphylaxis may occur only after ingestion of certain foods such as celery, shellfish, wheat, fruit, milk, and fish (food-dependent EIA).[45] Attacks occur when the patient exercises within 30 minutes after ingestion of the food; eating the food without exercising (and vice versa) causes no symptoms. Patients with wheat-associated EIA had positive skin tests to several wheat fractions.[46] Another precipitating factor includes drug intake; a familial tendency has been reported. The prognosis is not well defined, but a reduction of attacks occurs in 45% of patients by means of elimination diets and behavioral changes. The differential diagnosis includes exercise-induced asthma, idiopathic anaphylaxis, cardiac arrhythmias, and carcinoid syndrome.[47]

TREATMENT. H_1 antihistamines are recommended as pretreatment and acute therapy. Administration of epinephrine by auto-injector may be required. Exercising with a partner is prudent. Exercise should be stopped if itching, erythema, or whealing occur. Airway maintenance and cardiovascular support may be required. Prophylactic treatment includes avoidance of exercise, abstention from coprecipitating foods at least 4 hours before exercise, and pretreatment with antihistamines and cromolyn, or the induction of tolerance through regular exercise.

Cold urticaria

Cold urticaria syndromes are a group of disorders characterized by urticaria, angioedema, or anaphylaxis that develops after cold exposure.

PRIMARY ACQUIRED COLD URTICARIA. Primary acquired ("essential") cold urticaria occurs in children and young adults. Local whealing and itching occur within a few minutes of applying a solid or fluid cold stimulus to the skin. The wheal lasts for about a half hour. Dermographism and cholinergic urticaria are found relatively often in patients with cold urticaria. Urticaria may occur in the oropharynx after a cold drink. Systemic symptoms, occasionally severe and anaphylactoid, may occur after extensive exposure such as immersion in cold water. There may be a recent history of a virus infection (Mycoplasma pneumoniae). Spontaneous improvement occurs in an average of 2 to 3 years. Hives occur with a sudden drop in air temperature or during exposure to cold water. Many patients have severe reactions with generalized urticaria, angioedema, or both. Swimming in cold water is the most common cause of severe reactions and can result in massive transudation of fluid into the skin, leading to hypotension, fainting, shock, and possibly death. Like dermographism, cold urticaria often begins after infection, drug therapy, or emotional stress.

SECONDARY ACQUIRED COLD URTICARIA. Secondary acquired cold urticaria occurs in about 5% of patients with cold urticaria. Wheals are persistent, may have purpura, and demonstrate vasculitis on skin biopsy. Cryoglobulin, cold agglutinin, or cryofibrinogens are present. Order CBC, ESR, ANA, mononucleosis spot test, RPR, rheumatoid factor, total complement, cryoglobulins, cryofibrinogens, cold agglutinins, and cold hemolysins.[48] Demonstration of a cryoglobulin should prompt a search for chronic hepatitis B or C infection, lymphoreticular malignancy, or glandular fever. The cryoglobulins may be polyclonal (post infection) or monoclonal (IgG or IgM), and complement activation may be involved.[42]

DIAGNOSIS. The diagnosis is made by inducing a hive with a plastic wrapped ice cube held against the forearm for 3 to 5 minutes (Figure 6-15). Some patients require up to 20 minutes to elicit a response. A cold-water immersion test, in which the forearm is submerged for 5 to 15 minutes in water at 0° to 8° C, establishes the diagnosis when the results of the ice cube test are equivocal. The patient must be monitored closely because severe reactions are possible.

TREATMENT. Patients must learn to protect themselves from a sudden decrease in temperature. Cyproheptadine (Periactin) and doxepin (10 mg two or three times a day) are effective.[49] The dosage of cyproheptadine can be adjusted to as low as 2 mg orally once or twice a day to obtain optimum benefits with minimum side effects; side effects of cyproheptadine include sedation and increased appetite. Both loratadine and cetirizine may be effective.[50]

Systemic steroids are not effective.

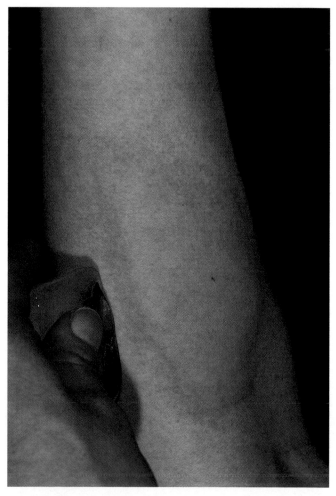

Figure 6-15 Cold urticaria. The hive occurred within minutes of holding an ice cube against the skin.

Solar urticaria

Hives that occur in sun exposed areas minutes after exposure to the sun and disappear in less than 1 hour are called solar urticaria. This photoallergic disorder is caused by both sunlight and artificial light. It is most common in young adults; females are more often affected. Systemic reactions that include syncope can occur. Previously exposed tanned skin may not react when exposed to ultraviolet light. Hives induced by exposure to ultraviolet light must be distinguished from the much more common sun-related condition of polymorphous light eruption. Lesions of polymorphous light eruption are rarely urticarial. They occur hours after exposure and persist for several days.

Pathogenesis

Evidence supports an immunologic IgE mediated mechanism for solar urticaria.[51] There are several different wavelengths that can cause solar urticaria.[52] The disease was classified into six types that correspond to six different wavelengths of light. An individual reacts to a specific wavelength or a narrow band of the light spectrum, usually within the range of 290 to 500 nm. The cause may be an allergic reaction to an antigen formed in the skin by light waves. Those reacting to light above 400 nm (visible light) develop hives even when exposed through glass. The wavelength responsible for solar urticaria is identified by phototesting. Antihistamines, sunscreens, and graded exposure to increasing amounts of light are effective treatments.

Heat, water, and vibration urticarias

Other physical stimuli such as heat, water of any temperature, or vibration are rare causes of urticaria. Aquagenic urticaria resembles the micropapular hives of cholinergic urticaria. Antihistamine and anticholinergic medication may not prevent the reaction. The mechanism of this phenomenon remains poorly understood.[53]

Aquagenic pruritus

Severe, prickling skin discomfort without skin lesions[54] occurs within 1 to 15 (or more) minutes after contact with water at any temperature and lasts for 10 to 120 minutes (average: 40 minutes). Histamine does not seem to play a key role in the pathogenesis of aquagenic pruritus. Capsaicin cream (Zostrix, Zostrix-HP) applied three times daily for 4 weeks resulted in complete relief of symptoms in the treated areas.[55] Ultraviolet B phototherapy and antihistamines provide some relief.[56] One paper reported that sodium bicarbonate (25 to 200 gm) added to the bath or applied as a paste prevented the symptoms.[57] Polycythemia rubra vera should be ruled out.

Angioedema

Angioedema (angioneurotic edema) is a hivelike swelling caused by increased vascular permeability in the subcutaneous tissue of the skin and mucosa and the submucosal layers of the respiratory and GI tracts. A similar reaction occurs in the dermis with hives. Hives and angioedema commonly occur simultaneously and can have the same etiology. All types are listed in Box 6-9. Suspect these types when recurrent angioedema occurs without hives.

CLINICAL CHARACTERISTICS. The deeper reaction produces a more diffuse swelling than is seen in hives. Itching is usually absent. Symptoms consist of burning and painful swelling. The lips, palms, soles, limbs, trunk, and genitalia are most commonly affected. Involvement of the GI and respiratory tracts produces dysphagia, dyspnea, colicky abdominal pain, and attacks of vomiting and diarrhea. GI symptoms are more common in the hereditary types of angioedema. Angioedema may occur as a result of trauma. Urticaria is rarely seen in hereditary or acquired angioedema.

In one report of 17 patients admitted during a 5-year period, 94% had angioedema in the head and neck; three required urgent tracheotomy or intubation, 35% had recent initiation of angiotensin-converting enzyme inhibitor therapy for hypertension, and 6% demonstrated classic hereditary angioedema. The majority (59%) had unclear etiologies for their symptoms.[58]

Box 6-9 Angioedema (all forms)
Acquired angioedema
Acute angioedema
Allergic IgE mediated (drugs, food, insect venom)
Contrast dyes
Serum sickness
Cold urticaria
Chronic recurrent angioedema
Idiopathic (most cases)
Acquired C1 inhibitor deficiency
Angioedema-eosinophilia syndrome
Hereditary angioedema
Type 1 (85%)—C1 inhibitor absent
Type 2 (15%)—C1 inhibitor not functional

Acquired forms of angioedema
Acute angioedema

Severe allergic type 1 immediate hypersensitivity IgE-mediated reactions can cause acute angioedema and urticaria (Figures 6-16, 6-17, and 6-18). IgE antibody cell surface unites with antigen (food, drug,[59] stinging insect venom, pollen) on the mast cell surface and precipitates an immediate and massive release of histamine and other mediators from mast cells. Angioedema occurs alone or with the other symptoms of systemic anaphylaxis (i.e., respiratory distress, hypotension). Some forms of cold urticaria are IgE mediated and occur initially as angioedema.

Contrast dyes used in radiology and drugs may also cause acute angioedema as a result of nonimmunologic mechanisms. Examples include nonsteroidal antiinflammatory drugs, such as aspirin and indomethacin, and angiotensin-converting enzyme–inhibiting drugs.

Angioedema occurs as part of serum sickness syndrome. Swelling, fever, arthralgias, and lymphadenopathy occur 7 to 10 days after exposure to heterologous serum or certain drugs.

Prescribe Epi-pen or Epi-pen Jr for patients who experience severe reactions with insect stings. The epinephrine in Epi-pen is packaged in an auto-injector to avoid manual needle insertion.

Advise affected patients to wear a bracelet that identifies the diagnosis; their reactions could be misdiagnosed as symptoms related to alcoholism, stroke, myocardial infarction, or a foreign body in the airway.

IDIOPATHIC ANGIOEDEMA. Most cases of angioedema are idiopathic. Angioedema can occur at any age but is most common in the 40- to 50-year-old age group. Women are most frequently affected. The pattern of recurrence is unpredictable, and episodes can occur for 5 or more years. Involvement of the GI and respiratory tracts occurs, but asphyxiation is not a danger. Treat with antihistamines. Long-term suppression may require corticosteroids. Alternate-day therapy is indicated (e.g., Prednisone 20 mg qod) with the lowest dosage of prednisone required to provide adequate control.

Acquired angioedema (acquired C1 inhibitor deficiency)

Acquired angioedema (AAE) is a rare disease that occurs in two forms, AAE-I and AAE-II. AAE-I is associated with malignancy (B-cell lineage, breast cancer, etc.); AAE-II is an autoimmune form. AAE-II patients have a C1-INH autoantibody (see Box 6-10, Acquired Angioedema). There is a lack of evidence of inheritance, and the onset of symptoms is in middle age.

LABORATORY DIAGNOSIS OF AAE I, II. (See Box 6-11, Hereditary and Acquired Angioedema—Laboratory Evaluation.) C4, C1q, and C1-INH levels are low. Search for lymphoproliferative disease and other neoplasms. Order serum protein electrophoresis, immunophoresis, peripheral blood lymphocyte immunophenotyping, and CT scans of the chest, abdomen, and pelvis. Initial studies may be negative. Angioedema can precede internal disease by up to 7 years. Follow-up is required.

TREATMENT. Acute attacks are treated with epinephrine and glucocorticoids. High dosages of antihistamines may be effective. Therapy of an underlying condition can control AAE-I. Androgens such as danazol are useful for frequent attacks. AAE-II has been treated with immunosuppressives.

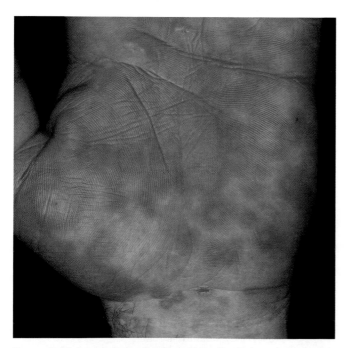

Figure 6-16 Angioedema. Swelling of the hands is a characteristic sign.

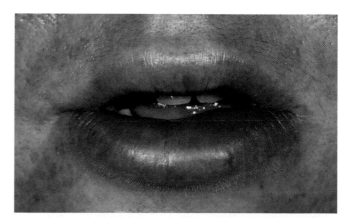

Figure 6-17 Angioedema. Swelling of the lips may be the only manifestation of angioedema.

ANGIOEDEMA

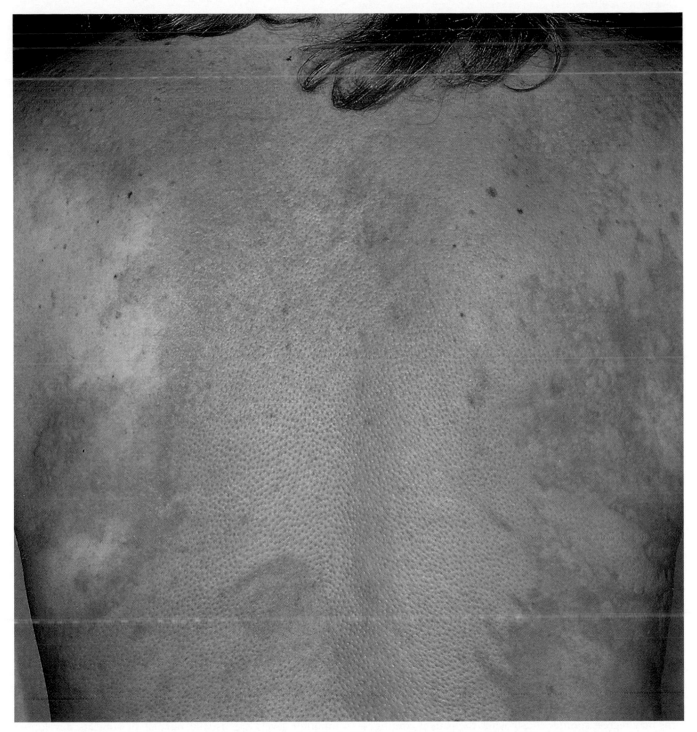

Figure 6-18 Wide areas of swelling occurred suddenly. There was discomfort from the swelling but no itching.

Box 6-10 Acquired Angioedema

Acquired C1 inhibitor deficiency

Swelling subcutaneous tissue, abdominal organs, upper airway

Onset middle age

	Etiology	C1-INH (normal amount produced) (levels are low)
AAE-I	Associated diseases B-cell lymphoproliferative disorders Other cancers (Angioedema precedes neoplasms) Connective tissue diseases Infections	Catabolism increases
AAE-II	Antibody directed against C1-INH molecule	Autoantibody cleaves C1-INH Blocks inhibitory capacity of C1-INH

C1-INH, C1 inhibitor.

Box 6-11 Hereditary and Acquired Angioedema—Laboratory Evaluation

	C4	C1q	C1-INH (Quantitative)	C1-INH (functional)
HAE-Type I	↓	Normal	↓	↓
HAE-Type II	↓	Normal	Normal	↓
AAE-Type I	↓	↓	↓	↓
AAE-Type II	↓	↓	Normal to mildly ↓	↓

C1-INH = C1 esterase inhibitor

HAE = Hereditary angioedema

AAE = Acquired angioedema

↓ = decreased

From: Green JJ, Heymann WR: Adv Dermatol 2001; 17:41.

ANGIOTENSIN-CONVERTING ENZYME INHIBITORS.
Angiotensin-converting enzyme inhibitors (ACEIs) are widely used for the treatment of mild forms of hypertension. They are the number one cause of acute angioedema in some hospitals.[60] Angioedema occurs in 0.1% to 0.2% of patients receiving an ACEI and it is a potentially life-threatening adverse effect.[61,62] The incidence may be higher in Black Americans.

The onset usually occurs within hours to 1 week after starting therapy. Angioedema may occur suddenly even though the drug has been well tolerated for months or years; symptoms may regress spontaneously while the patient continues the medication, erroneously prompting an alternative diagnosis. ACE-inhibitors seem to facilitate angioedema in predisposed subjects, rather than causing it with an allergic or idiosyncratic mechanism.

Most cases from the short-acting ACEI, captopril, present with mild angioedema that can be controlled with antihistamines and glucocorticosteroids. In contrast, the angioedema induced by the long-acting ACE inhibitors (lisinopril[63], enalapril) has been serious.[64]

The pathology has a special predilection for the tongue, a circumstance that renders orotracheal and nasotracheal intubation difficult; symptoms may progress rapidly despite aggressive medical therapy, necessitating emergency airway procedures.[65] Individuals with a history of idiopathic angioedema probably should not be given ACE inhibitors.[66] C1-inhibitor levels are usually normal in subjects developing ACE-inhibitor-dependent angioedema.

Treatment includes immediate withdrawal of the ACE inhibitor and acute symptomatic supportive therapy. Angioedema that results from ACEIs is probably not IgE mediated, and antihistamines and steroids may not alleviate the airway obstruction. Alternative therapy with other classes of drugs to manage hypertension and/or heart failure must be chosen. Angiotensin II receptor antagonists have a lower incidence of adverse effects than ACE inhibitors as they do not produce cough and appear much less likely to produce angioedema.

Continuing use of ACE inhibitors, in spite of angioedema, results in a markedly increased rate of angioedema recurrence with serious morbidity.

Hereditary angioedema

Hereditary angioedema (inherited C1 inhibitor deficiency) is transmitted as an autosomal dominant trait and is due to mutations in the C1 inhibitor (C1-INH) gene. The disease affects between 1 in 10,000 and 1 in 50,000 persons.

In most cases the disease begins in late childhood or early adolescence. Spontaneous occurrences occur in up to 25% of patients. Many have ancestors who died suddenly from asphyxia. In the past, the mortality rate for attacks involving the upper airways exceeded 25%. Patients live in constant dread of life-threatening laryngeal obstruction.

Persons with hereditary angioedema have one normal and one abnormal C1 inhibitor gene. Under normal circumstances, this defect is clinically silent. Minor trauma, mental stress, and other unknown triggering factors lead to the release of vasoactive peptides that produce episodic swelling. Histamine has no role in this type of edema.

CLINICAL MANIFESTATIONS. Swelling of the gastrointestinal mucosa results in nausea, vomiting, diarrhea, and severe pain that can mimic a surgical emergency. The swellings are not erythematous, pruritic, or painful. Attacks may be complicated by incapacitating cutaneous swelling, life-threatening upper airway impediment, and severe GI colic. There are episodes of acute subcutaneous or mucosal swelling, but hives do not occur.

During an episode, the swelling increases slowly over 12 to 18 hours, then slowly subsides over the next 48 to 72 hours. Swelling involves the extremities (96%), face (85%), oropharynx (64%), and intestinal mucosa (88%). Obstruction of the upper respiratory tract is responsible for the 30% mortality rate.

Hereditary angioedema results from a lack of functional C1 esterase inhibitor. There are two types. Type I is the most common and is characterized by an insufficient production of C1 inhibitor. This affects 85% of all patients with hereditary angioedema. Patients with type 2 have normal or elevated concentrations of C1 inhibitor but the protein is functionally deficient.

Patients usually experience attacks by the second decade of life. Angioedema occurs at three predominant sites: subcutaneous tissues (face, hands, arms, legs, genitalia, and buttocks); abdominal organs (stomach, intestines, bladder), which can mimic surgical emergencies; and the upper airway, which may result in life-threatening laryngeal edema. The extremities are the cutaneous site most commonly reported. Typically abdominal symptoms resolve within 12 to 24 hours, whereas the subcutaneous swellings resolve in 1 to 5 days.

LABORATORY DIAGNOSIS OF HAE. The diagnosis is suggested by the family and personal history. A laboratory workup confirms the diagnosis (see Box 6-11, Hereditary and Acquired Angioedema—Laboratory Evaluation). Both types of HAE have low serum levels of C4. The first step toward confirming the diagnosis of HAE is to order a serum C4 level test. C4 levels are markedly decreased during an episode and low between attacks. A normal C4 level during an episode suggests a different diagnosis. If the C4 level is abnormal, two more tests should be ordered: (1) a C1 esterase inhibitor test and (2) a C1 esterase inhibitor functional assay. C1 esterase inhibitor levels are 30% below normal levels in most type I patients. Order a C1-INH functional assay for patients with a low C4, but with normal C1-INH levels to establish the diagnosis of type II disease. C1q levels are normal in HAE and depressed in AAE. Family members of patients with hereditary angioedema may have markedly abnormal complement values despite being asymptomatic.

Evaluation

ACUTE ATTACKS. Antihistamines, corticosteroids, and adrenergic drugs are of little value. Replacement with a vapor-heated C1 inhibitor concentrate prevents and treats acute attacks and is the treatment of choice for unpredictable and dangerous acute episodes such as laryngeal edema and severe abdominal attacks.

Fresh frozen plasma, which contains C1-INH, can be used if C1-INH concentrate is not available. Laryngeal symptoms may require tracheostomy or intubation.

PROPHYLACTIC TREATMENT. Consider prophylactic treatment for patients with one or more attacks per month or for those with severe symptoms. The best drugs for prophylaxis are the attenuated androgens danazol (200 to 600 mg/day) and stanozolol (2 mg/day).[67] These drugs are not given to pregnant women and prepubertal patients. They prevent attacks triggered by manipulations of the oropharynx, such as those during dental surgery and intubation. They need to be taken for five days before they become effective. They correct the lowered C1 esterase inhibitor and C4 levels by inducing hepatic synthesis through the increase of serum levels of C1 esterase inhibitor, and they are effective in hereditary angioedema types I and II. Hepatocellular adenomas[68] and hepatocellular carcinoma[69] have been reported with long-term danazol treatment. Spontaneous improvement occurs and the need for prophylactic treatment may diminish with time.

ANGIOEDEMA-EOSINOPHILIA SYNDROME. This rare, non–life-threatening benign syndrome consists of periodic attacks of angioedema, urticaria, pruritus, myalgia, oliguria, and fever.[70] During attacks, body weights increase up to 18%, and leukocyte counts reach as high as 108,000/µl (88% eosinophils). Eosinophilia can persist between attacks. Attacks of angioedema last for about 6 to 10 days. Attacks resolve spontaneously or require short corticosteroids to control symptoms and normalize the blood count.[71]

Contact Urticaria Syndrome

Contact of the skin with various compounds can elicit a wheal and flare response. Most patients give a history of relapsing dermatitis or generalized urticarial attacks rather than a localized hive; others complain only of localized sensations of itching, burning, and tingling. This is in contrast to allergic contact dermatitis which is an eczematous reaction caused by cell-mediated immunity.

Contact urticaria is characterized by a wheal and flare that occur within 30 to 60 minutes after cutaneous exposure to certain agents. Direct contact of the skin with these agents may cause a wheal-and-flare response restricted to the area of contact, generalized urticaria, urticaria and asthma, or urticaria combined with an anaphylactoid reaction. There are nonimmunologic and immunologic forms.

NONIMMUNOLOGIC CONTACT URTICARIA. The nonimmunologic type is the most common and most benign. This form does not require prior sensitization. Nonimmunologic, histamine-releasing substances are produced by certain plants (nettles), animals (caterpillars, jellyfish), and medications (dimethyl sulfoxide [DMSO]).[72,73] Anaphylaxis may occur after application of bacitracin ointment.[74] Other implicated substances include cobalt chloride, benzoic acid, cinnamic aldehyde, cinnamic acid, and sorbic acid.

IMMUNOLOGIC CONTACT URTICARIA. Immunologic contact urticaria is due to an IgE immediate hypersensitivity reaction. Some patients experience rhinitis, laryngeal edema, and abdominal disturbances. Latex rubber, bacitracin, potato, apple, mechlorethamine, and henna have been implicated.

OTHER PRECIPITATING FACTORS. The mechanism by which wood, plants, foods, cosmetics, and animal hair and dander cause contact urticaria has not been defined. The term protein contact dermatitis is used when an immediate reaction occurs after eczematous skin is exposed to certain types of food (fish, garlic, onion, chives, cucumber, parsley, tomato), animal (cow hair and dander), or plant substances. Cooks who complain of burning or stinging when handling certain foods may have contact urticaria syndrome.

DIAGNOSIS. Because there is no standard test battery for routine evaluation of contact urticaria, a careful history concerning the occurrence of immediate reactions, whether localized or generalized, is essential. An open patch test may be performed by applying a drop of the suspected substance to the ventral forearm and observing the site for a wheal 30 to 60 minutes later. Closed tests may be associated with more intense or generalized reactions.

Prick testing (using fresh samples of the food suspected from the patient's history) is an accurate method of investigation for selected cases of hand dermatitis in patients who spend considerable time handling foods (e.g., catering workers, cooks).[75] Seafood is a common allergen. Radioallergosorbent (RAST) testing can confirm immunologic contact urticaria.

Pruritic Urticarial Papules and Plaques of Pregnancy

Pruritic urticarial papules and plaques of pregnancy (PUPPP),[75-82] or polymorphic eruption of pregnancy, is the most common gestational dermatosis affecting between 1 in 130 and 1 in 300 pregnancies. It is seen most frequently in primigravidas and begins late in the third trimester of pregnancy (mean onset, 35 weeks) or occasionally in the early postpartum period. The eruption appears suddenly, begins on the abdomen in 90% of patients (Figure 6-19, A), and in a few days may spread in a symmetric fashion to involve the buttock, proximal arms, and backs of the hands (Figure 6-19, B). The initial lesions may be confined to striae. The face is not involved. Itching is moderate to intense, but excoriations are rarely seen. The lesions begin as red papules that are often surrounded by a narrow, pale halo. They increase in number and may become confluent, forming edematous urticarial plaques or erythema multiforme-like target lesions that may look like the lesions of herpes gestationis. In other patients, the involved sites acquire broad areas of erythema, and the papules remain discrete. Papulovesicles have been reported. The mean duration is 6 weeks, but the rash is usually not severe for more than 1 week. Unlike urticaria, the eruption remains fixed and increases in intensity, clearing in most cases before or within 1 week after delivery. Recurrence with future pregnancies is unusual. There have been no fetal or maternal complications. Infants do not develop the eruption.

Significantly increased maternal weight gain, newborn birth weight, and twin birth rate have been reported in patients with PUPPP. It was postulated that abdominal distension or a reaction to it may play a role in the development of PUPPP.

The biopsy reveals a nonspecific perivascular lymphohistiocytic infiltrate. Eosinophils have also been noted in most biopsies. There are no laboratory abnormalities, and direct immunofluorescence of lesional and perilesional skin is negative.

Treatment is supportive. The expectant mother can be assured that pruritus will quickly terminate before or after delivery. Itching can be relieved with group V topical steroids; cool, wet compresses; oatmeal baths; and antihistamines. Antipruritic topical medications (menthol, doxepin) are useful. Prednisone (40 mg/day) may be required if pruritus becomes intolerable. Several patients were treated successfully with UVB therapy.[83]

PUPPP

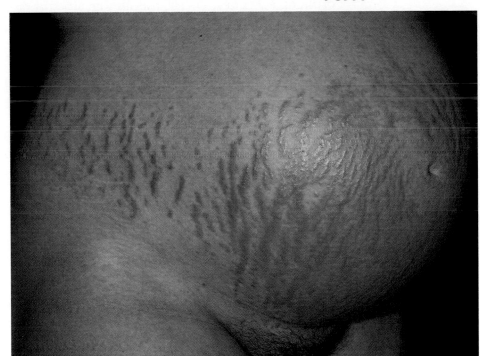

Figure 6-19 Pruritic urticarial papules and plaques of pregnancy.

A, The abdomen is often the initial site of involvement. Initial lesions may be confined to striae.

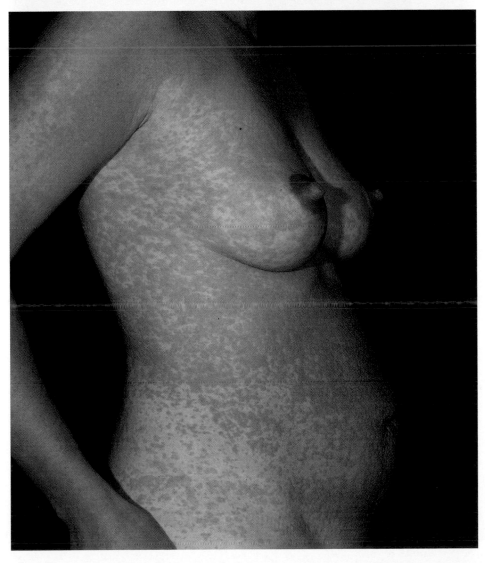

B, Fully evolved eruption.

Urticarial Vasculitis

Urticarial vasculitis (UV) is a subset of vasculitis characterized clinically by urticarial skin lesions and histologically by necrotizing vasculitis.[84]

Immune complexes are thought to lodge in small blood vessels with activation of complement, mast cell degranulation, infiltration by acute inflammatory cells, fibrin deposition, and blood vessel damage.

There is a spectrum of clinical and laboratory features.

Many patients have minimal signs or symptoms of systemic disease. Systemic symptoms include angioedema (42%), arthralgias (49%), pulmonary disease (21%), and abdominal pain (17%). Thirty-two percent have hypocomplementemia, 64% have lesions that last more than 24 hours, 32% have painful or burning lesions, and 35% have lesions that resolve with purpura or hyperpigmentation.[85]

CLINICAL FEATURES. Overall, patients with urticarial vasculitis tend to have a benign course. Urticarial plaques in most patients with typical chronic urticaria resolve completely in less than 24 hours and disappear while new plaques appear in other areas. Urticarial vasculitis plaques persist for 1 to 7 days and may have residual changes of purpura, scaling, and hyperpigmentation (Figure 6-20). The lesions are burning and painful rather than itchy.

Patients with urticarial vasculitis have been categorized into two subgroups: those with hypocomplementemia and those with normal complement levels.

NORMOCOMPLEMENT UV. Normocomplementemic urticarial vasculitis is usually idiopathic. This most common form has also been described in patients with monoclonal gammopathy, neoplasia, repeated cold exposure, and ultraviolet light sensitivity.[84]

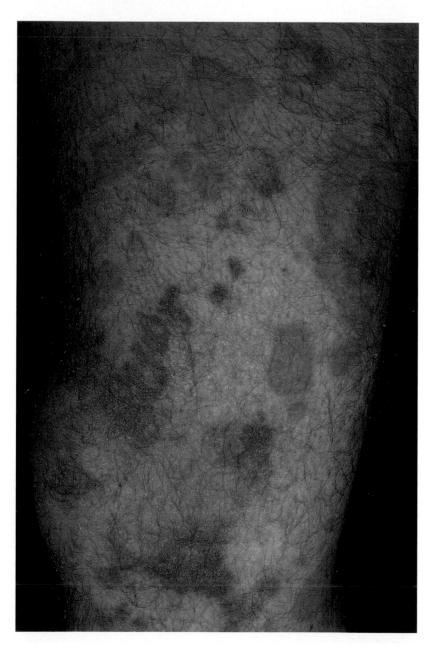

Figure 6-20 Urticarial vasculitis. Purpura occurs as the hive resolves.

HYPOCOMPLEMENT UV. Patients with hypocomplementemia are more likely to have systemic involvement than patients with normal complement levels. Hypocomplementemic urticarial vasculitis can present as or precede a syndrome that includes obstructive pulmonary disease and ureitis, systemic lupus erythematosus, Sjögren's syndrome, or cryoglobulinemia (which is closely linked with hepatitis B or C virus infection).[84]

LABORATORY TESTS. Order CBC, ESR, BUN, creatinine, ANA, anti-DNA, anti-Sm, complement assay, anti-C1q antibodies, cryoglobulins, a Schirmer's test, and pulmonary function tests.

As with typical cutaneous vasculitis, most patients have an elevated erythrocyte sedimentation rate. Anti-C1q autoantibody develops in disorders characterized by immune complex–mediated injury and appears in most patients with hypocomplementemic urticarial vasculitis syndrome.[86] Patients with more severe involvement have hypocomplementemia (hypocomplementemic urticarial vasculitis syndrome) with depressed CH_{50}, C_{1q}, C_4, or C_2.

BIOPSY. Biopsy shows a histologic picture that is indistinguishable from that seen in cutaneous necrotizing vasculitis (palpable purpura). Fragmentation of leukocytes and fibrinoid deposition occur in the walls of postcapillary venules, a pattern called leukocytoclastic vasculitis. There is an interstitial neutrophilic infiltrate of the dermis.

IMMUNOFLUORESCENCE. Patients with hypocomplementemia may have an immunofluorescent pattern of immunoglobulins or C_3 as determined by routine direct immunofluorescence. Direct immunofluorescence in patients with hypocomplementemia shows deposition of Ig and C_3; 87% have fluorescence of the blood vessels, and 70% have fluorescence of the basement membrane zone. Rule out other diseases in which cutaneous vasculitis may present as an urticarial-like eruption (e.g., viral illness, systemic lupus erythematosus, Sjögren's syndrome, and serum sickness).

TREATMENT. Prednisone in dosages exceeding 40 mg/day is effective. Other medications reported to be effective are indomethacin (25 mg three times daily to 50 mg four times daily),[87] colchicine (0.6 mg two or three times daily),[88,89] dapsone (up to 200 mg/day), low-dose oral methotrexate,[90,91] and antimalarial drugs.

Serum Sickness

Serum sickness is a disease produced by exposure to drugs,[92,93] blood products, or animal-derived vaccines. After exposure to these antigens, a strong host-antibody response occurs. These circulating antibodies react with the newly introduced antigen to form precipitating antigen-antibody complexes. This is a type III (immune complex) reaction, or Arthus reaction. These circulating immune complexes are trapped in vessel walls of various organs, where they activate complement. A rise in the level of immune complexes is accompanied by a decrease in serum levels of C_3 and C_4 and an increase in C_{3a}/C_{3a} des-arginine, a split product of C_3 whose presence indicates that the complement system has been activated by immune complexes. Inflammatory mediators are released. C_{3a}/C_{3a} des-arginine, a potent anaphylotoxin, induces mast cell degranulation to produce hives.

CLINICAL MANIFESTATIONS. Symptoms appear 8 to 13 days after exposure to the drug or antisera and last for 4 or more days. They include fever, malaise, skin eruptions, arthralgias, nausea, vomiting, occult blood in the stool, and lymphadenopathy. The disease resolves without sequelae in most cases. The skin eruption begins with the onset of other symptoms. A morbilliform rash or urticaria is limited to the trunk or may become generalized. The hands and feet may be involved.

DIAGNOSIS. The white blood count may be as high as 25,000. Serum C_3 and C_4 are below normal. Proteinuria occurs in 40% of patients. Direct immunofluorescence of skin lesions less than 24 hours old shows Ig deposits (IgM, IgE, IgA, or C_3) in the superficial small blood vessels.[94] Drugs are now the most common cause of serum sickness. Penicillin, sulfa drugs, thiouracils, cholecystographic dyes, hydantoins, aminosalicylic acid, and streptomycin are most often implicated.[95]

TREATMENT. The offending agent must be avoided. Antihistamines such as hydroxyzine control the hives. Prednisone 40 mg/day is used if symptoms are intense.

Mastocytosis

Mastocytosis is a disease in which there is an increased number of mast cells in various organs of the body.[96,97] The most frequent site of organ involvement with all forms of mastocytosis is the skin. In young children, the disease is usually confined to the skin; in adults, mastocytosis is usually systemic. Mast cells store histamine in granules. Histamine is released by scratching the lesions (Figure 6-21) or ingesting certain agents. The cause is unknown, and familial occurrence is only rarely documented.[98]

CLASSIFICATION. An older classification is shown in Box 6-12. New revisions have been proposed.[99] The first two categories represent the majority of cases in children and adults.

Cutaneous mastocytosis

There are several types of skin mast cell disease.[100]

SOLITARY MASTOCYTOMA. A larger solitary collection of mast cells is called a mastocytoma. Mastocytoma is the most common type of cutaneous mastocytosis. There are one or multiple lesions. They are reddish-brown nodules or plaques that can be several centimeters in diameter. Stroking induces whealing ("Darier's sign"). It is due to cutaneous mast cell degranulation and histamine release. They are either present at birth or developed within a median time of 1 week, most appear within the first 3 months of life. They are rare in adults. Bullae may be seen. Children rarely develop additional mastocytomas more than 2 months after onset of the initial lesions. Most occur on the extremities but not the palms or soles. Lesions may spontaneously involute. If it does not involute, it may be surgically removed. Transition to systemic involvement does not occur.

URTICARIA PIGMENTOSA. Urticaria pigmentosa is the second most frequent manifestation of mastocytosis in children. It may be present at birth and appears in infancy and childhood at a median age of 2.5 months and is present in 80% of affected individuals within 6 months. Cases gradually improve, and symptoms resolve in about 50% of patients by adolescence.[101] Urticaria pigmentosa that begins after age 10 usually persists and may be associated with systemic disease. After the age of 10 years, the median time of onset for urticaria pigmentosa is 26.5 years. Lesions are well demarcated, red-brown, slightly elevated plaques averaging 0.5 to 1.5 cm in diameter. They occur in small groups on the trunk and are often dismissed as variations of pigmentation (Figure 6-21). Large numbers can occur on any body surface. The palms and soles are spared. Mucous membranes may be involved. Lesions may increase in number for years. Infants may develop bullae and vesicles until the age of 2; bullae are rarely observed after age 2. Bullae heal without scarring. Pruritus, flushing, and dermatographism occur. Darier's sign (the wheal and flare reaction that is seen following brisk stroking of the lesions) can be elicited.

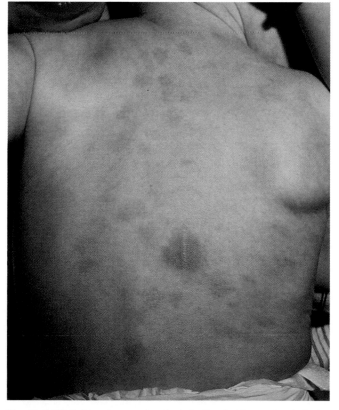

Figure 6-21 Cutaneous mastocytosis (urticaria pigmentosa). Red-brown, slightly elevated plaques averaging 0.5 to 3.5 cm in diameter typically occur in small groups on the trunk. One lesion turned red after being stroked.

Box 6-12 Classification of Mastocytosis
Cutaneous mastocytosis
Solitary or multiple mastocytoma(s)
Urticaria pigmentosa
Diffuse cutaneous mastocytosis
Telangiectasia macularis eruptiva perstans
Systemic mastocytosis
(with or without skin involvement)
Mast cell infiltration of at least one internal organ
(Bone marrow, GI tract, skeletal system)
Mastocytosis with hematological disorder
(with or without skin involvement)
Leukemia, lymphoma, myelodysplastic or myeloproliferative disorder
Lymphadenopathic mastocytosis with eosinophilia
(with or without skin involvement)
(aggressive mastocytosis)
Mast cell leukemia
Modified from: Metcalfe, DD: J Invest Dermatol 1991; 3(3):25.

DIFFUSE CUTANEOUS TYPES. There are two rare generalized forms of cutaneous disease. Diffuse erythrodermic cutaneous mastocytosis appears either as normal skin or as thickened, reddish-brown edematous skin with an orange-peel texture. These pediatric patients have a diffuse infiltration of the entire skin by mast cells. It presents before the age of 3. These patients have the highest frequency of systemic mastocytosis. Dermographism with hemorrhagic blisters is common. Diffuse cutaneous mastocytosis usually resolves spontaneously between the ages of 15 months and 5 years. Diffuse generalized infiltration of the skin is called pseudoxanthomatous mastocytosis, or xanthelasmoidea. It begins in childhood and persists throughout life.

TELANGIECTASIA MACULARIS ERUPTIVA PERSTANS (TMEP). TMEP is the rarest cutaneous form. It is limited to adults and consists of telangiectasias and sparse, widespread, mast cell infiltrates that resemble freckles. Pruritus, purpura, and blisters do not occur.

Systemic mastocytosis

Systemic mastocytosis can occur at any age but is generally seen in older children and adults.[102] The frequency of skin lesions ranges from 50% to 100%. Systemic mast cell disease occurs in approximately 50% of adult patients with urticaria pigmentosa.[103] There is flushing, syncope, and hypotension. Bone is the most common organ involved after the skin. Bone pain is a presenting symptom. Patients have diffuse or focal bony lesions that may be seen radiographically. Gastrointestinal tract involvement presents with nausea, vomiting, abdominal pain, diarrhea and weight loss. Infiltration of the liver, spleen, and lymph nodes causes hepatosplenomegaly and lymphadenopathy. Mast cell leukemia occurs in fewer than 2% of patients. It is the most aggressive form of mastocytosis. There is malignant transformation in 7% of patients with juvenile-onset systemic disease and in approximately 30% of patients with adult-onset systemic disease.[104]

DIAGNOSIS

Skin disease. Stroking a lesion with the wooden end of a cotton-tipped applicator induces intense erythema of the entire plaque and a wheal that is usually confined to the stroked site (Darier's sign) (Figures 6-22 through 6-26). This test is highly characteristic and is as reliable as a biopsy for establishing the diagnosis. Metachromatic stains (Giemsa or toluidine blue) stain cytoplasmic mast cell granules in biopsy specimens deep blue. Injecting anesthetic directly into the biopsy site can degranulate mast cells.

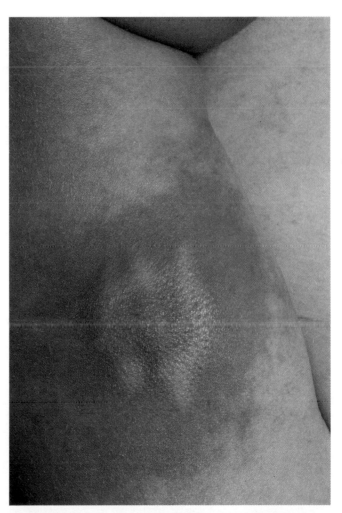

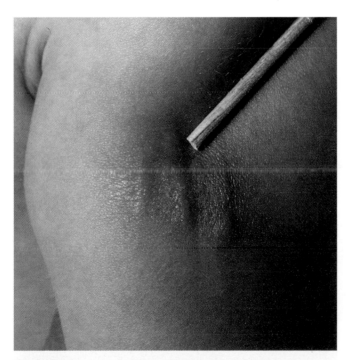

Figure 6-22 Cutaneous mastocytosis (urticaria pigmentosa): Darier's sign. Stroking a lesion with the wooden end of a cotton-tipped applicator produces a wheal that remains confined to the stroked site or enlarges.

Figure 6-23 Cutaneous mastocytosis (urticaria pigmentosa): Darier's sign. Same plaque as in Figure 6-21. Minutes later the wheal has extended and intense erythema has appeared.

MASTOCYTOSIS

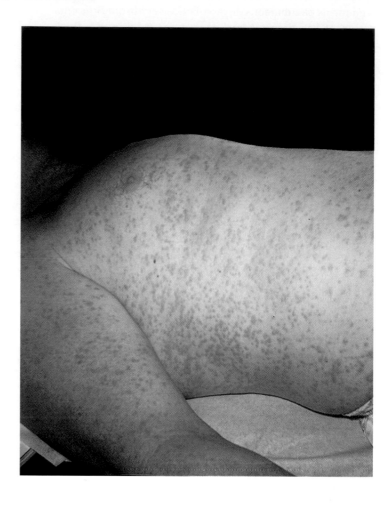

Figure 6-24 An adult with brown macules and papules in a widespread symmetric distribution. Lesions are typically located on the trunk. The face, palms, and soles were not involved.

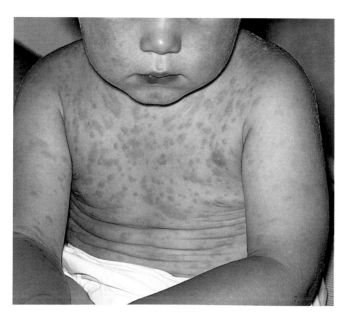

Figure 6-25 Yellow-brown papules and nodules located primarily on the trunk are the most common presentation in children. A wheal was produced by stroking (Darier's sign).

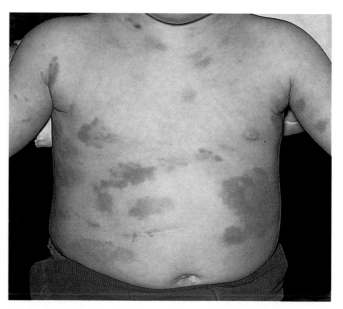

Figure 6-26 Large red-brown plaques are localized in the trunk. A wheal with surrounding erythema developed after stroking (Darier's sign) one of the lesions.

Systemic disease. The diagnosis of patients with systemic mast cell disease is accomplished by histologic examination of key tissues (skin, bone, bone marrow, GI tract) with analysis of chemical markers of the mast cell.

Blood and urine studies. Major urinary metabolites of histamine are elevated in patients who have systemic mastocytosis. Quantitation of urinary N-methyl-histamine or histamine is used as a measure of histamine release. Serum tryptase levels may be useful. Alpha-protryptase may be a very sensitive screening test for systemic mastocytosis. Call the Mayo Medical Labs (800-533-1710) for the latest tests available. Patients should not consume histamine-rich foods (e.g., wine, yogurt, cheese, sauerkraut, spinach, tomatoes, eggplant, chicken livers, sirloin steak) for 24 hours prior to the start of or during the 24-hour urine collection. Elevated plasma histamine levels have been demonstrated in most children with mastocytosis. High levels occur with diffuse cutaneous mastocytosis.

PROGNOSIS. Early-onset mastocytosis presenting by 3 years of age has a very favorable prognosis. Late-onset disease that presents between 7 and 10 years of age has a greater chance of continuing into adulthood. For approximately 50% of children who have cutaneous mastocytosis, symptoms and lesions will resolve during adolescence. Those whose mastocytosis continues into adulthood will have a 5% to 30% chance of systemic involvement.

MANAGEMENT

Cutaneous disease. Patients with urticaria pigmentosa and systemic disease may benefit from a combination of H_1 and H_2 histamine antagonists. Oral disodium cromoglycate reduces pruritus and whealing in patients with and without systemic disease. Application of 0.05% betamethasone dipropionate ointment (Diprolene), under plastic-film occlusion for 8 hours daily for 6 weeks, leads to control of pruritus and Darier's sign. Improvement lasts for an average of 1 year. Patients with urticaria pigmentosa may be treated with an intralesional injection of triamcinolone acetonide, 40 mg/ml. Control of pruritus, loss of Darier's sign, and cutaneous atrophy occurs within 4 weeks and may persist for 1 year. Patients must avoid triggers that induce systemic mast cell degranulation (see Box 6-13).

Systemic disease. Systemic mastocytosis is managed in a stepwise manner: an H_1 antihistamine for flushing and pruritus, an H_2 blocker or proton-pump inhibitor for gastric and duodenal manifestations, oral cromolyn sodium for diarrhea and abdominal pain, and a nonsteroidal antiinflammatory agent to block mast cell biosynthesis of prostaglandin D_2 for severe flushing that is associated with vascular collapse and is unresponsive to H_1 and H_2 antihistamines. Oral 8-methoxypsoralen plus ultraviolet A (PUVA) photochemotherapy in adults with urticaria pigmentosa with or without systemic manifestations decreases pruritus and whealing, lessens Darier's sign, and fades lesional pigmentary changes.[109]

Box 6-13 Triggers That Induce Systemic Mast Cell Degranulation

Cause	Source
Insect stings, poison	Hymenoptera Jellyfish Snakes

Drugs	Opiate analgesics
	  Codeine
	  Morphine
	Polymyxin B
	Vancomycin
	D-turbo curare
	Succinylcholine
	Iodinated radiocontrast media
	Aspirin
	Nonsteroidal antiinflammatory
	  agents
	Muscle relaxants
	Sympathomimetics
	Others

Temperature changes	Heat, cold
Ingestion of alcohol	
Mechanical irritation	Massage Friction
Infections	Bacterial Viral Ascaris
Bacterial toxins	Fish

Adapted from: Hartmann K, Metcalfe D: Hematol Oncol Clin North Am 2000; 14(3):625.

References

1. Mekkes J, Kozel M: New diagnostic and therapeutic possibilities in chronic idiopathic urticaria, Neth J Med 1998; 53(3):139.

2. Jacobson KW, Branch LB, Nelson HS: Laboratory tests in chronic urticaria, JAMA 1980; 243:1644.

3. Cooper KD: Urticaria and angioedema: diagnosis and evaluation, J Am Acad Dermatol 1991; 25:166.

4. Sorensen HT, Christensen B, Kjaerulff E: A two-year follow-up of children with urticaria in general practice, Scand J Prim Health Care 1987; 5:24.

5. Guillet MH, Guillet G: Food urticaria in children, review of 51 cases. Allerg Immunol 1993; 25:333-338.

6. Sampson H: Food allergy. Part 1: immunopathogenesis and clinical disorders, J Allergy Clin Immunol 1999; 103(5 Pt 1):717.

7. Warshaw E: Latex allergy. J Am Acad Dermatol 1998; 39(1):1; quiz: 25.

8. Katayama H: Adverse reactions to ionic and nonionic contrast media: a report from the Japanese Committee on the Safety of Contrast Media [see comments]. Radiology 1990; 175(3):621.

9. Grattan C, et al: Management and diagnostic guidelines for urticaria and angio-oedema. Br J Dermatol 2001; 144(4):708.

10. Barlow RJ, et al: Diagnosis and incidence of delayed pressure urticaria in patients with chronic urticaria, J Am Acad Dermatol 1993; 29:954.

11. Sabroe R, Greaves M: The pathogenesis of chronic idiopathic urticaria, Arch Dermatol 1997; 133(8):1003.

12. Tong L, et al: Assessment of autoimmunity in patients with chronic urticaria, J Allergy Clin Immunol 1997; 99(4):461.

13. Hide M, et al: Autoantibodies against the high-affinity IgE receptor as a cause of histamine release in chronic urticaria [see comments], N Engl J Med 1993; 328(22): 1599.

14. Zuraw B: Urticaria, angioedema, and autoimmunity, Clin Lab Med 1997; 17(3):559.

15. Asero R: Leukotriene receptor antagonists may prevent NSAID-induced exacerbations in patients with chronic urticaria, Ann Allergy Asthma Immunol 2000; 85(2):156.

16. Grattan C, et al: Randomized double-blind study of cyclosporin in chronic "idiopathic" urticaria, Br J Dermatol 2000; 143(2):365.

17. Fisherman EW, Cohen GN: Recurring and chronic urticaria: identification of etiologies, Ann Allergy 1976; 36:401.

18. Juhlin L: Recurrent urticaria: clinical investigation of 330 patients, Br J Dermatol 1981; 104:369.

19. Lanigan SW, Short P, Moult P: The association of chronic urticarial and thyroid autoimmunity, Clin Exp Dermatol 1987; 12:335.

20. Lanigan SW, et al: Association of urticaria and hypothyroidism, Lancet 1984; 1:1476.

21. Leznoff A, et al: Association of chronic urticaria with thyroid autoimmunity, Arch Dermatol 1983; 119:636.

22. Heymann W: Chronic urticaria and angioedema associated with thyroid autoimmunity: review and therapeutic implications, J Am Acad Dermatol 1999; 40(2 Pt 1):229.

23. Akers WA, Naverson DN: Diagnosis of chronic urticaria, Int J Dermatol 1978; 17:616.

24. Haas N, Toppe E, Henz B: Microscopic morphology of different types of urticaria, Arch Dermatol 1998; 134(1):41.

25. Kaplan A: Clinical practice: chronic urticaria and angioedema, N Engl J Med 2002; 346(3):175.

26. Goldsobel AB, et al: Efficacy of doxepin in the treatment of chronic idiopathic urticaria, J Allergy Clin Immunol 1986; 78:867.

27. Greene SL, Reed CE, Schroeter AL: Double-blind crossover study comparing doxepin with diphenhydramine for the treatment of chronic urticaria, J Am Acad Dermatol 1985; 12:669.

28. Paradis L, et al: Effects of systemic corticosteroids on cutaneous histamine secretion and histamine-releasing factor in patients with chronic idiopathic urticaria, Clin Exp Allergy 1996; 26(7):815.

29. O'Donnell B, et al: Intravenous immunoglobulin in autoimmune chronic urticaria, Br J Dermatol 1998; 138(1):101.

30. Loria M, et al: Cyclosporin A in patients affected by chronic idiopathic urticaria: a report of two cases, Br J Dermatol 2001; 145(2):340.

31. Toubi E, et al: Low-dose cyclosporin A in the treatment of severe chronic idiopathic urticaria, Allergy 1997; 52(3):312.

32. Gach J, et al: Methotrexate-responsive chronic idiopathic urticaria: a report of two cases, Br J Dermatol 2001; 145(2):340.

33. Weiner MJ: Methotrexate in corticosteroid-resistant urticaria, Ann Intern Med 1989; 110:848.

34. Wong RC, Fairley JA, Ellis CN: Dermographism: a review, J Am Acad Dermatol 1984; 11:643.

35. Dover JS, et al: Delayed pressure urticaria: clinical features, laboratory investigations, and response to therapy of 44 patients, J Am Acad Dermatol 1988; 18:1289.

36. Kontou-Fili K, et al: Therapeutic effects of cetirizine in delayed pressure urticaria: clinicopathologic findings, J Am Acad Dermatol 1991; 24(6 Pt 2):1090.

37. Zuberbier T, et al: Prevalence of cholinergic urticaria in young adults, J Am Acad Dermatol 1994; 31(6):978.

38. Jorizzo JL: Cholinergic urticaria, Arch Dermatol 1987; 123:455.

39. Lawrence CM, et al: Cholinergic urticaria with associated angioedema, Br J Dermatol 1981; 105:543.

40. Casale TB, Keahey TM, Kaliner M: Exercise-induced anaphylactic syndromes: insights into diagnostic and pathophysiologic features, JAMA 1986; 255:2049.

41. Zuberbier T, et al: Double-blind crossover study of high-dose cetirizine in cholinergic urticaria, Dermatology 1996; 193(4):324.

42. Greaves M: Chronic urticaria, J Allergy Clin Immunol 2000; 105(4):664.

43. Sheffer AL, Austen KF: Exercise-induced anaphylaxis, J Allergy Clin Immunol 1980; 60:106.

44. Sheffer AL, et al: Exercise-induced anaphylaxis: a distinct form of physical allergy, J Allergy Clin Immunol 1983; 11:311.

45. McNeil D, Strauss R: Exercise-induced anaphylaxis related to food intake, Ann Allergy 1988; 61(6):440.

46. Kushimoto H, Aoki T. Masked type I wheat allergy: relation to exercise-induced anaphylaxis, Arch Dermatol 1985; 121:355.

47. Nichols AW: Exercise-induced anaphylaxis and urticaria, Clin Sports Med 1992; 11:303.

48. Wanderer A: Cold urticaria syndromes: historical background, diagnostic classification, clinical and laboratory characteristics, pathogenesis, and management, J Allergy Clin Immunol 1990; 85(6):965.

49. Neittaanmaki H, Myohanen T, Fraki J: Comparison of cinnarizine, cyproheptadine, doxepin, and hydroxyzine in treatment of idiopathic cold urticaria: usefulness of doxepin, J Am Acad Dermatol 1984; 11(3):483.

50. Villas MF, et al: A comparison of new nonsedating and classical antihistamines in the treatment of primary acquired cold urticaria (ACU), J Investig Allergol Clin Immunol 1992; 2(5):258.

51. Leenutaphong V, Holzle E, Plewig G: Pathogenesis and classification of solar urticaria: a new concept, J Am Acad Dermatol 1989; 21(2 Pt 1):237.

52. Rauits M, Armstrong RB, Harber LC: Solar urticaria: clinical features and wavelength dependence, Arch Dermatol 1982; 118:228.

53. Luong K, Nguyen L: Aquagenic urticaria: report of a case and review of the literature, Ann Allergy Asthma Immunol 1998; 80(6):483.

54. Greaves MW, et al: Aquagenic pruritus, Br Med J 1981; 282:2008.

55. Lott T, et al: Treatment of aquagenic pruritus with topical capsaicin cream, J Am Acad Dermatol 1994; 30:232.

56. Steinman HK, Greaves MW: Aquagenic pruritus, J Am Acad Dermatol 1985; 13:91.

57. Bayoumi A-H, Highet AS: Baking soda baths for aquagenic pruritus, Lancet 1986; 23:464.

58. Megerian CA, et al: Angioedema: 5 years' experience, with a review of the disorder's presentation and treatment, Laryngoscope 1992; 102:256.

59. Saxon A, et al: Immediate hypersensitivity reactions to beta-lactam antibiotics, Ann Intern Med 1987; 107:204.

60. Agah R, Bandi V, Guntupalli K: Angioedema: the role of ACE inhibitors and factors associated with poor clinical outcome, Intensive Care Med 1997; 23(7):793.

61. Thompson T, Frable MA: Drug-induced, life-threatening angioedema revisited, Laryngoscope 1993; 103:10.

62. Israili ZH, Hall WD: Cough and angioneurotic edema associated with angiotensin-converting enzyme inhibitor therapy: a review of the literature and pathophysiology, Ann Intern Med 1992; 117:234.

63. Rees RS, et al: Angioedema associated with lisinopril, Am J Emerg Med 1992; 10:321.

64. Bielory L, et al: Long-acting ACE inhibitor-induced angioedema, Allergy Proc 1992; 13:85.

65. Roberts JR, Wuerz RC: Clinical characteristics of angiotensin-converting enzyme inhibitor-induced angioedema, Ann Emerg Med 1991; 20:555.

66. Orfan N, et al: Severe angioedema related to ACE inhibitors in patients with a history of idiopathic angioedema, JAMA 1990; 264:1287.

67. Cicardi M, et al: Long-term treatment of hereditary angioedema with attenuated androgens: a survey of a 13-year experience, J Allergy Clin Immunol 1991; 87:768.

68. Crampon D, et al: Danazol therapy: an unusual aetiology of hepatocellular carcinoma [letter], J Hepatol 1998; 29(6):1035.

69. Bork K, et al: Hepatocellular adenomas in patients taking danazol for hereditary angioedema [letter] [see comments], Lancet 1999; 353(9158):1066.

70. Chikama R, et al: Nonepisodic angioedema associated with eosinophilia: report of 4 cases and review of 33 young female patients reported in Japan, Dermatology 1998; 197(4):321.

71. Gleich GJ, et al: Episodic angioedema associated with eosinophilia, N Engl J Med 1984; 310:1621.

72. Von K, Maibach HI: The contact urticaria syndrome: an updated review, J Am Acad Dermatol 1981; 5:328.

73. Fisher AA: Contact urticaria due to medicants, chemicals and foods, Cutis 1982; 30:168.

74. Schechter JF, Wilkinson RD, Del CJ: Anaphylaxis following the use of Bacitracin ointment, Arch Dermatol 1984; 120:909.

75. Freeman S, Rosen RH: Urticarial contact dermatitis in food handlers, Med J Aust 1991; 155:91.

76. Holmes RC, Black MM: The specific dermatoses of pregnancy, J Am Acad Dermatol 1983; 8:405.

77. Lawley TJ, et al: Pruritic urticarial papules and plaques of pregnancy, JAMA 1979; 241:1696.

78. Winton GB, Lewis CW: Dermatosis of pregnancy, J Am Acad Dermatol 1982; 6:977.

79. Yancey KB, Hall RP, Lawley TJ: Pruritic urticarial papules and plaques of pregnancy: clinical experience in twenty-five patients, J Am Acad Dermatol 1984; 10:473.

80. Callen JP, Hanno R: Pruritic urticarial, papules, and plaques of pregnancy (PUPPP): a clinical experience in twenty-five patients, J Am Acad Dermatol 1981; 5:401.

81. Holmes RC, Black MM: The specific dermatoses of pregnancy: a reappraisal with special emphasis on a proposed simplified clinical classification, Clin Exp Dermatol 1982; 7:65.

82. Weiss R, Hull P: Familial occurrence of pruritic urticarial papules and plaques of pregnancy, J Am Acad Dermatol 1992; 26:715.

83. Krompouzos G, Cohen L: Dermatoses of pregnancy, J Am Acad Dermatol 2001; 45(1):1; quiz 19.

84. Wisnieski J: Urticarial vasculitis, Curr Opin Rheumatol 2000; 12(1):24.

85. Mehregan DR, et al: Urticarial vasculitis: a histopathologic and clinical review of 72 cases, J Am Acad Dermatol 1992; 26:441.

86. Wisnieski JJ, Jones SM: IgG autoantibody to the collagen-like region of C1q in hypocomplementemic urticarial vasculitis syndrome, systemic lupus erythematosus, and 6 other musculoskeletal or rheumatic diseases, J Rheumatol 1992; 19:884.

87. Millns JL, et al: The therapeutic response of urticarial vasculitis to indomethacin, J Am Acad Dermatol 1980; 3:349.

88. Wiles JC, Hansen RC, Lynch PJ: Urticarial vasculitis treated with colchicine, Arch Dermatol 1985; 121:802.

89. Muramatsu C, Tanabe E: Urticarial vasculitis: response to dapsone and colchicine, J Am Acad Dermatol 1985; 13:1055.

90. Fortson JS, et al: Hypocomplementemic urticarial vasculitis syndrome responsive to dapsone, J Am Acad Dermatol 1986; 15:1137.

91. Stack PS: Methotrexate for urticarial vasculitis, Ann Allergy 1994; 72:36.

92. Joubert G, et al: Selection of treatment of cefaclor-associated urticarial, serum sickness-like reactions and erythema multiforme by emergency pediatricians: lack of a uniform standard of care, Can J Clin Pharmacol 1999; 6(4):197.

93. Knowles S, Shapiro L, Shear N: Serious dermatologic reactions in children, Curr Opin Pediatr 1997; 9(4):388.

94. Lawley TJ, et al: A prospective clinical and immunologic analysis of patients with serum sickness, N Engl J Med 1984; 311:1407.

95. Berman BA, Ross RN: Acute serum sickness, Cutis 1983; 32:420.

96. Stein DH: Mastocytosis: a review, Pediatr Dermatol 1986; 3:365.

97. DiBacco RS, DeLeo VA: Mastocytosis and the mast cell, J Am Acad Dermatol 1982; 7:709.

98. Fowler JF, Parsley WM, Gotter PG: Familial urticaria pigmentosa, Arch Dermatol 1986; 122:80.

99. Hartmann K, Henz B: Classification of cutaneous mastocytosis: a modified consensus proposal, Leuk Res 2002; 26(5):483; discussion 485.

100. Assaf C, et al: Cutaneous mastocytosis, Lancet 2002; 359(9316):1465.

101. Carter M, Metcalfe D: Paediatric mastocytosis: Arch Dis Child 2002; 86(5):315.

102. Tebbe B, et al: Cutaneous mastocytosis in adults: evaluation of 14 patients with respect to systemic disease manifestations, Dermatology 1998; 197(2):101.

103. Czarnetzki BM, et al: Bone marrow findings in adult patients with urticaria pigmentosa, J Am Acad Dermatol 1988; 18:45.

104. Webb TA, Li C-Y, Yam LT: Systemic mast cell disease: a clinical and hematopathologic study of 26 cases, Cancer 1982; 49:927.

Acne, Rosacea, and Related Disorders

❑ **Acne**
  Classification
  Overview of diagnosis and treatment
  Etiology and pathogenesis
  Approach to acne therapy
  Acne treatment
  Therapeutic agents for treatment of acne

❑ **Acne surgery**
  Other types of acne

❑ **Perioral dermatitis**

❑ **Rosacea (acne rosacea)**
  Skin manifestations
  Ocular rosacea

❑ **Hidradenitis suppurativa**
  Clinical presentation
  Pathogenesis
  Management

❑ **Miliaria**
  Miliaria crystallina
  Miliaria rubra
  Miliaria profunda

Acne

Acne, a disease of the pilosebaceous unit, appears in males and females in westernized societies who are near puberty and in most cases becomes less active as adolescence ends. The intensity and duration of activity varies for each individual.

The disease may be minor, with only a few comedones or papules, or it may occur as the highly inflammatory and diffusely scarring acne conglobata. The most severe forms of acne occur more frequently in males, but the disease tends to be more persistent in females, who may have periodic flare-ups before menstrual periods, which continue until menopause.

PSYCHOSOCIAL EFFECTS OF ACNE. Acne is too often dismissed as a minor affliction not worthy of treatment. Believing it is a phase of the growing process and that lesions will soon disappear, parents of children with acne postpone seeking medical advice. Permanent scarring of the skin and the psyche can result from such inaction. The disease has implications far beyond the few marks that may appear on the face. Lesions cannot be hidden under clothing; each is prominently displayed and detracts significantly from one's personal appearance and self-esteem. Taunting and ridicule from peers is demoralizing. Appearing in public creates embarrassment and frustration. Because acne is perceived by adolescents to have important negative personal and social consequences, improvement in these areas accompanies medical treatment. Facial appearance then becomes more acceptable to peers, embarrassment diminishes, and patients feel less socially inhibited.[1]

THE PHYSICIAN-PATIENT RELATIONSHIP. Many acne sufferers expect to be disappointed with the results of treatment.[2] They may be sensitive to actual or supposed lack of acceptance on the part of their physicians. Adolescence is usually characterized by the challenge of parental rules, and this transfers to the relationship with the physician. Noncompliance can be decreased by carefully explaining the goals and techniques of treatment and leaving the choice of implementation to the adolescent. Parents who offer to make sure the adolescent follows the treatment plan may encourage noncompliance by placing the treatment within the context of existing parent-child struggles.[3] Greater consideration of adolescents' psychologic situations improves the therapeutic outcome, increases compliance, and leads to a greater confidence in the physician.

POSTADOLESCENT ACNE IN WOMEN. A low-grade, persistent acne is common in professional women. Closed comedones are the dominant lesions, with a few papulopustules. Premenstrual flare-ups are typical. Many of these patients passed through adolescence without acne. One author postulated that chronic stress leads to enhanced secretion of adrenal androgens, resulting in sebaceous hyperplasia and subsequent induction of comedones.[4] A survey was taken of adult premenopausal women treated for mild-to-moderate, nonscarring, inflammatory acne who had undergone standard acne treatments without success or who had a clinical presentation suggesting hyperandrogenism (premenstrual exacerbations, irregular menses, coexisting hirsutism, androgenetic alopecia, seborrhea, or acne distribution on the lower face area, mandibular line, or neck).[5]

The mean duration of acne was 20 years. A mean age at the time of the survey of 37 years and a mean age at onset of 16 years were documented. Acne was reported to be persistent in 80%.

Eighty-three percent reported exacerbation with menses, 67% with stress, and 26% by diet. Pregnancy affected acne in 65% of the women, with 41% reporting improvement and 29% reporting worsening with pregnancy.

Classification

The Consensus Conference on Acne Classification (1990) proposed that acne grading be accomplished by the use of a pattern-diagnosis system, which includes a total evaluation of lesions and their complications such as drainage, hemorrhage, and pain (Figure 7-1). It takes into account the total impact of the disease, which is influenced by the disfigurement it causes. Degree of severity is also determined by occupational disability, psychosocial impact, and the failure of response to previous treatment.

ACNE LESIONS. Acne lesions are divided into inflammatory and noninflammatory lesions. Noninflammatory lesions consist of open and closed comedones. Inflammatory acne lesions are characterized by the presence of one or more of the following types of lesions: papules, pustules, and nodules (cysts). Papules are less than 5 mm in diameter. Pustules have a visible central core of purulent material. Nodules are greater than 5 mm in diameter. Nodules may become suppurative or hemorrhagic. Suppurative nodular lesions have been referred to as cysts because of their resemblance to inflamed epidermal cysts. Recurring rupture and reepithelialization of cysts leads to epithelial-lined sinus tracks, often accompanied by disfiguring scars.

For inflammatory acne lesions, the Consensus Panel proposes that lesions be classified as papulopustular and/or nodular. A severity grade based on a lesion count approximation is assigned as mild, moderate, or severe. Illustrative examples of each category of severity are shown in Figure 7-2. Other factors in assessing severity include ongoing scarring, persistent purulent and/or serosanguineous drainage from lesions, and the presence of sinus tracks.

Overview of diagnosis and treatment

An overview of diagnosis and treatment is presented in Figures 7-1 to 7-3 and Box 7-1.

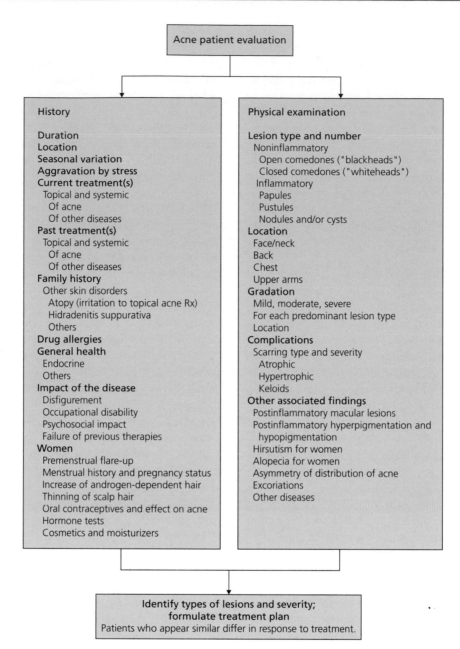

Figure 7-1 Patients who appear similar differ in response to treatment.

TYPE OF LESIONS

Noninflammatory lesions

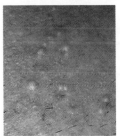
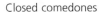

Closed comedones

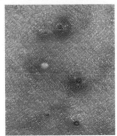

Open comedones

Inflammatory lesions

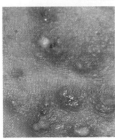

Papules/pustules

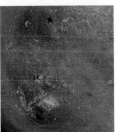

Nodules

ACNE CLASSIFICATION AND GRADING

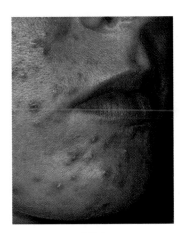

Mild
Papules/pustules +/++
Nodules 0

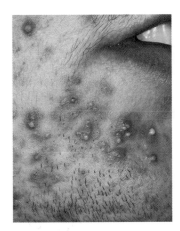

Moderate
Papules/pustules ++/+++
Nodules +/++

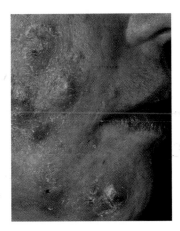

Severe
Papules/pustules +++/++++
Nodules +++

SEVERITY GRADING OF INFLAMMATORY LESIONS

Severity	Papules/pustules	Nodules	Additional factors tht determine severity
Mild	Few to several	None	Psychosocial circumstances
Moderate	Several to many	Few to several	Occupational difficulties
Severe	Numerous and/or extensive	Many	Inadequate therapeutic responsiveness

Figure 7-2 Acne classification of lesions.

ACNE TREATMENT

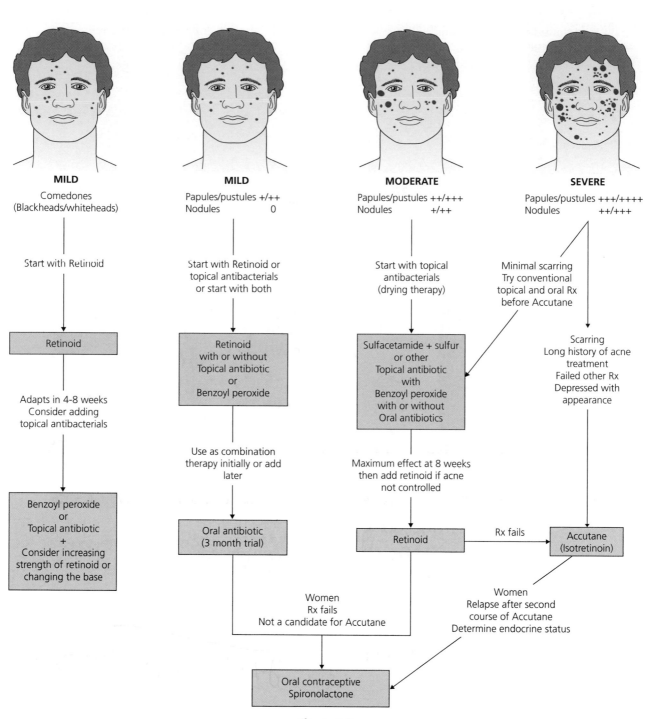

MILD
Comedones
(Blackheads/whiteheads)

Start with Retinoid

Retinoid

Adapts in 4-8 weeks
Consider adding
topical antibacterials

Benzoyl peroxide
or
Topical antibiotic
+
Consider increasing
strength of retinoid or
changing the base

MILD
Papules/pustules +/++
Nodules   0

Start with Retinoid or
topical antibacterials
or start with both

Retinoid
with or without
Topical antibiotic
or
Benzoyl peroxide

Use as combination
therapy initially or add
later

Oral antibiotic
(3 month trial)

Women
Rx fails
Not a candidate for Accutane

MODERATE
Papules/pustules ++/+++
Nodules   +/++

Start with topical
antibacterials
(drying therapy)

Sulfacetamide + sulfur
or other
Topical antibiotic
with
Benzoyl peroxide
with or without
Oral antibiotics

Maximum effect at 8 weeks
then add retinoid if acne
not controlled

Retinoid   Rx fails

SEVERE
Papules/pustules +++/++++
Nodules   ++/+++

Minimal scarring
Try conventional
topical and oral Rx
before Accutane

Scarring
Long history of acne
treatment
Failed other Rx
Depressed with
appearance

Accutane
(Isotretinoin)

Women
Relapse after second
course of Accutane
Determine endocrine status

Oral contraceptive
Spironolactone

Figure 7-3

Box 7-1 Acne Medications

Retinoids

Tazarotene
  Tazorac Gel, Cream

Tretinoin
  Retin-A: Gel, Cream, Solution, Micro

Adapalene
  Differin: Cream, Gel, Solution, Pledgets

Benzoyl peroxide

Brevoxyl-4, 8
  Creamy Wash, Cleansing Lotion, Gel

Benzaclin Gel
  Benzoyl Peroxide; Clindamycin

Benzamycin
  Benzoyl Peroxide; Erythromycin

Triaz
  Cleanser (3%, 6%, 9%)
  Gel (3%, 6%, 9%)

Many others

Topical antibiotics

Clindamycin
  Clindagel
  Clindets Pledgets
  Cleocin T (Gel, Lotion, Solution)

Azelaic acid
  Azelex, Finacea Gel, Cream

Erythromycin
  (Emgel Gel)

Topical antibiotics—cont'd

Sulfacetamide + Sulfur
  Sulfacet-R, Rosula,
  Klaron Lotion (no sulfur)
  Plexion (Topical Suspension, Cleanser)
  Rosanil (Cleanser)

Oral antibiotics

Tetracycline

Doxycycline

Minocycline

Amoxicillin

Trimethoprim

Cephalosporins

Clindamycin

Erythromycin

Azithromycin

Isotretinoin

Accutane, Amnesteen, Sotret, 10 mg, 20 mg, 40 mg

Antiandrogens

Oral Contraceptives
  Estrostep
  Ortho Tri-Cyclen 21 Tablets
  Ortho Tri-Cyclen 28 Tablets
  Others

Spironolactone

MODERATE-TO-SEVERE PUSTULAR ACNE

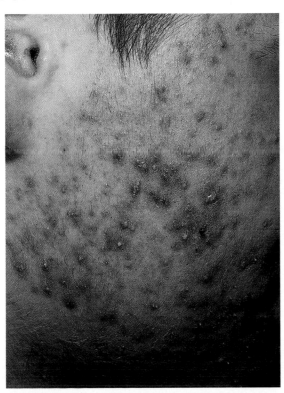

SEVERE NODULOCYSTIC ACNE

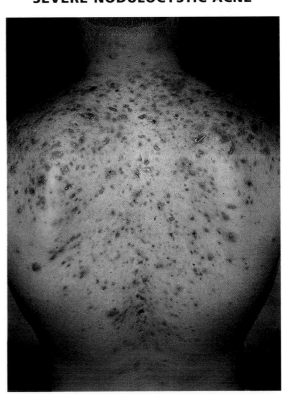

PATHOGENESIS OF ACNE

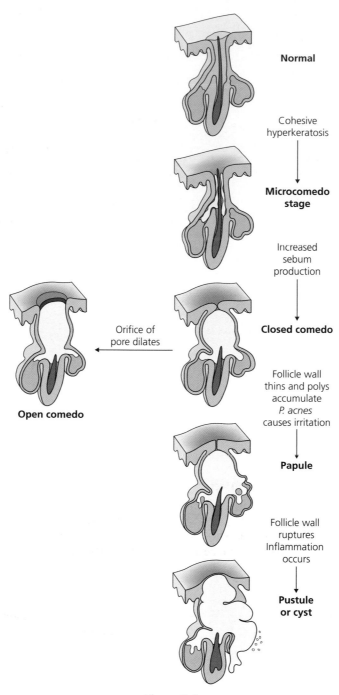

Figure 7-4

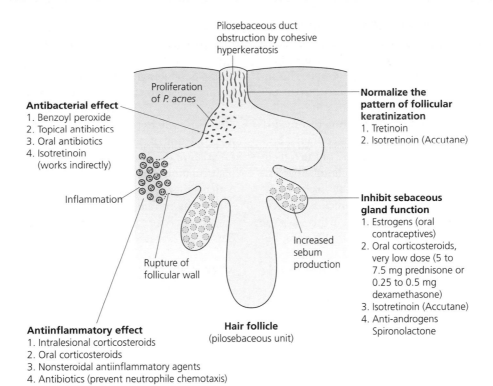

Pilosebaceous duct
obstruction by cohesive
hyperkeratosis

Proliferation
of *P. acnes*

Antibacterial effect
1. Benzoyl peroxide
2. Topical antibiotics
3. Oral antibiotics
4. Isotretinoin
   (works indirectly)

Inflammation

**Normalize the
pattern of follicular
keratinization**
1. Tretinoin
2. Isotretinoin (Accutane)

**Inhibit sebaceous
gland function**
1. Estrogens (oral
   contraceptives)
2. Oral corticosteroids,
   very low dose (5 to
   7.5 mg prednisone or
   0.25 to 0.5 mg
   dexamethasone)
3. Isotretinoin (Accutane)
4. Anti-androgens
   Spironolactone

Increased
sebum
production

Rupture of
follicular wall

Antiinflammatory effect
1. Intralesional corticosteroids
2. Oral corticosteroids
3. Nonsteroidal antiinflammatory agents
4. Antibiotics (prevent neutrophile chemotaxis)

Hair follicle
(pilosebaceous unit)

Figure 7-5 Mode of action of therapeutic agents.

Etiology and pathogenesis

Figure 7-4 illustrates the evolution of the different acne lesions, and Figure 7-5 illustrates the mechanism of action of therapeutic agents. Acne is a disease involving the pilosebaceous unit and is most frequent and intense in areas where sebaceous glands are largest and most numerous. Acne begins in predisposed individuals when sebum production increases. *Propionibacterium acnes* proliferates in sebum, and the follicular epithelial lining becomes altered and forms plugs called comedones. One study suggests that anxiety and anger are significant factors for patients who have severe acne.[6]

SEBACEOUS GLANDS. Sebum is the pathogenic factor in acne; it is irritating and comedogenic, especially when *P. acnes* proliferates and modifies its components. Most patients with acne have a higher-than-normal sebum level.

Sebaceous glands are located throughout the entire body except the palms, soles, dorsa of the feet, and lower lip. They are largest and most numerous on the face, chest, back, and upper outer arms. Clusters of glands appear as relatively large, visible, white globules on the buccal mucosa (Fordyce's spots), the vermilion border of the upper lip (Figure 7-6), the female areolae (Montgomery's tubercles), the labia minora, the prepuce, and around the anus.

Sebaceous glands are large in newborn infants, but regress shortly after birth. They remain relatively small in infancy

and most of childhood, but enlarge and become more active in prepuberty. Hormones influence sebaceous gland secretion. Testosterone is converted to dihydrotestosterone in the skin and acts directly on the sebaceous gland to increase its size and metabolic rate. Estrogens, through a less well-defined mechanism, decrease sebaceous gland secretion. Sebaceous gland cells produce a complex mixture of oily material. Sebaceous cells mature, die, fragment, and then extrude into the sebaceous duct, where they combine with the desquamating cells of the lower hair follicle and finally arrive at the skin surface as sebum.

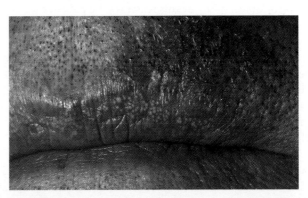

Figure 7-6 Cluster of sebaceous glands (tiny, white-yellow spots) are normally present on the vermillion border of the upper lip.

PILOSEBACEOUS DUCT OBSTRUCTION. The early acne lesion results from blockage in the follicular canal. Increased amounts of keratin result from hormonal changes and sebum modified by the resident bacterial flora *P. acnes.* The increased number of cornified cells remain adherent to the follicular canal (retention keratosis) directly above the opening of the sebaceous gland duct to form a plug (microcomedo). Factors causing increased sebaceous secretion (puberty, hormonal imbalances) influence the eventual size of the follicular plug. The plug enlarges behind a very small follicular orifice at the skin surface and becomes visible as a closed comedone (firm, white papule). An open comedone (blackhead) occurs if the follicular orifice dilates. Further increase in the size of a blackhead continues to dilate the pore, but usually does not result in inflammation. The small-pore, closed comedone is the precursor of inflammatory acne papules, pustules, and cysts.

BACTERIAL COLONIZATION AND INFLAMMATION. *P. acnes,* an anaerobic diphtheroid, is a normal skin resident and the principal component of the microbic flora of the pilosebaceous follicle. The bacteria are thought to play a significant role in acne. *P. acnes* generate components that create inflammation, such as lipases, proteases, hyaluronidase, and chemotactic factors. Lipases hydrolyze sebum triglycerides to form free fatty acids, which are comedogenic and primary irritants. Chemotactic factors attract neutrophils to the follicular wall. Neutrophils elaborate hydrolases that weaken the wall. The wall thins, becomes inflamed (red papule), and ruptures, releasing part of the comedone into the dermis. An intense, foreign-body, inflammatory reaction results in the formation of the acne pustule or cyst. Other bacteria substances possibly mediate inflammation by stimulation of immune mechanisms.

Approach to acne therapy
Initial visit

HISTORY. Many patients are embarrassed to ask for help. Any feeling of apathy or indifference on the part of the physician will be sensed, resulting in a loss of esteem and enthusiasm for the treatment. A careful history should be taken. Inquiring about many details reassures the patient that this is a disease to be taken seriously and managed carefully. Previous treatment should be documented—types of cleansers and lubricants, family history, and history of cyclic menstrual flareups. The potential for irritation can be determined by responses to drying therapy with over-the-counter benzoyl peroxide. This experience facilitates the choice of which strength and base of benzoyl peroxide, tretinoin, or other topical agents to start.

PATHOGENESIS AND COURSE. Acne is an inherited disease. It is not possible to predict which members of a family will inherit it. The severity of acne in persons developing the disease is not necessarily related to the severity of acne in their parents. Acne does not end at age 19 but can persist into a person's forties. Many women have their first episode after age 25. Several myths should be discussed. Acne is not caused by dirt. The pigment in blackheads is not dirt and may not be melanin as was once suspected.[7] Excessive washing is unnecessary and interferes with most treatment programs. Gentle manipulation of pustules is tolerated; aggressive pressure and excoriation produces permanent scarring. The erythema and pigmentation that follows resolution of acne lesions in some patients may take many months to fade.

Patients should not have inappropriate expectations. In most cases, acne can be controlled, but not cured. Stress is an important exacerbating factor.

ACNE AND DIET. In Western cultures, acne effects up to 95% of adolescents and persists into middle age in 12% of women and 3% of men. Two non-Westernized populations: the Kitavan Islanders of Papua New Guinea and the Ache hunter-gatherers of Paraguay do not have acne. They eat fruit, fish, game, and tubers but no cereals or refined sugars.[8]

This suggests that high-glycemic carbohydrates (bread, bagels, doughnuts, crackers, candy, cake, chips), those that substantially boost blood sugar levels, set off a series of hormonal changes that cause acne. Elevated blood sugar leads to increases in insulin production. This affects other hormones that can cause excess oil in the skin. Therefore low-glycemic diets, including fruits and vegetables, might offer a new treatment option for people with acne.

COSMETICS AND CLEANSERS. Moderate use of nongreasy lubricants and water-based cosmetics is usually well tolerated, but a gradual decrease in the use of cosmetics is encouraged as acne improves. Cream-based cleansers should be avoided.

ORAL CONTRACEPTIVES. If women patients are taking oral contraceptives, a change in estrogen and progestin combinations may be all that is necessary.

Initial evaluation

TYPE OF LESIONS. An overview of diagnosis and treatment is presented in the beginning of this chapter (see Figures 7-1 to 7-3). The types of lesions present are determined (i.e., comedones, papules, pustules, nodules, or cysts). The degree of severity (mild, moderate, severe) is also determined.

DEGREE OF SKIN SENSITIVITY. The degree of skin sensitivity can be determined by inquiring about experiences with topical medicines and soaps. Degree of pigmentation and hair color are not the sole determinants of skin sensitivity. Atopic patients with dry skin and a history of eczema generally do not tolerate aggressive drying therapy.

SELECTION OF THERAPY. Therapy appropriate to the type of acne is selected. (For initial orientation, refer to Figure 7-3.) If antibiotics are selected for initial therapy, it is best to start with "therapeutic dosages" (see section on oral antibiotics, p. 180).

COURSE OF TREATMENT. A program can be established for most patients after three visits, but some difficult cases require continual supervision. For maximum effect treatment must be continual and prolonged. Patients who had only a few lesions that quickly cleared may be given a trial period without treatment 6 to 8 weeks after clearing. In an attempt to suppress further activity, those patients who have numerous lesions should remain on continual topical treatment for several months. The patient's propensity to scar must be ascertained. Patients vary in their tendency to develop scars. Some demonstrate little scarring even after significant inflammation, whereas others develop a scar from nearly every inflammatory papular or pustular lesion. This latter group requires aggressive therapy to prevent further damage. The early use of isotretinoin may be justified in these patients.

Acne treatment

The following treatment programs are offered only as a guide. Modifications must be made for each individual (see Figure 7-3).

Comedonal acne

CLINICAL PRESENTATION. The earliest type of acne is usually noninflammatory comedones ("blackheads" and "whiteheads") (Figures 7-7 and 7-8). It develops in the pre-teenage or early teenage years and is caused by increased sebum production and abnormal desquamation of epithelial cells. There are no inflammatory lesions because colonization with *P. acnes* has not yet occurred.

TREATMENT. Closed comedone acne (whiteheads) responds slowly. A large mass of sebaceous material is impacted behind a very small follicular orifice. The orifice may enlarge during treatment, making extraction by acne surgery possible. Comedones may remain unchanged for months or evolve into a pustule or cyst.

Retinoids (Tazorac, Retin-A, Differin, Azelex) are applied at bedtime. The base and strength is selected according to skin sensitivity. Tazorac may be the most effective and most irritating. Start with a low concentration of the cream or gel (available in 0.05% and 0.1%) and increase the concentration if irritation does not occur. Retin-A and Differin are equally effective. Start with Retin-A cream (0.025%, 0.05%, 0.1%) or gel (0.01% and 0.025%) or Micro or Diffcrin (gel, cream, solution, pads). Azelex is less potent but is less irritating. It also has antibacterial activity. Medications are used more frequently if tolerated. Add benzoyl peroxide or topical antibiotics or combination medicines (e.g., Benzaclin) later to discourage *P. acne* and the formation of inflammatory lesions. The response to treatment is slow and discouraging. Several months of treatment are required. Large open comedones (blackheads) are expressed; many are difficult to remove. Several weeks of treatment facilitates easier extraction. Topical therapy may have to be continued for extended periods.

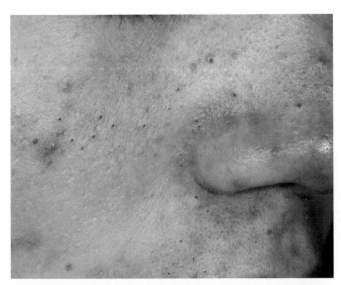

Figure 7-7 Comedones (blackheads) are occasionally inflamed.

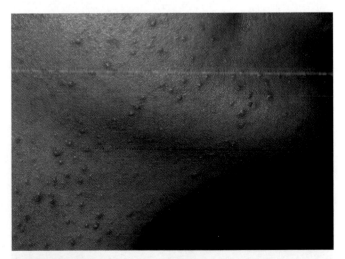

Figure 7-8 Closed comedones (whiteheads). Tiny, white, dome-shaped papules with a small follicular orifice. Stretching the skin accentuated these lesions.

Mild inflammatory acne

CLINICAL PRESENTATION. Mild pustular and papular inflammatory acne is defined as fewer than 20 pustules. Inflammatory lesions occur in comedones after proliferation of *P. acnes.* Papules or pustules with a minimum of comedones may develop after comedonal acne (Figure 7-9).

TREATMENT. Benzoyl peroxide, a topical antibiotic, or combination medicine (e.g., Benzaclin) and a retinoid are initially applied on alternate evenings. The lowest concentrations are initially used. After the initial adjustment period, the retinoid is used each night and benzoyl peroxide or antibiotic each morning. The strength of the medications is increased if tolerated. Oral antibiotics are introduced if the number of pustules does not decrease. Topical therapy may have to be continued for extended periods.

Moderate-to-severe inflammatory acne

CLINICAL PRESENTATION. Patients who have moderate-to-severe acne (more than 20 pustules) are temporarily disfigured (Figures 7-10 through 7-13).

Their disease may have been gradually worsening or may be virulent at the onset. The explosive onset of pustules can sometimes be precipitated by stress. There may be few to negligible visible comedones. Affected areas should not be irritated during the initial stages of therapy.

TREATMENT. Moderate inflammation is treated with twice-daily application of a topical antibiotic, benzoyl peroxide, or combination medicine (e.g., Benzaclin) or the combination of benzoyl peroxide and sulfacetamide/sulfur. This drying agent program can be very effective. Patients using drying agents should adjust the frequency of application to induce a mild, continuous peel. Response to treatment may occur in 2 to 4 weeks. Oral antibiotics (tetracycline or doxycycline) are used for patients with more than ten pustules. Treatment should be continued until no new lesions develop (2 to 4 months) and then should be slowly tapered. If there are any signs of irritation, the frequency and strength of topical medicines should be decreased. Irritation, particularly around the mandibular areas and neck, worsens pustular acne.

A retinoid can be introduced if the number of pustules and the degree of inflammation have decreased. Start minocycline at full dosage if there is no response to tetracycline or doxycycline after 3 months. Pustules are gently incised and expressed. Injecting each pustule with a very small amount of triamcinolone acetonide (Kenalog 2.5 to 5.0 mg/cc) can give immediate and very gratifying results.

Those who have responded well may begin to taper and eventually discontinue oral antibiotics.

Some patients respond very well to lower dosages of oral antibiotics and require tetracycline, 250 mg/day or even every other day for control. Those patients may be safely maintained on low-dose oral antibiotics for extended periods. Patients who do not respond to conventional therapy may have lesions that are colonized by gram-negative organisms. Culture of pustules and cysts are obtained and an appropriate antibiotic such as ampicillin is started. The response may be dramatic.

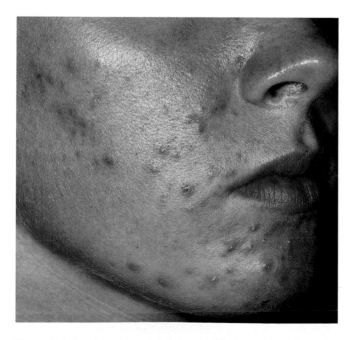

Figure 7-9 Papular and pustular acne (mild). Several papules are localized on the cheeks.

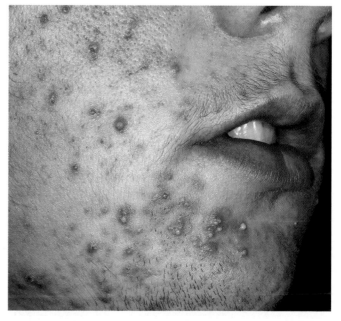

Figure 7-10 Papular and pustular acne (moderate). Many pustules are present, and several have become confluent on the chin area.

MODERATE-TO-SEVERE INFLAMMATORY ACNE

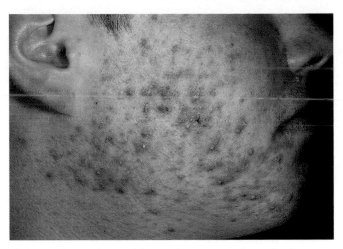

Figure 7-11 Papules, nodules, and cysts cover the entire face. Scarring is extensive.

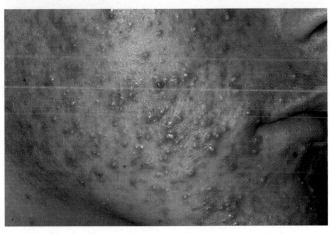

Figure 7-12 All forms of conventional therapy failed to control these numerous pustules. Isotretinoin cleared the acne.

Figure 7-13 Localized nodular and cystic acne. Cystic and nodular lesions appeared in this patient, who has chronic comedo and pustular acne.

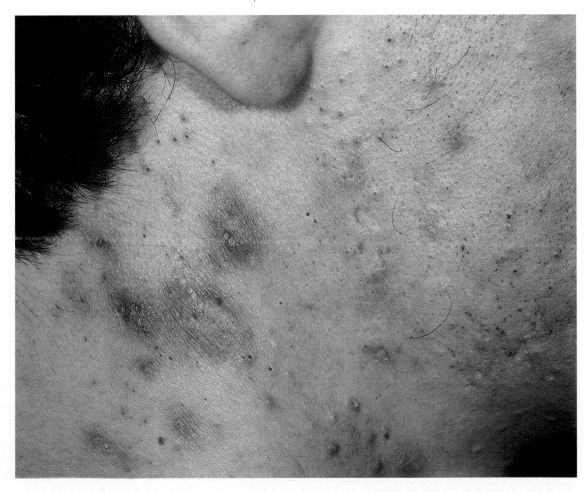

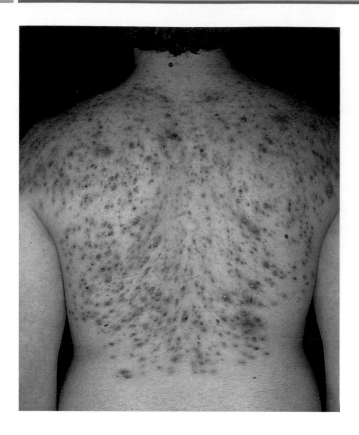

Severe: Nodulocystic acne

CLINICAL PRESENTATION. Nodulocystic acne includes localized cystic acne (few cysts on face, chest, or back), diffuse cystic acne (wide areas of face, chest, and back) (Figures 7-14 through 7-19), pyoderma faciale (inflamed cysts localized on the face in females) (Figure 7-20), and acne conglobata (highly inflammatory, with cysts that communicate under the skin, abscesses, and burrowing sinus tracts) (Figures 7-21 and 7-23).

Cystic acne

Cystic acne is a serious and sometimes devastating disease that requires aggressive treatment. The face, chest, back, and upper arms may be permanently mutilated by numerous atrophic or hypertrophic scars. Patients sometimes delay seeking help, hoping that improvement will occur spontaneously; consequently, the disease may be quite advanced when first viewed by the physician.

Figure 7-14 Nodular and cystic acne (severe). Active nodular and cystic acne covering the entire back.

Figure 7-15 Nodular and cystic acne (severe). Granulation tissue and crusts suddenly occurred after starting treatment with isotretinoin (high doses) 2 mg/kg/day.

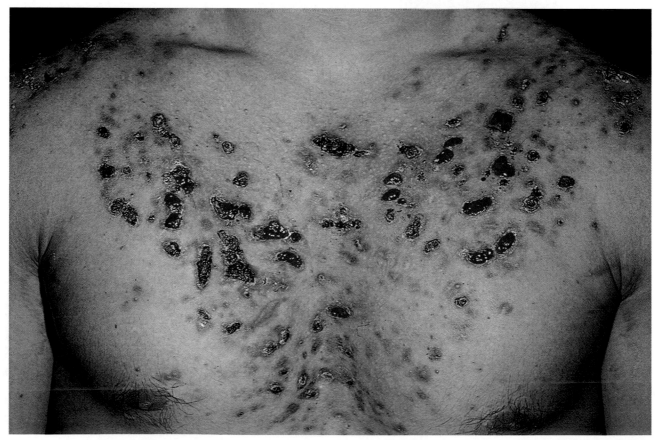

SEVERE INFLAMMATORY CYSTIC ACNE

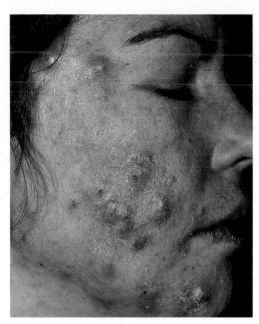

Figure 7-16 Cystic acne. The lesions in this patient are primarily cystic. Only a few pustules and comedones are present.

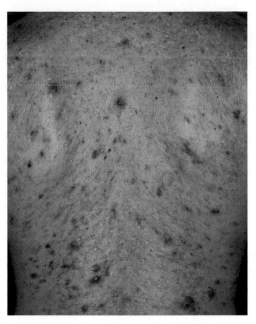

Figure 7-17 Nodular and cystic acne. Years of activity have left numerous scars over the entire back. Several active cysts are present.

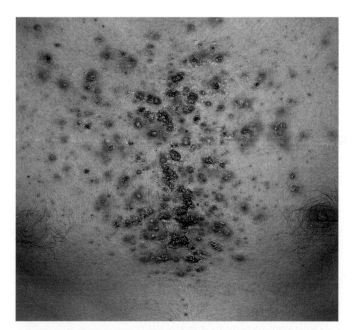

Figure 7-18 Nodular and cystic acne (severe). Many cysts have opened and drained.

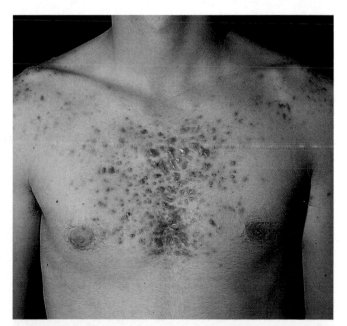

Figure 7-19 Nodular and cystic acne (severe). Patient in Figure 7-18 six months after stopping isotretinoin. There are numerous atrophic and hypertrophic scars with postinflammatory pigmentation.

Patients are often embarrassed by and preoccupied with their disease. They may experience anxiety, depression, insecurity, psychic suffering, and social isolation. The physical appearance may be so unattractive that teenagers refuse to attend school and adults fear going to work. Patients report difficulty securing employment when afflicted and problems being accepted in the working environment. Patients with a few inflamed cysts can be treated with a program similar to that outlined for moderate-to-severe inflammatory acne. Oral antibiotics, conventional topical therapy, and periodic intralesional Kenalog injections may keep this problem under adequate control.

Extensive cystic acne requires a different approach. There are three less common variants of cystic acne.

PYODERMA FACIALE. Pyoderma faciale is a distinctive variant of cystic acne that remains confined to the face (Figure 7-20).[9] It is a disease of adult women ranging in age from the teens to the forties. They experience the rapid onset of large, sore, erythematous-to-purple cysts, predominantly on the central portion of the cheeks. Erythema may be intense. Purulent drainage from cysts occurs spontaneously or with minor trauma. Comedones are absent and scarring occurs in most cases. A traumatic emotional experience has been associated with some cases. Many patients do not have a history of acne.

Cultures help to differentiate this condition from gram-negative acne. Highly inflamed lesions can be managed by starting isotretinoin and oral corticosteroids. A study reported effective management with the following. Treatment was begun with prednisolone (1.0 mg/kg daily for 1 to 2 weeks). Isotretinoin was then added (0.2 to 0.5 mg/kg/day [rarely, 1.0 mg/kg in resistant cases]), with a slow tapering of the corticosteroid over the following 2 to 3 weeks. Isotretinoin was continued until all inflammatory lesions resolved. This required 3 to 4 months. None of the patients had a recurrence.[9] This group of patients were "flusher and blushers," and it was suggested that pyoderma faciale is a type of rosacea. The investigators proposed the term *rosacea fulminans*. Another review showed that the disease could be effectively managed by omitting prednisone and using Vlem Dome (sulfur solution compresses) and oral antibiotics.[10]

Acne fulminans

Acne fulminans is a rare ulcerative form of acne of unknown etiology with an acute onset and systemic symptoms. It most commonly affects adolescent white boys. A genetic predisposition is suspected.[11] An ulcerative, necrotic acne with systemic symptoms develops rapidly. There are arthralgias or severe muscle pain, or both, that accompany the acne flare.[12] Painful bone lesions occur in approximately 40% of patients. Weight loss, fever, leukocytosis, and elevated erythrocyte sedimentation rate (ESR) are common findings.

Antibiotic therapy is not effective. Oral corticosteroids (e.g., prednisolone, 0.5 to 1.0 mg/kg) are the primary therapy. They quickly control the skin lesions and systemic symptoms. Isotretinoin (0.5 to 1.0 mg/kg) is started simultaneously and, as in the therapy of severe cystic acne, is continued for 5 months.[13] The duration of steroid therapy is often at least 2 months. The bone lesions have a good prognosis; chronic sequelae are rare.

Acne conglobata

Acne conglobata is a chronic, highly inflammatory form of cystic acne in which involved areas contain a mixture of double comedones (two blackheads that communicate under the skin), papules, pustules, communicating cysts, abscesses, and draining sinus tracts (Figures 7-21 and 7-23). The disease may linger for years, ending with deep atrophic or keloidal scarring. Acne conglobata is part of the rare follicular occlusion triad syndrome of acne conglobata, hidradenitis suppurativa, and dissecting cellulitis of the scalp (Figure 7-22).[14] Musculoskeletal symptoms have been reported in some of these patients; 85% were black. There is no fever or weight loss as is seen in acne fulminans.

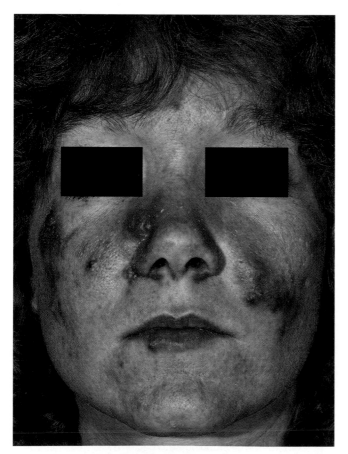

Figure 7-20 Pyoderma faciale. Confluent cysts remain localized to the face. The disease occurs almost exclusively in females.

Treatment of nodulocystic acne

The patient is assured that effective treatment is available. Patients should be told that they will be observed closely and, if the disease becomes very active, they will be seen at least weekly until the condition is adequately controlled. A primary therapeutic goal is to avoid scarring by terminating the intense inflammation quickly; prednisone is sometimes required. Cysts with thin roofs are incised and drained. Deeper cysts are injected with triamcinolone acetonide (Kenalog 2.5 to 10 mg/mL).

Patients who show little tendency to scar can be treated as patients with moderate-to-severe inflammatory acne. Most patients will require the rapid introduction of isotretinoin. The simultaneous use of tetracyclines (tetracycline, doxycycline, or minocycline) and isotretinoin is avoided, because a higher incidence of pseudotumor cerebri may occur with this combination. For highly active cases, prednisone (adult dosage is 20 to 30 mg two times a day) is used.

Intralesional triamcinolone acetonide injections and incision and drainage of cysts are important in the early weeks of management. Patients taking isotretinoin are usually not treated with other oral or topical agents.

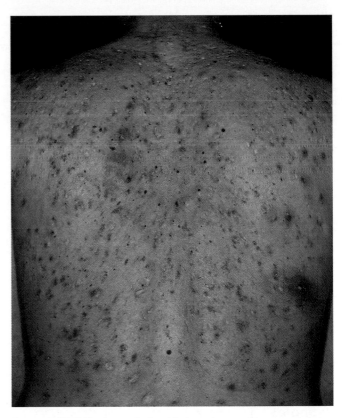

Figure 7-22 Follicular occlusion triad syndrome. Acne conglobata is part of the rare follicular occlusion triad syndrome of acne conglobata, hidradenitis suppurativa, and dissecting cellulitis of the scalp. Note the huge blackheads.

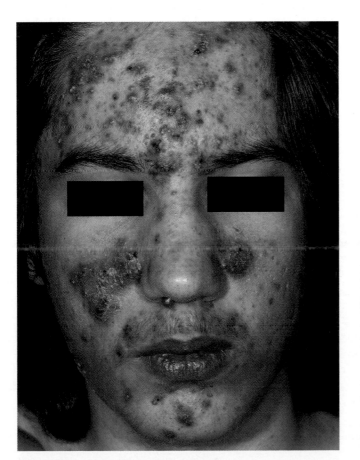

Figure 7-21 Acne congloblata. Large communicating cysts are present on the cheeks; scarring is extensive.

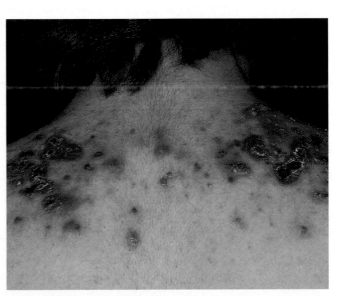

Figure 7-23 Acne conglobata. Abscesses and ulcerated cysts are found over most of the upper shoulder area.

Therapeutic agents for treatment of acne

There are four pathogenetic factors responsible for the development of acne. These are hyperkeratinization (plugging) of the pilosebaceous follicles, increased testosterone levels (producing hyperseborrhea), bacterial colonization with *P. acnes,* and inflammation. Topical agents influence at least one of these factors. More than 50% of patients present with comedones and papulopustular acne. These patients are initially treated with topical treatment. Combination regimens that include an antibiotic and a retinoid to reduce follicular plugging are the mainstay of topical treatment. Pustular acne may respond quickly to drying therapy with a combination of benzoyl peroxide and sulfacetamide and sulfur lotion. Systemic therapy with antibiotics or isotretinoin is used when scarring occurs or for cystic acne.

Topical and oral agents act at various stages (see Figure 7-5) in the evolution of an acne lesion and may be used alone or in combination to enhance efficacy. Topical agents should be applied to the entire affected area to treat existing lesions and to prevent the development of new ones. Potent topical steroid creams produce no short-term improvement in patients with moderate acne.[15]

Retinoids

Retinoids reverse the abnormal pattern of keratinization seen in acne vulgaris. Agents that act in a comedolytic and anticomedogenic manner to reduce follicular plugging are the retinoids tretinoin, adapalene and tazarotene, azelaic acid, and isotretinoin. Azelaic acid has strong antibacterial potency without inducing bacterial resistance similar to benzoyl peroxide. Adapalene has antiinflammatory activity. Retinoids may cause an increase in facial dryness and erythema.

Mechanism of action. Retinoids initiate increased cell turnover in both normal follicles and comedones and reduces the cohesion between keratinized cells. They act specifically on microcomedones (the precursor lesion of all forms of acne), causing fragmentation and expulsion of the microplug, expulsion of comedones, and conversion of closed comedones to open comedones.[16] New comedone formation is prevented by continued use. Inflammation may occur during this process, temporarily making acne worse. Continual topical application leads to thinning of the stratum corneum, making the skin more susceptible to sunburn; sun damage; and irritation from wind, cold, or dryness. Irritants such as astringents, alcohol, and acne soaps will not be tolerated as they were previously. The incidence of contact allergy is very low. Because of the direct action of retinoids on the microcomedone, many clinicians believe retinoids are appropriate for all forms of acne.

Combination therapy—synergism. Vitamin A acid enhances the penetration of other topical agents such as topical antibiotics and benzoyl peroxide. The enhanced penetration results in a synergistic effect with greater overall drug efficacy and a faster response to treatment.

Application techniques. The skin should be washed gently with a mild soap (e.g., Purpose, Basis) no more than two to three times each day, using the hands rather than a washcloth. Special acne or abrasive soaps should be avoided. To minimize possible irritation, the skin should be allowed to dry completely by waiting 20 to 30 minutes before applying retinoids. The retinoid is applied in a thin layer once daily. Medication is applied to the entire area, not just to individual lesions. A pea-sized amount is enough for a full facial application. Patients with sensitive skin or those living in cold, dry climates may start with an application every other or every third day. The frequency of application can be gradually increased to as often as twice each day if tolerated. The corners of the nose, the mouth, and the eyes should be avoided; these areas are the most sensitive and the most easily irritated. Retinoids are applied to the chin less frequently during the initial stages of therapy; the chin is sensitive and is usually the first area to become red and scaly. Sunscreens should be worn during the summer months if exposure is anticipated.

Response to treatment. One to 4 weeks: During the first few weeks, patients may experience redness, burning, or peeling (Figure 7-24). Those with excessive irritation should use less frequent applications (i.e., every other or every third day.) Most patients adapt to treatment within 4 weeks and return to daily applications. Those tolerating daily applications may be advanced to a higher dosage or to the more potent solution.

Figure 7-24 Response to treatment with retinoids.

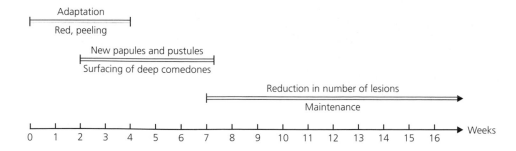

Three to 6 weeks: New papules and pustules may appear because comedones become irritated during the process of being dislodged. Patients unaware of this phenomenon may discontinue treatment. Some patients never get worse and sometimes begin to improve dramatically by the fifth or sixth week.

After 6 weeks: Most patients improve by the 9th to 12th week and exhibit continuous improvement thereafter. Some patients never adapt to retinoids and experience continuous irritation or continue to worsen. An alternate treatment should be selected if adaptation has not occurred by 6 to 8 weeks. Some patients adapt but never improve. Retinoids may be continued for months to prevent appearance of new lesions.

TRETINOIN. Tretinoin (Retin-A) is effective for noninflammatory acne consisting of open and closed comedones. It is available in various preparations: Retin-A solution (0.05%) is the strongest and most irritating. Retin-A gel (0.025% and 0.01%) and Retin-A microgel (0.04% and 0.1%) are for oily skin. Retin-A cream (0.1%, 0.05%, and 0.025%) is lubricating and is for dry skin.

TAZAROTENE. Tazarotene (Tazorac) is a new retinoid. It is available as a gel (0.05%, 0.1%) and cream (0.05%, 0.1%). Tazarotene 0.1% gel (once daily) is more effective than tretinoin 0.025% gel (once-daily) in reducing the numbers of papules and open comedones, and achieves a more rapid reduction in pustules in mild-to-moderate facial acne.[17] Alternate-day tazarotene 0.1% gel is as effective as once-daily adapalene 0.1% gel.[18] The tolerability of tazarotene gel is comparable to that of tretinoin 0.025% gel, tretinoin 0.1% gel microsphere (Retin-A micro), and adapalene 0.1% gel. Tolerability of tazarotene is better when initiating therapy with an alternate-day regimen.

A short contact method may be effective. Apply the gel for just a few minutes, then wash it off.

ADAPALENE. Adapalene (Differin) is available as a gel, solution, and in pads. It has tretinoin-like activity in the terminal differentiation process of the hair follicle. Adapalene has antiinflammatory activity. Adapalene gel 0.1% is as effective as 0.025% tretinoin gel for mild-to-moderate acne. It is better tolerated than tretinoin gel.[19,20] It does not cause sun sensitivity.

AZELAIC ACID. Azelaic acid cream (Azelex) is a naturally occurring compound that has antikeratinizing, antibacterial, and antiinflammatory properties. It is effective for noninflammatory and inflammatory acne. It is an effective monotherapy in mild-to-moderate forms of acne, with an overall efficacy comparable to that of tretinoin (0.05%), benzoyl peroxide (5%), and topical erythromycin (2%).[21] Its efficacy can be enhanced when it is used in combination with other topical medications such as benzoyl peroxide 4% gel, clindamycin 1% gel, tretinoin 0.025% cream, and erythromycin 3%/benzoyl peroxide 5% gel.[22] Azelaic acid cream may be combined with oral antibiotics for the treatment of moderate-to-severe acne and may be used for maintenance therapy when antibiotics are stopped. It does not cause sun sensitivity or significant local irritation. It does not induce resistance in *P. acnes*.

Benzoyl peroxide

The primary effect of benzoyl peroxide is antibacterial; therefore it is most effective for inflammatory acne consisting of papules, pustules, and cysts, although many patients with comedone acne respond to it. Benzoyl peroxide is less effective than vitamin A acid at disrupting the microcomedo. Benzoyl peroxide and isotretinoin significantly reduce noninflamed lesions in 4 weeks. In one study, benzoyl peroxide had a more rapid effect on inflamed lesions with significant reductions at 4 weeks, whereas the use of isotretinoin showed a significant improvement at 12 weeks.[23]

Benzoyl peroxide is available over the counter and by prescription. Some examples of benzoyl peroxide preparations are water-based gel (Benzac AC 2.5%, 5%, and 10%), alcohol-based gel (Benzagel 5% and 10%), and acetone-based gel (Persa-Gel 5% and 10%) (see the Formulary). Water-based gels are less irritating, but alcohol-based gels, if tolerated, might be more effective. Benzoyl peroxide is also available in a soap base in strengths from 2.5% to 10%.

BENZOYL PEROXIDE/ANTIBIOTIC FORMULATIONS. The combinations of erythromycin/benzoyl peroxide (Benzamycin) and clindamycin/benzoyl peroxide (BenzaClin) are superior for inflammatory and noninflammatory acne versus either ingredient used alone.[24] The clindamycin/benzoyl peroxide combination gel has an advantage over erythromycin/benzoyl peroxide gel because the former does not require refrigeration. The two products have similar efficacy.[25]

Benzoyl peroxide produces a drying effect that varies from mild desquamation to scaliness, peeling, and cracking. Patients should be reassured that drying does not cause wrinkles. It causes a significant reduction in the concentration of free fatty acids via its antibacterial effect on *P. acnes*. This activity is presumably caused by the release of free radical oxygen, which is capable of oxidizing bacterial proteins. Benzoyl peroxide seems to reduce the size of the sebaceous gland, but whether sebum secretion is suppressed is still unknown. Patients should be warned that benzoyl peroxide is a bleaching agent that can ruin clothing.

PRINCIPLES OF TREATMENT. Benzoyl peroxide should be applied in a thin layer to the entire affected area. Most patients experience mild erythema and scaling during the first few days of treatment, even with the lowest concentrations, but adapt in a week or two. It was previously held that vigorous peeling was necessary for maximum therapeutic effect; although many patients improved with this technique, others became worse. An adequate therapeutic result can be obtained by starting with daily applications of the 2.5% or 5% gel and gradually increasing or decreasing the frequency of applications and strength until mild dryness and peeling occur.[26]

ALLERGIC REACTION. Allergic contact dermatitis develops in approximately 2% of patients who must discontinue its use. The sudden appearance of diffuse erythema and vesiculation suggests contact allergy to benzoyl peroxide.

Drying and peeling agents

The oldest technique for treating acne is to use agents that induce a continuous mild drying and peeling of the skin. In selected patients, especially those with pustular acne, this technique may provide fast and effective results. Prescription and over-the-counter products used for this purpose contain sulfur, salicylic acid, resorcinol, and benzoyl peroxide. Before the use of tretinoin and antibiotics, this approach secured very acceptable results for many patients.

The goal is to establish a mild continuous peel by varying the frequency of application and strength of the agent. Treatment is stopped temporarily if dryness becomes severe. The drying and peeling technique can be recommended to patients who are reluctant to visit the physician or to parents inquiring about children who are beginning to develop acne. If improvement is negligible after an 8-week trial, the patient should consider evaluation by a physician. Two effective agents are benzoyl peroxide and sulfacetamide 10%, sulfur 5% lotion (Sulfacet-R). One is used in the morning and the other in the evening or as often as tolerated.

Topical antibiotics

Topical antibiotics are useful for mild pustular and comedone acne. They can be prescribed initially or as adjunctive therapy after the patient has adapted to tretinoin or benzoyl peroxide. Clinical trials have demonstrated that application twice a day is as effective as oral tetracycline,[26] 250 mg taken twice daily or minocycline 50 mg taken twice daily.[27] Most solutions are alcohol-based and may produce some degree of irritation. Cleocin T lotion does not contain propylene glycol and for some patients may be less irritating. Clindamycin (Cleocin-T pads, solution, and lotion) is a commonly used topical antibiotic.

Oral antibiotics

Antibiotics have been used for approximately three decades for the treatment of papular, pustular, and cystic acne (Table 7-1).

MECHANISM OF ACTION AND DOSAGE. The major effect of antibiotics is believed to ensue from their ability to decrease follicular populations of *P. acnes*. The role of *P. acnes* in the pathogenesis of acne is not completely understood. Neutrophil chemotactic factors are secreted during bacterial growth, and these may play an important role in initiating the inflammatory process. Because several antibiotics used to treat acne can inhibit neutrophil chemotaxis *in vitro*, they are

Table 7-1 Antibiotics Used to Treat Acne

Antibiotic	Dosage available	Starting dosage	Adverse effects	Comments
Tetracycline	250, 500 mg	500 mg bid	GI intolerance Photosensitivity *Candida* vaginitis Pseudotumor cerebri	Most widely prescribed antibiotic for acne Take on empty stomach
Erythromycin	250, 333, 400, 500 mg	500 mg bid	GI intolerance *Candida* vaginitis	Many forms absorbed with food Safe during pregnancy Erythromycin-resistant *P. acnes* is a significant problem
Minocycline	50, 100 mg	50 or 100 mg bid	Vertigo	Expensive More effective than tetracycline Adequate absorption with food Rare serious side effects
Doxycycline	50, 100 mg	50 or 100 mg bid	Photosensitivity	As effective as minocycline Less expensive than minocycline
Clindamycin	75, 150, 300 mg	75 or 150 mg bid	Pseudomembranous colitis	Highly effective
Ampicillin, amoxicillin	250, 500 mg	500 mg bid	Maculopapular rash	Alternative to tetracycline Gram-negative acne Safe during pregnancy
Cephalosporins (e.g., Cephalexin)	500 mg	500 mg bid	Urticaria Pseudomembranous colitis	Consider for resistant pustular acne
Trimethoprim/ sulfamethoxazole	Double strength (DS) tablets	One DS tablet bid Photosensitivity	Rash, hives	Consider for resistant pustular acne, gram-negative acne
Trimethoprim	300 mg	300 mg bid		Considered if other antibiotics fail

thought to act as an antiinflammatory agent. Subliminal inhibitory concentrations of minocycline were shown to have an antiinflammatory effect by inhibiting the production of neutrophil chemotactic factors in comedonal bacteria.[28] Antibiotic-resistant strains of *P. acnes* have been discovered.

ANTIBIOTIC-RESISTANT PROPIONIBACTERIA AND LONG-TERM THERAPY. *P. acnes* are sensitive to several antibiotics but the prevalence of *P. acnes* resistant to antibiotics is increasing. Resistance genes are easily transferred among different bacteria. After treatment with both systemic and oral antibiotics, *P. acnes* develops resistance in more than 50% of cases, and it is estimated that one in four acne patients harbors strains resistant to tetracycline, erythromycin, and clindamycin. Resistance to minocycline is rare. Carriage of resistant strains results in therapeutic failure of some but not all antibiotic regimens. In many patients with acne, continued treatment with antibiotics can be inappropriate or ineffective. It is important to recognize therapeutic failure and alter treatment accordingly. The use of long-term rotational antibiotics is outdated and will only exacerbate antibiotic resistance.[29]

LONG-TERM TREATMENT. Patients may express concern about long-term use of oral antibiotics but experience has shown that this is a safe practice.[30,31] Routine laboratory monitoring of patients who receive long-term oral antibiotics for acne rarely detects an adverse drug reaction and does not justify the cost of such testing. Laboratory monitoring should be limited to patients who may be at higher risk for an adverse drug reaction.[32]

DOSAGE AND DURATION. Better clinical results and a lower rate of relapse after stopping antibiotics are achieved by starting at higher dosages and tapering only after control is achieved.[33] Typical starting dosages are tetracycline 500 mg twice daily, doxycycline 100 mg once daily or twice daily, minocycline 100 mg twice daily, and amoxicillin 500 mg twice daily. Antibiotics are prescribed in divided doses; there is better compliance with twice-a-day dosing. Antibiotics must be taken for weeks to be effective and are used for many weeks or months to achieve maximum benefit. Attempts to control acne with short courses of antibiotics, as is often tried to prevent premenstrual flare-ups of acne, are usually not effective.[34]

TETRACYCLINE. Tetracycline is widely prescribed for acne. One major disadvantage is the requirement that tetracycline not be taken with food (particularly dairy products), certain antacids, and iron, all of which interfere with the intestinal absorption of the drug. Failure to adhere to these restrictions accounts for many of the reported therapeutic failures of tetracycline.

Dosing. Efficacy and compliance are obtained by starting tetracycline administration at 500 mg twice each day and continuing this dosage until a significant decrease in the number of inflamed lesions occurs, usually in 3 to 6 weeks.[35]

Thereafter the dosage may be decreased to 250 mg twice each day, or oral therapy may be discontinued in favor of topical antibiotics. Patients who do not respond after 6 weeks of adequate dosages of oral tetracycline should be introduced to an alternative treatment. For unknown reasons a significant number of patients who take tetracycline exactly as directed do not respond to high dosages, whereas others respond very favorably to 250 mg once a day or once every other day and experience flare-ups when attempts are made to discontinue treatment.

Adverse effects. The incidence of photosensitivity to tetracycline is low, but it increases when higher dosages are used. All females should be warned about the increased incidence of *Candida albicans* vaginitis. The package labeling of oral contraceptives warns that reduced efficacy and increased incidence of breakthrough bleeding may occur with tetracycline and other antibiotics. Although this association has not been proven, it is prudent to inform patients of this potential risk.[36] Pseudotumor cerebri, a self-limited disorder in which the regulation of intracranial pressure is impaired, is a rare complication of tetracycline treatment.[37] Increased intracranial pressure causes papilledema and severe headaches. Increased intraocular pressure can lead to progressive visual impairment and eventually blindness.

DOXYCYCLINE. Doxycycline is a safe and effective medication. It is commonly prescribed for acne. Studies of doxycycline (50 mg and 100 mg) showed no significant difference between its clinical efficacy and that of minocycline in treating acne.[38] Doxycycline is less expensive than minocycline. The incidence of photosensitivity is low but increases with increasing dose levels.

Dosing. Start at 100 mg once daily or twice daily and decrease the dosage once control is obtained. Doxycycline can be taken with food.

MINOCYCLINE. Minocycline (50-mg and 100-mg capsules and scored tablets) is a tetracycline derivative that has proved valuable in cases of pustular acne that have not responded to conventional oral antibiotic therapy. Minocycline is expensive; generic forms are available. One study comparing minocycline (50 mg three times a day) with tetracycline (250 mg four times a day) revealed that minocycline resulted in significant improvement in patients who did not respond to tetracycline. Patients who responded to tetracycline had significantly advanced improvement when switched to minocycline.[39] The inhibitory effect on gastrointestinal absorption with food and milk is significantly greater for tetracycline than for minocycline. Food causes a 13% inhibition of absorption with minocycline and a 46% inhibition with tetracycline, milk a 27% inhibition with minocycline and a 65% inhibition with tetracycline.[40] The simpler regime and early onset of clinical improvement are likely to result in better patient compliance. There is therefore justification for the use of minocycline as first-line oral therapy.

Dosing. The usual initial dosage is 50 to 100 mg twice each day. The dosage is tapered when a significant decrease in the number of lesions is observed, usually in 3 to 6 weeks.

Adverse effects. Minocycline is highly lipid-soluble and readily penetrates the cerebrospinal fluid, causing dose-related ataxia, vertigo, nausea, and vomiting in some patients. In susceptible individuals, central nervous system (CNS) side effects occur with the first few doses of medication. If CNS adverse reactions persist after the dosage is decreased or after the capsules are taken with food, alternative therapy is indicated. Penetration of the blood-brain barrier may cause pseudotumor cerebri. Pseudotumor cerebri syndrome associated with minocycline therapy is reported in daily doses of 50 to 200 mg. The duration of treatment ranged from less than 1 week to 1 year. Symptoms were headache (75%), transient visual disturbances (41%), diplopia (41%), pulsatile tinnitus (17%), and nausea and vomiting (25%).[41] Cases of drug hepatitis and lupus-like reactions have been reported. Warn patients to report any symptoms.

A blue-gray pigmentation of the skin, oral mucosa, nails, sclera, bone and thyroid gland has been found in some patients, usually those taking high dosages of minocycline for extended periods. Skin pigmentation has been reported in depressed acne scars, at sites of cutaneous inflammation, as macules resembling bruises on the lower legs, and as a generalized discoloration suggesting an off-color suntan.[42] Pigmentation may persist for long periods after minocycline has been discontinued.[43] The consequences of these deposits are unknown. Tooth staining (lasting for years) located on the incisal one half to three fourths of the crown has been reported in adults, usually after years of minocycline therapy.[44] In contrast, tooth staining produced by tetracycline occurs on the gingival third of the teeth in children treated before age 7. Autoimmune hepatitis, serum-sickness-like reactions and drug-induced lupus have been reported in rare instances.

CLINDAMYCIN. Clindamycin (75 mg and 150 mg capsules) is a highly effective oral antibiotic for the control of acne.[45] Its use has been curtailed in recent years because of its association with severe pseudomembranous colitis caused by *Clostridium difficile*, which fortunately responds in most cases to oral or intravenous antibiotics. Clindamycin is effective in dosages ranging from 75 to 300 mg twice daily.

AMPICILLIN OR AMOXICILLIN. Long-term use of oral antibiotics for treatment of acne may result in the appearance of cysts and pustules that yield gram-negative organisms when cultured.[46] Ampicillin (250 mg and 500 mg capsules) is effective for this so-called gram-negative acne. Ampicillin is often effective for the treatment of conventional mild-to-moderate inflammatory acne and is a safe alternative for patients who do not respond to tetracycline.[47] Ampicillin may be prescribed for acne during pregnancy or during lactation. A dosage of 500 mg twice each day is maintained until satisfactory control is achieved. The dosage is then decreased. Some patients experience a flare-up of activity at lower dosages and must resume taking 500 mg twice each day.

CEPHALOSPORINS. There are several anecdotal reports extolling the efficacy of cephalosporins.[48] These drugs may be considered for antibiotic-resistant pustular acne.

TRIMETHOPRIM AND SULFAMETHOXAZOLE. Trimethoprim and sulfamethoxazole (Bactrim, Septra) or trimethoprim are useful for treating gram-negative acne and acne that is resistant to tetracycline.[49] The adult dosage is 160 mg of trimethoprim combined with 800 mg of sulfamethoxazole once or twice daily.

TRIMETHOPRIM. Trimethoprim 300 mg twice daily may be considered if other antibiotics fail.[50]

MACROLIDE ANTIBIOTICS. Erythromycin (e.g., E-Mycin 250 mg or 333 mg; ERYC 250 mg; EES 400 mg) is not first-line drug treatment as it was in the past. Erythromycin-resistant *P. acnes* is a significant problem. Some patients may still, however, respond to erythromycin or related drugs such as azithromycin (Zithromax). Azithromycin has a very long half-life and is given in a single 250-mg dose three times a week. Many other schedules have been tried.

Hormonal treatment

Acne can be the presenting sign of the overproduction of androgens. Polycystic ovary syndrome, anovulation, Cushing's disease, and androgen-secreting tumors cause acne and hirsutism.

ANDROGENS. Androgens are produced in response to pituitary hormones (luteinizing hormone, adrenocorticotropic hormone [ACTH]). Testosterone is produced by the testes and, to a lesser extent, by the ovaries. Dehydroepiandrosterone (DHEAS) is produced in the adrenal glands and converted to testosterone. Testosterone is converted at target tissues by 5-alpha-reductase to DHT. Testosterone and dihydrotestosterone DHT bind to the same androgen receptor on sebocytes. DHT has ten times the affinity for the receptor than does testosterone. Acne is seen only in the presence of DHT. A combination of the effects of circulating androgens and the effects of their metabolism at the hair follicle modulates sebum production and acne severity. Androgens (free testosterone [f T], dehydroepiandrosterone sulfate [DHEAS]) are the most important hormones in the pathogenesis of acne. Plasma-free testosterone is the active fraction of testosterone and determines plasma androgenicity.

PATIENT POPULATION. There is a group of women with treatment-resistant, late-onset, or persistent acne. Some of these women have signs suggesting hyperandrogenism, such as hirsutism, irregular menses, or menstrual dysfunction, but others are normal. Serum androgens may or may not be elevated.

OVULATION ABNORMALITIES. Ovulation disturbances have been found in 58.3% of women with acne, with a preva-

Table 7-2 Hormonal Treatment Of Acne

Drug	Indication (also see box above)	Mechanism of action	Dose
Oral contraceptives	Failed antibiotics No response to dexamethasone or prednisone fT elevated	Inhibit ovarian androgen secretion	(see Table 7-3)
Spironolactone	Failed antibiotics	Androgen receptor blockade	25-200 mg/d usually taken in 2 divided doses
Dexamethasone or prednisone	DHEAS elevated DHEAS normal but fails Rx with antibiotics or Accutane Not responsive to oral contraceptives or spironolactone	Inhibits adrenal androgen secretion	0.25-0.5 mg in the evening 5-10 mg qd or qod evenings

fT, Free testosterone; *DHEAS*, dehydroepiandrosterone sulfate.

lence of anovulation in juvenile acne and of luteal insufficiency in late-onset/persistent acne.[51] Women affected by late-onset or persistent acne have a high incidence of polycystic ovary disease.[52] Polycystic ovaries are not necessarily associated with menstrual disorders, obesity, or hirsutism. The presence of polycystic ovaries in acne patients does not correlate with acne severity, infertility, menstrual disturbance, hirsuties, or biochemical endocrinologic abnormalities.

WHEN TO ORDER HORMONE TESTS. Most women with acne have normal serum androgen concentrations and do not require serum evaluation. Women presenting with rapid onset (1 to 4 months) of acne, hirsutism, androgenetic alopecia, or signs of virilization, such as low voice, increased muscle mass, increased libido, or clitoromegaly, require screening to rule out a tumor. Total testosterone levels of greater than 200 ng/dL (7 nmol/L) suggest a possible tumor, usually ovarian in origin. Serum testosterone levels of 170 ng/dL (6 nm/L) can be seen in polycystic ovarian disease, and imaging can confirm this diagnosis. Adrenal tumor (rare) should be suspected if plasma DHEAS is greater than 800 μg/dL (normal value, 350 μg/dL).[53] A second indication for hormone evaluation is when there is obesity, acanthosis nigricans, or concern about diabetes or Cushing's syndrome. Insulin resistance is common in hyperandrogenemic women with polycystic ovary syndrome.

TESTS TO ORDER. Tests include total testosterone and fT, DHEAS, ACTH stimulation, prolactin, luteinizing hormone, follicle-stimulating hormone, lipid profiles, and glucose tolerance tests. fT and DHEAS are the most practical ways of evaluating hormonal influences in the female. DHEAS is the best index of adrenal androgen activity.

TREATMENT INDICATIONS. Antiandrogenic therapy is reserved for women with acne who have clinical signs of androgen excess and for those in whom other treatments have failed (Box 7-2). Women who have had incomplete responses

to systemic antibiotics may be treated with oral contraceptives, spironolactone or both. The majority of patients with acne do not have serum androgen abnormalities. The profound sebum suppression produced by isotretinoin has to a large extent eliminated the need for antiandrogenic therapy. Patients with abnormal serum androgen levels can be managed as outlined in Table 7-2.

TREATMENT OPTIONS. Acne hormonal treatment is accomplished by androgen receptor blockade or suppression of androgen production. There are three options for treating acne systemically with hormone manipulation. Estrogens (oral contraceptives) suppress ovarian androgens, antiandrogens (spironolactone, cyproterone acetate) act at the peripheral level (hair follicle, sebaceous gland), and glucocorticoids (prednisone, dexamethasone) suppress adrenal androgen. Five alpha-reductase inhibitors are not commonly used to treat acne. The recommended treatment is shown in Table 7-2.

Box 7-2 Women Best Suited for Hormonal Treatment

Most likely to respond to hormonal treatment
Increased facial oiliness (seborrhea)
Premenstrual acne flare-ups
Inflammatory acne on mandibular line and neck
Other indications
Acne onset as adult
Acne worsening as adult
Treatment failures with intolerance to standard therapies
Treatment failure with Accutane
History of irregular menses
History of ovarian cysts
Hirsutism by history or examination
Androgenetic alopecia

Adapted from Shaw JC: Dermatol Clin. 2001; 19:169.

ORAL CONTRACEPTIVES. Ovarian hypersecretion of androgens can be suppressed with oral contraceptives. Most oral contraceptives (Table 7-3) contain combinations of estrogens and progestational agents. Oral contraceptives with estrogen (e.g., ethynyl estradiol) and progestins of low androgenic activity are the most useful. Most synthetic progesterones have some degree of androgenic activity, which is undesirable in patients who already have signs of androgen excess.

Combination oral contraceptives reduce cutaneous androgen effect by suppressing gonadotropin release (luteinizing hormone), which results in suppression of ovarian androgen production. Oral contraceptives also regulate menstrual cycles in oligomenorrheic women and reduce side effects of androgen receptor blockers.

In many instances, acne flares after the use of oral contraceptives is discontinued. Selection of an appropriate agent may provide the benefit of effective acne therapy for women who have chosen an oral contraceptive for birth control. Women in their thirties and forties without risk factors such as smoking or a family history of premature cardiovascular disease can safely use low-dose oral contraceptives to reduce ovarian androgen secretion.

Antibiotics and oral contraceptives. Available scientific and pharmacokinetic data do not support the hypothesis that antibiotics (with the exception of rifampin) lower the contraceptive efficacy of oral contraceptives. The American College of Obstetricians and Gynecologists has stated that tetracycline, doxycycline, ampicillin, and metronidazole do not affect oral contraceptive steroid levels. In a legal action, a court stated there was no evidence of causation between the use of antibiotics and decreased effectiveness of oral contraceptives. The evidence suggests that back-up contraception is not necessary for women who reliably use oral contraceptives during oral antibiotic use.[36]

SPIRONOLACTONE. Spironolactone (SPL) is an androgen receptor blocker that has antiandrogenic properties and is used to treat acne, hirsutism, and androgenic alopecia. Men do not tolerate the high incidence of endocrine side effects; therefore it is only used in women. SPL decreases steroid production in adrenal and gonadal tissue. In women, total serum testosterone decreases and dehydroepiandrosterone sulfate is either decreased or remains unchanged. Free testosterone levels are unchanged or decreased. SPL acts as an antiandrogen peripherally by competitively blocking receptors for dihydrotestosterone in the sebaceous glands.

Indications. Treatment failures are common in adult women. Spironolactone is successful in treating many adult women with acne.

Spironolactone can be used with antibiotics or oral contraceptives or as a single drug therapy. Therefore it can be used when the source of androgen is either adrenal or ovarian or when screening for serum androgens is normal. Cyproterone acetate has similar effects (available outside the United States). A formulation of cyproterone acetate, in combination with 50 or 35 mg of estradiol, is available outside the United States. These drugs (Diane and Dianette) serve as an oral contraceptive and as an inhibitor of androgen receptors.

Acne. Spironolactone causes a significant reduction in sebum secretion and a decrease in the lesion counts of patients. Studies show that SPL at a dosage of 200 mg/day suppresses sebum production by 75% and can reduce lesion counts by up to 75% over a 4-month period.[54,55] Indications for its use are listed in Box 7-3. Spironolactone can be used in low doses (50 to 100 mg/day) as a single drug or as an adjunct to standard acne therapies. Clearing of acne occurred in 33% of patients treated with low doses of spironolactone; 33% had marked improvement, 27.4% showed partial improvement, and 7% showed no improvement. The treatment regimen was well tolerated, with 57.5% reporting no adverse effects.[56]

Table 7-3 Oral Contraceptives With Potential Use in Androgen-Mediated Skin Disease

Brand Name	Estrogen	Progestin	Androgenic activity
Estrostep	Ethinyl estradiol 20, 30, 35 μg	Norethindrone, 1 mg	0.53
Norinyl	Ethinyl estradiol, 35 μg	Norethindrone, 1 mg	0.34
Ortho-Novum 1/35	Ethinyl estradiol, 35 μg	Norethindrone, 1 mg	0.34
Triphasil/Tri-Levlen	Ethinyl estradiol, 30, 40, 30 μg	Levonorgestrel, 0.05, 0.075, 0.125 mg	0.29
Ortho-Novum 10-11	Ethinyl estradiol, 35 μg	Norethindrone, 0.5, 1 mg	0.25
Ortho-Novum 7/7/7	Ethinyl estradiol, 35 μg	Norethindrone, 0.5, 0.75, 1 mg	0.25
Demulen 1/35	Ethinyl estradiol, 35 μg	Ethynodiol diacetate, 1 mg	0.21
Ortho-Cept	Ethinyl estradiol, 30 μg	Desogestrel, 0.15 mg	0.17
Desogen	Ethinyl estradiol, 30 μg	Desogestrel, 0.15 mg	0.17
Ortho-Cyclen	Ethinyl estradiol, 35 μg	Norg 20/1, 30/1, 35/1 estimate, 0.25 mg	0.18
Ovcon 35			0.15
Ortho Tri-Cyclen	Ethinyl estradiol, 35 μg	Norgestimate, 0.18, 0.215, 0.25 mg	0.15

Adapted from Shaw JC: Dermatol Clin 1996;14:803.
*Listed in order of relative decreasing androgenicity.

The incidence of side effects increases with higher doses. In another study, spironolactone, 50 mg twice daily, was given on days 5 through 21 of the menstrual cycle. The most common adverse effect was metrorrhagia, which appears to be well tolerated.[57] The incidence of metrorrhagia can be significantly decreased by adding birth control pills to patients' regimens.

Adverse reactions. Side effects are dose-related. The incidence is high, but the severity is generally mild and most women tolerate treatment. Menstrual irregularities (80%) such as amenorrhea, increased or decreased flow, midcycle bleeding and shortened length of cycle occur. Oral contraceptives reduce the incidence and severity of menstrual irregularities. Breast tenderness or enlargement and decreased libido are infrequent. Other effects include mild hyperkalemia, headache, dizziness, drowsiness, confusion, nausea, vomiting, anorexia, and diarrhea. There are no documented cases of spironolactone-related tumors in human beings. The safety of spironolactone use during pregnancy is unknown.

CORTICOSTEROIDS. Corticosteroids can be considered in recalcitrant cases of acne not responsive to oral contraceptives or spironolactone and for patients with elevated DHEAS. Corticosteroids can be used alone or in combination with oral contraceptives and antiandrogens. Elevated DHEAS indicates adrenal androgen overproduction. Either dexamethasone (0.25 to 0.5 mg at bedtime) or prednisone (5 to 7.5 mg at bedtime qd or qod) is prescribed.[58] Low-dose steroids administered at bedtime prevent the pituitary from producing extra ACTH and thereby reduce the production of adrenal androgens. Dexamethasone may be the more rational choice for adrenal suppression with its longer duration of action. The drug is given at bedtime so that effective levels will be present during the early morning hours when ACTH secretion is most active. Initial dosage should be dexamethasone 0.25 mg or prednisone 2.5 mg, and the dosage should be increased to dexamethasone 0.5 mg or prednisone 5.0 to 7.5 mg if the DHEAS level has not been decreased after 3 to 4 weeks of treatment.[59] Therapy is continued for 6 to 12 months, but the benefits may persist beyond that. This low dosage produces a clinical improvement and suppresses DHEAS levels. At these dosages, few patients experience shutdown of the adrenal-pituitary axis or other adverse effects of the drug. ACTH stimulation tests or early morning cortisol levels may be performed every few months to make sure that there is no adrenal suppression. Not all patients respond.

CYPROTERONE. The antiandrogen cyproterone acetate (CPA) is available outside the United States. It is the most widely used hormonal antiandrogen. Cyproterone is a potent androgen receptor blocker, has progestin activity, and is used as the progestin in oral contraceptives outside the United States. Low doses (2 mg/d) as part of oral contraceptives (Dianette, Diane) are highly effective in improving acne.

Box 7-3 Guidelines for Treatment of Acne With Spironolactone (Aldactone 25-, 50-, 100-mg Tablets)

A. INDICATIONS

1. Adult women with inflammatory facial acne
2. Hormonal influence suggested by
   a. Premenstrual flares
   b. Onset after age 25 years
   c. Distribution on the lower face, including the mandibular line and chin
   d. Increase in oiliness on the face
   e. Coexistent facial hirsutism
3. Inadequate response or intolerance to standard treatment with topical therapies, systemic antibiotics, or isotretinoin
4. Presence of coexisting symptoms such as irregular menses, premenstrual weight gain, or other symptoms of premenstrual syndrome

B. PRETREATMENT EVALUATION

1. Evaluation of serum androgens generally is not required because most women with acne have normal serum levels. In the clinical setting of new onset of acne with other signs of virilization, evaluation by an endocrinologist may be required
2. Determination of adequate birth control measures
3. Discussion of potential side effects with oral spironolactone
4. Obtaining baseline blood pressure

C. GUIDELINES FOR STARTING TREATMENT

1. Begin with 1 or 2 mg/kg/day (50-100 mg/day) as a single daily dose to minimize side effects. It is not known whether twice-daily dosing has an advantage over a single daily dose
2. Check serum potassium levels and blood pressure in 1 month. Obtaining a CBC is optional because hematologic abnormalities occur only rarely
3. Topical therapies and systemic antibiotics may be continued while spironolactone treatment is initiated. Tapering of the standard therapies may then be possible as a beneficial response to spironolactone is noted
4. Oral contraceptives, if not contraindicated, may be given concomitantly at the start of treatment with spironolactone, or they can be considered if menstrual irregularities develop
5. If no clinical response is seen in 1 to 3 months, consider increasing the dosage to 150 or 200 mg/day as tolerated. Good clinical responses can be followed by a reduction of the dosage to the lowest effective daily dose
6. If adverse effects develop, consider lowering the dose; consider adding an oral contraceptive for menstrual irregularities
7. Effective treatment of hirsutism usually requires longer treatment periods and higher dosages to obtain clinical benefit than is seen in the treatment of acne

From Shaw JC: J Am Acad Dermatol 1991;24:236.

Box 7-4 Guidelines for the Treatment of Acne With Isotretinoin (Isotretinoin 10-, 20-, 40-mg Capsules)

INDICATIONS

Severe, recalcitrant cystic acne

Severe, recalcitrant nodular and inflammatory acne

Moderate acne unresponsive to conventional therapy

Patients who scar

Excessive oiliness

Severely depressed or dysmorphic patients

Unusual variants

Acne fulminans

Gram-negative folliculitis

Pyoderma faciale

DOSAGE

Total cumulative dose determines remission rate

Cumulative dose 120 to 150 mg/kg

88% of patients have a stable, complete remission when treated in this dosage range

No therapeutic benefit from doses >150 mg/kg

0.5 to 1.0 mg/kg/day for 4 months—typical course of Rx

Optimal long-term benefit: 1.0 mg/kg/day for initial course of Rx

1.0 mg/kg/day × 120 days = 120 mg/kg

Treat with 1 mg/kg/day especially in

Young patients

Males

Severe acne

Truncal acne

Treat with 0.5 mg/kg/day

Older patients, especially men

Double dosage at end of 2 months if no response

DURATION

Usually 85% clear in 4 months at 0.5 to 1.0 mg/kg/day; 15% require longer Rx

May treat at lower dosage for longer period to arrive at the optimum total cumulative dosage

RELAPSE

39% relapse (usually within 3 years, most within 18 months)

23% require antibiotics

16% require additional isotretinoin

ADDITIONAL COURSES OF ISOTRETINOIN

Appears to be safe

Response is predictable

Some patients require three to five courses

Cumulative dosage for each course should not exceed 150 mg/kg

Adapted from Layton AM, Cunliffe WJ: J Am Acad Dermatol 1992; 27:S2; and Lehucher-Ceyrac D, Weber-Buisset MJ: Dermatology 1993; 186:123.

Isotretinoin

Isotretinoin (Accutane, Amnesteen, Sotret 10-, 20-, 40-mg capsules; 13-cis retinoic acid), an oral retinoid related to vitamin A, is a very effective agent for control of acne and in the induction of long-term remissions, but it is not suitable for all types of acne. Isotretinoin affects all major etiologic factors implicated in acne. It dramatically reduces sebum excretion, follicular keratinization, and ductal and surface *P. acnes* counts. These effects are maintained during treatment and persist at variable levels after therapy. A full list of indications and guidelines for treatment are found in Table 7-4 and Box 7-4. A number of side effects occur during treatment.[60] Isotretinoin is a potent teratogen; pregnancy must be avoided during treatment. Isotretinoin is not mutagenic; female patients should be assured that they may safely get pregnant but should wait for at least 1 month after stopping isotretinoin. Age is not a limiting factor in patient selection.

INDICATIONS

Severe, recalcitrant cystic or nodular and inflammatory acne. A few patients with severe disease respond to oral antibiotics and vigorous drying therapy with a combination of agents such as benzoyl peroxide and sulfacetamide/sulfur lotion. Those who do not respond after a short trial of this conventional therapy should be treated with isotretinoin to minimize scarring.

Moderate acne unresponsive to conventional therapy. Moderate acne usually responds to antibiotics (e.g., tetracycline or doxycycline) plus topical agents. Change to a different antibiotic (e.g., minocycline 100 mg twice daily) if response is poor after 3 months. Change to isotretinoin if response is unsatisfactory after two consecutive 3-month courses of antibiotics. Patients who have a relapse during or after two courses of antibiotics are also candidates for isotretinoin.

Patients who scar. Any patient who scars should be considered for isotretinoin therapy. Acne scars leave a permanent mark on the skin and psyche.

Excessive oiliness. Excessive oiliness is disturbing and can last for years. Antibiotics and topical therapy may provide some relief, but isotretinoin's effect is dramatic. Relief may last for months or years; some patients require a second or third course of treatment. Some patients respond

Table 7-4 Dosage of Isotretinoin by Body Weight				
Body weight		**Total mg/day**		
Kilograms	**Pounds**	**0.5 mg/kg**	**1 mg/kg**	**2 mg/kg**
40	88	20	40	80
50	110	25	50	100
60	132	30	60	120
70	154	35	70	140
80	176	40	80	160
90	198	45	90	180
100	220	50	100	200

to a long-term low-dose regimen such as 10 mg every other or every third day.

Severely depressed or dysmorphophobic patients. Some patients, even with minor acne, are depressed. Those who do not respond to conventional therapy are candidates for isotretinoin. They respond well to isotretinoin, although some may relapse quickly and require repeat courses.[61]

Sebaceous hyperplasia. Patients with numerous facial lesions of sebaceous hyperplasia may experience a dramatic clearing with a low dosage of isotretinoin. A typical patient is age 40 to 50 and has more than 50 lesions on the forehead and cheeks. Start with 10 mg qd and lower the dosage once control is achieved. Many patients are maintained on 10 mg every other or every third day. Lesions reappear weeks or months after stopping treatment.

DOSAGE. The severity of the side effects of isotretinoin is proportional to the daily dose. Start with lower dosages and progressively increase the dosage in accordance with the tolerance. Treatment is usually begun at 0.5 mg/kg a day and increased to 1.0 mg/kg a day.

The cumulative dose may be more important than the duration of therapy. A cumulative dose of greater than 120 mg/kg is associated with significantly better long-term remission.[62] This dosage level can be achieved by either 1 mg/kg/day for 4 months or a smaller dosage for a longer period. The therapeutic benefit from a total cumulative dose of more than 150 mg/kg is virtually nonexistent.[63] Analysis of 9 years of experience demonstrated that 1 mg/kg/day of isotretinoin for 4 months resulted in the longest remissions Relapse rates in patients receiving 0.5 mg/kg/day were approximately 40% and those receiving 1.0 mg/kg/day were approximately 20%. Younger patients, males, and patients with truncal acne derive maximum benefit from the higher dosages. In these patients, dosages less than 0.5 mg/kg/day for a standard 4-month course are associated with a high relapse rate. Treat older patients with facial acne with a dosage of 0.5 mg/kg/day. Double the dosage if there is no response at the end of 2 months. Intermittent dosing may be useful for patients over the age of 25 with mild-to-moderate facial acne that is unresponsive to or that relapses rapidly after conventional antibiotic therapy. Treat with isotretinoin, 0.5 mg/kg a day, for 1 week in every 4 weeks for a total of 6 months.[64] Very low-dose isotretinoin may be a useful therapeutic option in rare patients who continue to suffer with acne into their 60s and 70s. Isotretinoin, 0.25 mg/kg a day, for 6 months is well tolerated and effective.[65] Side effects in all patients depend on the dosage and can be controlled through reduction.

DURATION OF THERAPY. A standard course of isotretinoin therapy is 16 to 20 weeks. Approximately 85% of patients are clear at the end of 16 weeks; 15% require longer treatment. Side effects are related to the dosage. Treat for a longer duration at a lower dosage if mucocutaneous side effects become troublesome. Patients with large, closed comedones may respond slowly and relapse early with inflammatory papules. Another ill-defined group responds slowly and requires up to 9 months until the condition begins to clear.

RELAPSE AND REPEAT COURSES OF ISOTRETINOIN. Approximately 39% of patients relapse and require oral antibiotics (23%) or additional isotretinoin (16%). Relapse usually occurs within the first 3 years after isotretinoin is stopped; most often during the first 18 months after therapy. Some patients require multiple courses of therapy. The response to repeat therapy is consistently successful, and side effects are similar to those of previous courses. Repeat courses of isotretinoin seem to be safe.

ISOTRETINOIN THERAPY. Patients are seen every 4 weeks. Isotretinoin is given in two divided doses daily, preferably with meals. Many patients experience a moderate to severe flare of acne during the initial weeks of treatment. This adverse reaction can be minimized by starting at 10 to 20 mg twice each day and gradually increasing the dosage during the first 4 to 6 weeks. Treatment is discontinued at the end of 16 to 20 weeks, and the patient is observed for 2 to 5 months. Those with persistently severe acne may receive a second course of treatment after the posttreatment observation period.

Response to therapy. At dosages of 1 mg/kg/day, sebum production decreases to approximately 10% of pretreatment values and the sebaceous glands decrease in size.[66] Maximum inhibition is reached by the third or fourth week. Within a week, patients normally notice drying and chapping of facial skin and skin oiliness disappears quickly. These effects persist for an indefinite period when therapy is discontinued.

During the first month, there is usually a reduction in superficial lesions such as papules and pustules. New cysts evolve and disappear quickly. A significant reduction in the number of cysts normally takes at least 8 weeks. Facial lesions respond faster than trunk lesions.

RESISTANT PATIENTS. Younger patients (14 to 19 years of age) and those who have severe acne relapse more often.[67] Truncal acne relapses more often than facial acne. A return of the reduced sebum excretion rate to within 10% of the pretreatment level is a poor prognostic factor.[60] Patients with microcystic acne (whiteheads) and women with gynecoendocrinologic problems are resistant to treatment. Women who do not clear after a total cumulative dose of 150 mg/kg need laboratory and clinical evaluation of their endocrinologic status. They may benefit from antiandrogen therapy.

PSYCHOSOCIAL IMPLICATIONS. Patients successfully treated with isotretinoin have significant posttreatment gains in social assertiveness and self-esteem.[69] There is also a significant reduction in anxiety and depression.[70]

Patients with minimal facial acne but with symptoms of dysmorphophobia (inappropriate depression and/or anxiety response to mild acne) are often treated with long-term antibiotic therapy with no perceived improvement. These patients respond to isotretinoin in that they are satisfied with the cosmetic results achieved. The incidence of relapse is greater than that of other acne patients and often requires additional therapy in the form of antibiotics or further isotretinoin.[61]

LABORATORY STUDIES. Pregnancy tests, triglyceride tests, complete blood cell counts, and liver function tests are performed on patients taking isotretinoin (Table 7-5); pregnancy tests are performed at each 4-week follow-up.

SIDE EFFECTS. Side effects occur frequently, are dose-dependent, and are reversible shortly after discontinuing treatment. Patients with side effects can be managed at a lower dosage for a period long enough to reach the 120 mg/kg cumulative dose level. Explain to patients that the long-term benefit is related to the cumulative dosage, not to the duration of therapy.

The incidence of side effects was documented in a large study (Table 7-6). Patients in that study stopped isotretinoin for the following reasons: mucous/skin effects (2.5%), elevated triglyceride levels (2.0%), musculoskeletal effects (1.3%), headaches (1.1%), elevated liver enzyme levels (0.6%), amenorrhea (0.4%), and other (0.5%).

Teratogenicity. PREGNANCY PREVENTION PROGRAM. Isotretinoin is a potent teratogen primarily involving craniofacial, cardiac, thymic, and central nervous system structures.[71] A number of physicians inadvertently prescribed isotretinoin to pregnant women, which resulted in birth defects.[72]

Women should be educated about the risks to the fetus and the need for adequate contraception. Some physicians will not prescribe isotretinoin to women of child-bearing age unless they are taking oral contraceptives. Others withhold isotretinoin if abortion is not an option. Isotretinoin is not mutagenic, nor is it stored in tissue. It is recommended that contraception be continued for 1 month after stopping isotretinoin. Patients can be reassured that conception is safe after this 1-month period. One study showed that from the fourth month of treatment onward, a statistically significant increase in the mean sperm density, sperm morphology, and motility were not affected. One year after treatment there was no evidence of any negative influence of 6 months of treatment with isotretinoin on spermatogenesis.[73]

The S.M.A.R.T. Guide to Best Practices (System to Manage Accutane Related Teratogenicity) is a program developed to assist the clinician and patient in fulfilling the requirements for Accutane pregnancy prevention risk management and in understanding contraindications and warnings. Female patients are qualified under the guidelines of this program to receive an isotretinoin prescription. Physicians must register with Roche Laboratories to receive yellow Accutane Qualification Stickers that are placed on each prescription. A similar program is available for the branded generic forms of isotretinoin (Amnesteen, Sotret).

Plasma lipid abnormalities. Isotretinoin therapy induces an elevation of plasma triglycerides. In one study of patients (ages 14 to 40 years) treated for 20 weeks with 1 mg/kg/day, the maximum mean triglyceride levels increased 46.3 mg/dL in men and 52.3 mg/dL in women. In that study, two of 53 patients had a triglyceride elevation over 500 mg/dL, and eight had elevations of 200 to 500 mg/dL. Triglyceride levels increase after 6 weeks of therapy and continue to increase while therapy continues.[74] Age, gender, and

Table 7-5 Laboratory Tests with Isotretinoin	
Test	**Comments**
Pregnancy	Two urine or serum pregnancy tests before a prescription is given. The first is performed at the office, the second performed on the second day of her next menstrual cycle or 11 days after her last unprotected act of sexual intercourse, whichever is later. Additional tests are conducted monthly during treatment.
Triglyceride level*	Performed during pretreatment, after 2-3 weeks of treatment, and then at 4-week intervals. If levels exceed 350 to 400 mg/dL, repeat blood lipids at 2- to 3-week intervals. Stop if the value exceeds 700 to 800 mg/dL to reduce the risk of pancreatitis
Complete blood cell count	Performed before treatment and after 4-6 weeks of treatment
Liver function*	Performed before treatment and after 4-6 weeks of treatment
* Liver and lipid abnormalities rarely necessitate dosage reduction.	

Table 7-6 Frequency of Mucocutaneous and Musculoskeletal Events in 404 Subjects*	
Event	**Frequency, No**
Cheilitis	96
Dry skin	87
Pruritus	23
Dry mouth	29
Dry nose	40
Epistaxis	33
Conjunctivitis	40
Musculoskeletal symptoms	42
Rash	16
Hair thinning	6
Peeling	6

From McElwee NE, et al: Arch Dermatol 1991; 127:341.
*Mean initial isotretinoin dose was 1 mg/kg. Most commonly used initial dosage regimen for males is 80 or 120 mg/day, and 80 or 40 mg/day for females.

weighted dose do not appear to be risk factors for triglyceride elevations. Overweight subjects are six times more likely to develop significant elevations in serum triglyceride, and subjects with elevated baseline triglyceride levels are 4.3 times more likely to develop significant elevations.[75] Plasma lipid and lipoprotein levels return to baseline by 8 weeks after treatment.[76]

Bony changes. Asymptomatic hyperostoses (spurs) of the spine and extremities can be documented radiographically in some patients but do not seem to be of concern with a standard course of isotretinoin therapy.[77-79] This toxicity is common and related to dose and to duration of treatment and age. It increases with age. Approximately 10% of patients who are treated for acne with standard courses develop detectable changes.[80] With higher doses, changes are more prominent. After long-term treatment (5 years), they can be found in most patients. Premature epiphyseal closure is rare. It has occurred at the higher doses and decreases with age, occurring only in children. Studies verified that there are no lasting changes in calcium homeostasis or bone mineralization as a result of a single course of isotretinoin for acne.[81]

Cheilitis. Cheilitis is the most common side effect, occurring in virtually all patients. Application of emollients should be started with the initiation of therapy to minimize drying.

OTHER EFFECTS. Approximately 40% of patients develop an elevated sedimentation rate during treatment. Isotretinoin does not specifically affect skeletal or myocardial muscles, although 28% of patients complain of musculoskeletal symptoms.[81] Isotretinoin contains the preservative parabens; those patients with a proven allergy to parabens cannot receive isotretinoin. Exuberant granulation tissue may occur at the sites of healing acne lesions and is more likely to develop in patients who have preexisting crusted, draining, or ulcerated lesions. Granulation tissue can be controlled with intralesional steroid injections or silver nitrate sticks. Severe dry skin or eczema commonly occurs on the backs of the hands. Routine use of moisturizers and infrequent washing is recommended. Group V topical steroids treat the eczema.

Depression. In 1998, the manufacturers of isotretinoin, in conjunction with the FDA, announced a new warning. "Psychiatric disorders: isotretinoin may cause depression, psychosis and rarely, suicidal ideation, suicide attempts and suicide. Discontinuation of isotretinoin therapy may be insufficient; further evaluation may be necessary. No mechanism of action has been established for these events." The product labeling now states, "Of the patients reporting depression, some reported that the depression subsided with discontinuation of therapy and recurred with reinstitution of therapy." No cause-and-effect relationship between isotretinoin and depression has been demonstrated in the literature. Clinicians should be aware of this potential side effect, particularly in patients at risk, such as those with a history of depression.

Prednisone

Prednisone has a limited but definite place in the management of acne. Nodulocystic acne can be resistant to all forms of conventional topical and antibiotic therapy. Nodulocystic acne can be destructive, producing widespread disfigurement through scarring. Intervention with powerful antiinflammatory agents should not be postponed in the case of rapidly advancing disease. Deep cysts improve only slowly with isotretinoin, and much permanent damage can be done while waiting for an effect.

PREDNISONE THERAPY. The dosage and duration of prednisone treatment is determined by the patient's response. The following program has been successful for treating extensive, rapidly advancing, painful cystic acne. Prednisone should be started at 40 to 60 mg per day given in divided doses twice daily. This dosage is maintained until the majority of lesions are significantly improved. Dosage is tapered. The dosage is lowered to 30 mg given as a single dose in the morning. The dosage can be tapered by 5 mg each week until 20 mg is reached, at which point prednisone can be further tapered to 30 mg every other day and withdrawn in 5-mg increments every 4 days. Patients with acne severe enough to require prednisone usually require isotretinoin for lasting control. Both drugs can be started simultaneously.

Intralesional corticosteroids

Individual nodulocystic and large pustular lesions can be effectively treated with a single injection of triamcinolone acetonide delivered with a 27- or 30-gauge needle. Commercial preparations include Kenalog (10 mg/mL) and Tac-3 (3 mg/mL). The 10 mg/mL suspension can be used at full strength or diluted with 1% lidocaine or physiologic saline. Saline is preferred because injections of Xylocaine mixtures are painful. A 2.5 to 5.0 mg/mL concentration is usually an adequate injection for suppressing inflammation.

INTRALESIONAL CORTICOSTEROID THERAPY. The bottle of steroid solution needs to be shaken thoroughly to disperse the white suspension. The syringe should be shaken immediately before injection. The needle is inserted through the thinnest portion of the cyst root and 0.1 to 0.3 mL of solution is deposited into the cyst cavity. This quantity momentarily blanches most cysts. Atrophy may occur if steroids are injected into the base of the cyst. Patients should be assured that if skin depression does occur, in most cases it is temporary and gradually resolves in 4 to 6 months. Multiple cysts can be injected in the course of one session. Intralesional injection is used specifically to supplement other programs.

It is comforting for patients to know that if a large, painful cyst appears, fast relief is available with this relatively painless procedure. Occasionally, intralesional steroid injections may be given for small papules and pustules when rapid resolution is desired. Prolonged, continual use of intralesional steroids has resulted in adrenal suppression.

Acne Surgery

Acne surgery is the manual removal of comedones and the drainage of pustules and cysts. When done correctly, acne surgery speeds resolution and rapidly enhances cosmetic appearance. Three instruments are used: the round loop comedone extractor; the oval loop acne extractor, or the Schamberg extractor; and the no. 11 pointed-tip scalpel blade.

Comedones

Removal of open comedones (blackheads) enhances the patient's appearance and discourages self-manipulation. By use of either type of extractor, most comedones can easily be expressed with uniform, smooth pressure. Lesions that offer resistance are loosened and sometimes disengaged by inserting the point of a no. 11 blade into the blackhead and elevating. The orifice of the closed comedone must be enlarged before pressure can be applied. Following the angle of the follicle, the scalpel point is inserted with the sharp edge up approximately 1 mm into the tiny orifice. The blade is drawn slightly forward and up, then pressure is applied with the extractor to remove the sometimes surprisingly large quantity of soft, white material. Macrocomedones (whiteheads, microcystic acne) can also be treated with light cautery.[82]

Pustules and cysts

After the head of the white pustule is nicked with the no. 11 blade, pustules are easily drained by pressing the material with the acne extractor. Cysts are preferably managed by intralesional injection because incision and drainage may cause scarring. Pustules and cysts that have a thin, effaced roof in which fluid contents are easily felt are drained through a small incision by manual pressure. To prevent scarring, a short incision (approximately 3 mm) should be made. After drainage, a no. 1 curette may be inserted through the incision on the cyst to dislodge chunks of necrotic tissue.

Scar revision

Many patients are very self-conscious about the pitted and craterlike scars (Figure 7-25) that remain as a permanent record of previous inflammation. Some people will endure any procedure and spare no expense to rid themselves of the most minute scar. A new acne scar classification system identifies three scar types: icepick, rolling, and boxcar.[83] Treatments include punch excision, punch elevation, subcutaneous incision (Subcision), scar excision, and laser skin resurfacing. A dermatologic or plastic surgeon is best equipped to perform such procedures.

Generally, it is advisable to wait until disease activity has been low or absent for several months. Scars improve as they atrophy. The color contrast is often the most troublesome aspect of acne. Inflamed lesions may leave a flat or depressed red scar that is so obvious patients mistake the mark for an active lesion. The color will fade and approach skin tones in 4 to 12 months.

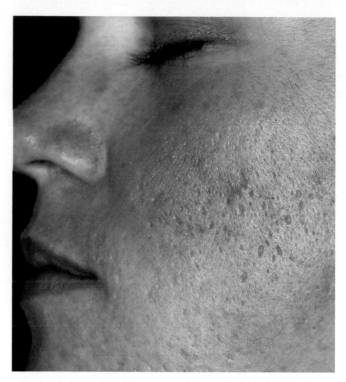

Figure 7-25 Pitted acne scars. The dermatologic and plastic surgeons have a number of techniques (e.g., dermabrasion, punch grafting, laser resurfacing) for treating this difficult problem.

Other types of acne
Gram-negative acne

Patients with a long history of treatment with oral antibiotics for acne may have an increased carriage rate of gram-negative rods in the anterior nares. There are three presentations. The most common is the sudden development of superficial pustules around the nose and extending to the chin and cheeks. Others present with the sudden development of crops of pustules. Some patients develop deep nodular and cystic lesions. Cultures of these lesions and the anterior nares reveal *Escherichia aerogenes, Proteus mirabilis, Klebsiella pneumoniae, Escherichia coli, Serratia marcescens,* and other gram-negative organisms.[84,85] Selection of the appropriate antibiotic is made after antibiotic culture and sensitivities.

Ampicillin or trimethoprim and sulfamethoxazole (Bactrim, Septra) are generally the appropriate drugs. Gram-negative acne responds quickly to the proper antibiotic, usually within 2 weeks. A quick relapse is common when antibiotics are stopped, even if given for 6 months. Elimination of the gram-negative organisms is difficult. Isotretinoin (1 mg/kg/day for 20 weeks) is successful for resistant cases of gram-negative acne.[84,86]

Steroid acne

In predisposed individuals, sudden onset of follicular pustules and papules may occur 2 to 5 weeks after starting oral corticosteroids.[87] The lesions of steroid acne (Figure 7-26) differ from acne vulgaris by being of uniform size and symmetric distribution, usually on the neck, chest, and back. They are 1- to 3-mm, flesh-colored or pink-to-red, dome-shaped papules and pustules.[88] Comedones may form later. There is no scarring. Steroid-induced acne is rare before puberty and in the elderly. There is no residual scarring. This drug eruption is not a contraindication to continued or future use of oral corticosteroids. Topical therapy with benzoyl peroxide and/or sulfacetamide/sulfur lotion (Sulfacet-R, Plexion TS, Rosula) is effective. The eruption clears when steroids are stopped.

Neonatal acne

Acneiform lesions (Figure 7-27) confined to the nose and cheeks may be present at birth or may develop in early infancy. The lesions clear without treatment as the large sebaceous glands stimulated by maternal androgens become smaller and less active.

INFANTILE ACNE. Infantile acne is uncommon. The age at onset is 6 to 16 months. There is a male predominance. The acne is mild, moderate, or severe. It is predominantly inflammatory. A mixed pattern is present in 17% of cases and nodular in 7%. Treatment is similar to that of adult acne, with the exclusion of the use of tetracyclines. Patients with mild acne respond to topical treatment (benzoyl peroxide and retinoids). Most infants with moderate acne respond to oral erythromycin 125 mg twice daily and topical therapy. Patients with erythromycin-resistant *P. acnes* require oral antibiotics such as trimethoprim 100 mg twice daily. Most patients are able to stop oral antibiotics within 18 months. In 38% of children, long-term oral antibiotics (>24 months) is required. The time for clearance of the acne is 6 to 40 months (median, 18 months). Oral isotretinoin may be used in severe cases. Scarring is possible.[89]

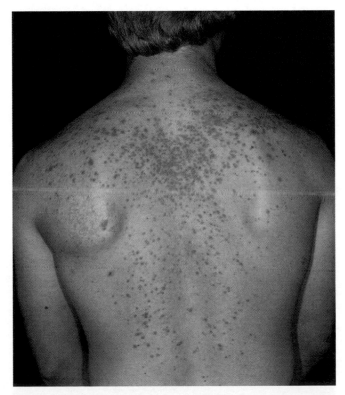

Figure 7-26 Steroid acne. Numerous papules and pustules are of uniform size and symmetrically distributed.

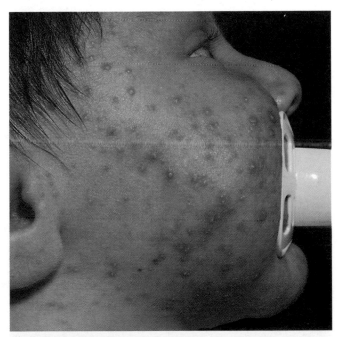

Figure 7-27 Neonatal acne. Small papules and pustules commonly occur on the cheeks and nose of infants.

Occupational acne

An extensive, diffuse eruption of large comedones and pustules (Figure 7-28) may occur in some individuals who are exposed to certain industrial chemicals. These include chlorinated hydrocarbons[90] and other industrial solvents, coal tar derivatives, and oils. Lesions occur on the extremities and trunk where clothing saturated with chemicals has been in prolonged close contact with the skin. Patients predisposed to this form of acne must avoid exposure by wearing protective clothing or finding other work. Treatment is the same as for inflammatory acne.

Acne mechanica

Mechanical pressure may induce an acneiform eruption (Figure 7-29). Common causes include forehead guards and chin straps on sports helmets and orthopedic braces.

Acne cosmetica

Closed and open comedones, papules, and pustules may develop in postadolescent women who regularly apply layers of cosmetics. This may be the patient's first experience with acne. Trials with specific cosmetics on women have revealed that some formulations cause acne, some have no effect, and some may possibly result in decreasing the number of comedones. Until specific formulations are tested and their comedogenic potential is known, patients should be advised to use light, water-based cosmetics and to avoid cosmetic programs that advocate applying multiple layers of cream-based cleansers and coverups. Many patients are under the false impression that "facials" performed in beauty salons are therapeutic and deep clean pores. The various creams and cosmetics used during a facial are tolerated by most people, but acne can be precipitated by this practice.

One alternative to cosmetics is the use of tinted acne preparations (e.g., Sulfacet-R) (see the Formulary). These are generally very well received by patients.

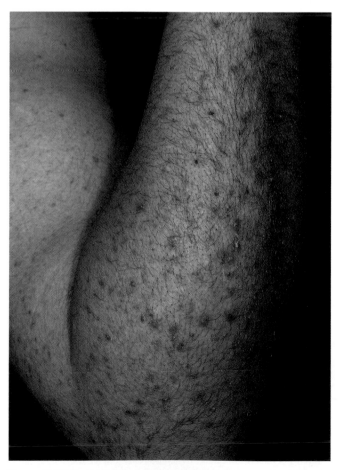

Figure 7-28 Comedones, papules, and pustules occur in areas exposed to oils and industrial solvents.

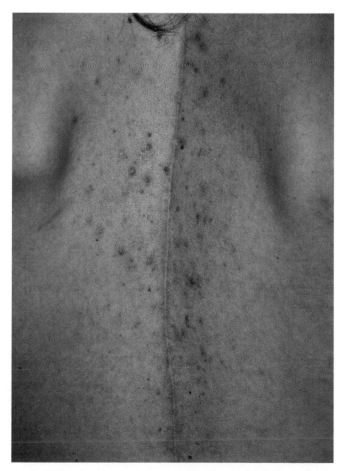

Figure 7-29 Acne mechanica. Comedones, papules, and pustules occurred after a few weeks of wearing a back brace.

Excoriated acne

Most acne patients attempt to drain comedones and pustules with moderate finger pressure. Occasionally, a young woman with little or no acne develops several deep, linear erosions on the face (Figures 7-30 through 7-33). The skin has been picked vigorously with the fingernail and eventually forms a crust. These broad, red erosions with adherent crusts are obvious signs of manipulation and can easily be differentiated from resolving papules and pustules. This inappropriate attempt to eradicate lesions causes scarring and brown hyperpigmentation. Women may deny or be oblivious to their manipulation. It should be explained that such lesions can occur only with manipulation, and that the lesions may be unconsciously created during sleep. Once confronted, many women are capable of exercising adequate restraint. Those unable to refrain from excoriation may benefit from psychiatric care. A patient improved on olanzapine 2.5 mg for 6 months.[91]

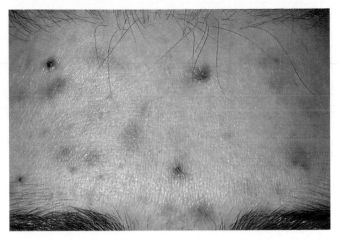

Figure 7-31 Excoriations with no primary lesion on the forehead.

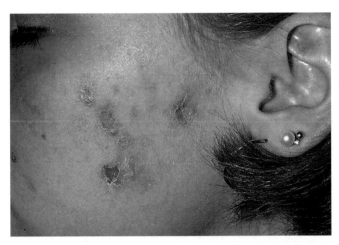

Figure 7-32 Linear and jagged ulcers occur with violent attempts to drain lesions.

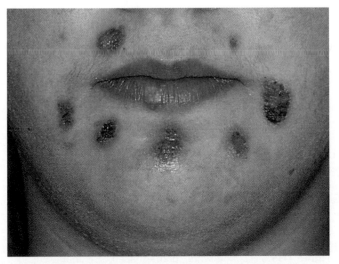

Figure 7-30 Acne excorieé des jeunes filles. Erosions and ulcers are created by inappropriate attempts to drain acne lesions.

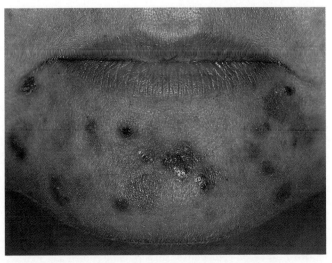

Figure 7-33 Excoriated acne. There are no primary lesions. Erosions have healed with postinflammatory hyperpigmentation.

Senile comedones

Excessive exposure to sunlight in predisposed individuals causes large open and closed comedones around the eyes and on the temples (Figure 7-34). Inflammation rarely occurs, and comedones can easily be expressed with acne surgery techniques. Topical retinoids (Retin-A, Tazorac) may be used to loosen impacted comedones and continued to discourage recurrence. Once cleared, the comedones may not return for months or years and retinoids may be discontinued. Lesions that recur can be effectively treated with a 2-mm curette. The skin is held taut, and the comedone is lifted out with a quick flick of the wrist.[92] It is important to go deep enough to remove the entire lesion. Bleeding is controlled with Monsel's solution; electrocautery causes scars and should be avoided.

Solid facial edema

Solid, persistent, inflammatory edema of the face may occur in rare instances in patients with acne and last for years. The edema is often resistant to conventional treatment, including isotretinoin. The therapeutic combination of oral isotretinoin (0.5 mg/kg body weight daily) and ketotifen (2 mg daily) led to complete resolution of all facial lesions in one reported case.[93] Surgical treatment of this problem has been reported.[94]

The pathogenesis of persistent edema remains mysterious but may be related to chronic inflammation that results in obstruction of lymph vessels or fibrosis induced by mast cells.

Milia

Milia are tiny, white, pea-shaped cysts that commonly occur on the face, especially around the eyes (Figure 7-35). A distinction is made between primary and secondary milia. Primary milia arise spontaneously, most often on the eyelids and cheeks. They are derived from the lowest portion of the infundibulum of the vellus hairs. They are small cysts that differ from epidermal cysts only in size.

Secondary milia may represent retention cysts following injury to the skin. Milia may occur spontaneously or after habitual rubbing of the eyelids. They are seen in blistering dermatoses, such as epidermolysis bullosa, porphyria cutanea tarda, and bullous pemphigoid, after dermabrasion or topical treatment with fluorouracil, in areas of chronic corticosteroid-induced atrophy, and after burns and radiation therapy. Secondary milia are morphologically and histologically identical to primary milia.[95]

These tiny structures annoy patients, and drainage is frequently requested.

Milia have no opening on the surface and cannot be expressed like blackheads. A no. 11 pointed surgical blade tip is inserted with the sharp edge up and advanced laterally approximately 1 mm. Apply pressure with the Schamberg extractor to remove the soft, white material. Other treatments are laser ablation or electrodesiccation.

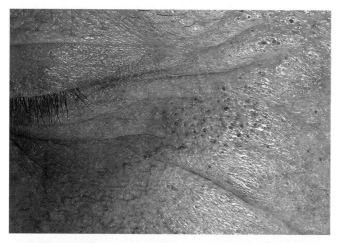

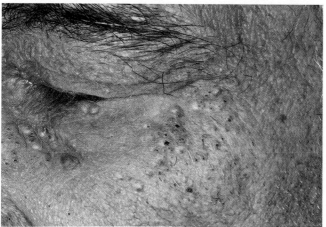

Figure 7-34 Senile comedones. Small or large comedones may appear around the eyes and temples in middle-aged and older individuals. Sunlight is a predisposing factor.

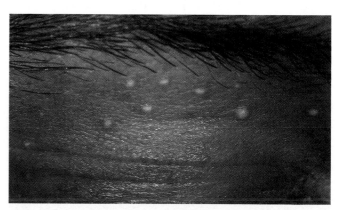

Figure 7-35 Milia. Tiny, white, dome-shaped cysts that occur about the eyes and cheeks. There is no obvious follicular opening like that seen in closed comedones.

Perioral Dermatitis

Perioral dermatitis is a distinctive eruption. It occurs in young women and resembles acne. Papules and pustules on an erythematous and sometimes scaling base are confined to the chin and nasolabial folds while sparing a clear zone around the vermilion border (Figure 7-36). There are varying degrees of involvement. Patients may develop a few pustules on the chin and nasolabial folds. These cases resemble acne. Pustules on the cheeks adjacent to the nostrils are highly characteristic initially (Figures 7-37 and 7-38), and sometimes the disease remains confined to this area. Pustules and papules may also be seen lateral to the eyes (Figure 7-39).

Perioral dermatitis has been reported in children. Perioral dermatitis is a unique skin disorder of childhood. The age ranged from 7 months to 13 years. Boys and girls, blacks and whites are equally affected. There are perioral, perinasal, and periorbital flesh-colored or erythematous inflamed papules and micronodules. Pustules are rare. The disease waxes and wanes for weeks and months.

Prolonged use of fluorinated steroid creams (Figures 7-40 and 7-41) was thought to be the primary cause when this entity was described more than 25 years ago. However, in recent years, most women have denied using such creams. Perioral dermatitis occurs in an area where drying agents are poorly tolerated; topical preparations such as benzoyl peroxide, tretinoin, and alcohol-based antibiotic lotions aggravate the eruption.

The pathogenesis is unknown. A group of authors proposed that the dermatitis is a cutaneous intolerance reaction linked to constitutionally dry skin and often accompanied by a history of mild atopic dermatitis. It is precipitated by the habitual, regular, and abundant use of moisturizing creams. This results in persistent hydration of the horny layer, impairment of barrier function, and proliferation of the skin flora.[96] Another study showed that application of foundation, in addition to moisturizer and night cream resulted in a 13-fold increased risk for perioral dermatitis. The combination of moisturizer and foundation was associated with a lesser but significantly increased risk. Moisturizer alone was not associated with an increased risk. These findings suggest that cosmetic preparations play a vital role in the etiology of perioral dermatitis, perhaps by an occlusive mechanism.[97]

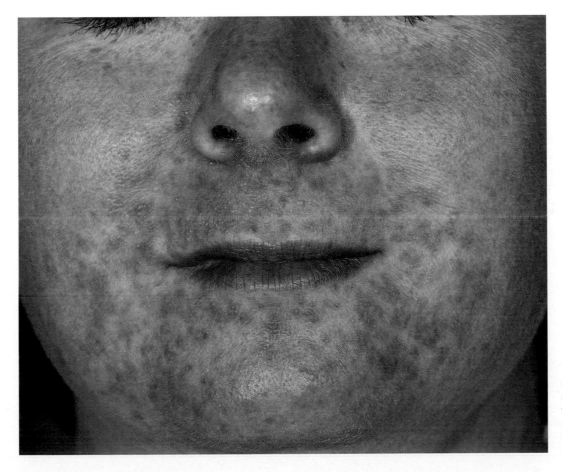

Figure 7-36 Perioral dermatitis. A florid case with numerous tiny papules and pustules located around the mouth.

PERIORAL DERMATITIS

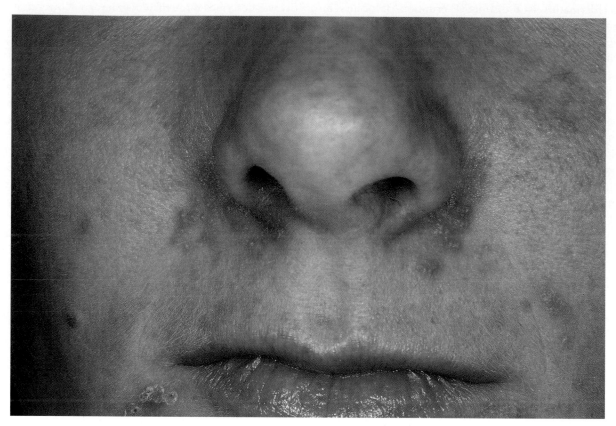

Figure 7-37 Perioral dermatitis. Pinpoint pustules next to the nostrils may be the first sign or the only manifestation of the disease.

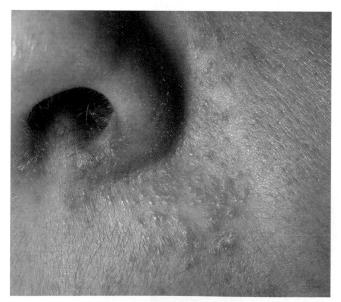

Figure 7-38 Pinpoint papules in a cluster next to the nostrils. These lesions resist topical therapy and often require short courses of oral antibiotics (e.g., tetracycline, doxycycline, minocycline, azithromycin) for control.

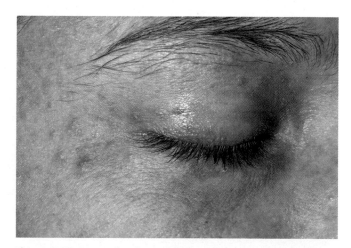

Figure 7-39 Grouped red papules may be found on the lateral portions of the lower lids.

Treatment

Perioral dermatitis uniformly responds in 2 to 3 weeks to 1 gm per day of tetracycline or erythromycin. Doxycycline 100 mg once or twice daily is also effective. Once cleared, the dosage may be stopped or tapered and discontinued in 4 to 5 weeks. Patients with renewed activity should have an additional course of antibiotics. Long-term maintenance therapy with oral antibiotics is sometimes required. Topical antibiotics are frequently prescribed but are not very effective. The twice-daily topical application of 1% metronidazole cream (Metrogel) reduces the number of papules, but oral antibiotics are more effective.[98] Short courses of group VII nonfluorinated steroids, such as hydrocortisone, may occasionally be required to suppress erythema and scaling. Stronger steroids should be avoided. A preliminary study demonstrates that tacrolimus ointment may be effective.[99] Encourage patients to discontinue or limit the use of moisturizing creams and cosmetics.

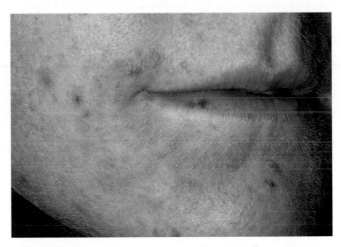

Figure 7-40 Perioral dermatitis. Intermittent use of a group V topical steroid resulted in the appearance of papules and pustules that flared after each attempt at stopping treatment. The topical steroids were finally stopped; the patient flared but recovered after 5 weeks.

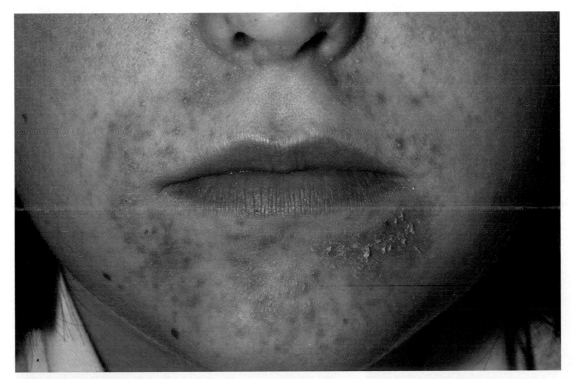

Figure 7-41 Perioral dermatitis. Self-treatment with a group I topical steroid once or twice a week for months resulted in the appearance of papules, pustules, scaling, and swelling. The flaring persisted for 8 weeks after stopping the steroid cream and did not respond to oral antibiotics.

Rosacea (Acne Rosacea)

W.C. Fields drank excessively and had clusters of papules and pustules on red, swollen, telangiectatic skin of the cheeks and forehead. The red, bulbous nose completed the full-blown syndrome of active rosacea. Many patients with rosacea are defensive about their appearance and must explain to unbelieving friends that they do not imbibe. Rosacea with the same distribution and eye changes occurs in children but is rare.[100,101] The etiology is unknown. Alcohol may accentuate erythema, but does not cause the disease. Sun exposure may precipitate acute episodes, but solar skin damage is not a necessary prerequisite for its development.[102] Coffee and other caffeine-containing products once topped the list of forbidden foods in the arbitrarily conceived elimination diets previously recommended as a major part of the management of rosacea. It is the heat of coffee, not its caffeine content, that leads to flushing.[103] Hot drinks of any type should be avoided. A significant increase in the hair follicle mite, *Demodex folliculorum,* is found in rosacea.[104,105]

Mite counts before and after a 1-month course of oral tetracycline showed no significant difference. Increased mites may play a part in the pathogenesis of rosacea by provoking inflammatory or allergic reactions, by mechanical blockage of follicles, or by acting as vectors for microorganisms.

Skin Manifestations

Rosacea occurs after the age of 30 and is most common in people of Celtic origin. The resemblance to acne is at times striking. A new classification system has been established (Box 7-5).[106] The cardinal features are erythema and edema, papules and pustules, and telangiectasia (Figures 7-42 through 7-45). One or all of these features may be present. The disease is chronic, lasting for years, with episodes of activity followed by quiescent periods of variable length. Eruptions appear on the forehead, cheeks, nose, and occasionally about the eyes. Most patients have some erythema, with less than ten papules and pustules at any one time. At the other end of the spectrum are those with numerous pustules, telangiectasia, diffuse erythema, oily skin, and edema, particularly of the cheeks and nose (Figure 7-46).

Granuloma formation occurs in some patients (granulomatous rosacea). It is characterized by hard papules or nodules that may be severe and lead to scarring.[107,108] Chronic, deep inflammation of the nose leads to an irreversible hypertrophy called rhinophyma (Figure 7-47).[109]

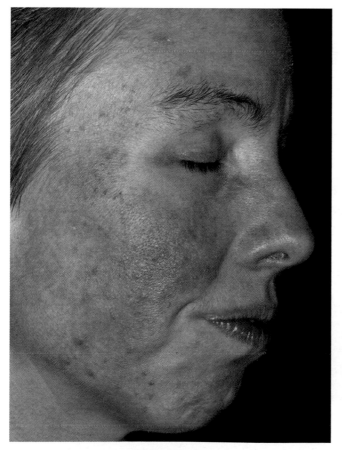

Figure 7-42 Rosacea. Persistent erythema, with a few pustules.

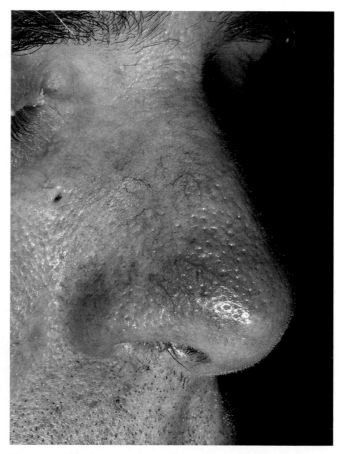

Figure 7-43 Rosacea. Persistent erythema and flushing. There were no pustules.

Box 7-5 Guidelines for the Diagnosis of Rosacea

Primary features (presence of one or more of the following)

    Flushing (transient erythema)

    Nontransient erythema

    Papules and pustules

    Telangiectasia

Secondary features (one or more of the following)

    Burning or stinging

    Plaque

    Dry appearance

    Edema

    Ocular manifestations

    Peripheral location

    Phymatous changes

Adapted from Wilkin J, et al: J Am Acad Dermatol 2002; 46:584.

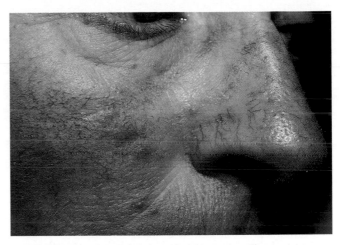

Figure 7-44 Rosacea. Telangiectasia is extensive. There were no papules or pustules. Oral or topical antibiotics will not affect telangiectasia. Laser surgery may provide a very satisfactory result.

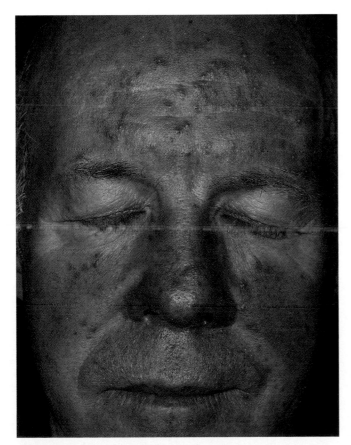

Figure 7-45 Rosacea. Pustules and erythema occur on the forehead, cheeks, and nose.

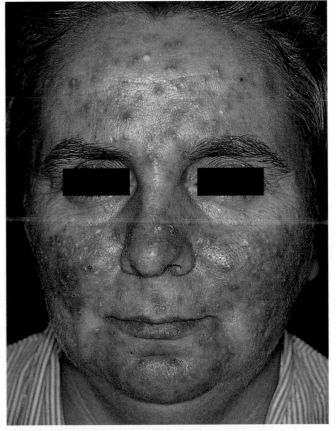

Figure 7-46 Severe rosacea. Oral antibiotics failed. Prednisone followed by isotretinoin cleared the eruption.

Ocular Rosacea

Ocular rosacea is a common disease. It is widely underdiagnosed by many ophthalmologists.[110] Manifestations of this disease range from minor to severe (Box 7-6). Symptoms frequently go undiagnosed because they are too nonspecific. The prevalence in patients with rosacea is as high as 58%, with approximately 20% of those patients developing ocular symptoms before the skin lesions. The diagnosis should be considered when a patient's eyes have one or more of the signs and symptoms listed in Box 7-6.

A common presentation is a patient with mild conjunctivitis with soreness, foreign body sensation and burning, grittiness, and lacrimation. Patients with ocular rosacea have been reported to have subnormal tear production (dry eyes)[111]; and they frequently have complaints of burning that are out of proportion to the clinical signs of disease.[112] The reported signs are conjunctival hyperemia (86%), telangiectasia of the lid (63%), blepharitis (47%) (Figure 7-48), superficial punctate keratopathy (41%), chalazion (22%), corneal vascularization and infiltrate (16%), and corneal vascularization and thinning (10%).[113] Visual acuity less than 20/400 may result from long-standing disease. Conjunctival epithelium is infiltrated by chronic inflammatory cells.[114] Doxycycline, 100 mg daily, will improve ocular disease and increase the tear break-up time.[115]

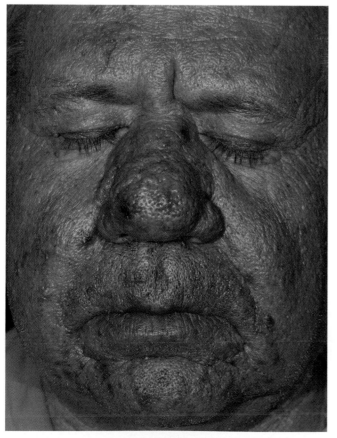

Figure 7-47 Rosacea and rhinophyma. Chronic rosacea of the nose has caused irreversible hypertrophy (rhinophyma).

Treatment
Oral antibiotics and isotretinoin

Both the skin and eye manifestations of rosacea respond to doxycycline (100 to 200 mg/day) or tetracycline or erythromycin (1 gm/day in divided doses). Resistant cases can be treated with 100 to 200 mg/day of minocycline or with 200 mg of metronidazole twice daily.[116] Medication is stopped when the pustules have cleared. The response after treatment is unpredictable. Some patients clear in 2 to 4 weeks and stay in remission for weeks or months. Others flare and require long-term suppression with oral antibiotics. Treatment should be tapered to the minimum dosage that provides adequate control. Patients who remain clear should periodically be given a trial without medication. However, many patients promptly revert to the low-dose oral regimen. Isotretinoin, 0.5 mg/kg/day for 20 weeks, was effective in treating severe, refractory rosacea[117]; 85% had no relapse at the end of a year.[118] Patients resistant to conventional treatment were treated with oral isotretinoin, 10 mg/day, for 16 weeks. Papular and pustular lesions, telangiectasia and erythema were significantly reduced at the end of 16 weeks.[119]

Topical therapy

Patients with mild, moderate, to severe rosacea may respond to 0.75% metronidazole (Metrogel) applied twice each day or 1% metronidazole (Noritate cream) applied once each day. Topical metronidazole may be used for initial treatment for mild cases or for maintenance after stopping oral antibiotics.[120] Clindamycin in a lotion base is less effective.[121]

Sulfacetamide/sulfur lotion (Sulfacet-R, Plexion TS, Rosula) controls pustules. Sulfacet-R is flesh-colored and hides redness. Sulfacet-R is also available tint-free. They are effective alone or when used with oral antibiotics. Azelaic acid 20% cream (Azelex) is effective and well tolerated in the treatment of papulo-pustular rosacea.[122,123]

Patients with rhinophyma may benefit from specialized procedures performed by plastic or dermatologic surgeons. These include electrosurgery, carbon dioxide laser, and surgery. Unsightly telangiectatic vessels can be eliminated with careful electrocautery or laser.

Patients who do not respond to antibiotics may have *D. folliculorum* mite infestation or tinea, in which the facial pustules and scales are usually localized to one cheek; a potassium hydroxide examination confirms the diagnosis. Crotamiton (Eurax) is reported to be effective.[124] Lindane lotion or sulfur and salicylic acid soap should also be effective.

Box 7-6 Ocular Rosacea: Signs and Symptoms

Watery or bloodshot appearance
   (interpalpebral conjunctival hyperemia)

Foreign body sensation

Burning or stinging

Dryness

Itching

Light sensitivity

Blurred vision

Telangiectases of the conjunctiva and lid margin

Lid and periocular erythema

Blepharitis, conjunctivitis, and irregularity of the eyelid
   margins

Chalazion

Hordeolum (stye)

Decreased visual acuity

Punctate keratitis

Corneal infiltrates/ulcers

Marginal keratitis

Adapted from Wilkin J, et al: J Am Acad Dermatol 2002; 46:584.

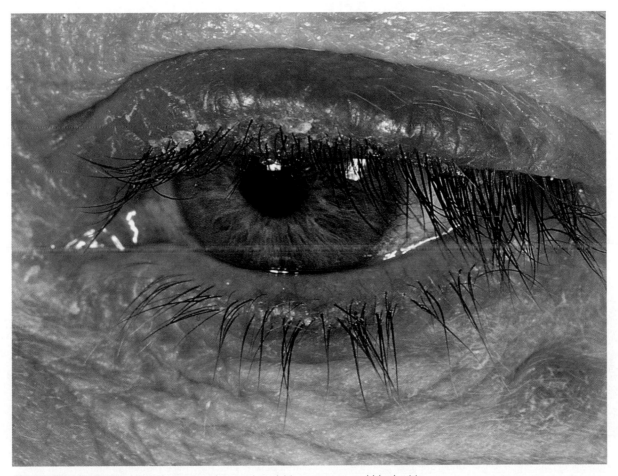

Figure 7-48 Ocular rosacea. The patient has conjunctivitis, soreness, and blepharitis.

Hidradenitis Suppurativa

Hidradenitis suppurativa is a chronic suppurative and scarring disease of the skin and subcutaneous tissue occurring in the axillae, the anogenital regions, and under the female breast (Figures 7-49 through 7-54). Those patients who gain weight will often develop lesions between newly formed folds of fat. There is a great variation in clinical severity. Many cases, especially of the thighs and vulva, are mild and misdiagnosed as recurrent furunculosis. The disease is worse in the obese. Inflammatory arthropathy may occur in patients with hidradenitis suppurativa and acne conglobata.

Clinical presentation

A hallmark of hidradenitis is the double comedone, a blackhead with two or sometimes several surface openings that communicate under the skin (Figures 7-51 and 7-54). This distinctive lesion may be present for years before other symptoms appear. Unlike acne, once the disease begins it becomes progressive and self-perpetuating. Extensive, deep, dermal inflammation results in large, painful abscesses (Figures 7-49 and 7-53). The healing process permanently alters the dermis. Cordlike bands of scar tissue criss-cross the axillae and groin (Figure 7-49). Reepithelialization leads to meandering, epithelial-lined sinus tracts in which foreign material and bacteria become trapped. A sinus tract may be small and misinterpreted as a cystic lesion. The course varies among individuals from an occasional cyst in the axillae to diffuse abscess formation in the inguinal region.

Pathogenesis

Hidradenitis suppurativa is now believed to be a disease of the follicle rather than one beginning in the apocrine apparatus.[125] Like acne, the initial event may be the formation of a keratinous follicular plug. Like acne, the plugged structure dilates, ruptures, becomes infected, and progresses to abscess formation, draining, and fistulous tracts. In the chronic state, secondary bacterial infection probably is a major cause of exacerbations.

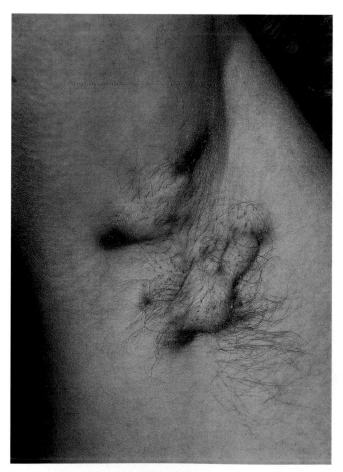

Figure 7-49 Hidradenitis suppurativa. A chronic suppurative and scarring disease occurs in the axillae, under the breast, in the groin, and on the buttocks.

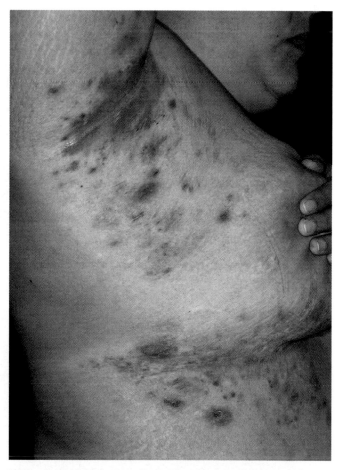

Figure 7-50 Hidradenitis suppurativa. An extensive case with cysts and postinflammatory hyperpigmentation.

The disease does not appear until after puberty, and most cases develop in the second and third decades of life.

Studies show clustering in families. A familial form with autosomal dominant inheritance has been described.[126] As with acne, there may be an excessive rate of conversion of androgens within the gland to a more active androgen metabolite or an exaggerated response of the gland to a given hormonal stimulus.[127]

Hidradenitis is part of the rare follicular occlusion triad syndrome of acne conglobata, hidradenitis suppurativa, and dissecting cellulitis of the scalp.[14]

Management

Antiperspirants, shaving, chemical depilatories, and talcum powder are probably not responsible for the initiation of the disease.[128] Tretinoin cream (0.05%) may prevent duct occlusion, but it is irritating and must be used only as tolerated. Large cysts should be incised and drained, whereas smaller cysts respond to intralesional injections of triamcinolone acetonide (Kenalog, 2.5 to 10 mg/m). Weight loss helps to reduce activity.

Actively discharging lesions should be cultured. Repeated bacteriologic assessment is advisable in all cases. The laboratory should be instructed to look specifically for sensitivity to erythromycin and tetracycline in particular.[129] Oral contraceptives do not seem to work nearly as well as they do with acne.

Cigarette smoking has been identified as a major triggering factor.

Smoking cessation should be encouraged. It is unknown whether this improves the course of the disease.[130]

Antibiotics

Antibiotics are the mainstay of treatment, especially for the early stages of the disease. Long-term oral antibiotics such as tetracycline (500 mg twice daily), erythromycin (500 mg twice daily), doxycycline (100 mg twice daily) or minocycline (100 mg twice daily) may prevent disease activation. High dosages are effective for active disease. Lower doses may be effective for maintenance once control is established. Topical clindamycin has been shown to be as effective as systemic therapy with tetracyclines.[131]

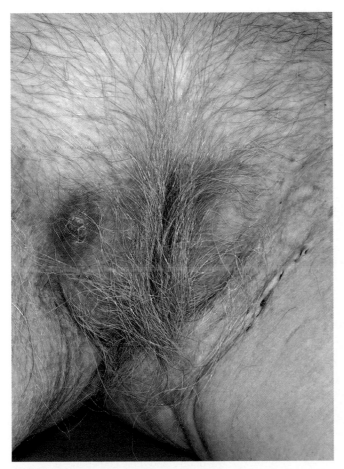

Figure 7-51 Hidradenitis suppurativa. Linear scars and comedones are present in the right groin.

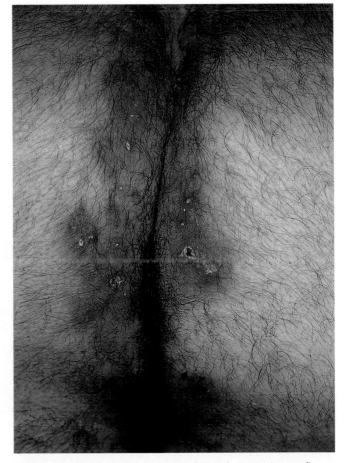

Figure 7-52 Hidradenitis suppurativa buttock. Extensive confluent cysts.

Isotretinoin

Isotretinoin (1 mg/kg/day for 20 weeks) may be effective in selected cases. The response is variable and unpredictable, and complete suppression or prolonged remission is uncommon. Early cases with only inflammatory cystic lesions in which undermining sinus tracts have not developed have the best chance of being controlled,[132] but severe cases have also responded.[133,134]

Monotherapy with isotretinoin has a limited therapeutic effect. Retrospective data of patients treated with isotretinoin for 4 to 6 months was analyzed. In 23.5%, the condition completely cleared during initial therapy and 16.2% maintained their improvement. Treatment was more successful in the milder forms of disease.[135]

Surgery

Surgical excision is at times the only solution. Residual lesions, particularly indolent sinus tracts, are a source of recurrent inflammation. Local excision is often followed by recurrence.

Early radical excision is the operative treatment of choice. Intraoperative color-marking of sinus tracts with methylviolet solution is used. The rate of recurrence within the operated fields is 2.5%. The method of reconstruction (wide excision of affected skin, and healing by granulation[136] or applying split skin grafts or transposed or pedicle flaps) has no influence on recurrence and should be chosen with respect to the size and location of the excised area.[137] Local recurrence after wide excision varies greatly with the disease site. The reported recurrence rates in one study were axillae (3%), inguinoperineal area (37%), and submammary area (50%). There were no recurrences in the perianal region. Treatment of the axillae by local excision and suture was found to result in a high rate (54%) of reoperation for recurrence at the same site when compared with groups treated by either wide excision and split skin grafting (13%), or excision and local flap cover (19%).[138]

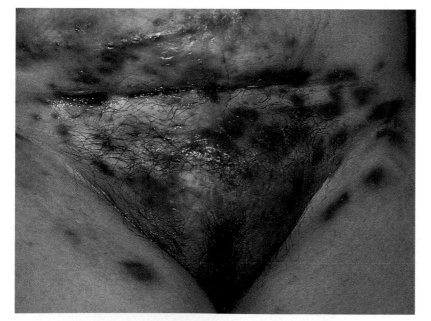

Figure 7-53 The disease may remain localized or involve large areas of the groin or anal area. The inflammation in this case is severe.

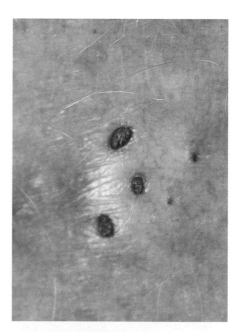

Figure 7-54 A hallmark of hidradenitis is the double and triple comedone, a blackhead with two or sometimes several surface openings that communicate under the skin.

Miliaria

Miliaria, or heat rash, is a common phenomenon occurring in predisposed individuals during periods of exertion or heat exposure. Eccrine sweat duct occlusion is the initial event. The duct ruptures, leaks sweat into the surrounding tissues, and induces an inflammatory response. Occlusion occurs at three different levels to produce three distinct forms of miliaria. The papular and vesicular lesions that resemble pustules of folliculitis have one major distinguishing feature: They are not follicular and therefore do not have a penetrating hair shaft. Follicular pustules are likely to be infectious, whereas nonfollicular papules, vesicles, and pustules, such as those seen in miliaria, are usually noninfectious.

Miliaria crystallina

In miliaria crystallina (Figure 7-55), occlusion of the eccrine duct at the skin surface results in accumulation of sweat under the stratum corneum. The sweat-filled vesicle is so near the skin surface that it appears as a clear dew drop. There is little or no erythema and the lesions are asymptomatic. The vesicles appear individually or in clusters and are most frequently seen in infants or bedridden, overheated patients. Rupture of a vesicle produces a drop of clear fluid. A cool water compress and proper ventilation are all that is necessary to treat this self-limited process.

Miliaria rubra

Miliaria rubra (prickly heat, heat rash) (Figure 7-56), the most common of the sweat-retention diseases, results from occlusion of the intraepidermal section of the eccrine sweat duct. Papules and vesicles surrounded by a red halo or diffuse erythema develop as the inflammatory response develops. Instead of itching, the eruption is accompanied by a stinging or "prickling" sensation. The eruption occurs underneath clothing or in areas prone to sweating after exertion or overheating; the palms and soles are spared. The disease is usually self-limited, but some patients never adapt to hot climates and must therefore make a geographic change to aid their condition.

Treatment consists of removing the patient to a cool, air-conditioned area. Frequent application of a mild antiinflammatory lotion (e.g., Desonide lotion) relieves symptoms and shortens the duration of inflammation.

Miliaria profunda

Miliaria profunda is observed in the tropics in patients who have had several bouts of miliaria rubra. Occlusion of the dermal section of the eccrine duct is followed by a white papular eruption. Anhydrous lanolin and isotretinoin are described as effective treatment.[139]

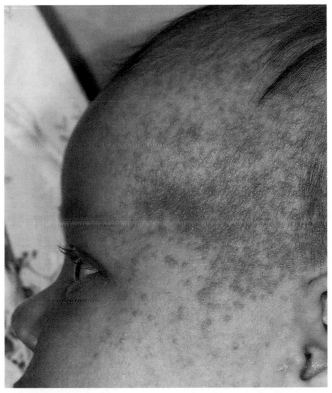

Figure 7-55 Miliaria crystallina. Eccrine sweat duct occlusion at the skin surface results in a cluster of vesicles filled with clear fluid.

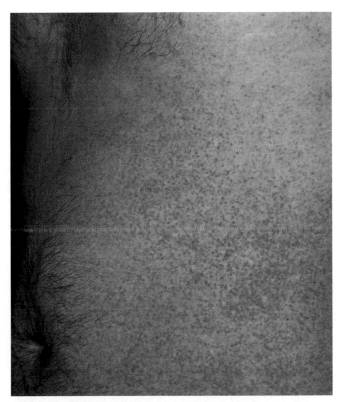

Figure 7-56 Miliaria (prickly heat). A diffuse eruption of tiny papules and vesicles occurs after exertion or overheating.

References

1. Krowchuk DP, et al: The psychosocial effects of acne on adolescents. Pediatr Dermatol 1991; 8:332.

2. Korczak D: The psychological status of acne patients. Personality structure and physician-patient relations. Fortschr Med 1989; 107:309.

3. Rauch PK, Jellinek MS: Pediatric dermatology: developmental and psychological issues. Adv Dermatol 1989; 4:143.

4. Kligman AM: Postadolescent acne in women. Cutis 1991; 48:75.

5. Shaw J, White L: Persistent acne in adult women. Arch Dermatol 2001; 137(9):1252.

6. Wu SF, et al: Role of anxiety and anger in acne patients: a relationship with the severity of the disorder. J Am Acad Dermatol 1988;18:325.

7. Zelickson AS, Mottaz JH: Pigmentation of open comedones. Arch Dermatol 1983; 119:567.

8. Cordain L, Lindeberg S, Hurtado M, Hill K, Eaton SB: Acne vulgaris: a disease of western civilization. Arch Dermatol 2002; 138:1584.

9. Plewig G, et al: Pyoderma faciale. A review and report of 20 additional cases: is it rosacea? Arch Dermatol 1992; 128:1611.

10. Massa MC, Daniel WP: Pyoderma faciale: a clinical study of twenty-nine patients. J Am Acad Dermatol 1982; 6:85.

11. Wong SS, et al: Familial acne fulminans. Clin Exp Dermatol 1992; 17:351-353.

12. Reunala T, Pauli S-L, Rasasen L: Musculoskeletal symptoms and bone lesions in acne fulminans. J Am Acad Dermatol 1990; 22:44.

13. Karvonen S-L: Acne fulminans: report of clinical findings and treatment of twenty-four patients. J Am Acad Dermatol 1993; 28:572.

14. Chicarilli ZN: Follicular occlusion triad: hidradenitis suppurativa, acne conglobata, and dissecting cellulitis of the scalp. Ann Plast Surg 1987; 18:230.

15. Hull SM, Cunliffe WJ: The use of a corticosteroid cream for immediate reduction in the clinical signs of acne vulgaris. Acta Derm Venereol 1989; 69:452.

16. Thomas JR, Doyle JA: The therapeutic uses of topical vitamin A acid. J Am Acad Dermatol 1981; 4:505.

17. Webster G, et al: Efficacy and tolerability of once-daily tazarotene 0.1% gel versus once-daily tretinoin 0.025% gel in the treatment of facial acne vulgaris: a randomized trial [In Process Citation]. Cutis 2001; 67(6 Suppl):4.

18. Leyden J, et al: Comparison of treatment of acne vulgaris with alternate-day applications of tazarotene 0.1% gel and once-daily applications of adapalene 0.1% gel: a randomized trial [In Process Citation]. Cutis 2001; 67(6 Suppl):10.

19. Cunliffe W, et al: Clinical efficacy and safety comparison of adapalene gel and tretinoin gel in the treatment of acne vulgaris: Europe and U.S. multicenter trials. J Am Acad Dermatol 1997; 36(6 Pt 2):S126.

20. Cunliffe W, et al: A comparison of the efficacy and tolerability of adapalene 0.1% gel versus tretinoin 0.025% gel in patients with acne vulgaris: a meta-analysis of five randomized trials. Br J Dermatol 1998; 139 Suppl 52:48.

21. Graupe K, et al: Efficacy and safety of topical azelaic acid (20 percent cream): an overview of results from European clinical trials and experimental reports. Cutis 1996; 57(1 Suppl):20.

22. Webster G: Combination azelaic acid therapy for acne vulgaris. J Am Acad Dermatol 2000; 43(2 Pt 3):S47.

23. Hughes BR, et al: A double-blind evaluation of topical isotretinoin 0.05%, benzoyl peroxide gel 5% and placebo in patients with acne. Clin Exp Dermatol 1992; 17:165.

24. Ellis C, et al: Therapeutic studies with a new combination benzoyl peroxide/clindamycin topical gel in acne vulgaris. Cutis 2001; 67(2 Suppl):13.

25. Leyden J, et al: The efficacy and safety of a combination benzoyl peroxide/clindamycin topical gel compared with benzoyl peroxide alone and a benzoyl peroxide/erythromycin combination product [In Process Citation]. J Cutan Med Surg 2001; 5(1):37.

26. Mills OH, Jr, et al: Comparing 2.5%, 5%, and 10% benzoyl peroxide on inflammatory acne vulgaris. Int J Dermatol 1986; 25:664.

27. Sheehan-Dare RA, et al: A double-blind comparison of topical clindamycin and oral minocycline in the treatment of acne vulgaris. Acta Derm Venereol 1990; 70:534.

28. Akamatsu H, et al: Effects of subminimal inhibitory concentrations of minocycline on neutrophil chemotactic factor production in comedonal bacteria, neutrophil phagocytosis and oxygen metabolism. Arch Dermatol Res 1991; 283:524.

29. Cooper A: Systematic review of *Propionibacterium acnes* resistance to systemic antibiotics. Med J Aust 1998; 169(5):259.

30. Ad Hoc Committee Report: Systemic antibiotics for treatment of acne vulgaris: efficacy and safety. Arch Dermatol 1975; 111:1630.

31. Sauer GC: Safety of long-term tetracycline therapy for acne. Arch Dermatol 1976; 112:1603.

32. Driscoll MS, et al: Long-term oral antibiotics for acne: is laboratory monitoring necessary? J Am Acad Dermatol 1993; 28:595.

33. Greenwood R, Burke B, Cunliffe WJ: Evaluation of a therapeutic strategy for the treatment of acne vulgaris with conventional therapy. Br J Dermatol 1986; 114:353-358.

34. Rajka G: On therapeutic approaches to some special types of acne. Acta Dermatovener 1986, 120(suppl).39.

35. Cunliffe WJ: Evolution of a strategy for the treatment of acne. J Am Acad Dermatol 1987; 16:591.

36. Archer JSM, Archer DF: Oral contraceptive efficacy and antibiotic interaction: a myth debunked. J Am Acad Dermatol 2002; 46:917.

37. Pierog SH, Al-Salihi FL, Cinotti D: Pseudotumor cerebri: a complication of tetracycline treatment of acne. J Adolescent Health Care 1986; 7:139.

38. Laux B: Treatment of acne vulgaris. A comparison of doxycycline versus minocycline. Hautarzt 1989; 40:577.

39. Rossman RE: Minocycline treatment of tetracycline-resistant and tetracycline-responsive acne vulgaris. Cutis 1981; 27:196.

40. Leyden JJ: Absorption of minocycline hydrochloride and tetracycline hydrochloride. J Am Acad Dermatol 1985; 12:308.

41. Chiu A, et al: Minocycline treatment and pseudotumor cerebri syndrome. Am J Ophthalmol 1998; 126(1):116.

42. Basler RSW: Minocycline-related hyperpigmentation. Arch Dermatol 1985; 121:606.

43. Pepine M, et al: Extensive cutaneous hyperpigmentation caused by minocycline. J Am Acad Dermatol 1993; 28:295.

44. Poliak SC, et al: Minocycline-associated tooth discoloration in young adults. JAMA 1985; 254:2930.

45. Christian GL, Krueger GG. Clindamycin vs placebo as adjunctive therapy in moderately severe acne. Arch Dermatol 1975; 111:997.

46. Leyden JJ, et al: Gram-negative folliculitis: a complication of antibiotic therapy in acne vulgaris. Br J Dermatol 1973; 88:583.

47. Shore RN: Usefulness of ampicillin in treatment of acne vulgaris. J Am Acad Dermatol 1983; 9:604.

48. Sheeler RD: Cephalosporin for acne vulgaris. J Am Acad Dermatol 1986; 14:1091.

49. Nordin K, et al: A clinical and bacteriological evaluation of the effect of sulfamethoxazole trimethoprim in acne vulgaris, resistant to prior therapy with tetracyclines. Dermatologica 1978; 157:245.

50. Bottomley W, Cunliffe W: Oral trimethoprim as a third-line antibiotic in the management of acne vulgaris. Dermatology 1993; 187(3):193.

51. Noto G, et al: Ovulatory patterns in women with juvenile and late-onset/persistent acne vulgaris. Acta Eur Fertil 1990; 21:293.

52. Bunker CB, et al: Most women with acne have polycystic ovaries. Br J Dermatol 1989; 121:675.

53. Shaw J: Hormonal therapy in dermatology. Dermatol Clin 2001; 19(1):169, ix.

54. Goodfellow A, et al: Oral spironolactone improves acne vulgaris and reduces sebum excretion. Br J Dermatol 1984; 111:209.

55. Burke BM, Cunliffe WJ: Oral spironolactone therapy for female patients with acne, hirsutism or androgenic alopecia. Br J Dermatol 1985;112:124.

56. Shaw J: Low-dose adjunctive spironolactone in the treatment of acne in women: a retrospective analysis of 85 consecutively treated patients. J Am Acad Dermatol 2000; 43(3):498.

57. Lubbos H, et al: Adverse effects of spironolactone therapy in women with acne. Arch Dermatol 1998; 134(9):1162.

58. Redmond GP, Bergfeld WF: Treatment of androgenic disorders in women: acne, hirsutism, and alopecia. Cleve Clin J Med 1990; 57:428.

59. Nader S, et al: Acne and hyperandrogenism: impact of lowering androgen levels with glucocorticoid treatment. J Am Acad Dermatol 1984; 11:256.

60. McLane J. Analysis of common side effects of isotretinoin. J Am Acad Dermatol 2001; 45(5):S188.

61. Hull SM, et al: Treatment of the depressed and dysmorphophobic acne patient. Clin Exp Dermatol 1991; 16:210.

62. Falk ES, Stenvold SE: Long-term effects of isotretinoin in the treatment of severe nodulocystic acne. Riv Eur Sci Med Pharmacol 1992; 14:215.

63. Lehucher-Ceyrac D, Weber-Buisset MJ: Isotretinoin and acne in practice: a prospective analysis of 188 cases over 9 years. Dermatology 1993; 186:123.

64. Goulden V, et al: Treatment of acne with intermittent isotretinoin. Br J Dermatol 1997; 137(1):106.

65. Seukeran D, Cunliffe W: Acne vulgaris in the elderly: the response to low-dose isotretinoin. Br J Dermatol 1998; 139(1):99.

66. Strauss JS, Stranier AM: Changes in long-term sebum production from isotretinoin therapy. J Am Acad Dermatol 1982; 6:751.

67. Chivot M, Midoun H: Isotretinoin and acne-a study of relapses. Dermatologica 1990; 180:240.

68. Cunliffe WJ, Norris JFB: Isotretinoin: an explanation for its long-term benefit. Dermatologica 1987; 175(suppl 1):133.

69. Myhill JE, Leichtman SR, Burnett JW. Self-esteem and social assertiveness in patients receiving isotretinoin treatment for cystic acne. Cutis 1988; 41:171.

70. Rubinow DR, et al: Reduced anxiety and depression in cystic acne patients after successful treatment with oral isotretinoin. J Am Acad Dermatol 1987; 17:25.

71. Lammer EJ, et al. Retinoic acid embryopathy. N Engl J Med 1985; 313:837-841.

72. Dai WS, et al: Epidemiology of isotretinoin exposure during pregnancy. J Am Acad Dermatol 1992; 26:599.

73. Hoting VE, et al: Isotretinoin treatment of acne conglobata. Andrologic follow-up. Fortschr Med 1992; 110:427.

74. Walker BR, Mac K: Serum lipid elevation during isotretinoin therapy for acne in the west of Scotland. Br J Dermatol 1990; 122:531.

75. McElwee NE, et al: An observational study of isotretinoin recipients treated for acne in a health maintenance organization. Arch Dermatol 1991; 127:341.

76. Bershad S, et al: Changes in plasma lipids and lipoproteins during isotretinoin therapy for acne. N Engl J Med 1985; 313:981.

77. Tangrea JA, et al: Skeletal hyperostosis in patients receiving chronic, very-low-dose isotretinoin. Arch Dermatol 1992; 128:921.

78. Ellis CN, et al: Long-term radiographic follow-up after isotretinoin therapy. J Am Acad Dermatol 1988; 18:1252.

79. Kilcoyne RF, et al: Minimal spinal hyperostosis with low-dose isotretinoin therapy. Invest Radiol 1986; 21:41.

80. Di GJ : Isotretinoin effects on bone. J Am Acad Dermatol 2001; 45(5):S176.

81. Margolis D, Attie M, Leyden J: Effects of isotretinoin on bone mineralization during routine therapy with isotretinoin for acne vulgaris. Arch Dermatol 1996; 132(7):769.

82. Pepall LM, Cosgrove MP, Cunliffe WJ: Ablation of white-heads by cautery under topical anesthesia. Br J Dermatol 1991; 125:256.

83. Jacob C, Dover J, Kaminer M: Acne scarring: a classification system and review of treatment options. J Am Acad Dermatol 2001; 45(1):109.

84. James WD, Leyden JJ: Treatment of gram-negative folliculitis with isotretinoin: positive clinical and microbiologic response. J Am Acad Dermatol 1985; 12:319.

85. Mostafa WZ: Citrobacter freundii in gram-negative folliculitis. J Am Acad Dermatol 1989; 20:504.

86. Plewig G, Nikolowski J, Wolff HH: Action of isotretinoin in acne rosacea and gram-negative folliculitis. J Am Acad Dermatol 1982; 6:766.

87. Hitch JM: Acneiform eruptions induced by drugs and chemicals. JAMA 1967; 200:879.

88. Hurwitz RM: Steroid acne. J Am Acad Dermatol 1989; 21:1179.

89. Cunliffe W, et al: Comedogenesis: some new aetiological, clinical and therapeutic strategies. Br J Dermatol 2000; 142(6):1084.

90. Bond GG, et al: Incidence of chloracne among chemical workers potentially exposed to chlorinated dioxins. J Occup Med 1989; 31:771.

91. Gupta M, Gupta A: Olanzapine may be an effective adjunctive therapy in the management of acne excoriee: a case report. J Cutan Med Surg 2001; 5(1):25.

92. Mohs FE, McCall MW, Greenway HT: Curettage for removal of the comedones and cysts of the Favre-Racouchot syndrome. Arch Dermatol 1982; 118:365.

93. Jungfer B, et al: Solid persistent facial edema of acne: successful treatment with isotretinoin and ketotifen. Dermatology 1993; 187:34.

94. Mendez-Fernandez M: Surgical treatment of solid facial edema: when everything else fails. Ann Plast Surg 1997; 39(6):620.

95. Alapati U, Lynfield Y: Multiple papules on the eyelids. Primary milia. Arch Dermatol 1999; 135(12):1545, 1548.

96. Fritsch P, et al: Perioral dermatitis. Hautarzt 1989; 40:475.

97. Malik R, Quirk C: Topical applications and perioral dermatitis. Aust J Dermatol 2000; 41(1):34.

98. Veien NK, et al: Topical metronidazole in the treatment of perioral dermatitis. J Am Acad Dermatol 1991; 24:258.

99. Goldman D: Tacrolimus ointment for the treatment of steroid-induced rosacea: a preliminary report. J Am Acad Dermatol 2001; 44(6):995.

100. Drolet B, Paller AS: Childhood rosacea. Pediatr Dermatol 1992; 9:22.

101. Erzurum SA, et al: Acne rosacea with keratitis in childhood. Arch Ophthalmol 1993; 111:228.

102. Dupont C: The role of sunshine in rosacea. J Am Acad Dermatol 1986; 15:713.

103. Wilkin JK: Oral thermal-induced flushing in erythematotelangiectatic rosacea. J Invest Dermatol 1981; 76:15.

104. Bonnar E, et al: The Demodex mite population in rosacea. J Am Acad Dermatol 1993; 28:443.

105. Sibenge S, Gawkrodger DJ: Rosacea: a study of clinical patterns, blood flow, and the role of Demodex folliculorum. J Am Acad Dermatol 1992; 26:590.

106. Wilkin J, et al. Standard classification of rosacea: Report of the National Rosacea Society Expert Committee on the Classification and Staging of Rosacea. J Am Acad Dermatol 2002; 46(4):584.

107. Helm KF, et al: A clinical and histopathologic study of granulomatous rosacea. J Am Acad Dermatol 1991; 25:1038.

108. Patrinely JR, et al: Granulomatous acne rosacea of the eyelids. Arch Ophthalmol 1990; 108:561.

109. Black AA, et al: Prevalence of acne rosacea in a rheumatic skin disease subspecialty clinic. Lupus 1992; 1:229.

110. Akpek E, et al: Ocular rosacea: patient characteristics and follow-up. Ophthalmology 1997; 104(11):1863.

111. Gudmundsen KJ, et al: Schirmer testing for dry eyes in patients with rosacea. J Am Acad Dermatol 1992; 26:211.

112. Browning DJ, Proia AD: Ocular rosacea. Surv Ophthalmol 1986; 31:145.

113. Jenkins MA, et al: Ocular rosacea. Am J Ophthalmol 1979; 88:618.

114. Hoang-Xuan T, et al: Ocular rosacea: a histologic and immunopathologic study. Ophthalmology 1990; 97:1468.

115. Quarterman M, et al: Ocular rosacea: signs, symptoms, and tear studies before and after treatment with doxycycline. Arch Dermatol 1997; 133(1):49.

116. Nielsen PG: Metronidazole treatment in rosacea. Int J Dermatol 1988 (review); 27:1.

117. Hoting E, Paul E, Plewig G: Treatment of rosacea with isotretinoin. Int J Dermatol 1986; 25:660.

118. Turjanmaa K, Reunala T: Isotretinoin treatment of rosacea. Acta Derm Venereol 1987; 67:89.

119. Erdogan F, et al: Efficacy of low-dose isotretinoin in patients with treatment-resistant rosacea. Arch Dermatol 1998; 134(7):884.

120. Dahl M, et al: Topical metronidazole maintains remissions of rosacea. Arch Dermatol 1998; 134(6):679.

121. Wilkin JK, De WS: Treatment of rosacea: topical clindamycin versus oral tetracycline. Int J Dermatol 1993; 32:65.

122. Bjerke R, Fyrand O, Graupe K: Double-blind comparison of azelaic acid 20% cream and its vehicle in treatment of papulo-pustular rosacea. Acta Derm Venereol 1999; 79(6):456.

123. Maddin S: A comparison of topical azelaic acid 20% cream and topical metronidazole 0.75% cream in the treatment of patients with papulopustular rosacea. J Am Acad Dermatol 1999; 40(6 Pt 1):961.

124. Shelley WB, et al: Unilateral demodectic rosacea. J Am Acad Dermatol 1989; 20:915.

125. Jemec G, Hansen U: Histology of hidradenitis suppurativa. J Am Acad Dermatol 1996; 34(6):994.

126. Von DWJ, Williams H, Raeburn J: The clinical genetics of hidradenitis suppurativa revisited. Br J Dermatol 2000; 142(5):947.

127. Mortimer PS, et al: Mediation of hidradenitis suppurativa by androgens. BMJ 1986; 292:245.

128. Morgan WP, Leicester G. The role of depilation and deodorants in hidradenitis suppurativa. Arch Dermatol 1982; 118:101.

129. Highet AS, Warren RE, Weekes AJ: Bacteriology and antibiotic treatment of perineal suppurative hidradenitis. Arch Dermatol 1988; 124:1047.

130. Konig A, et al: Cigarette smoking as a triggering factor of hidradenitis suppurativa. Dermatology 1999; 198(3):261.

131. Jemec G, Wendelboe P: Topical clindamycin versus systemic tetracycline in the treatment of hidradenitis suppurativa. J Am Acad Dermatol 1998; 39(6):971.

132. Dicken CH, Powell ST, Spear KL: Evaluation of isotretinoin treatment of hidradenitis suppurativa. J Am Acad Dermatol 1984; 11:500.

133. Shalita AR, et al: Isotretinoin treatment of acne and related disorders: an update. J Am Acad Dermatol 1983; 9:629.

134. Brown CF, Gallup DG, Brown VM: Hidradenitis suppurativa of the anogenital region: response to isotretinoin. Am J Obstet Gynecol 1988; 158:12.

135. Boer J, van GM: Long-term results of isotretinoin in the treatment of 68 patients with hidradenitis suppurativa. J Am Acad Dermatol 1999; 40(1):73.

136. Banerjee AK: Surgical treatment of hidradenitis suppurativa. Br J Surg 1992; 79:863.

137. Rompel R, Petres J: Long-term results of wide surgical excision in 106 patients with hidradenitis suppurativa. Dermatol Surg 2000; 26(7):638.

138. Harrison BJ, Mudge M, Hughes LE: Recurrence after surgical treatment of hidradenitis suppurativa. BMJ 1987; 294:487.

139. Kirk J, et al: Miliaria profunda. J Am Acad Dermatol 1996;35 (5 Pt 2):854.

Psoriasis and Other Papulosquamous Diseases

❏ **Psoriasis**
   Chronic plaque psoriasis
   Guttate psoriasis
   Generalized pustular psoriasis
   Erythrodermic psoriasis
   Light-sensitive psoriasis
   Psoriasis of the scalp
   Psoriasis of the palms and soles
   Pustular psoriasis of the palms and soles
   Keratoderma blennorrhagicum (Reiter's
      syndrome)
   Psoriasis of the penis and Reiter's syndrome
   Pustular psoriasis of the digits
   Psoriasis inversus
   Human immunodeficiency virus (HIV)-induced
      psoriasis
   Psoriasis of the nails
   Psoriatic arthritis

❏ **Pityriasis rubra pilaris**

❏ **Seborrheic dermatitis**
   Infants (cradle cap)
   Young children (tinea amiantacea and
      blepharitis)
   Adolescents and adults (classic seborrheic
      dermatitis)
   Acquired immunodeficiency syndrome

❏ **Pityriasis rosea**

❏ **Lichen planus**
   Localized papules
   Hypertrophic lichen planus
   Generalized lichen planus and lichenoid drug
      eruptions
   Lichen planus of the palms and soles
   Follicular lichen planus
   Oral mucous membrane lichen planus
   Erosive vaginal lichen planus
   Nails

❏ **Lichen sclerosus et atrophicus**

❏ **Pityriasis lichenoides**

Papulosquamous diseases are a group of disorders characterized by scaly papules and plaques. These entities have little in common except the clinical characteristics of their primary lesion. A complete list of diseases characterized by scaly plaques appears in the section on primary lesions in Chapter 1. The major papulosquamous diseases are described here.

Psoriasis

Psoriasis occurs in 1% to 3% of the population. The disease is transmitted genetically, most likely with a dominant mode with variable penetrance; the origin is unknown. The disease is lifelong and characterized by chronic, recurrent exacerbations and remissions that are emotionally and physically debilitating.

There may be many millions of people with the potential to develop psoriasis, with only the correct combination of environmental factors needed to precipitate the disease. Stress, for example, may precipitate an episode. Environmental influences may modify the course and severity of disease. Extent and severity of the disease vary widely. Psoriasis frequently begins in childhood, when the first episode may be stimulated by streptococcal pharyngitis (as in guttate psoriasis).

"THE HEARTBREAK OF PSORIASIS." Psoriasis for most patients is more emotionally than physically disabling. Psoriasis erodes the self-image and forces the victim into a life of concealment and self-consciousness. Patients may avoid activities, including sunbathing, the very activity that can clear the disease, for fear of being discovered.[1] Therefore, even when a patient has only a few asymptomatic, chronic plaques, the disease is more serious than it appears.

Clinical manifestations

The lesions of psoriasis are distinctive. They begin as red, scaling papules that coalesce to form round-to-oval plaques, which can easily be distinguished from the surrounding normal skin (Figure 8-1). The scale is adherent, silvery white, and reveals bleeding points when removed (Auspitz's sign). Scale may become extremely dense, especially on the scalp. Scale forms but is macerated and dispersed in intertriginous areas; therefore the psoriatic plaques of skin folds appear as smooth, red plaques with a macerated surface. The most common site for an intertriginous plaque is the intergluteal fold; this is referred to as gluteal pinking (Figure 8-2). The deep rich red color is another characteristic feature and remains constant in all areas.

Psoriasis can develop at the site of physical trauma (scratching, sunburn, or surgery), the so-called isomorphic or Köebner's phenomenon (Figure 8-3; see also Figures 8-8 and 8-10). Pruritus is highly variable. Although psoriasis can affect any cutaneous surface, certain areas are favored and should be examined in all patients in whom the diagnosis of psoriasis is suspected. Those areas are the elbows, knees, scalp, gluteal cleft, fingernails, and toenails.

The disease affects the extensor more than the flexor surfaces and usually spares the palms, soles, and face. Most patients have chronic localized disease, but there are several other presentations. Localized plaques may be confused with eczema or seborrheic dermatitis, and the guttate form with many small lesions can resemble secondary syphilis or pityriasis rosea.

Drugs that precipitate or exacerbate psoriasis

LITHIUM. Exacerbation of preexisting psoriasis during lithium treatment is well documented, but preexisting psoriasis is not a general contraindication to lithium treatment.[2] The disease does not worsen in many lithium-treated patients. Lithium dosage reduction or more intensive psoriasis treatment is indicated when lithium must be continued.

BETA-BLOCKING AGENTS. Beta-blockers may worsen psoriasis and should be carefully evaluated in the management of these patients.[3]

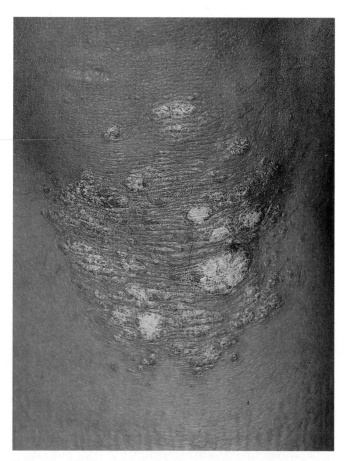

Figure 8-1 Psoriasis. Typical oval plaque with well-defined borders and silvery scale.

ANTIMALARIAL AGENTS. Exfoliative dermatitis and exacerbation of psoriasis is reported in psoriatic patients treated with antimalarials,[4] but the incidence is low. Antimalarials are not contraindicated in psoriasis patients who need prophylactic treatment for malaria.[5]

SYSTEMIC STEROIDS. Systemic steroids rapidly clear psoriasis; unfortunately, in many instances the disease worsens, occasionally evolving into pustular psoriasis, when corticosteroids are withdrawn.[6] For this reason systemic corticosteroids have been abandoned as a routine treatment for psoriasis.

Histology
The psoriatic epidermis contains a large number of mitoses. There is epidermal hyperplasia and scale, the final product of the abnormally functioning epidermis. The dermis contains enlarged and tortuous capillaries that are very close to the skin surface and impart a characteristic erythematous hue to the lesions. Bleeding occurs (Auspitz's sign) when the capillaries are ruptured as scale is removed.

Clinical presentations
Variations in the morphology of psoriasis
Chronic plaque psoriasis
Guttate psoriasis (acute eruptive psoriasis)
Pustular psoriasis
Erythrodermic psoriasis
Light-sensitive psoriasis
HIV-induced psoriasis
Keratoderma blennorrhagicum (Reiter's syndrome)

Variations in the location of psoriasis
Scalp psoriasis
Psoriasis of the palms and soles
Pustular psoriasis of the palms and soles
Pustular psoriasis of the digits
Psoriasis inversus (psoriasis of flexural areas)
Psoriasis of the penis and Reiter's syndrome
Nail psoriasis
Psoriatic arthritis

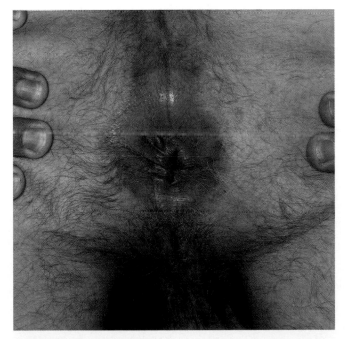

Figure 8-2 Psoriasis. Gluteal pinking, a common lesion in patients with psoriasis. Intertriginous psoriatic plaques retain the rich red color typical of skin lesions but do not retain scale.

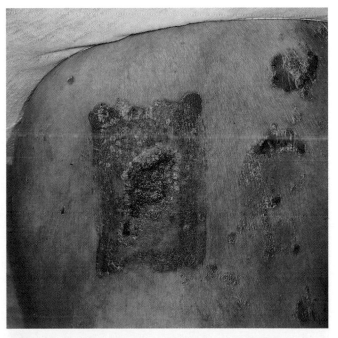

Figure 8-3 Psoriasis. Köebner's phenomenon. Psoriasis has appeared on the donor site of the skin graft.

Chronic plaque psoriasis

Chronic, noninflammatory, well-defined plaques are the most common presentation of psoriasis. Lesions can appear anywhere on the cutaneous surface. They enlarge to a certain size and then tend to remain stable for months or years (Figure 8-4). A temporary brown, white, or red macule remains when the plaque subsides.

Guttate psoriasis

More than 30% of psoriatic patients have their first episode before age 20; in many instances, an episode of guttate psoriasis is the first indication of the patient's propensity for the disease. Streptococcal pharyngitis or a viral upper respiratory infection may precede the eruption by 1 or 2 weeks.[7] Scaling papules suddenly appear on the trunk and extremities, not including the palms and soles (Figure 8-5, A and B). Their number ranges from a few to many, and their size may be that of a pinpoint up to 1 cm. Lesions increase in diameter with time. The scalp and face may also be involved. Pruritus is variable. Guttate psoriasis may resolve spontaneously in weeks or months; it responds more readily to treatment than does chronic plaque psoriasis. Throat cultures should be taken to rule out streptococcal infection. There is a high incidence of positive antistreptolysin O titers in this group.

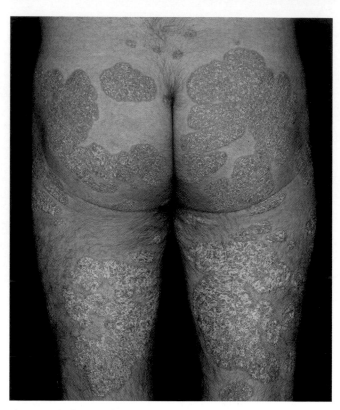

Figure 8-4 Chronic plaque psoriasis. Noninflamed plaques tend to remain fixed in position for months.

Figure 8-5 Guttate psoriasis.

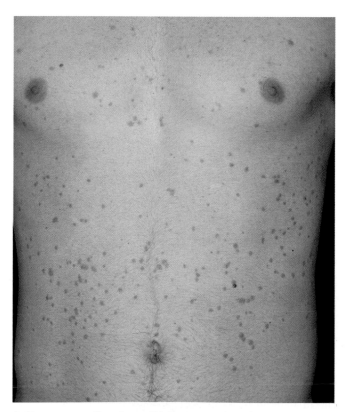

A, Numerous, uniformly small lesions may abruptly occur following streptococcal pharyngitis.

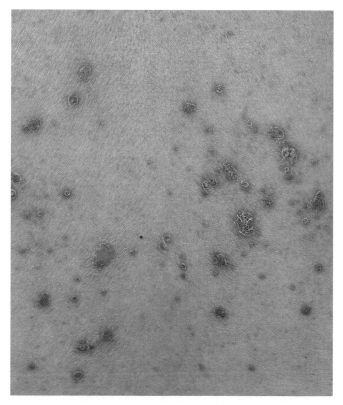

B, Numerous pinpoint to 1-cm lesions develop typical psoriatic scale soon after appearance.

Generalized pustular psoriasis

This rare form of psoriasis (also called von Zumbusch psoriasis) is a serious and sometimes fatal disease. Erythema suddenly appears in the flexural areas and migrates to other body surfaces. Numerous tiny, sterile pustules evolve from an erythematous base and coalesce into lakes of pus (Figure 8-6). The superficial, upper epidermal pustules are easily ruptured. The patient is toxic, febrile, and has leukocytosis. Topical medications such as tar and anthralin may precipitate episodes in patients with unstable or labile psoriasis. Withdrawal of both topical and systemic steroids has precipitated flares. Relapses are common. Wet dressings and group V topical steroids provide initial control. Systemic therapy may be necessary for severe cases. Acitretin yields rapid control. Methotrexate and cyclosporine are also effective.[8]

Erythrodermic psoriasis

Generalized erythrodermic psoriasis, like generalized pustular psoriasis, is a severe, unstable, highly labile disease that may appear as the initial manifestation of psoriasis but usually occurs in patients with previous chronic disease (Figure 8-7). Precipitating factors include the administration of systemic corticosteroids; the excessive use of topical steroids; overzealous, irritating topical therapy; phototherapy complications; severe emotional stress; and preceding illness, such as an infection. Treatment includes bed rest, initial avoidance of all UV light, Burrow's solution compresses, colloidal oatmeal baths, the liberal use of emollients, increased protein and fluid intake, antihistamines for pruritus, avoidance of potent topical steroids, and, in severe cases, hospitalization.[9] Methotrexate, cyclosporine, or acitretin is used if rapid control is not obtained with topical therapy. Tar and anthralin may exacerbate the disease and should be avoided.

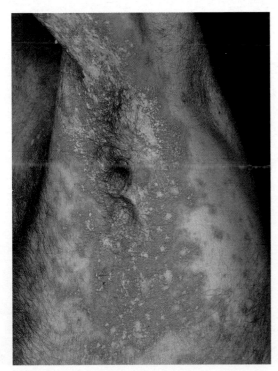

Figure 8-6 Generalized pustular psoriasis. An erythematous plaque has evolved into numerous sterile pustules, which have coalesced in many areas.

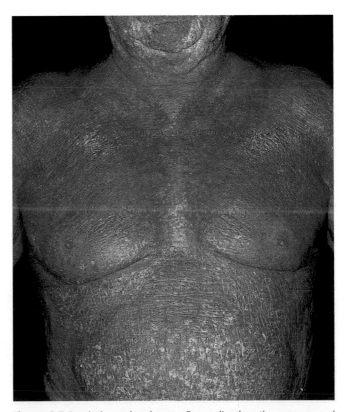

Figure 8-7 Psoriatic erythroderma. Generalized erythema occurred shortly after this patient discontinued use of methotrexate.

Light-sensitive psoriasis

Psoriatic patients wait for sunny summer months when, in most cases, the disease responds predictably to ultraviolet light. However, too much of a good thing can be dangerous, especially for the patient who gets sunburned in an anxious attempt to clear the disease rapidly. As a result of Köebner's phenomenon, guttate lesions or a painful, diffusely inflamed plaque forms in the burned areas (Figure 8-8). Plaques subsequently converge onto the clear, previously protected sites. Some patients do not tolerate ultraviolet light of any intensity.

Psoriasis of the scalp

The scalp is a favored site for psoriasis and may be the only site affected. Plaques are similar to those of the skin except that the scale is more readily retained; it is anchored by hair. Extension of the plaques onto the forehead is relatively common (Figure 8-9). A dense, tight-feeling scale can cover the entire scalp. Even in the most severe cases, the hair is not permanently lost. A distinct scaling eruption of the scalp observed in children is described in this chapter in the section concerning seborrheic dermatitis.

Psoriasis of the palms and soles

The palms and soles may be involved as part of a generalized eruption, or they may be the only locations involved in the manifestation of the disease. There are several presentations. Superficial red plaques with thick brown scale may be indistinguishable from chronic eczema (Figure 8-10). Smooth, deep red plaques are similar to those found in the flexural area (Figure 8-11).

Pustular psoriasis of the palms and soles

Deep pustules first appear on the middle portion of the palms and insteps of the soles; they may either remain localized or spread (Figure 8-12, A and B). The pustules do not rupture but turn dark brown and scaly as they reach the surface. The surrounding skin becomes pink, smooth, and tender. A thick crust may later cover the affected area. The course is chronic, lasting for years while the patient endures periods of partial remission followed by exacerbations so painful that mobility is affected. There is a considerably higher prevalence of smoking in these patients.[10] Acitretin, methotrexate, psoralen ultraviolet light A (PUVA), and intermittent courses of topical steroids under plastic occlusions are therapeutic alternatives.

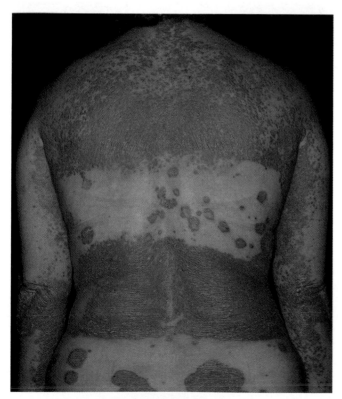

Figure 8-8 Light-induced psoriasis. Overexposure to sunlight precipitated this diffuse flare of psoriasis. The mid back was protected by a wide halter strap.

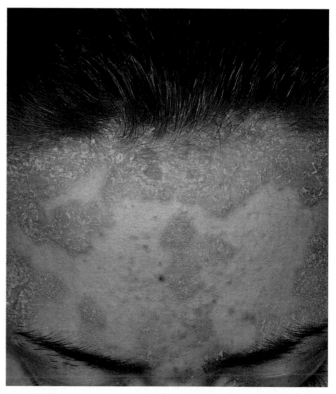

Figure 8-9 Psoriasis of the scalp. Plaques typically form in the scalp and along the hair margin. Occasionally plaques occur on the face.

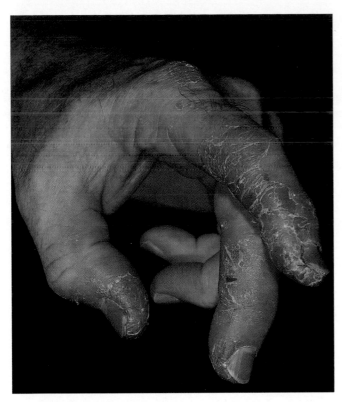

Figure 8-10 Psoriasis of the fingertips. The eruption appears eczematous, but the rich red hue is typical of psoriasis. This eruption occurred as a Köebner's phenomenon in a surgeon.

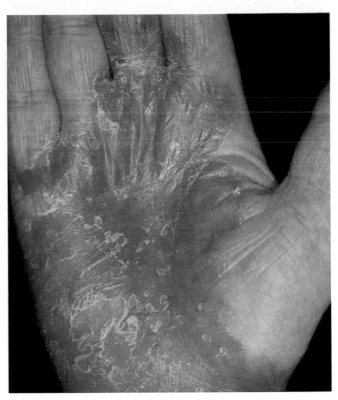

Figure 8-11 Psoriasis of the hand. Deep red, smooth plaque in a patient with typical lesions on the body.

Figure 8-12 Pustular psoriasis of the soles.

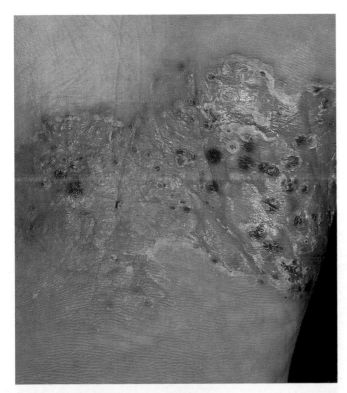

A, An early case in a typical location.

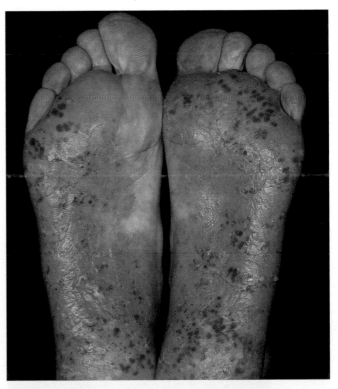

B, This is a chronic disease in which the soles may remain inflamed for years.

Keratoderma blennorrhagicum (Reiter's syndrome)

Reiter's syndrome appears to be a reactive immune response that is usually triggered in a genetically susceptible individual (60% to 90% of patients are HLA-B27 positive) by any of several different infections, especially those that cause dysentery or urethritis, such as *Yersinia enterocolitica* and *Y. pseudotuberculosis*. Psoriasiform skin lesions develop in patients with Reiter's syndrome (urethritis and/or cervicitis, peripheral arthritis of more than 1 month's duration) usually 1 to 2 months after the onset of arthritis; conjunctivitis develops in 25%. The distinctive lesions, keratoderma blennorrhagica, typically appear on the soles (Figure 8-13, A) and extend onto the toes (Figure 8-13, B) but also occur on the legs, scalp, and hands. Nail dystrophy, thickening, and destruction occur. The plaques are psoriasiform with a distinctive circular, scaly border. The scaly, scalloped-edged plaques develop from coalescence of expanding papulovesicular plaques with thickened yellow, heaped-up scale. Similar lesions occur on the penis. Skin and joint symptoms have responded to methotrexate, acitretin,[11] and ketoconazole.[12]

Psoriasis of the penis and Reiter's syndrome

Typical psoriatic scaling plaques with white scale can appear on the body and circumcised penis (Figure 8-15). Scale does not form when the penis is covered by a foreskin. A highly characteristic psoriasiform lesion, balanitis circinata, occurs in Reiter's syndrome when erosions covered by scale and crust on the corona and glans coalesce to form a distinctive winding pattern (Figure 8-16). A biopsy helps confirm the diagnosis. A potassium hydroxide examination excludes *Candida*.

Pustular psoriasis of the digits

This severe localized variant of psoriasis, also known as acrodermatitis continua, may remain localized to one finger for years. Vesicles rupture, resulting in a tender, diffusely eroded, and fissured surface that continually exudes serum. The loosely adherent, moist crust is easily shed, but recurs (Figure 8-17). Localized pustular psoriasis is very resistant to therapy.

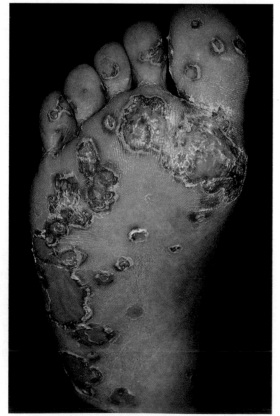

A

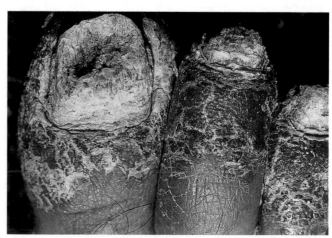

B

Figure 8-13 Keratoderma blenorrhagicum (Reiter's syndrome). **A,** The palms and soles are commonly involved. There are keratoic papules, plaques, and pustules that coalesce to form circular borders like those seen on the penis. (see Figure 8-16). **B,** Psoriasiform plaques develop from coalescence of expanding papulovesicular plaques and are typically found on the soles and toes.

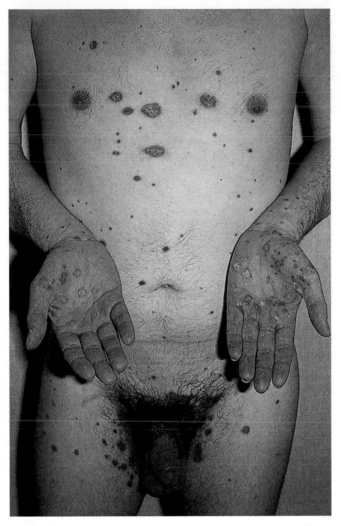

Figure 8-14 Patients with Reiter's syndrome develop psoriasiform skin lesions (keratoderma blenorrhagica) with a distinctive circular, scaly border. These distinctive lesions occur most frequently on the soles and toes.

Psoriasis inversus (psoriasis of the flexural or intertriginous areas)

The gluteal fold, axillae, groin, submammary folds, retroauricular fold, and the glans of the uncircumcised penis may be affected. The deep red, smooth, glistening plaques may extend to and stop at the junction of the skin folds, as with intertrigo or *Candida* infections. The surface is moist and contains macerated white debris. Infection, friction, and heat may induce flexural psoriasis, a Köbner's phenomenon. Cracking and fissures are common at the base of the crease, particularly in the groin, gluteal cleft, and superior and posterior auricular fold (Figure 8-18). As with typical psoriatic plaques, the margin is distinct. Pustules beyond the plaque border suggest secondary yeast infection. Infants and young children may develop flexural psoriasis of the groin that extends onto the diaper area.

Human immunodeficiency virus (HIV)–induced psoriasis

Psoriasis may be the first or one of the first signs of acquired immunodeficiency syndrome (AIDS). Psoriasis in the setting of HIV disease may be mild, moderate, or severe.[13] It can be atypical and unusually severe with involvement of the groin, axilla, scalp, palms, and soles. An explosive onset with erythroderma or pustular lesions that rapidly become confluent should lead one to suspect AIDS. The disease is difficult to treat. PUVA, ultraviolet light B, and topical steroids are immunosuppressive and should be avoided. It is not clear that use of methotrexate adversely affects the natural course of HIV disease.[14] Acitretin is the drug of choice for severe disease. Zidovudine is effective and cleared an acitretin-resistant case.[15]

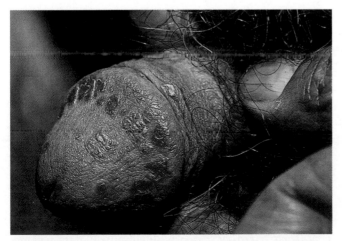

Figure 8-15 Psoriasis. Typical psoriatic scaling plaques with white scale can appear on the circumcised penis. Scale does not form when the penis is covered by a foreskin.

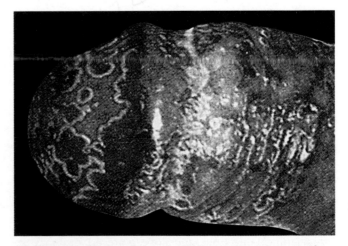

Figure 8-16 Reiter's syndrome. A highly characteristic psoriasiform lesion, balanitis circinata, occurs in Reiter's syndrome when erosions covered by scale and crust on the corona and glans coalesce to form a distinctive winding pattern.

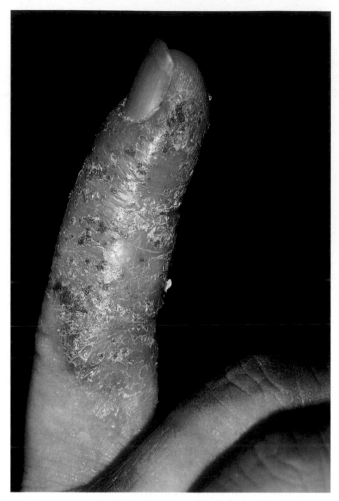

Figure 8-17 Pustular psoriasis of the digits. The eruption has remained localized in this one finger for years.

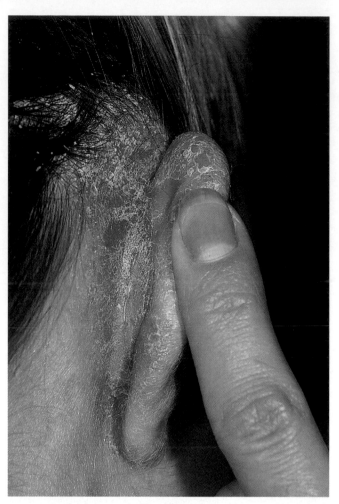

Figure 8-18 Psoriasis of the posterior auricular fold.

Psoriasis of the nails

Nail changes are characteristic of psoriasis and the nails of patients should be examined (see Chapter 25). These changes offer supporting evidence for the diagnosis of psoriasis when skin changes are equivocal or absent.

Pitting. Nail pitting is the best known and possibly the most frequent psoriatic nail abnormality (Figures 8-19 and 8-20). Nail plate cells are shed in much the same way as psoriatic scale is shed, leaving a variable number of tiny, punched-out depressions on the nail plate surface. They emerge from under the cuticle and grow out with the nail. Many other cutaneous diseases may cause pitting (e.g., eczema, fungal infections, and alopecia areata), or it may occur as an isolated finding as a normal variation.

Oil spot lesion. Psoriasis of the nail bed may cause lo-calized separation of the nail plate. Cellular debris and serum accumulates in this space. The brown yellow color observed through the nail plate looks like a spot of oil (see Figure 8-19).

Onycholysis. Psoriasis of the nail bed causes separation of the nail from the nail bed. Unlike the uniform separation caused by pressure on the tips of long nails, the nail detaches in an irregular manner. The nail plate turns yellow, simulating a fungal infection (Figure 8-21).

Subungual debris. This is analogous to fungal infection; the nail bed scale is retained, forcing the distal nail to separate from the nail bed (Figure 8-21).

Nail deformity. Extensive involvement of the nail matrix results in a nail losing its structural integrity, resulting in fragmentation and crumbling (Figure 8-22).

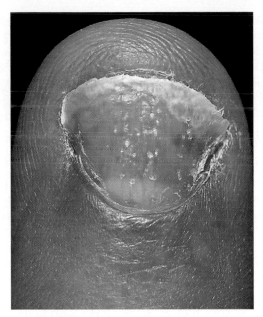

Figure 8-19 Pitting psoriasis of the proximal nail matrix results in loss of parakeratotic cells from the surface of the nail plate. This is a process analogous to the shedding of psoriatic skin scale.

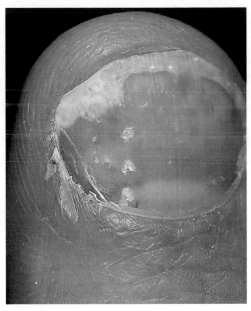

Figure 8-20 Oil spot lesion. A translucent yellow-red discoloration resembles a drop of oil beneath the nail plate. It occurs from psoriasis of the nail bed, which causes serum to be trapped under the nail plate.

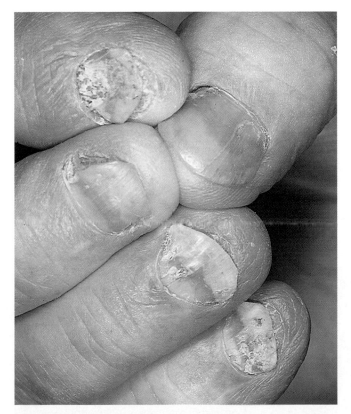

Figure 8-21 Separation of the nail, or onycholysis, is accompanied by yellow discoloration. Scaly debris elevates the nail plate. The debris is commonly mistaken for nail fungus infection.

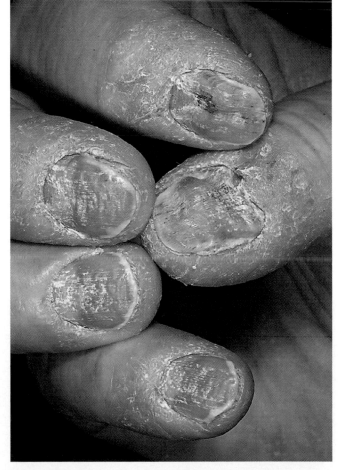

Figure 8-22 Malformed nails. Severe psoriasis of the matrix and nail bed results in grossly malformed nails.

Psoriatic arthritis

Psoriatic arthritis is a distinct form of arthritis in which the rheumatoid factor is usually negative. It may precede, accompany, or, more often, follow the skin manifestations. Onset may occur at any age, but peak occurrence is between ages 20 and 40; women and men are equally affected. The incidence in the psoriatic population is approximately 5% to 8%, but up to 53% of psoriatic patients suffer from arthralgia.[16,17] The prevalence of psoriatic arthritis is higher among patients with more severe cutaneous disease. Nail involvement occurs in more than 80% of patients with psoriatic arthritis, compared with 30% of patients with uncomplicated psoriasis. The prevalence of nail psoriasis is highest among patients with psoriatic arthritis who have arthritic involvement of their fingers, but the presence of nail disease does not have predictive value in determining if a patient is at risk for psoriatic arthritis. Cases of arthritis have been reported to develop following trauma. Patients with psoriatic arthritis who become pregnant improve or even remit in 80% of cases.[18] Despite active treatment and a reduction in joint inflammation and the rate of damage, psoriatic arthritis may be a progressively deforming arthritis.[19]

DIAGNOSIS. Laboratory tests are most useful to exclude other arthritic diseases. Although tests for antinuclear antibody (ANA) levels, erythrocyte sedimentation rate (ESR), white blood cell (WBC) counts, and uric acid sometimes identify elevated levels, they have little predictive value in diagnosing psoriatic arthritis. ESR is the best laboratory guide to disease activity. Rheumatoid factor levels are typically normal, but are elevated in a small percentage of patients.

CLINICAL FEATURES. There are five recognized presentations of psoriatic arthritis (Table 8-1).[20]

Asymmetric arthritis. The most common pattern is an asymmetric arthritis involving one or more joints of the fingers and toes (Figure 8-23). Usually one or more proximal interphalangeal (PIP), distal interphalangeal (DIP), metatarsophalangeal, or metacarpophalangeal joints are involved.

During the acute phase, the joint is red, warm, and painful. Continued inflammation promotes soft-tissue swelling on either side of the joint ("sausage finger") and restricts mobility. HLA-DR7 is significantly increased in this group with peripheral arthritis.[21]

Symmetric arthritis. A symmetric polyarthritis resembling rheumatoid arthritis occurs, but the rheumatoid factor is negative. The small joints of the hands and feet, wrists, ankles, knees, and elbows may be involved.

Distal interphalangeal joint disease. Perhaps the most characteristic presentation of arthritis with psoriasis is the involvement of the DIP joints of the hands and feet with associated psoriatic nail disease. The disease is chronic but mild, is not disabling, and is responsible for approximately 5% of cases of psoriatic arthritis.

Arthritis mutilans. The most severe form of psoriatic arthritis involves osteolysis of any of the small bones of the hands and feet. Gross deformity and subluxation are attributed to this condition. Severe osteolysis leads to digital telescoping, producing the "opera glass" deformity. This deformity may be seen in rheumatoid arthritis.

Ankylosing spondylitis. This condition occurs as an isolated phenomenon or in association with peripheral joint disease. The association of HLA-B27 and spondylitis is well known. The strongest association is in males with sacroiliitis. Asymptomatic sacroiliitis occurs in as many as one third of cases of psoriasis. It is usually asymmetrical and may be associated with spondylitis.

TREATMENT OF PSORIATIC ARTHRITIS. Management is similar to that of other chronic inflammatory joint diseases. Nonsteroidal antiinflammatory agents are the mainstay of therapy and usually provide adequate control, but they do not induce remissions. Intraarticular injections with corticosteroids may be effective.

Methotrexate controls advanced joint and skin diseases. Sulfasalazine and cyclosporine are also effective. Anti-tumor necrosis factor (TNF)-α therapy (etanercept, infliximab) may be very effective.

Table 8-1 Psoriatic Arthritis

Type	Percentage of all psoriatic arthritis	Features
Asymmetric arthritis (one or more joints)	60-70	Joints of fingers and toes ("sausage finger")
Symmetric polyarthritis	15	Clinically resembles rheumatoid arthritis, rheumatoid factor negative
Distal interphalangeal joint disease	5	Mild, chronic, associated with nail disease
Destructive polyarthritis (arthritis mutilans)	5	Osteolysis of small bones of hands and feet; gross deformity; joint subluxation
Ankylosing spondylitis	5	With or without peripheral joint disease

Modified from Moll JMH: Clin Orthop 1979;143:66.

Methotrexate. Methotrexate is an effective second-line agent for psoriatic arthritis.[22] Pain and function improve dramatically 2 to 6 weeks after starting methotrexate therapy with 5 mg every 12 hours in three consecutive doses once a week. Lower dosages may not be effective.[23] Methotrexate may also be given as a single dose or divided into two doses taken 12 hours apart. The amount is increased to 25 to 30 mg/week, until control is obtained, and then tapered to a maintenance dose of around 5 to 15 mg/week.

The risk of liver toxicity in patients undergoing long-term, low-dose methotrexate therapy for psoriatic arthritis is substantial, and that risk increases with the total cumulative dose and with heavy consumption of alcohol. Liver biopsies should be done periodically to monitor for liver toxicity.[24]

Etanercept (Embrel) and Infliximab (Remicade). These anti-tumor necrosis factor (anti-TNF agents) agents bind and inhibit the activity of TNF. Etanercept is given twice a week as a subcutaneous injection. Infliximab is given as an intravenous infusion at intervals dependent on the state of the disease. Both are highly effective for psoriatic arthritis. The cost is very high.

Antimalarial agents, particularly hydroxychloroquine, are usually avoided in psoriatic patients for fear of precipitating exfoliative dermatitis or exacerbating psoriasis. Two studies showed that these reactions did not occur in patients treated with hydroxychloroquine[25] or chloroquine.[26]

Hydroxychloroquine is inadequately effective for psoriatic arthritis. Systemic corticosteroids are usually avoided because of possible rebound of the skin disease on withdrawal.

Cyclosporine at daily doses ranging usually from 1.5 to 5.0 mg/kg provides impressive relief from arthralgias and improvement of joint function.[27] Although mild-to-moderate relapses occur, rebound phenomena is not observed after discontinuation of treatment.[28] Renal toxicity limits its use.

Acitretin (1 mg/kg/day) has a beneficial effect on objective symptoms. The dosage is decreased after the initial response in an attempt to minimize side effects.[29] Sulfasalazine (2 gm/day) is a safe and effective second-line agent for psoriatic arthritis.[30,31]

Some psoriatic patients treated with photochemotherapy (PUVA) experience improvement in joint symptoms.

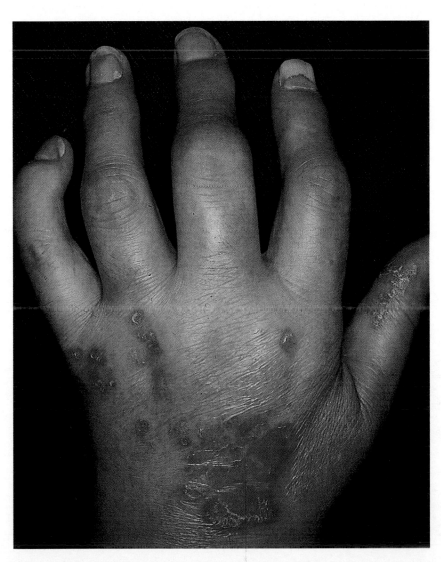

Figure 8-23 Psoriatic arthritis. Asymmetric arthritis pattern.

Treatment of psoriasis

Many topical and systemic agents are available. None of the topical medications are predictably effective. All require lengthy treatment to give relief that is often temporary. Compliance is a problem. Patients become discouraged with moderately effective expensive topical treatment that lasts weeks or months. Limited disease can be managed with topical therapy (Table 8-2). One intralesional steroid injection can heal a small plaque and keep it in remission for months. This is an ideal treatment for patients with a few small plaques. Topical steroid creams and ointments, calcipotriol (Dovonex), tazarotene (Tazorac), anthralin, and tar are the mainstays of topical treatment. These agents are used with or without ultraviolet light exposure. Effective programs can be designed for patients who do not have access to a therapeutic light source and for patients who have limited disease. Without light, tar is moderately effective, but persistent use of calcipotriol, tazarotene, or anthralin can clear the disease and offers the patient substantial remission periods. Topical steroids work quickly, but total eradication of the plaques is difficult to accomplish; remission times are short, and the creams become less effective with continued use.

Patients with psoriasis covering more than 20% of the body need special treatment programs (Table 8-3).

DETERMINING THE DEGREE OF INFLAMMATION. The most common form of psoriasis is the localized chronic plaque disease involving the skin and scalp (see Figures 8-1 and 8-4). It must be determined whether the plaque is inflamed prior to instituting therapy (Figure 8-24). Red, sore plaques can be irritated by tar, calcipotriol, and anthralin. Irritation can induce further activity. Inflammation should be suppressed with topical steroids and/or antibiotics before initiating other treatments.

DETERMINING THE END OF TREATMENT. The plaque is effectively treated when induration has disappeared. Residual erythema, hypopigmentation, or brown hyperpigmentation is common when the plaque clears; patients frequently mistake the residual color for disease and continue treatment. If the plaque cannot be felt by drawing the finger over the skin surface, treatment may be stopped.

CONTROL STRESS. A study demonstrated a positive correlation between the severity of psoriatic symptoms and psychologic distress.[32] Stress reduction techniques may be appropriate for certain patients.[33]

Table 8-2 Therapeutic Options for Persons with Psoriasis on Less than 20% of the Body

Treatment	Advantages	Disadvantages	Comments
Topical steroids	Rapid response, controls inflammation and itching, best for intertriginous areas and face, convenient, not messy	Temporary relief (tolerance occurs), less effective with continued use, atrophy and telangiectasia occur with continued use, brief remissions, very expensive	Best results occur with pulse dosing (e.g., 2 weeks of medication and 1 week of lubrication only); plastic occlusion is very effective
Calcipotriol (Dovonex)	Well tolerated, long remissions possible	Burning, skin irritation, expensive	Best for moderate plaque psoriasis
Tazarotene (Tazorac)	Effective, long remissions possible	Irritating, expensive	Topical steroids can control irritation and enhance effectiveness
Anthralin	Convenient short contact programs, long remissions, effective for scalp	Purple-brown staining, irritating, careful application (only to plaque) required	Used on chronic (not inflamed) plaques; best results occur when used with UVB light
Tar	New preparations are pleasant	Only moderately effective in a few patients	Most effective when combined with UVB (Goeckerman regimen)
UVB and lubricating agents or tar	Insurance may cover part or all of treatment, effective for 70% of patients, no need for topical steroids	Expensive, office-based therapy	Used only on plaque and guttate psoriasis, travel and time required
Tape or occlusive dressing	Convenient, no mess	Expensive; only for limited disease	May be used to occlude topical steroids
Intralesional steroids	Convenient, rapidly effective, long remissions	Only for limited areas, atrophy and telangiectasia occur at injection site	Ideal for chronic scalp and body plaques when small and few in number

DURATION OF REMISSION. Among topical monotherapy, anthralin and tazarotene induce longer remissions than calcipotriene and corticosteroids; among systemic agents, longer remissions occur with acitretin than cyclosporine or methotrexate, but compared with the remission rate of phototherapeutic modalities, the remission rates are much less (see Tables 8-2 and 8-3). Traditional Goeckerman therapy, conducted in a day treatment setting, is more likely to induce prolonged remissions than simple UVB phototherapy, "home Goeckerman therapy" using LCD, or heliotherapy. PUVA phototherapy also induces prolonged remissions.[34]

Some treatments are better suited for rapid clearing; others are better suited to be maintenance treatment.[35] The optimal management involves the sequential use of therapeutic agents involving three steps, namely the clearing phase, the transitional phase, and the maintenance phase.

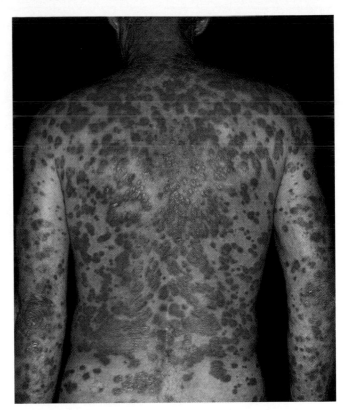

Figure 8-24 Inflammatory plaque psoriasis. A patient with such highly inflamed disease must not be treated initially with irritating medicines such as anthralin, tar, or calcipotriol.

Table 8-3 Therapeutic Options for Persons with Psoriasis on More than 20% of the Body		
Treatment	**Advantages**	**Disadvantages**
UVB and tar administered in physician's office	More effective than UVB alone	More expensive and carcinogenic than UVB alone; requires many office visits
PUVA	Allows patient to be ambulatory; effective	Many treatments needed; many office visits required
Methotrexate	"Gold standard" for efficacy, helps arthritis	Hepatotoxicity, liver biopsy periodically required
Hydrea	Effective in the few for whom it works at all	Hematopoietic toxicity; flulike syndrome
Acitretin (Soriatane)	Effective for palmar-plantar-pustular, erythrodermic, and pustular types of psoriasis; fast, effective; helps arthritis	Teratogenic; may be as effective as monotherapy for plaque psoriasis
Cyclosporine	Fast, effective; helps arthritis	Nephrotoxic; immunosuppressive; expensive
Biologic therapies	No multiorgan adverse effects	Very expensive No long term experience
Alefacept (Amevive), Etanercept (Embrel), Infliximab (Remicade)	Very effective	Give by injection or intravenously
Many others in development	Potential for interaction with other drugs is very low	

Topical therapy
Calcipotriene (Dovonex)

Calcipotriene (Dovonex) 0.005% ointment and cream is a vitamin D3 analog that inhibits epidermal cell proliferation and enhances cell differentiation. It is effective and safe and well tolerated for the short- and long-term treatment of psoriasis. Up to 100 gm/week can be used. The cream base is often preferred, but it is slightly less effective than ointment. Calcipotriene is more effective than the group II corticosteroid ointments fluocinonide 0.05% and anthralin.[36] Tachyphylaxis (tolerance) does not occur with calcipotriene. Calcipotriene solution is used for scalp psoriasis. It is not as effective as betamethasone valerate, but it does not have the corticosteroid side effects of atrophy. It is valuable for long-term scalp treatment programs.

Calcipotriene is not as effective as group I corticosteroids, but regimens using calcipotriene and group I corticosteroids are superior over either agent alone. Most patients now use the following regimen. Calcipotriene is applied in the morning and a group I corticosteroid is applied in the evening for 2 weeks.[37] Then a maintenance regimen is begun using group I corticosteroids twice daily on weekends and calcipotriene twice daily on weekdays. Application for 6 to 8 weeks gives a 60% to 70% improvement in plaque-type psoriasis. Remission is maintained with long-term use of this program. Application of calcipotriene twice a day is much more effective than once a day application. Encourage patients to comply with this program for optimal efficacy. Topical steroid use is limited and side effects such as atrophy do not occur. Occlusion improves the response to calcipotriol by enhancing its penetration but many patients will not tolerate the irritation.[38]

Calcipotriene treatment can produce a mild irritant contact dermatitis at the site of application. The face and intertriginous areas are prone to this side effect.

Calcipotriene is very effective for treating the face and intertriginous sites. Dilution of calcipotriene with petrolatum is one method of avoiding the irritant dermatitis. Treatment with a low- to mid-potency topical steroid is another.

Calcipotriene is not very effective at improving the response to UVB or narrowband UVB.[39] UVB does not inactivate calcipotriene. Calcipotriene combined with PUVA is very effective.[40] Calcipotriene treated patients required fewer treatments and lower cumulative doses of UVA to clear. Calcipotriene is applied after UVA exposures because UVA inactivates calcipotriene.[41] Hypercalcemia is reported with excessive quantities of calcipotriene applied over large surface areas.[42] Parameters of calcium metabolism do not change when less than 100 gm per week is used.

Retinoids

Tazarotene (0.05%, 0.1%) is available as a gel and cream. Irritation develops in most patients. The stronger formulation is more effective but more irritating.

Topical steroids can control irritation and enhance effectiveness. Group I, II, and IV topical steroids are all effective when used in combination with tazarotene. The retinoid may prevent corticosteroid atrophy. Treatment consists of application of tazarotene once a day and a topical steroid approximately 12 hours later.

Remission of psoriasis was maintained for at least 5 months with a regimen of tazarotene gel 0.1% applied Mondays, Wednesdays, and Fridays and clobetasol ointment applied Tuesdays and Thursdays.[43]

Some clinicians think that a short-contact regimen is effective. Tazarotene is applied for 5 minutes and then washed off. This regimen minimizes irritation but maintains efficacy.

Patients treated with UVB and tazarotene responded more favorably than patients treated with UVB alone. Tazarotene thins the stratum corneum of the epidermis, allowing patients to burn more easily. UV doses are reduced by at least one third if tazarotene is added to a course of phototherapy.[44] Tazarotene remained chemically stable when used in conjunction with UVB or UVA phototherapy.[45]

Topical steroids

Topical steroids (see Chapter 2) give fast but temporary relief. They are most useful for reducing inflammation and controlling itching. Initially, when the patient is introduced to topical steroids, the results are most gratifying. However, tachyphylaxis, or tolerance, occurs, and the medication becomes less effective with continued use. Patients remember the initial response and continue topical steroids in anticipation of continued effectiveness. Long-term use of topical steroids results in atrophy and telangiectasia. Topical steroids are useful for treating inflamed and intertriginous plaques.

A group I through V steroid applied one to four times a day in a cream or ointment base is required for best results. Plastic occlusion of topical steroids is much more effective than simple application. Diprolene, Cormax, and Olux foam are extremely potent, and occlusion is not used with these drugs. Group V topical steroids applied once or twice a day should be used in the intertriginous areas and on the face. Some plaques resolve completely, but most remain only partially reduced with continued application. Continual application for more than 3 weeks should be discouraged. Remissions are usually brief and the plaques may return shortly after treatment is terminated. Topical steroid creams applied under an occlusive plastic dressing promote more rapid clearing, but remissions are not extended.

The rapid appearance of atrophy and telangiectasia occurs when the group I topical steroids are occluded. Topical steroid solutions are useful for scalp psoriasis. Intralesional injection of small plaques with triamcinolone acetonide (Kenalog, 5 to 10 mg/mL) almost invariably clears the lesion and accords long-term remission. Atrophy may occur with the 10 mg/mL concentration.

Betamethasone valerate foam (Luxiq) and clobetasol propionate foam (Olux) are available in 50-gm and 100-gm containers. The foam becomes a liquid upon contact with the skin. These formulations are very effective and preferred by many patients to creams, ointments, and solutions for treating scalp lesions and plaque psoriasis on the trunk and extremities. Transient stinging occurs in some patients. Moisturizers can be applied soon after application of the foam.

Intralesional steroids

Patients with a few, small, chronic psoriatic plaques of the scalp or body can be effectively treated with a single intralesional injection of triamcinolone acetonide (Kenalog, 5 to 10 mg/mL). The 10 mg/mL solution may be diluted with saline. Most injected plaques clear completely and remain in remission for months. Atrophy and telangiectasias may appear at the injection site. The face and intertriginous areas are avoided.

Anthralin

Anthralin is used only for chronic plaques. For years anthralin has been used effectively in the hospital to treat psoriasis. The principal objections were to the mess, long treatment times, and staining. Maximum patient compliance can be achieved with the new, short-treatment time schedules and commercially available preparations. There are several effective treatment programs. Psoriasis clears faster when UVB radiation is used in combination with anthralin.[46]

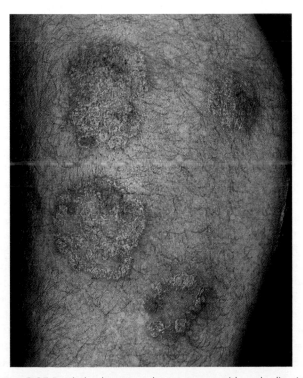

Figure 8-25 Psoriatic plaques under treatment with anthralin. As with all forms of treatment, plaques first clear in the center.

PREPARATIONS AND USE. Anthralin is commercially available in concentrations of 0.1%, 0.25%, 0.5%, and 1.0% (3% outside United States). Patients must be cautioned about irritation and staining. Hands should be washed carefully after application, with care to avoid eye contact. Care must also be taken to protect normal skin, and anthralin should not be applied to intertriginous areas or to the face. Ointment is removed with a shower with soap. Lubricants are applied to avoid dryness and to remove the last traces of anthralin. If irritation occurs, anthralin should be discontinued, and the patient should be treated with group II through V topical steroids until improvement is noted.

Skin stains fade in a matter of weeks, but purple clothing stains are permanent (Figure 8-25). Anthralin is also used for scalp psoriasis. Triethanolamine, applied when anthralin is removed, prevents irritation and staining of the skin. Hypochlorite detergents have been used successfully to remove anthralin stains from materials, and mild acid soaps wash off anthralin skin stains.

Short-contact therapy. Apply the medication and wash it off in 20 minutes. Contact time can be increased to an hour; longer times are probably no more effective and become inconvenient.[48] The goal is to maintain a daily schedule using the highest concentration of anthralin that can be tolerated without inducing inflammation.

Ultraviolet light B

The most effective topical programs use ultraviolet light in combination with tar or tazarotene. The addition of tazarotene to a regimen of UVB phototherapy results in faster and more effective clearing. Several studies have indicated that the duration of remission is shortened when UVB is administered with topical corticosteroids.[49] When UVB phototherapy is used in conjunction with short-contact anthralin therapy, studies have shown little additional benefit from the combination in comparison to UVB alone, and patients disliked using anthralin. When calcipotriene is used in conjunction with UVB, there is slightly more clearing with the combination of treatments compared with UVB alone.

Ultraviolet light in intensities high enough to be effective can be obtained from natural sunlight or commercially available light cabinets. Inexpensive single-bulb tanning lights and long-wave ultraviolet light (UVA) tanning salon lights are sometimes effective. Most dermatologists have phototherapy units; many patients are best treated in that setting. There is a significant positive correlation between patients' responses to sunbathing and their responses to short-wave ultraviolet light (UVB) phototherapy. Sunlight nonresponders have a 70% chance of failure with UVB phototherapy; sunlight responders have an 80% chance that clearance treatment will succeed.[50]

ULTRAVIOLET LIGHT B AND LUBRICATING AGENTS. Tar enhances the effectiveness of ultraviolet light,[51] but studies suggest that application of lubricants before UVB exposure provides results similar to those achieved with tar and UVB.[52] The ideal schedules for treatment frequency and increasing UVB dosages have not been established. Data suggest that aggressive treatment with UVB exposures intense enough to produce erythema (maximally erythemogenic UVB) at each treatment results in clearing with fewer treatments and less total UVB dosage.[53] Practically speaking, these aggressive techniques may be difficult to manage for routine office use; acceptable results have been achieved using suberythemogenic doses.[52] Optimal, long-term management may be achieved by continuing UVB phototherapy after initial clearing (average—six treatments per month).[54] Treatment with UVB and lubricating agents is just as effective as UVB and topical steroids; therefore costly topical steroids can be avoided during light therapy.[55] If not removed before phototherapy, preparations containing tar or thickly applied petrolatum or emollients can block UVB.[56]

ULTRAVIOLET LIGHT B AND TAR. Despite several studies that show lubricating agents are as effective as tar for treatment before UVB exposure, the final answer is not yet known. Tar and UVB phototherapy have been used for years with gratifying results, and this method continues to be used. Tar preparations are applied 2 or more hours before ultraviolet light exposure. There are several commercially available tar preparations (see the Formulary, p. 945). Some of these preparations cause drying, whereas others, particularly those with a lubricating base (e.g., T-Derm and Fototar), are well tolerated.

GOECKERMAN REGIMEN. This regimen combines the daily application of tar with UVB exposure; it is safe, highly effective, and possibly produces the longest remissions.[57] However, a major commitment of time and money is required. Many larger hospitals used to provide inpatient facilities for this program but these treatment options have been stopped in the health-maintenance organization insurance environment. The Goeckerman regimen can be used on an outpatient basis. The addition of topical steroids to the Goeckerman regimen may interfere with treatment by shortening the duration of remission.[58] A tar concentrate such as Balnetar can be added to the bath water as a substitute for tar ointments and lotions. Tar-solution soaks are useful for psoriasis of the palms and soles. The feet can be soaked for 1 hour each day in a basin of warm water and one or two capfuls of Balnetar.

ULTRAVIOLET LIGHT B AND SYSTEMIC AGENTS. The combination of UVB phototherapy with systemic agents can be very effective. Combining methotrexate and UVB resulted in clearing of extensive psoriasis.[59] Patients with extensive psoriasis were treated with a 3-week course of methotrexate followed by a combination of UVB therapy and methotrexate. When lesions cleared to less than 5% of body involvement, the methotrexate was stopped, and UVB therapy alone was used as maintenance therapy. This protocol achieved clearance of disease in all patients in a mean of 7 weeks. The combination therapy of methotrexate and UVB allows for clearing of psoriasis at relatively low doses of UVB and methotrexate and thus may reduce the long-term cumulative toxicity of both agents. Similarly, the combination of acitretin with UVB results in more rapid and more effective clearing than monotherapy with either agent alone.[60]

NARROWBAND ULTRAVIOLET LIGHT B. The spectrum of UV light most effective for the treatment of psoriasis is in a narrow range (approximately 311 nm). Treatment with these narrowband bulbs is superior to treatment with broadband UVB. Narrowband UVB is not as effective as PUVA. Burns with narrowband UVB can be more severe. This treatment is not available in all dermatologists' offices. The bulbs are very expensive.

Photochemotherapy

Complete prescribing information is in the Formulary.

The treatment, known as PUVA, is so designated because of the use of a class of drugs called psoralens (P), along with exposure to long-wave ultraviolet light (UVA). Oxsoralen-Ultra capsules are an encapsulated liquid formulation of methoxsalen (available in 10-mg capsules). Patients ingest a prescribed dose of methoxsalen approximately 2 hours before being exposed to a carefully measured amount of UVA in a uniquely designed enclosure. A major advantage of PUVA is that it controls severe psoriasis with relatively few maintenance treatments, and it can be done on an outpatient basis. Light does not penetrate hair: scalp psoriasis must be treated with conventional therapy.

Indications. PUVA is an effective method of controlling but not curing psoriasis. Patients should be selected only by physicians who are experienced in the treatment of all forms of psoriasis. PUVA is indicated for the symptomatic control of severe, recalcitrant, and disabling plaque psoriasis that is not adequately responsive to other forms of therapy. Erythrodermic and pustular psoriasis are best treated with acitretin. Pustular psoriasis of the palms and soles responds best to PUVA-acitretin.[61,62] Because of the concerns about long-term toxicity, PUVA is most appropriate for severe psoriasis in patients older than 50 years of age. The American Academy of Pediatrics has disapproved the use of PUVA therapy in children.

Psoriatic arthropathy of the nonspondylitic type may respond to PUVA with improvement in erythema, tenderness, and inflammation of the peripheral joints.[50]

Treatment regimen. The treatment regimen is divided into two phases: the clearance phase, in which continual treatment is given until clearing occurs, followed by the maintenance phase, in which treatments are given less frequently but in numbers sufficient to prevent a flare-up of the disease.

Response to treatment. After the initial clearing phase, patients require a mean of 30 treatments per year during the first 1½ years.[63] Most patients who are clear after the initial 2- to 3-month maintenance period remain clear for at least 6 to 12 months. Disease control lasts longer after PUVA than after UVB therapy. Continued use of PUVA after initial clearing affords good disease control for prolonged periods. The recurrence rate is higher in patients who do not continue maintenance treatment; however, long-term maintenance results in high cumulative doses of energy.

PUVA COMBINED WITH OTHER MODALITIES. Combining PUVA with other modalities (UVB,[64] Calcipotriene,[65] tazarotene, acitretin,[66] and methotrexate[67]) reduces the number of PUVA treatments required to maintain remission, results in fewer adverse effects from treatment, increases efficacy, and reduces cost.

PUVA plus acitretin. Combination therapy of psoriasis with acitretin and phototherapy (psoralen-ultraviolet A [PUVA] or ultraviolet B [UVB]) offers multiple advantages over use of either modality alone.

LONG-TERM SIDE EFFECTS. Most long-term side effects of PUVA are dose-dependent. Methods should be sought to control disease using the minimum amount of PUVA therapy. These include the use of appropriate dosage regimens, the avoidance of maintenance therapy as far as possible, and the use of combination therapies.

Skin tumors. PUVA promotes skin aging, actinic keratoses, and squamous cell carcinoma (SCC),[68] especially in patients previously treated with arsenic or ionizing radiation and in patients with a history of skin cancer.[69-71] The risk of cutaneous SCC from PUVA is dose related. There is a strong, dose-dependent increase in the risk of genital tumors associated with exposure to PUVA and ultraviolet B radiation. Men should use genital protection when they are exposed to PUVA and to other forms of ultraviolet radiation for therapeutic, recreational, or cosmetic reasons.[72]

Approximately 15 years after the first treatment with PUVA, the risk of malignant melanoma increases, especially among patients who receive 250 treatments or more (Table 8-4).[73]

Lentigines. Lentigines develop in many patients after long-term treatment with PUVA. These small black macules occur in PUVA-exposed sites.[77,78]

Cataracts. Concern has been expressed that PUVA therapy may cause cataracts, but the incidence seems to be very low if eye protection is used.[79] During the first day of PUVA treatment, patients should wear UVA-blocking, plastic, wraparound glasses when they are outdoors from the time they ingest the drug until bedtime. While indoors or in dim light, either wraparound glasses or clear UVA-blocking glasses should be worn. During the second day, either plastic wraparound or clear UVA-blocking glasses should be worn the entire day.

SHORT-TERM SIDE EFFECTS. Short-term side effects include dark tanning, pruritus, nausea, and severe sunburn.

Nausea. Nausea is the most common side effect. It develops shortly after methoxsalen is taken. Nausea is prevented by dividing the psoralen dose over 15 minutes and take it with food. Fifteen hundred milligrams of ginger ingested 20 minutes before the psoralen may also prevent nausea. PUVA treatments later in the day are less likely to result in nausea than those administered in the morning.

Phototoxicity. Avoid sun exposure on the days of treatment to prevent burns. PUVA burns begin 24 hours after exposure and peak at 48 hours. PUVA is not administered 2 days in a row because the second treatment might be given to a patient who is not aware that a burn will occur from the first day's treatment.

Tape or occlusive dressings

One study showed that adhesive occlusive dressings applied and changed every week were therapeutically superior to a group V topical steroid and comparable to UVB therapy.[80] Complete clearing occurred in 47% of the cases in an average of 5 weeks; another 41% improved. Waterproof tape with low-moisture vapor transmission applied continually for 1 week gave similar results. Two or more applications were required.[81] This treatment may be appropriate for treating localized chronic plaques. Actiderm and DuoDerm are self-adhesive patches that are applied alone or over topical steroids and changed every 1 to 7 days.

Table 8-4 PUVA Cancer Risks		
Malignant melanoma[73]	Squamous cell carcinoma[72,74]	Basal cell cancer
15 years after the first PUVA Rx, risk increases in patients with > 250 treatments	Persistent, dose-related increase in the risk	No increase risk within a decade of beginning treatment
Number of patients small	11-fold increase in patients treated with more than 260 PUVA sessions	
From Morison W, et al: Arch Dermatol 1998; 134(5):595.		

Treating the scalp

The scalp is difficult to treat because hair interferes with the application of medicine and shields the skin from ultraviolet light. Symptoms of tenderness and itching vary considerably. The goal is to provide symptomatic and cosmetic relief. It is unnecessary and impractical to attempt to keep the scalp constantly clear.

REMOVING SCALE. Scale must be removed first to facilitate penetration of medicine. Superficial scale can be removed with shampoos that contain tar and salicylic acid (e.g., T-gel). Thicker scale is removed by applying Baker's P & S or 10% liquor carbonis detergens (LCD) in Nivea oil to the scalp and washing 6 to 8 hours later with shampoo or Dawn dishwashing liquid. Combing during the shampoo helps dislodge scale.

Baker's P & S liquid (phenol, sodium chloride, and liquid paraffin) applied to the scalp at bedtime and washed out in the morning is moderately effective in reducing scale. Baker's liquid is pleasant and well tolerated for extended periods.

LCD (10%), a tar extract of crude oil tar, is mixed with Nivea oil by the pharmacist. The unpleasant mixture is liberally massaged into the scalp at bedtime. Warming the mixture before application enhances scale penetration. A shower cap protects pillows and also encourages scale penetration. An impressive amount of scale is removed in the first few days. Nightly applications are continued until the scalp is acceptably clear.

MILD TO MODERATE SCALP INVOLVEMENT. When used at least every other day, tar shampoos (see the Formulary, p. 945) may be effective in controlling moderate scaling. Corticosteroid solutions are very expensive, but a few drops can cover a wide area. Steroid gels (e.g., Lidex gel, Temovate gel, Topicort gel), which have a keratolytic base and penetrate hair, are effective for localized plaques. Derma-Smoothe FS lotion (peanut oil, fluocinolone acetonide 0.01%) is an effective topical steroid that can be applied to the entire scalp and occluded with a shower cap. The scalp is dampened before application. The oil base penetrates and loosens scale. Treatment is repeated each night for 1 to 3 weeks until itching and erythema are controlled.

Betamethasone valerate foam (Luxiq) and clobetasol foam (Olux) are available in 50-gm and 100-gm containers. The foam becomes a liquid upon contact with the skin. This formulation is effective, pleasant, and easily penetrates through hair. Temporary stinging may occur during application.

Small plaques are effectively treated with intralesional steroid injections of triamcinolone acetonide (Kenalog, 10 mg/mL). Remissions following use of intralesional steroids are much longer than those following topical steroids.

Ketoconazole cream is sometimes useful. Oral ketoconazole (400 mg daily) may be effective in some cases.[82] The possibility of drug toxicity limits its usefulness.

TREATMENT OF DIFFUSE AND THICK SCALP PSORIASIS. Three different programs can be implemented, all of which use oil or ointment-based preparations for scale penetration. They are applied at bedtime and washed out each morning with strong detergents such as Dawn dishwashing liquid. Topical steroid solutions can be applied during the day.

Tar and oil. Ten percent LCD in Nivea oil applied to the scalp, covered with a shower cap and washed out each morning removes scale and suppresses inflammation.

Anthralin. Anthralin ointment applied each evening and removed in the morning is another method for treating resistant scalp psoriasis. A short-contact method similar to that previously described for anthralin is used. Apply 0.25% to 0.5% anthralin ointment and wash completely 10 to 20 minutes after application. Dritho-Scalp (0.25% and 0.5%) is packaged in a tube with a long nozzle for hair penetration.

Systemic therapy

Topical treatment has its limits. Many patients do not respond to the most vigorous topical programs, or the disease may be so extensive that topical treatment is not practical.

Moderate-to-severe psoriasis, variably defined as patients with 20% or more involvement of body surface area or patients unresponsive to topical therapy, can be treated with several modalities including phototherapy, photochemotherapy (PUVA), retinoids, methotrexate, or biologic agents.[83]

A number of systemic drugs are available, some of which have potentially serious side effects. Methotrexate is highly effective, relatively safe, and well tolerated, but the need for periodic liver biopsies discourages some patients and physicians. Photochemotherapy (PUVA) is effective and relatively safe. Acitretin is used to potentiate the effects of PUVA and as a monotherapy for plaque, pustular, and erythrodermic forms of psoriasis. Acitretin has many annoying side effects. Hydrea is not hepatotoxic, but it is rarely used because it is effective in only a few patients. Cyclosporine is rapidly effective, but long-term use may be associated with loss of kidney function.

Rotational therapy

A rotational approach to therapy has been suggested (see the diagram on p. 229). Rotation of available therapies (UVB plus tar, PUVA, methotrexate, acitretin, cyclosporine, and biologic therapy) for moderate to severe psoriasis may minimize long-term toxicity and allow effective treatments to be maintained for many years. Patients may receive each form of therapy for 1 to 2 years and then switch to the next form of treatment. By rotating each of the treatments at these intervals, it may be 4 or 5 years before the patient needs to return to the first therapy, thereby minimizing the cumulative toxicity by long periods off each treatment.[83,84,85]

The physician and patient must make the final decision about which therapeutic modality is appropriate based on the unique features of each individual case.

ROTATIONAL THERAPY

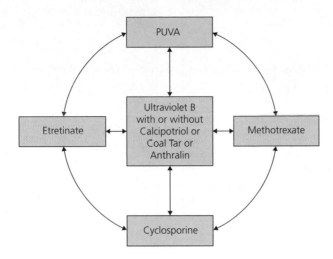

Rotational therapy. For moderate-to-severe psoriasis to minimize toxic effects from any one therapy. A reasonable sequence would start with phototherapy (PUVA or ultraviolet B), followed by methotrexate, then the other form of radiation, then another oral agent, and so on. Patients who do not tolerate radiation therapy rotate oral agents.

Methotrexate

INDICATIONS. Methotrexate (MTX) has been used to treat psoriasis for over 30 years. It is the "gold standard" for the treatment of severe psoriasis and is particularly effective in controlling erythrodermic and generalized pustular psoriasis.[86] It induces remissions in the majority of treated patients and maintains remissions for long periods with continued therapy. MTX is also effective for psoriatic arthritis. It is relatively safe and well tolerated,[87] but the need for periodic liver biopsies discourages many patients and physicians from using it. Guidelines for the use of MTX are listed in Boxes 8-1 to 8-3.

MECHANISM OF ACTION. MTX is a folic acid antagonist that inhibits dihydrofolate reductase. DNA synthesis is inhibited as the concentrations of thymidine and purines fall after treatment with MTX.[88] MTX suppresses psoriatic epidermal cell reproduction and has antiinflammatory and immunomodulatory effects. Methotrexate is immunosuppressive; use should be avoided in patients with active infections.

DOSING. The oral triple-dose regimen is the most common method used (Box 8-3). A dose is taken at 12-hour intervals during a 36-hour period once each week. An initial test dose of 2.5 to 5 mg is given, and complete blood cell counts and liver function tests are obtained 1 week later. If this dose was well tolerated, start with one 2.5-mg tablet at 12-hour intervals for three doses. The next week the dosage is increased by one to two tablets. In the following weeks, titrate up or down by a 2.5-mg tablet to the most effective and best-tolerated dosage. Most patients are controlled and tolerate 15 mg/week (two-tablet, two-tablet, two-tablet dosage). Once the desired degree of clearing is obtained, the dosage is decreased by one tablet per week every few weeks to arrive at a maintenance regimen (i.e., 2.5 to 5.0 mg/week). The goal is not necessarily 100% clearance, but to reach 80% improvement. This is safer than pushing higher, more toxic dosages to obtain 100% clearance.

Discontinue the drug for several months of rest; the summer months are a good time to attempt this, when sunlight may control the disease. Gradually tapering to withdraw MTX seems to present fewer problems of rebound than does a sudden discontinuance of the drug.

MONITORING. See Boxes 8-4 and 8-5. The responses to abnormal test results are listed in Box 8-6. Bone marrow toxicity is the most serious short-term side effect, hepatotoxicity is the most common long-term adverse effect. MTX is excreted mainly via the kidney. Older individuals tend to have reduced renal function and require lower dosages of MTX.

Box 8-1 Indications for Methotrexate in Psoriasis

Severe psoriasis that may be life-ruining physically, emotionally, or economically.

1. Patients with moderate to severe psoriasis
2. Psoriatic erythroderma
3. Psoriatic arthritis, moderate to severe
4. Acute pustular psoriasis, von Zumbusch type
5. More than 20% involvement of body surface
6. Localized pustular psoriasis
7. Psoriasis that affects certain areas of body so that normal function and employment are prevented
8. Lack of response to phototherapy, PUVA, and retinoids

From Roenigk H, et al: J Am Acad Dermatol 1998; 38(3):478.

Box 8-2 Relative Contraindications for Methotrexate in Psoriasis

- Any abnormalities in renal function may require other therapy or a marked reduction in the dose
- Significant abnormalities in liver function
- Pregnancy or nursing (absolute contraindications)
- Male or female fertility (conception must be avoided during methotrexate therapy and afterward for at least 3 months in the male or one ovulatory cycle in the female)
- Hepatitis, active or recent
- Cirrhosis
- Severe anemia, leukopenia, or thrombocytopenia
- Excessive alcohol consumption
- Active infectious disease (e.g., tuberculosis, pyelonephritis)
- Unreliability on the part of the patient

Circumstances may arise in which contraindications must be waived, such as when benefits can be expected to outweigh the risks of methotrexate therapy in an individual patient.

From Roenigk H, et al: J Am Acad Dermatol 1998; 38(3):478.

Box 8-3 Methotrexate Dosage

- Test dose: 2.5-5.0 mg (to detect any predisposition to toxic effects—obtain CBC, and liver function test 1 wk later)
- Average dose: 7.5-15 mg/wk
- Increased gradually (2.5 to 5.0 mg)
- Maximum dose oral: 30 mg/wk
- Maximum dose parenteral: 50-75 mg/wk
- When improved, taper by 2.5 mg/mo

Methotrexate dosing schedules

The following two dosage schedules are commonly used:

- Single weekly oral, intravenous, intramuscular, or subcutaneous administration. Intravenous drips of methotrexate should not be used.
- Intermittent oral schedule of three divided doses each week (every 12 hours three times in 1 week). The average dose is 2.5 to 5.0 mg at 12-hour intervals for three doses each week.

Gradually increase by 2.5 mg/wk. The total oral dose usually does not exceed 30 mg/wk. The oral administration can be tablets or parenteral solution. (0.1 ml of 50 mg/2 ml parenteral solution is equivalent to 2.5 mg oral.)

There are fewer toxic effects when the drug is given in one dose than when the same total amount is dispensed in daily doses over an extended period of 5 to 7 days.

Adapted from Lebwohl M, Ali S: J Am Acad Dermatol 2001; 45(5): 649; and Roenigk H, et al: J Am Acad Dermatol 1998; 38(3):478.

Box 8-4 Methotrexate: Baseline and Follow-up Monitoring

Baseline monitoring

- History and physical examination
- CBC, platelet count
- Renal function: serum creatinine, blood urea nitrogen, urinalysis, and creatinine clearance, particularly in elderly patients
- Liver chemistry: AST (SGOT), ALT (SGPT), alkaline phosphatase, bilirubin, albumin, and hepatitis A, B, and C serology test
- HIV antibody in patients at risk for AIDS

Follow-up monitoring

- Complete blood cell count with differential and platelet counts weekly for the first 2 weeks then biweekly for the next month, and then approximately monthly depending on leukocyte count and stability of patient
- Liver chemistries: ALT, AST, alkaline phosphatase, and serum albumin levels every 4 to 8 weeks (more frequent liver chemistry monitoring in lieu of an initial liver biopsy)
- Renal function studies: BUN and serum creatinine levels at 3- to 4-month intervals
- Repeat blood work 7 d after dose escalation

Adapted from Lebwohl M, Ali S: J Am Acad Dermatol 2001; 45(5): 649; and Roenigk H, et al: J Am Acad Dermatol 1998; 38(3):478.

Box 8-5 Abnormal Laboratory Studies and Management

Reduction in WBC or platelet counts. Maximum depression occurs 7 to 10 days after a dose of MTX.	Reduce or stop MTX.
Leukocyte count <3500/mm³ continuing beyond 1 week. Platelet count <100,000/mm³.	Discontinue MTX for 2 to 3 weeks. Treat with folinic acid (20 mg).
Increasing mean cell volume may signal the development of megaloblastic anemia.	Folic acid 1 to 5 mg qd will reverse this side effect.
Obtain liver chemistries at least 1 week after the last MTX dose.	Values are frequently elevated 1 to 2 days after MTX therapy.
Persistent abnormal liver chemistry.	Withhold MTX for 1 to 2 weeks and then repeat tests. Liver chemistry values should return to normal in 1 to 2 weeks.
Abnormal liver chemistry values persist for 2 to 3 months.	Consider liver biopsy.

Box 8-6 Adverse Reactions To Methotrexate In Doses Used To Treat Psoriasis

1. General fatigue: Headaches, chills and fever, dizziness
2. Skin: Pruritus, pain, urticaria, mild reversible alopecia, ecchymosis, acute ulcerations of psoriatic lesions, reactivation of phototoxic responses. Methotrexate, when given within a few days after UV irradiation, may reactivate an acute sunburn response.
3. Blood: Bone marrow depression, leukopenia leading to decreased resistance to infection, anemia, thrombocytopenia, bleeding, and megaloblastic anemia
4. Gastrointestinal system: Ulcerative stomatitis, nausea and anorexia; less frequently, hepatotoxicity, pharyngitis, diarrhea, vomiting, enteritis
5. Urogenital system: Azotemia, microscopic hematuria, cystitis, transient oligospermia, defective spermatogenesis, defective oogenesis, teratogenesis, menstrual dysfunction, nephropathy
6. Nervous system: Headaches, dizziness, drowsiness, blurred vision, acute depression

Box 8-7 Risk Factors for Liver Disease

- History of or current excessive alcohol consumption (methotrexate toxicity is associated with a history of total lifetime alcohol intake before methotrexate therapy. The exact amount of alcohol that confers risk is unknown and differs among persons.)
- Persistent abnormal liver chemistry studies
- History of liver disease including chronic hepatitis B or C
- Family history of inheritable liver disease
- Diabetes mellitus (probably of secondary importance)
- Obesity (probably of secondary importance)
- History of significant exposure to hepatotoxic drugs or chemicals (probably of secondary importance)

The presence of any of these factors to a significant degree would be important in considering an early treatment liver biopsy.

Leukocyte and platelet counts are depressed maximally approximately 7 to 10 days after treatment. A drop in these counts below normal levels necessitates reducing or stopping therapy. LFTs are obtained at 3- to 4-month intervals, but at least 1 week after the last dose of the drug. MTX causes transient elevations in LFTs for 1 to 3 days after its administration, so a false-positive elevation might be seen if the patient is tested too soon.

SIDE EFFECTS. Short-term side effects (Box 8-6) include nausea, anorexia, fatigue, oral ulcerations and stomatitis, mild leukopenia, thrombocytopenia, and macrocytic anemia. These are dose-related and rapidly reversible and related to renal and hematologic function. Switching among triple dosing, weekly oral dosing and intramuscular dosing may decrease these reactions.[89] Hepatic fibrosis or cirrhosis can develop with long-term treatment. Extensive alcohol intake, daily dosing, prior liver disease, and cumulative MTX intake predispose patients to fibrosis and cirrhosis. Male and female patients should discontinue MTX for 3 to 4 months before attempting conception.[90]

FOLIC AND FOLINIC ACID SUPPLEMENTS. Gastrointestinal symptoms and megaloblastic anemia can be controlled with folic acid, 1 to 5 mg daily.[91] The therapeutic result may be better if folic acid is not given on the day MTX is taken.[92] An increase in the erythrocyte mean corpuscular volume may be a useful indicator of folate deficiency and impending toxicity. Folinic acid administered on days when methotrexate is not given may also reduce side effects.

LIVER FIBROSIS, CIRRHOSIS, AND BIOPSY INTERVAL. Methotrexate is liver toxic and is avoided if possible in patients with liver disease or in those with risk factors for liver disease (Box 8-7). Active alcoholics must not take methotrexate. Patients who are obese or diabetic can have an increased risk of cirrhosis. Serum LFTs are not reliable indicators of liver disease. Patients receiving long-term methotrexate therapy should be followed up with liver biopsies.

LIVER BIOPSY. Guidelines for obtaining a liver biopsy are listed in Table 8-5.

Data suggest that at 1.5 gm of cumulative drug usage, cirrhosis can occur in approximately 3% of patients.[93] Cumulative doses of 4 gm or more have led to an incidence as high as 25%.[94] MTX-induced cirrhosis may be of a "low aggressive" type.

If the patient has normal liver chemistry values, a normal history, a normal physical examination, and no risk factors, a liver biopsy is recommended after a cumulative MTX dose of approximately 1.5 gm. If the first postmethotrexate liver biopsy shows no significant abnormalities, repeat liver biopsies are recommended at 1.0- to 1.5-gm intervals of further cumulative doses. Patients taking 15 mg of MTX each week reach the 1.5-gm cumulative dose in 25 months (Table 8-6).

Repeat biopsies are done approximately every 1 to 1.5 gm thereafter if liver function tests and biopsy findings are normal. Patients with a history of liver disease have the first liver biopsy after 2 to 4 months of therapy, when it is determined that methotrexate is tolerated and effective.

The management of abnormal liver biopsy findings is found in Box 8-8. Cirrhosis is more common in patients with psoriasis than patients with rheumatoid arthritis. Therefore rheumatologists do not require routine liver biopsies.

LUNG TOXICITY. Methotrexate-induced lung injury can be sudden and severe. The presenting symptom is usually a new onset of cough and shortness of breath. It is most often a subacute process, in which symptoms are commonly present for several weeks before diagnosis. Approximately 50% of the cases are diagnosed within 32 weeks from initiation of MTX treatment. A patient who recovers from MTX lung injury should not be re-treated. Earlier recognition and drug withdrawal may avoid the serious and sometimes fatal outcome.[95]

The strongest predictors of lung injury were older age, diabetes, rheumatoid pleuropulmonary involvement, previous use of disease-modifying antirheumatic drugs, and hypoalbuminemia.[96]

Table 8-5 Liver Biopsy: Patients With and Without Hepatic Risk Factors

	Cumulative methotrexate dose (gm)
Patients with hepatic risk factors (Liver disease, active alcoholism, diabetes, obesity)	
• First biopsy	0.12-0.24 (2-4 mo of therapy)
• Repeat biopsy	1.0-1.5
• Next repeat biopsy	3.0
• After repeat biopsy	4.0
Patients with no risk factors (normal liver function tests and no history of liver disease or alcoholism)	
• First biopsy	1.0-1.5
• Repeat biopsy	3.0
• Repeat biopsy	4.0

From Lebwohl M, Ali S: J Am Acad Dermatol 2001; 45(5):649-61.

Table 8-6 Duration of Methotrexate Treatment to Achieve a Cumulative Dose of 1.5 gm

Weekly dose (mg)	Months to 1.5 gm
7.5	50
15.0	25
22.5	17

Box 8-8 Classification of Liver Biopsy Findings and Management

Grade I: Normal; fatty infiltration, mild; nuclear variability, mild; portal inflammation, mild	Continue MTX
Grade II: Fatty infiltration, moderate to severe; nuclear variability, moderate to severe; portal tract expansion, portal tract inflammation, and necrosis moderate to severe	Continue MTX
Grade IIIA: Fibrosis, mild (portal fibrosis here denotes formation of fibrotic septa extending into the lobules; slight enlargement of portal tracts without disruption of limiting plates or septum formation does not classify the biopsy specimen as grade III	Continue MTX Repeat biopsy after approximately 6 months of MTX therapy Consider alternative Rx
Grade IIIB: Fibrosis, moderate to severe	Stop MTX Exceptional circumstances, however, may require continued methotrexate therapy, with thorough follow-up liver biopsies
Grade IV: Cirrhosis (regenerating nodules, as well as bridging of portal tracts, must be demonstrated)	Stop MTX Exceptional circumstances, however, may require continued methotrexate therapy, with thorough follow-up liver biopsies

Adapted from Roenigk H, et al: J Am Acad Dermatol 1998; 38(3):478.

RECALL OF SUNBURN. Patients taking methotrexate with a previous history of radiation burns or sunburns may experience a flare-up of symptoms in the areas that had been burned. This reaction is distinct from true photosensitivity.[97,98]

PREGNANCY. Methotrexate is teratogenic and not prescribed for pregnant women. The drug may temporarily affect fertility in males. There are reports of normal infants born to the partners of males who had been treated with methotrexate around the time of conception.[99] Although the risk to the fetus may be low, it has been suggested that methotrexate be discontinued several months before conception.

DRUG INTERACTIONS. Potentially interacting drugs are listed in Table 8-7. Drug interactions are most likely to be a problem in patients with low renal function. Neutropenia is a major problem; life-threatening bone marrow toxicity can occur. Blood counts should be monitored after changes in therapy, especially in patients with impaired renal function, such as the elderly.[100,101] Nonsteroidal anti-inflammatory drugs can reduce renal clearance of methotrexate, resulting in toxic levels. Methotrexate can increase serum levels of some agents (e.g., naproxen). Patients with psoriatic arthritis can be safely treated with ketoprofen, fluorobiprofen, and piroxicam. Avoid trimethoprim-sulfamethoxazole. It is commonly associated with severe methotrexate toxicity. It competes with methotrexate for renal tubular secretion. Plasma prothrombin times should be monitored for patients receiving warfarin anticoagulants.

Table 8-7 Drugs That May Interact With Methotrexate to Increase Toxicity	
Mechanism	**Drugs***
Decreased renal elimination of methotrexate	Nephrotoxins (e.g., aminoglycosides, cyclosporine)
	Salicylates
	Phenylbutazone
	Sulfonamides
	Probenecid
	Cephalothin
	Penicillins
	Colchicine
	Many nonsteroidal antiinflammatory drugs (e.g., naproxen, ibuprofen)
Additive or synergistic toxicity	Trimethoprim/sulfamethoxazole
	Ethanol
	Pyrimethamine
Displacement of methotrexate from protein binding	Probenecid
Salicylates	Barbiturates
	Phenytoin
	Retinoids
	Sulfonamides (absolute contraindication)
	Sulfonylureas
	Tetracycline
Intracellular accumulation of methotrexate	Dipyridamole
Hepatotoxicity	Retinoids
	Ethanol
For a more complete list, see Evans and Christensen: J Rheumatol 1985; 12(Suppl 12):15-20.	
From Lebwohl M, Ali S: J Am Acad Dermatol 2001; 45(5):649.	

Retinoids

ACITRETIN. Acitretin (Soriatane) is an oral retinoid and one of the safest systemic psoriasis therapies. A summary of the characteristics of acitretin are found in Box 8-9. As monotherapy, acitretin is most effective in treating pustular and erythrodermic psoriasis. Monotherapy is less effective for plaque psoriasis. Acitretin in combination with PUVA or UVB is more effective for plaque psoriasis than monotherapy. Efficacy and side effects vary among patients. Acitretin is started at a low dose (10 to 25 mg/day) and increased to find the proper balance between efficacy and tolerance of side effects.

Indications. Pustular and erythrodermic psoriasis are very responsive to acitretin. Plaque psoriasis is less responsive with monotherapy, higher more toxic doses are often required for control. Improvement is gradual, taking more than 3 months to reach optimum dose.

Dosing strategy. Therapeutic and toxic responses to acitretin vary greatly. Some patients are very retinoid-responsive. A single "correct" dose cannot be recommended. Dose escalation is the optimal strategy for establishing the dosage. Start with a low dose of acitretin (10 to 25 mg/day) and escalate as needed to enhance efficacy while minimizing side effects. Start with 25 mg/day for most patients. This regimen allows gradual onset of "tolerance" to side effects and avoids use of higher doses than needed.

Acitretin and ultraviolet light B and PUVA. Compared with either acitretin or UV light monotherapy alone, combination regimens enhance efficacy and limits treatment frequency, duration, and cumulative doses.[66,102] Lower doses of acitretin are usually effective when used in combination with phototherapy. Acitretin can often be used at the dose range of 10 to 25 mg daily. This results in faster and more complete responses to PUVA and to UVB. Significantly lower ultraviolet doses are required when retinoids are added to a phototherapy regimen. Review the guidelines for treatment in reference 103.

Laboratory changes. The monitoring schedule is listed in Box 8-10. Elevation of serum lipids, particularly triglycerides, can be prevented by concomitant administration of gemfibrozil (Lopid) or atorvastatin calcium (Lipitor). Elevation of liver function tests can occur.

Side effects. Acitretin is teratogenic. In the presence of ethanol, acitretin is esterified to etretinate.[104] Etretinate persists in tissue for years. Therefore acitretin is not prescribed to women of childbearing potential who may become pregnant within 3 years. In doses of 50 mg per day or higher, mucocutaneous side effects are common and include cheilitis, conjunctivitis, hair loss, failure to develop normal nail plates, dry skin, and "sticky skin." Periungual pyogenic granulomas can develop. Headache is a possible sign of pseudotumor cerebri. High dose for long-term treatment may produce calcification of ligaments and skeletal hyperostoses. These are often asymptomatic.[105]

Isotretinoin

Isotretinoin is highly effective for pustular psoriasis[83] and is beneficial when combined with PUVA[106] or UVB for plaque psoriasis.[107]

Box 8-9 Summary of Studies on Acitretin Therapy for Psoriasis

- Acitretin monotherapy is very effective for pustular and erythrodermic psoriasis. Combination regimens with UVB or PUVA are preferred for plaque psoriasis; in these cases, it is even more advantageous to start with lower doses of acitretin (10-25 mg/day).
- Optimal dose range for monotherapy is 25-50 mg/day.
- Improvement occurs gradually, requiring up to 3-6 months for peak response.
- Overall rate of complete remission is generally <50%.
- Higher doses (50-75 mg/day) result in more rapid, and possibly more complete, responses but are associated with significantly increased side effects.
- Mucocutaneous side effects, hepatotoxicity, and alterations in serum lipid profile are dose-dependent.
- Initial flare involving increased surface area of psoriatic lesions despite decreased erythema and scaling may occur, lasting 1-2 months after initiation of therapy.

Box 8-10 Retinoids: Baseline and Follow-up Monitoring

Baseline monitoring

- History and physical examination
- Pregnancy test
- Complete blood cell and platelet counts
- Liver function tests, blood urea nitrogen level, creatinine level
- Cholesterol, high-density lipoprotein, triglyceride levels
- Urinalysis

Follow-up monitoring

- History and monthly physical examination
- Liver function tests, cholesterol and triglyceride levels at 2 wk; then monthly for 4 to 6 mo; then every 3 mo
- Complete blood cell and platelet counts, blood urea nitrogen and creatinine levels, urinalysis monthly; then every 3 mo
- Pregnancy test monthly or as indicated

Adapted from Lebwohl M, Ali S: J Am Acad Dermatol 2001; 45(5):649.

Cyclosporine

Cyclosporine (CS) at dosages of 2.5 to 5.0 mg/kg/day administered to reliable, carefully selected patients who are closely monitored for both clinical and laboratory parameters produces fast and favorable results for severe plaque psoriasis. Cyclosporine is indicated for the treatment of severe, recalcitrant, plaque psoriasis in adults who are immunocompetent. Cyclosporine microemulsion (Neoral) is available in soft gelatin capsules (25 mg, 100 mg) and oral solution (50-mL bottle to 100 mg/mL). The cyclosporine consensus conference report provides the guidelines for using this medication.[108]

BASELINE MONITORING. The key to monitoring is to obtain accurate baseline values before therapy is started (Box 8-11).

Adverse events are summarized in Box 8-12.

KIDNEY FUNCTION AND CREATININE. Renal changes are functional and anatomic. They are caused by changes in renal blood flow patterns and cytotoxic effects on renal cells. Anatomic changes that include interstitial fibrosis, tubular atrophy, and arteriolopathy occur. They occur in nearly all patients treated for at least 1 year. More severe effects occur with increasing age, decreased renal function, and hypertension at baseline. Some loss in renal function occurs in many patients; it is usually mild and reversible.

Elevated creatinine levels usually occur in the first 16 weeks of treatment and stabilize after that. Biweekly visits are suggested for at least the first 12 weeks of therapy. If the serum creatinine level increases by more than 30% above the baseline, another determination is done within 2 weeks. If the second level confirms the increase, the dosage should be decreased by at least 1 mg/kg/d, and the level rechecked in 1 month. If the level decreases to less than 30% above the baseline, treatment can be continued. If the level remains greater than 30% above the baseline, therapy should be stopped and not resumed until the level returns to within 10% of the baseline. Routine measurements of glomerular filtration rate and creatinine clearance are not necessary. Routine kidney biopsies are not done.

HYPERTENSION. Hypertension develops in 8% to 30% of patients. Antihypertensive therapy can control the blood pressure elevation. The best response is achieved with calcium channel antagonists such as nifedipine, isradipine, or felodipine. Angiotensin-converting enzyme inhibitors are not as effective, and beta blockers may occasionally worsen psoriasis. Decreased renal function and hypertension are somewhat reversible with a decrease in dose or discontinuation of cyclosporine, but there is irreversible kidney damage in many patients. In a few patients hypertension remains after the discontinuation of cyclosporine. A decrease in dosage of 25% to 50% is recommended if hypertension develops.

LIVER FUNCTION. Serum bilirubin usually is increased. Isolated elevations of bilirubin should not cause alarm. Only in the presence of other consistent and significant abnormalities of liver function does the patient need referral for further evaluation. The safety of cyclosporine in patients with chronic active hepatitis is unknown.

OTHER CHEMISTRIES. Uric acid may increase and rarely requires anti-gout therapy. Serum magnesium may decline; if blood levels are below the normal range, replacement with magnesium tablets is indicated. Cholesterol and triglyceride levels may increase.

Box 8-11 Cyclosporine: Monitoring

Baseline monitoring

History, including medication history

Physical examination, including blood pressure

Serum creatinine (measured at least twice before therapy is started with the expectation that the repeated measures will be within 10% of each other)

Chemistry screening, including electrolytes, magnesium, blood urea nitrogen, lipids, liver function tests, uric acid

Complete blood cell count

Follow-up monitoring (at 2 weeks, 4 weeks, and monthly thereafter)

History including new medications

Physical examination including blood pressure

Chemistry screen including electrolytes, blood urea nitrogen, creatinine, magnesium, lipids, liver function tests, uric acid

From Lebwohl M, et al: J Am Acad Dermatol 1998; 39(3):464.

Box 8-12 Adverse Reactions

Renal dysfunction	Dizziness
Hypertension	Abdominal pain
Hirsutism	Diarrhea
Tremor	Dyspepsia
Gingival hyperplasia	Hyperkalemia
Musculoskeletal pain	Hypomagnesemia
Paresthesia	Hyperuricemia
Microangiopathic hemolytic anemia	Hypoglycemia
Thrombocytopenia	Bilirubinemia
Headache	Leukopenia
Leg cramps	Hyperlipidemia

From Lebwohl M, et al: J Am Acad Dermatol 1998; 39(3):464.

OTHER SIDE EFFECTS. Side effects occur in proportion to the dose. Malaise or fatigue, nausea, headaches, and general achiness may occur. Hand tremors, paresthesias, or sensitivity to hot and cold in the fingers and toes tend to occur at higher doses. These symptoms tend to resolve as therapy proceeds. Hypertrichosis may occur. Patients who develop gingival hyperplasia are sent to a dentist. Increased uric acid may precipitate gout. Elevations of triglycerides (>750 mg/dL) occur in 15% of patients; elevations of cholesterol levels (>300 mg/dL) occur in less than 3%. Most laboratory abnormalities are reversible when cyclosporine is stopped.

DOSAGE. The starting dose depends on the clinical state (Box 8-13). There are two approaches to determine the starting dosage. The speed of improvement and the success rate are proportional to the dosage.

Low-dose approach. Start at 2.5 mg/kg/d, and wait at least 1 month before considering increasing the dosage. This approach with slow increments in dosages is for patients with stable, generalized psoriasis or for patients in whom the severity lies between moderate and severe. Increase the dosage by 0.5- to 1.0-mg/kg/d increments every 2 weeks, up to a maximum of 5 mg/kg/d if needed. Higher doses are rarely necessary.

High-dose approach. Start at 5 mg/kg/d dose when rapid improvement is critical. Patients with severe, inflammatory flares, recalcitrant cases that have failed to respond to other modalities, or distressed patients in a crisis situation are candidates for the high dose approach. High doses are usually well tolerated for short-term use. As soon as there is a response, the dosage is decreased by 0.5 to 1 mg/kg/d, but no more than 1 step in the decrement of dosage per week, until the minimum effective maintenance dosage is defined.

Intermittent short courses. A new therapeutic strategy to manage moderate to severe plaque psoriasis with cyclosporine is the use of intermittent short courses of treatment.[109] It is effective, well tolerated and reduces the risk of side effects. Cyclosporine is initially given at a dose of 2.5 mg/kg per day in two divided doses. This dosage could be increased by increments of 0.5 to 1.0 mg/kg per day each week up to a maximum of 5 mg/kg per day. Treatment is continued until clearance of psoriasis, defined as 90% or more reduction in the area affected, or for a maximum of 12 weeks. Cyclosporine is stopped abruptly. On relapse, patients are given another course of cyclosporine, commencing at the optimal dose from the previous treatment period. Intermittent short courses for up to 2 years appear safe and well tolerated.

RESPONSE TO TREATMENT. Clearance is usually maintained as long as the clearing dose is held constant. Relapse may occur during attempts to adjust to a maintenance dose.

CONTRAINDICATIONS. Contraindications are listed in Table 8-8.

Vaccination with live vaccines should be avoided; other vaccinations may be less effective during cyclosporine treatment. Patients with prostate or cervical cancer that has been completely removed may take cyclosporine.

DRUG INTERACTIONS. Patients taking drugs that are also metabolized by the cytochrome P-450 complex must be cautioned that the concurrent use of cyclosporine may raise or lower blood levels of the interacting drug (Table 8-9).

COMBINATION THERAPY. Topical agents (superpotent corticosteroids, tazarotene, calcipotriene) can be used to treat resistant plaques. Topical medication can also be used to maintain clearing. Common programs of treatment include the morning application of a superpotent corticosteroid and an evening application of either tazarotene or calcipotriene to each new erupting lesion. Other agents that can be considered to keep the acute and/or the cumulative dose of cyclosporine as low as possible are listed in Box 8-14. There is not much experience with these combination therapies. The combination of PUVA or UVB and cyclosporine is rarely used because of the concern about the higher incidence of skin cancer in immunosuppressed patients. The use of cyclosporine with acitretin is well-tolerated. Switching from cyclosporine to acitretin may be a useful way of withdrawing cyclosporine treatment.

Box 8-13 Cyclosporine/Neoral Dosage
Capsules (25 mg, 100 mg)
Oral solution (50 mL bottle-100 mg/mL)
Starting dose: 2.5-5 mg/kg/d in 1 or 2 divided doses
Adjust by 0.5-1 mg/kg/d each week as needed

Table 8-8 Contraindications

Absolute contraindications	Relative contraindications
Renal disease	Internal malignancy
Poorly controlled hypertension	Immunodeficiency
Severe infections	Noncompliant patient
	Concomitant nephrotoxic drugs
	Interacting drugs
	Gout
	Liver disease
	Pregnancy

From Lebwohl M, et al:, J Am Acad Dermatol 1998; 39(3):464.

Table 8-9 Drugs That May Affect Serum Cyclosporine Levels

Drugs that may potentiate renal dysfunction	Drugs that increase cyclosporine concentrations	Drugs that decrease cyclosporine concentrations
Antibiotics	Calcium channel blockers	Antibiotics
Gentamicin	Diltiazem	Nafcillin
Tobramycin	Nicardipine	Rifampin
Vancomycin	Verapamil	Anticonvulsants
Trimethoprim-sulfamethoxazole	Antifungals	Carbamazepine
Antineoplastics	Fluconazole	Phenobarbital
Melphalan	Itraconazole	Phenytoin
Antiinflammatory drugs	Ketoconazole	Other drugs
Diclofenac	Antibiotics	Octreotide
Antifungals	Clarithromycin	Ticlopidine
Amphotericin B	Erythromycin	
Ketoconazole	Glucocorticoids	
Gastrointestinal agents	Methylprednisolone	
Cimetidine	Other drugs	
Ranitidine	Allopurinol	
Immunosuppressives	Bromocriptine	
Tacrolimus	Danazol	
	Metoclopramide	

The metabolism of cyclosporine may be decreased in patients with severe liver disease.

From Lebwohl M, Ellis C, Gottlieb A, et al: J Am Acad Dermatol 1998; 39(3):464.

Rotational therapy

Rotational therapy is a standard approach to limit side effects associated with long-term use of single agents. This involves rotating between UVB, PUVA, methotrexate, retinoids, biologic agents, and cyclosporine at intervals of approximately 1 to 2 years. The use of cyclosporine immediately before or, especially after, PUVA should be avoided because of the possible synergistic effects in the production of skin cancers.[110]

Box 8-14 Possible Combination Therapies for Psoriasis

Cyclosporine plus topical agents

Corticosteroids

Anthralin

Calcipotriene

Tazarotene

Cyclosporine plus systemic drugs

Acitretin

Methotrexate

Hydroxyurea

Thioguanine

Sulfasalazine

Mycophenolic acid

Adapted from Lebwohl M, et al: J Am Acad Dermatol 1998; 39(3): 464.

Biologic therapy for psoriasis

Psoriasis is driven by activated memory T cells. Many biologic agents are being studied or are available to selectively target the immune system. Biologic agents are proteins that can be synthesized using recombinant DNA techniques (genetic engineering).[111] Recently, immune-mediated diseases including Crohn's disease and rheumatoid arthritis have been treated with biologic agents to inhibit immunity. Biologic agents bind to specific cells and do not have multiorgan adverse effects as seen with acitretin, cyclosporine, and methotrexate. The potential for interaction with other drugs is very low. The risk of immunosuppression is unlikely to be worse than other commonly used dermatological drugs.

Alefacept (Amevive)

Alefacept is a fusion protein that binds to T cells expressing CD2. These cells are important in the propagation of psoriasis. Alefacept reduces the number of these cells in the circulation. Patients remain in remission for weeks or months after treatment. Alefacept is given by IM injection or IV bolus weekly for 12 weeks.

Table 8-10 Other Systemic Agents for Psoriasis

	Tacrolimus	Mycophenolate Mofetil
Characteristics	Very effective for psoriasis Immunosuppressive agent Prevention of organ transplant rejection Inhibits T-cell activation	Immunosuppressive agent Prevention of organ transplant rejection Can be administered with cyclosporine[114] Not as effective as cyclosporine[115] Effective for psoriatic arthritis[116]
Baseline monitoring	• H&P • Blood pressure • Creatinine and blood urea nitrogen levels every 2 wk • Chemistry screen, including glucose and electrolytes • CBC and platelet counts • HIV testing, if at risk	• H&P • CBC • Chemistry screen • Urinalysis • Pregnancy test
Follow-up monitoring	Every 2 to 4 wk, then monthly: • H&P, blood pressure • Creatinine and blood urea nitrogen levels • Complete blood cell count and chemistry screen	• H&P monthly • CBC at weeks 1, 2, 3, 4, 6, 8, and then monthly
Dosage	• Initial dosage: 0.05 mg/kg daily Depending on response: • Can be increased to 0.10 mg/kg daily at 3 wk • Can be increased to 0.15 mg/kg daily at 6 wk	• 500 mg po 4 times/d for 12 wk based on clinical response • Can be increased or reduced by 250 mg/d each month up to a maximum of 4 g/d • Available in 250-mg capsules and 500-mg tablets
Adverse effects	Diarrhea, paresthesias, and insomnia Risks like cyclosporine; hypertension, nephrotoxicity, immunosuppression No hypertrichosis or gingival hyperplasia	Leukopenia at high doses Gastrointestinal side effects can be minimized by lowering the dose or by dividing the dose so that it is administered 4 times daily Herpes zoster 11% Opportunistic infections 1% to 2% incidence of lymphoproliferative disease Other noncutaneous malignancies 5.5%

Adapted from Lebwohl M, et al: J Am Acad Dermatol 1998; 39(3):464.

H&P, History and physical examination; *CBC*, complete blood cell count; *LFT*, liver function tests.

Etanercept (Embrel) and infliximab (Remicade)

These anti-TNF agents bind and inhibit the activity of TNF. Etanercept is given twice a week as a subcutaneous injection. Infliximab is given as an intravenous infusion at intervals dependent on the state of the disease. They are both effective for psoriasis.

Other systemic drugs for psoriasis

Several other drugs have been used to treat patients who experience toxicity or fail to respond to retinoids, methotrexate, or cyclosporine. Experience with all of these medications is limited (Table 8-10).

Hydroxyurea	6-Thioguanine[112]	Sulfasalazine[113]
Antimetabolite Used for psoriasis for 3 decades Can be effective as monotherapy	Purine analog Highly effective for psoriasis (see ref. 117) Determine thiopurine methyltransferase levels to predict predisposition for myelosuppression	Somewhat effective for psoriasis Limited experience
• H&P • CBC and platelet counts, weekly for 4 wk; then every 2 to 4 wk for at least 12 wk • Chemistry screen; repeat LFT every 3 mo	• H&P • CBC and platelet counts • Chemistry screen	• H&P • CBC and platelet counts • Chemistry screen • Urinalysis
• H&P, monthly • CBC and platelet counts, weekly for 4 wk; then every 2 to 4 wk for at least 12 wk • Repeat LFT every 3 mo	• Repeat baseline tests weekly during dose escalation; then every 2 wk • Hold if white blood cell count is $<4.0 \times 10^9$/L, platelet count is $<125 \times 10^9$/L, or hemoglobin is <110 g/L	• Repeat every 2 wk for 3 mo; during the next 3 mo repeat labs, monthly then every 3 mo or as clinically indicated
• 1 g po daily • Can be increased by 500-mg daily increments each month; doses up to 2.0 g/d have been used. After dose increases, repeat CBC and platelet counts weekly. Hold dosage if white blood cell count is $<2.5 \times 10^9$/L, platelet count is $<100 \times 10^9$/L, or severe anemia occurs • Available in 500-mg capsules	Daily dosing and pulse dosing used, from 20 mg two times a week to 120 mg daily.[117] • Starting dose: 80 mg po twice weekly • Increase by 20 mg every 2-4 wk • Maximum dose 160 mg po 3 times weekly	• Starting dose: 500 mg po 3 times/d • If tolerated, after 3 d, increase dose to 1 g po 3 times/d • If tolerated after 6 wk, increase dose to 1 g po 4 times/d • Efficacy, or lack thereof, should be apparent by 4 to 6 wk
Nearly 50% develop bone marrow toxicity with leukopenia or thrombocytopenia; megaloblastic anemia is common but rarely requires treatment Leg ulcers are the most troublesome	Bone marrow suppression Nausea Diarrhea Elevated LFT	High incidence of headache, gastrointestinal symptoms, rash

Pityriasis Rubra Pilaris

Pityriasis rubra pilaris (PRP) is a rare, chronic disease of unknown etiology with a unique combination of features. PRP often has a devastating impact on the lives of patients. Descriptions of its histopathologic features are not uniform.[118] Finding a successful therapy can be challenging. PRP may occur at any age, but most cases occur in the first and fifth or sixth decades of life. PRP has been divided into adult and childhood forms. Griffiths subclassified the disease into five groups, separating adult disease into classic and atypical types and the juvenile form into classic, circumscribed, and atypical types.[119] Classic adult PRP (type I) and juvenile PRP are the most common.

A severe form of PRP may be unmasked, precipitated, or otherwise associated with HIV infection.[120,121]

Clinical manifestations

Classic adult PRP begins insidiously, usually in the fifth or sixth decade, with a small, indolent, red scaling plaque on the face or upper body. The plaque slowly enlarges over days and weeks, the palms and soles begin to thicken, and bright red-orange follicular papules appear on the dorsal aspects of the proximal phalanges, elbows, knees, and trunk as the disease evolves and progresses into a grotesque generalized eruption (Figures 8-26, 8-27, and 8-28). The follicular keratotic papules coalesce on many areas of the trunk to produce a complex pattern of discrete papules and sharply bordered, red plaques with islands of normal skin ("skip spots") (Figures 8-26 and 8-27). The eruption may spread to involve almost the entire cutaneous surface. Scaling is coarse on the lower half of the body and fine and powdery on the upper half. Ectropion is present with extensive facial involvement. The nails show

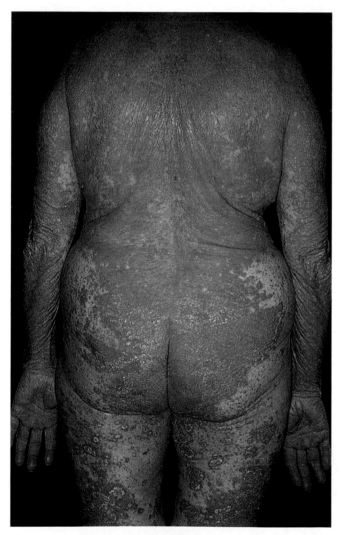

Figure 8-26 Pityriasis rubra pilaris. Red-orange scaling plaques with sharp borders have expanded to involve the entire body. The areas of uninvolved skin or islands of sparing "skip spots" are characteristic.

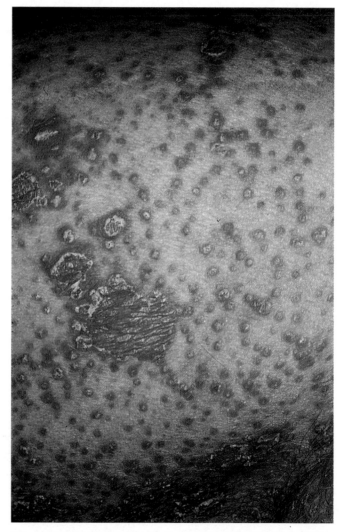

Figure 8-27 Pityriasis rubra pilaris, the classic presentation. Bright red follicular papules merge to form large, bright red-orange plaques.

distal yellow-brown discoloration, subungual hyperkeratosis, nail thickening, and splinter hemorrhages. Psoriatic nails show onycholysis (particularly marginal), oil spots, small pits, and larger indentations of the nail plate.[122]

There is little or no itching. The patient is impaired by the thick, tight scales of the scalp, face, and palms and the painful fissures that develop on the soles. The diffuse, red, tight-scaling face destroys the self-image, and these patients remain isolated. The eruption lasts for months and years; 80% are clear within 3 years.

CHILDHOOD PITYRIASIS RUBRA PILARIS. Childhood PRP begins on the scalp and face and simulates seborrheic dermatitis. The disease becomes more widespread and follicular keratotic papules develop. The childhood form tends to recur for years, which is not characteristic of the adult form. The circumscribed form is characterized by red-orange plaques, usually on the elbows and knees, consisting of sharply demarcated areas of follicular hyperkeratosis and erythema. The 3-year remission rate is 32%.[123]

Diagnosis

The distinctive clinical picture is the most valuable diagnostic feature. The disease looks like psoriasis when localized to the scalp, elbows, and knees. The biopsy shows thick scale and dense, keratotic, follicular plugs an increased granular cell layer, and acantholysis. Many other features are reported.[118]

Treatment

Frequent use of lubricants such as Lac-Hydrin (12% lactic acid) and Eucerin, Aquaphor, or Vaseline keeps the skin supple. Vanamide (40% urea cream) applied to the feet and covered with a plastic bag at bedtime is an effective approach for removing scale. Application of heavy moisturizers, such as equal parts Aquaphor and Unibase, followed by occlusion with a plastic suit for several hours also makes the skin supple. Dovonex (Calcipotriene) may be effective.

RETINOIDS. Retinoids are effective systemic agents.[124] Isotretinoin provides symptomatic improvement of erythema, pruritus, scaling, ectropion, and keratoderma in 4 weeks, while significant improvement or clearing takes 16 to 24 weeks. Remission or maintained improvement persists after stopping therapy in many patients. Dosages in the range of 0.5 to 2.0 mg/kg/day are used for up to 6 months.[125] Acitretin with or without light therapy may be superior to isotretinoin in the treatment of adult-onset disease.[126,127]

Initial oral retinoids plus concurrent or later low-dose weekly methotrexate resulted in 25% to 75% improvement of PRP in 17 of 24 patients after 16 weeks of therapy.[128]

Megadose vitamin A (1 million IU/day) given for 5 to 14 days clears the skin in days in some reports but has been less effective in others.[129,130]

METHOTREXATE. Daily methotrexate (2.5 mg/day) is more effective than the standard weekly regimen used for psoriasis and may be more effective than retinoids. Improvement may be noted in the second or third week, and there may be marked improvement in 10 to 12 weeks, at which time the dose can be tapered.

Cyclosporine should be considered in the treatment of classical adult-type PRP.[131]

Penicillin, stanozolol,[132] and the Goeckerman regimen (UVB and crude coal tar) are probably not effective. Patients with PRP are photosensitive and the majority flare with either psoralens and ultraviolet A (PUVA) or ultraviolet B therapy.

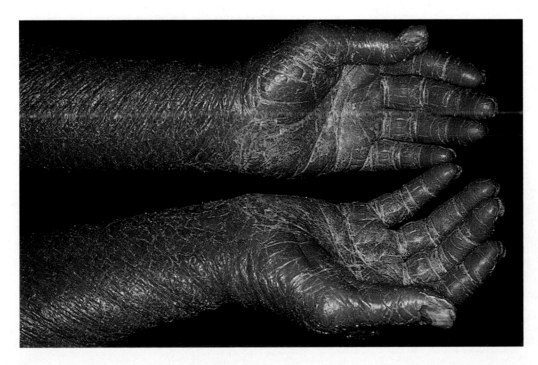

Figure 8-28 Pityriasis rubra pilaris. The entire surface of the palms and soles becomes thick (hyperkeratotic) and yellow.

Seborrheic Dermatitis

Seborrheic dermatitis is a common, chronic, inflammatory disease with a characteristic pattern for different age groups. The yeast *Pityrosporum ovale* probably is a causative factor, but both genetic and environmental factors seem to influence the onset and course of the disease. Many adult patients have an oily complexion, the so-called seborrheic diathesis. In adults, seborrheic dermatitis tends to persist, but it does undergo periods of remission and exacerbation. The extent of involvement among patients varies widely. Most cases can be adequately controlled.

Infants (cradle cap)

Infants commonly develop a greasy adherent scale on the vertex of the scalp. Minor amounts of scale are easily removed by frequent shampooing with products containing sulfur, salicylic acid, or both (e.g., Sebulex shampoo, T-Gel shampoo). Scale may accumulate and become thick and adherent over much of the scalp and may be accompanied by inflammation (Figure 8-29). Secondary infection can occur.

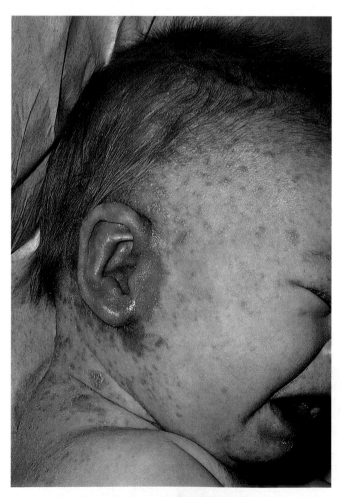

Figure 8-29 Seborrheic dermatitis (cradle cap). Diffuse inflammation with secondary infection. Much of the scale from this child's scalp was removed with shampoos.

TREATMENT. Patients with serum and crust are treated with oral antistaphylococcal antibiotics. Once infection is controlled, erythema and scaling can be suppressed with group VI or VII topical steroid creams or lotions. Dense, thick, adherent scale is removed by applying warm mineral oil, olive oil, or Derma-Smoothe FS lotion (peanut oil, mineral oil, fluocinolone acetonide 0.01%) to the scalp and washing several hours later with detergents such as Dawn dishwashing liquid. Remissions possibly can be prolonged with frequent use of salicylic acid or tar shampoos (see the Formulary, p. 945). Carmol scalp solution (sulfacetamide) may also be effective. It is applied once or twice each day.

Young children (tinea amiantacea and blepharitis)

Tinea amiantacea is a characteristic eruption of unknown etiology. Mothers of afflicted children often recall the child experiencing episodes of cradle cap during infancy. Some authors believe that tinea amiantacea is a form of eczema or psoriasis. One patch or several patches of dense scale appear anywhere on the scalp and may persist for months before the parent notices temporary hair loss or the distinctive large, oval, yellow-white plates of scale firmly adhered to the scalp and hair (Figure 8-30). Characteristically, the scale binds to the hair and is drawn up with the growing hair. Patches of dense scale range from 2 to 10 cm. The scale suggests fungal scalp disease, which explains the designation tinea. Amiantacea, meaning asbestos, refers to the plate-like quality of the scale, which resembles genuine asbestos.

TREATMENT. Warm 10% liquor carbonis detergens (LCD) in Nivea oil (prescription is for 8 oz; it must be prepared by the pharmacist) is applied to the scalp at bedtime and removed by shampooing each morning with Dawn dishwashing liquid. Derma-Smoothe FS lotion (peanut oil, mineral oil, fluocinolone acetonide 0.01%) is an effective topical steroid that can be applied to the entire scalp and occluded with a shower cap. The scalp is dampened before application. Treatments are repeated each night for 1 to 3 weeks until itching and erythema is controlled. The scale is completely removed in 1 to 3 weeks, and tar shampoos such as T-gel or Tarsum are used for maintenance. Periodic recurrences are similarly treated.

White scale adherent to the eyelashes and lid margins with variable amounts of erythema is characteristic of seborrheic blepharitis (Figure 8-31). The disease produces some discomfort and is unbecoming. The disease persists for years and is resistant to treatment. Scale may be suppressed by frequent washing with zinc- or tar-containing antidandruff shampoos (see the Formulary, p. 945). Although topical steroid creams and lotions suppress this disease, prolonged use of such preparations around the eyes may cause glaucoma and must be avoided. Ketoconazole (Nizoral cream) applied once a day is worth a trial in resistant cases.

SEBORRHEIC DERMATITS

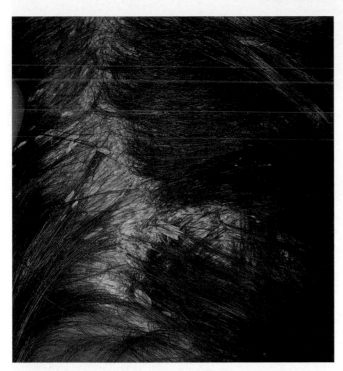

Figure 8-30 Seborrheic dermatitis (tinea amiantacea). The scalp contains dense patches of scale. Large plates of yellow-white scale firmly adhere to the hair shafts.

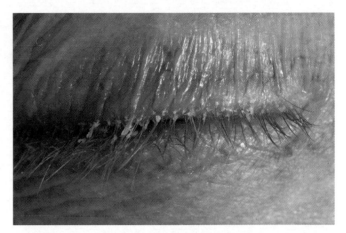

Figure 8-31 Seborrheic dermatitis (blepharitis). Scale accumulates and adheres to the lashes. A few drops of baby shampoo mixed in a cap of warm water can be used as a cleanser. Sulfacetamide ointments may control inflammation and scale.

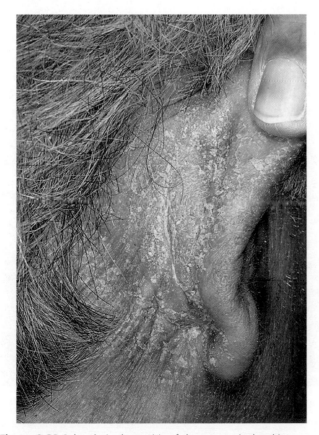

Figure 8-32 Seborrheic dermatitis of the postauricular skin.

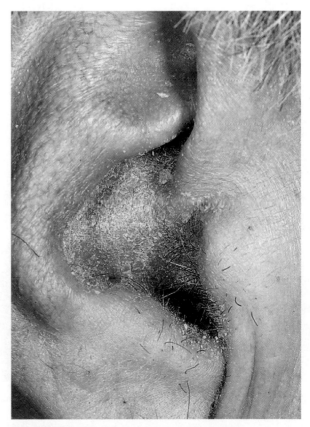

Figure 8-33 Seborrheic dermatitis of the ear canal.

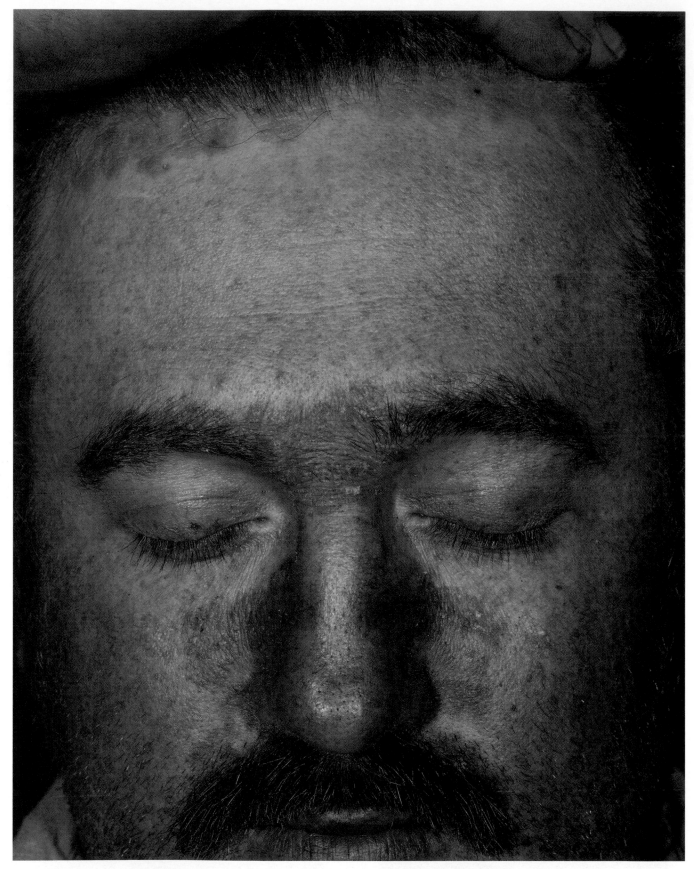

Figure 8-34 Seborrheic dermatitis in an adult with extensive involvement in all of the characteristic sites.

Adolescents and adults (classic seborrheic dermatitis)

Most individuals periodically experience fine, dry, white scalp scaling with minor itching; this is dandruff. They tend to attribute this condition to a dry scalp and consequently avoid hair washing. Avoidance of washing allows scale to accumulate and inflammation may occur. Patients with minor amounts of dandruff should be encouraged to wash every day or every other day with antidandruff shampoos (see the Formulary, p. 945). Fine, dry, white or yellow scale may occur on an inflamed base. The distribution of scaling and inflammation may be more diffuse and occur in the seborrheic areas: scalp and scalp margins, eyebrows, base of eyelashes, nasolabial folds, external ear canals (Figures 8-32 and 8-33), posterior auricular fold, and presternal area (Figure 8-34).

The axillae, inframammary folds, groin, and umbilicus are affected less frequently. Scaling of the ears may be misjudged as eczema or fungus infection. Its presence in association with characteristic scaling in other typical areas assists in supporting the diagnosis. Scaling may appear when a beard is grown and disappear when it is shaved (Figure 8-35). Once established, the disease tends to persist to a variable degree. Older patients, particularly those who are bedridden or those with neurologic problems such as Parkinson's disease, tend to have a more chronic and extensive form of the disease. Occasionally the scalp scale may be diffuse, thick, and adherent. Differentiation from psoriasis may be impossible.

Patients should be reassured that seborrheic dermatitis does not cause permanent hair loss. Tinea capitis caused by *Trichophyton tonsurans* has a dry, white, diffuse scale in the adult that does not fluoresce under Wood's light. Fungal culture and potassium hydroxide examination are indicated for atypical or resistant cases of scalp scaling.

Acquired immunodeficiency syndrome

Seborrheic dermatitis is one of the most common cutaneous manifestations of AIDS. The onset usually occurs before the development of AIDS symptoms. The severity of the seborrheic dermatitis correlates with the degree of clinical deterioration.

Treatment of seborrheic dermatitis

SHAMPOOS. Treatment consists of frequent washing of all affected areas, including the face and chest, with an antiseborrheic shampoo. Zinc soaps (Head & Shoulders shampoo, ZNP bar soap), selenium lotions (Head & Shoulders Intensive Care, Selsun), Tar (Tarsum, T-Gel) or Sal acid (T-Sal) suppresses activity and maintains remission.

TOPICAL STEROIDS. Remaining inflamed areas respond quickly to group V through VII topical steroid creams. Steroid lotions may be applied to the scalp twice daily. Patients must be cautioned that topical steroids should not be used as maintenance therapy.

ANTIYEAST MEDICATIONS. Ketoconazole (Nizoral cream) or ciclopirox olamine (Loprox cream or gel) applied once or twice a day is effective against even the most difficult and diffuse cases.[133] Patients with widespread disease involving the face, ears, chest, and upper back can now be treated effectively by using Nizoral or Loprox to clear the scale and erythema. Curiously, minor seborrheic dermatitis of the face may not respond as well and may require the addition of group V through VII topical steroids for control.

Dense, diffuse scalp scaling is treated with Derma-Smoothe FS lotion (peanut oil, mineral oil, fluocinolone acetonide 0.01%) or 10% LCD in Nivea oil as previously described for treating young children. Adults may apply oil preparations at bedtime and cover with a shower cap. Treatment is repeated each night until the scalp is clear, in approximately 1 to 3 weeks. Shampoo is then used for maintenance.

OTHER TOPICALS. Sulfacetamide (Carmol Scalp Treatment Lotion) applied once or twice each day can be very effective for active disease, especially if pustules are present. One percent metronidazole gel (Noritate) may be effective. Significant improvement occurred in 2 weeks. There was marked improvement or complete clearance at 8 weeks.[134] Anecdotal reports claim that tacrolimus ointment (Protopic) and Elidel cream (pimecrolimus) are effective.

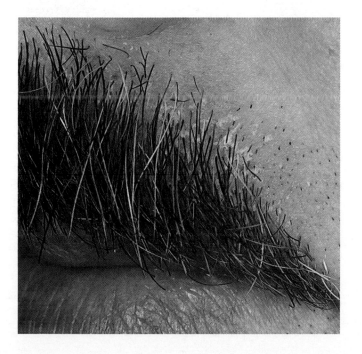

Figure 8-35 Seborrheic dermatitis. Redness and scaling can appear when a mustache or beard is grown. The scaling spontaneously clears when the hair is cut.

Pityriasis Rosea

Pityriasis rosea is a common, benign, usually asymptomatic, distinctive, self-limiting skin eruption of unknown etiology.[135] There is some evidence that it is viral in origin. Small epidemics have occurred in fraternity houses and military bases. The incidence in men and women varies in different studies. More than 75% of patients are between the ages of 10 and 35 years, with a mean age of 23 years and an age range of 4 months to 78 years. Two percent of patients have a recurrence.[136,137] The incidence of disease is higher during the colder months. Twenty percent of patients have a recent history of acute infection with fatigue, headache, sore throat, lymphadenitis, and fever; the disease may be more common in atopic patients. Upper respiratory tract infection before the appearance of skin lesions was reported in 68.8%.[138]

Differential diagnosis

Pityriasis rosea has several unique features, but variant patterns do exist; these may create confusion between pityriasis rosea and secondary syphilis, guttate psoriasis, viral exanthems, tinea, nummular eczema, and drug eruptions.

Clinical manifestations

Typically, a single 2- to 10-cm round-to-oval lesion, the herald patch, abruptly appears in 17% of patients. It may occur anywhere, but is most frequently located on the trunk or proximal extremities. The herald patch retains the same features as the subsequent oval lesions. At this stage, many patients are convinced that they have ringworm.

Within a few days to several weeks (average, 7 to 14 days) the disease enters the eruptive phase. Smaller lesions appear and reach their maximum number in 1 to 2 weeks (Figure 8-36). They are typically limited to the trunk and proximal extremities, but in extensive cases they develop on the arms, legs, and face (Figure 8-37). An inverse distribution involving mainly the extremities is seen in 6% of cases.[139] Lesions are typically benign and are concentrated in the lower abdominal area (Figure 8-38). Individual lesions are salmon pink in whites and hyperpigmented in blacks. Many of the earliest lesions are papular, but in most cases the typical 1- to 2-cm oval plaques appear (Figure 8-39). A fine, wrinkled, tissue-like scale remains attached within the border of the plaque giving the characteristic ring of scale, called collarette scale (Figure 8-40). The long axis of the oval plaques is oriented along skin lines. Numerous lesions on the back, oriented along skin lines, give the appearance of drooping pine-tree branches, which explains the designation "Christmas-tree distribution." The number of lesions varies from a few to hundreds.

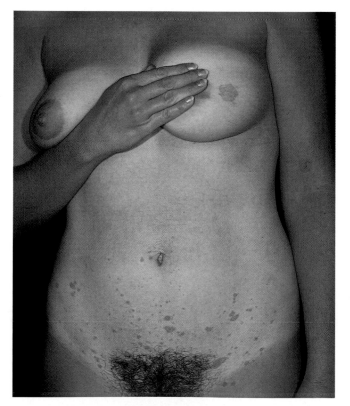

Figure 8-36 Pityriasis rosea. A herald patch is present on the breast. Subsequent lesions commonly begin in the lower abdominal region.

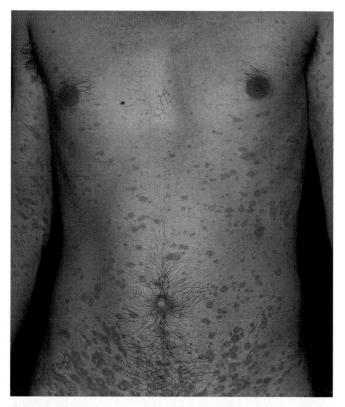

Figure 8-37 Pityriasis rosea. The fully evolved eruption 2 weeks after onset.

PITYRIASIS ROSEA

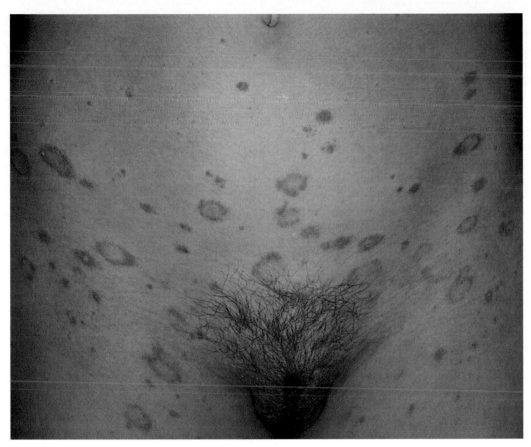

Figure 8-38 Lesions are typically concentrated in the lower abdominal area.

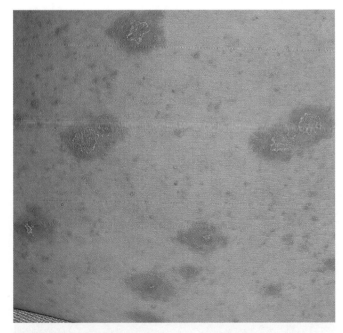

Figure 8-39 Both small, oval plaques and multiple, small papules are present. Occasionally the eruption consists only of small papules.

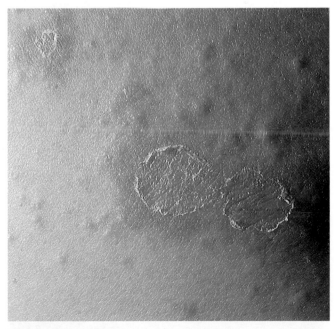

Figure 8-40 A ring of tissuelike scale (collarette scale) remains attached within the border of the plaque.

In some cases, other types of lesions predominate. The papular variety is more common in young children, pregnant women, and blacks (Figures 8-41 and 8-42). Vesicular and, rarely, purpuric lesions are seen in infants and children.[142] Eczematized lesions were noted in 5.4% of cases.[139] In rare instances the lesions seem to cover the entire skin surface (Figure 8-43). A variety of oral lesions have been reported.[140,141]

Most lesions are asymptomatic, but many patients complain of mild transient itching. Severe itching may accompany extensive inflammatory eruptions. The disease clears spontaneously in 1 to 3 months. There may be postinflammatory hyperpigmentation, especially in blacks.

Diagnosis

The experienced observer can rely on a clinical impression to make the diagnosis. Tinea can be ruled out with a potassium hydroxide examination. Secondary syphilis may be indistinguishable from pityriasis rosea, especially if the herald patch is absent. A serologic test for syphilis should be ordered if a clinical diagnosis cannot be made.[143] A biopsy is useful in atypical cases; it reveals extravasated erythrocytes within dermal papillae and dyskeratotic cells within the dermis. Pityriasis rosea may also be mimicked by psoriasis and nummular eczema.

Management

Whether or not PR is contagious is unknown. The disease is benign and self-limited and does not appear to affect the fetus; therefore isolation is unnecessary. Oral erythromycin stearate daily (1 gm in four equally divided doses for 2 weeks in adults and 25 to 40 mg/kg in four divided doses in children) was used in a study to treat PR. In this study 33 patients achieved complete response in 2 weeks, four patients showed complete disappearance of lesions by the end of 6 weeks, and 8 patients did not respond.[138] Group V topical steroids and oral antihistamines may be used as needed for itching. The rare extensive case with intense itching responds to a 1- to 2-week course of prednisone (20 mg twice a day). Direct sun exposure hastens the resolution of individual lesions, whereas those in protected areas, such as under bathing suits, remain (see Figure 8-36). Ultraviolet light B (UVB), administered in five consecutive daily erythemogenic exposures, results in decreased pruritus and hastens the involution of lesions. Therapy is most beneficial within the first week of the eruption.[144] UVB phototherapy five times per week for 2 weeks resulted in decreased severity of disease during the treatment period. However, the itching and the course of the disease were unchanged.[145]

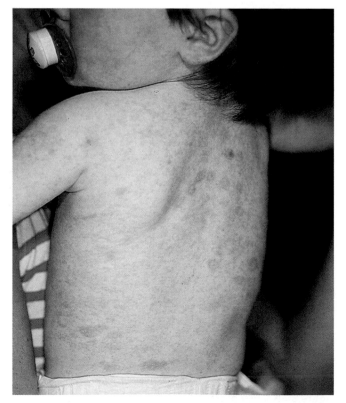

Figure 8-41 Pityriasis rosea. Papular lesions are seen in children, pregnant women, and blacks.

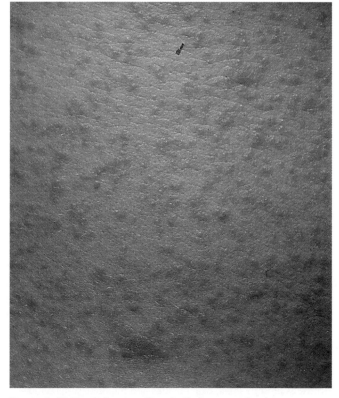

Figure 8-42 Pityriasis rosea. Papular lesions may be the predominant lesion in children.

PITYRIASIS ROSEA

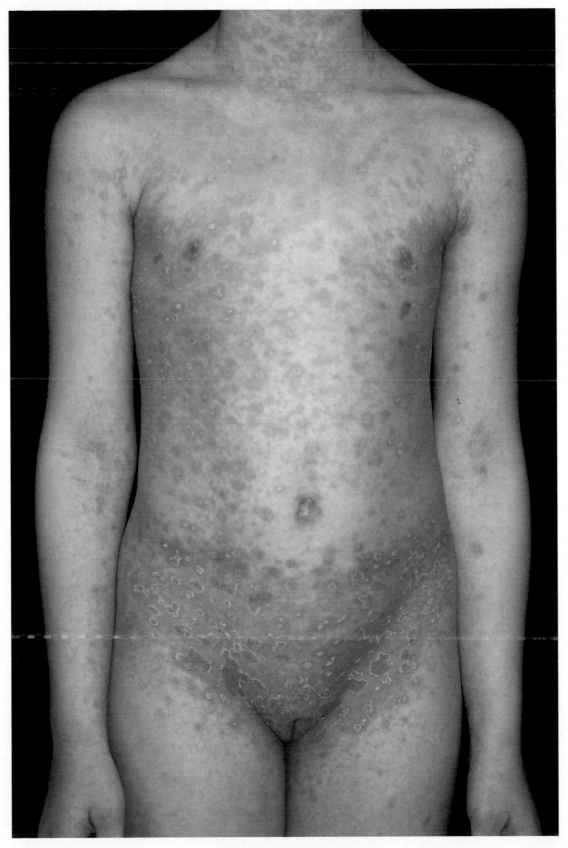

Figure 8-43 A rare generalized eruption.

Lichen Planus

Lichen planus (LP) is a unique inflammatory cutaneous and mucous membrane reaction pattern of unknown etiology. The mean age of onset is 40.3 years in males compared with 46.4 years in females. The main eruption clears within 1 year in 68% of patients, but 49% recur.[146] Although the disease may occur at any age, it is rare in children younger than 5 years. Approximately 10% of patients have a positive family history. This supports the hypothesis that genetic factors are of etiologic importance.[147] Liver disease is a risk factor for LP although not a specific marker of it. LP may be associated with hepatitis C virus–related, chronic, active hepatitis. The virus may play a potential pathogenic role by replicating in cutaneous tissue and triggering lichen planus in genetically susceptible HCV-infected patients.

There are several clinical forms, and the number of lesions varies from a few chronic papules to acute generalized disease (Table 8-11).

Eruptions from drugs (e.g., gold, chloroquine, methyldopa, penicillamine), chemical exposure (film processing), bacterial infections (secondary syphilis), and post–bone marrow transplants (graft-versus-host reaction) that have a similar appearance are referred to as lichenoid.

Primary lesions

The morphology and distribution of the lesions are characteristic (Figure 8-44). The clinical features of lichen planus can be remembered by learning the five Ps of lichen planus: pruritic, planar (flat-topped), polyangular, purple papules. The primary lesion is a 2- to 10-mm flat-topped papule with an irregular angulated border (polygonal papules). Close inspection of the surface shows a lacy, reticular pattern of crisscrossed, whitish lines (Wickham's striae) that can be accentuated by a drop of immersion oil (Figures 8-45 and 8-46). Histologically, Wickham's striae are areas of focal epidermal thickening.

Table 8-11 Various Patterns of Lichen Planus

Various patterns of lichen planus	Most common site
Actinic	Sun-exposed areas
Annular	Trunk, external genitalia
Atrophic	Any area
Erosioulcerative	Soles of feet, mouth
Follicular (lichen plano pilaris)	Scalp
Guttate (numerous) small papules	Trunk
Hypertrophic	Lower limbs (especially ankles)
Linear	Zosteriform (leg), scratched area
Nail disease	Fingernails
Papular (localized)	Flexor surface (wrists and forearms)
Vesiculobullous	Lower limbs, mouth

Newly evolving lesions are pink-white, but over time they assume a distinctive violaceous, or purple, hue with a peculiar waxy luster. Lesions that persist for months may become thicker and dark red (hypertrophic lichen planus). Papules aggregate into different patterns. Patterns are usually haphazard clusters, but they may be annular, diffusely papular (guttate), or linear, appearing in response to a scratch (Köebner's phenomenon). Rarely, a line of papules may extend the length of extremity. Vesicles or bullae may appear on preexisting lesions or on normal skin. Many patients have persistent brown staining many years after the rash has cleared.

Localized papules

Papules are most commonly located on the flexor surfaces of the wrists and forearms, the legs immediately above the ankles (Figure 8-47), and the lumbar region. Itching is variable; 20% of patients with lichen planus do not itch. Some patients with generalized involvement have minimal symptoms, whereas others display intolerable pruritus. The course is unpredictable. Some patients experience spontaneous remission in a few months, but the most common localized papular form tends to be chronic and endures for an average of approximately 4 years.

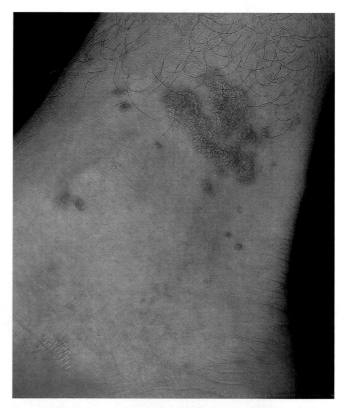

Figure 8-44 Lichen planus. A characteristic lesion of planar, polyangular, purple papules with lacy, reticular, criss-crossed whitish lines (Wickham's striae) on the surface.

LICHEN PLANUS

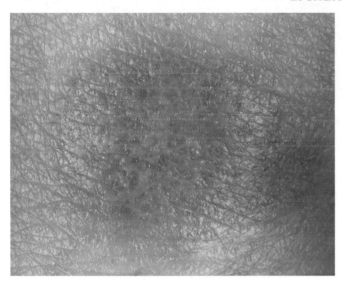

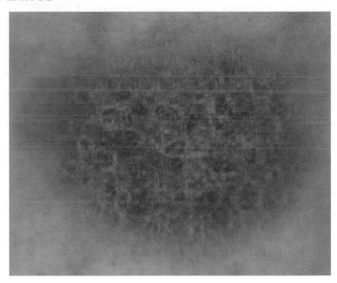

A, The primary lesion is a flat-topped papule with an irregular, angulated border (polygonal papules).

B, Close inspection of the surface shows a lacy, reticular pattern of criss-crossed whitish lines (Wickham's striae), accentuated here by a drop of immersion oil.

Figure 8-45 Primary lesions.

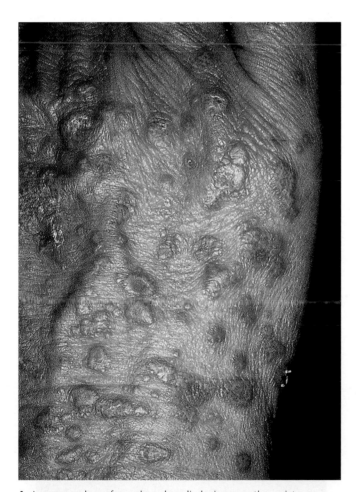

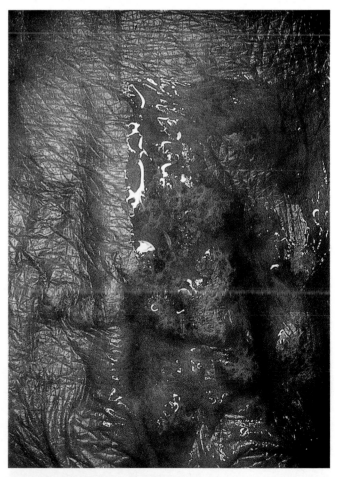

A, Large number of purple polycyclic lesions on the wrists.

B, Oil accentuates the lacy, white Wickham's striae and helps confirm the clinical diagnosis.

Figure 8-46 Localized lesions.

Hypertrophic lichen planus

This second most common cutaneous pattern may occur on any body region, but it is typically found on the pretibial areas and ankles (Figures 8-48 and 8-50). After a long time, papules lose their characteristic features and become confluent as reddish-brown or purplish, thickened, round-to-elongated (bandlike) plaques with a rough or verrucose surface; itching may be severe. Lesions continue for months or years, averaging approximately 8 years, and may be perpetuated by scratching. After the lesions clear, a dark-brown pigmentation remains.

Generalized lichen planus and lichenoid drug eruptions

Lichen planus may occur abruptly as a generalized, intensely pruritic eruption (Figure 8-49). Initially, the papules are pinpoint, numerous, and isolated. The papules may remain discrete or become confluent as large, red, eczematous-like, thin plaques. A highly characteristic, diffuse, dark brown, postinflammatory pigmentation remains as the disease clears. Before resolving spontaneously, untreated generalized lichen planus continues for approximately 8 months. Lichenoid drug eruptions are frequently of this diffuse type.[148] Low-grade fever may be present in the first few days, and lesions appear on the trunk, extremities, and lower back. The disease is seldom seen on the face or scalp and is rare on the palms and soles. Widespread inflammation can occur after sun exposure.

Lichen planus of the palms and soles

Lichen planus of the palms and soles generally occurs as an isolated phenomenon, but may appear simultaneously with disease in other areas. The lesions differ from classic lesions of lichen planus in that the papules are larger and aggregate into semitranslucent plaques with a globular waxy surface (Figure 8-51). Itching may be intolerable. Ulceration may occur and lesions of the feet may be so resistant to treatment that surgical excision and grafting is required.[149] The disease may last indefinitely.

Follicular lichen planus

Follicular lichen planus is also known as lichen planopilaris.[150] Lesions localized to the hair follicles may occur alone or with papular lichen planus. Follicular lichen planus, manifested as pinpoint, hyperkeratotic, follicular projections, is the most common form of lichen planus found in the scalp, where papular lesions are rarely observed. Hair loss occurs and may be permanent if the disease is sufficiently active to cause scarring. Lichen planus of the scalp is a cause of scarring alopecia. Patients with scarring alopecia should be evaluated histologically and with direct immunofluorescence. The immunofluorescence abnormalities differ from those associated with lichen planus, suggesting that lichen planopilaris and lichen planus are two different diseases.[151,152]

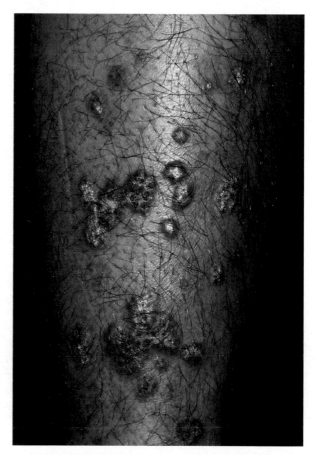

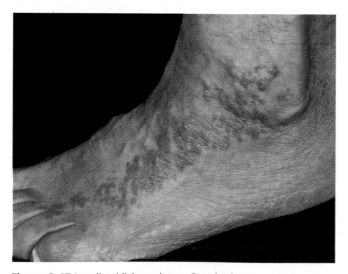

Figure 8-47 Localized lichen planus. Papules become thicker and confluent with time.

Figure 8-48 Hypertrophic lichen planus. Thick, reddish-brown plaques are most often present on the lower legs.

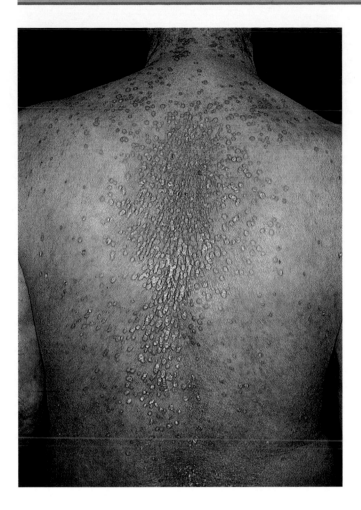

Figure 8-49 Generalized lichen planus. These discrete (guttate) lesions range from 1 mm to 1 cm in size. This generalized eruption occurred after starting antimalarial drugs.

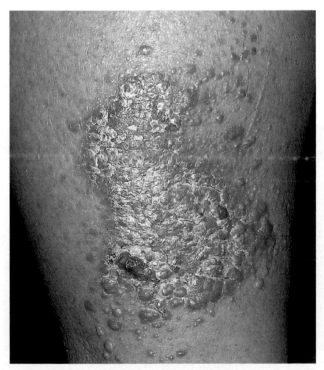

Figure 8-50 Confluent hypertrophic lichen planus. Lesions are extremely pruritic.

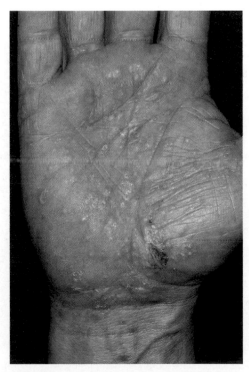

Figure 8-51 Lichen planus of the palms. Papules are large and become aggregated.

Oral mucous membrane lichen planus

Oral lichen planus can occur without cutaneous disease. Onset before middle age is rare; the mean age of onset is in the sixth decade.[153] Women outnumber men by more than 2:1.[154] Mucous membrane involvement is observed in more than 50% of patients with cutaneous lichen planus (Figures 8-52, 8-53, and 8-54). Lesions may be located on the tongue and lips, but the most common site is the buccal mucosa (see Figure 8-52). There are two stages of severity. The most common form is the nonerosive, generally asymptomatic, dendritic branching or lacy, white network pattern seen on the buccal mucosa; papules and plaques may appear with time. The oral cavity should always be examined if the diagnosis of cutaneous lichen planus is suspected. The presence of this dendritic pattern is solid supporting evidence for the diagnosis of cutaneous lichen planus.

A more difficult form is erosive mucosal lichen planus (see Figure 8-53). Localized or extensive ulcerations may involve any area of the oral cavity. Candidal infection was found in 17% to 25% of ulcerated and nonulcerated cases of lichen planus.[155] Oral squamous cell carcinoma developed in 0.8% patients at sites previously diagnosed by clinical examination as erosive or erythematous lichen planus.[156]

Superficial and erosive lesions are less commonly found on the glans penis (Figure 8-55), vulvovaginal region (Figure 8-56), and anus.[157]

A small number of oral lichen planus patients have hepatitis C virus infection.[158]

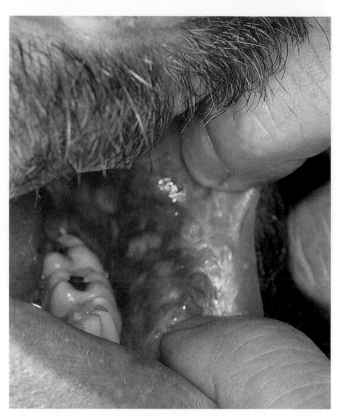

Figure 8-53 Erosive oral lichen planus. Localized or extensive ulcerations may involve any area of the oral cavity.

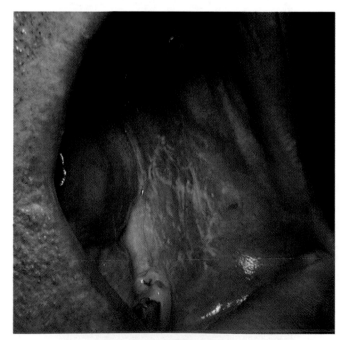

Figure 8-52 Mucous membrane lichen planus. A lacy, white pattern is present on the buccal mucosa. *(Courtesy Gerald Shklar, B.Sc., D.D.S., M.S., Harvard School of Dental Medicine.)*

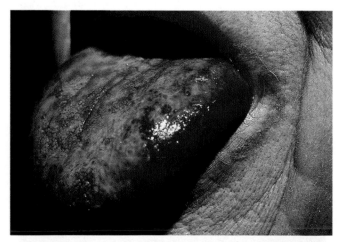

Figure 8-54 Lichen planus tongue. The surface is red and smooth with loss of papillae. White striae are an almost constant feature. Candida has a similar appearance.

Erosive vaginal lichen planus

Lichen planus usually involves skin and oral cavity lesions, but erosive vaginal disease may be the first sign. Lichen planus may be the most common cause of desquamative vaginitis. There are flares and partial remissions but no tendency for complete remission. There is marked vaginal mucosal fragility and erythema (see Figure 8-56). Agglutination of the labia minora may occur, and vaginal adhesions may render a patient unable to engage in sexual intercourse. Vaginal histology may be nonspecific, showing only a loss of epithelium. A biopsy taken from a white hyperkeratotic area on the labial skin may provide a specific histologic picture. Vaginal desquamation is not associated with lichen sclerosus. Topical and oral steroids are the most effective treatment. Topical tacrolimus (Protopic ointment) or pimecrolimus (Elidel cream) may be effective. Some patients respond to dapsone. Many other systemic agents have been used.[159,160]

The vulvovaginal-gingival syndrome is a variant of mucosal lichen planus characterized by erosions and desquamation of the vulva, vagina, and gingiva. Gingival lichen planus is present in all patients and is characterized by erosions, erythema and white, reticulated lesions. Vulvovaginal lichen planus also displayed erosions in most patients. Concomitant use of several drugs is usually required to achieve beneficial results.[161] Estrogens are not effective.

Nails

Nail changes frequently accompany generalized lichen planus but may occur as the only manifestation of disease. Approximately 25% of patients with nail LP have LP in other sites before or after the onset of nail lesions. Nail LP usually appears during the fifth or sixth decade of life. The changes include proximal to distal linear depressions or grooves and partial or complete destruction of the nail plate. The development of severe and early destruction of the nail matrix characterizes a small subset of patients with nail LP.[162] Long-term observation indicates that permanent damage to the nail is rare even in patients with diffuse involvement of the matrix (see Figure 25-10).

Diagnosis

The diagnosis can be made clinically, but a skin biopsy eliminates any doubt. Direct immunofluorescence may help to establish the diagnosis.[163] The skin shows ovoid globular deposits of IgG, IgM, IgA, and complement. Basement membrane zone deposits of fibrin and fibrinogen are present in a linear pattern in both cutaneous and oral lesions in almost all patients. Circulating antibodies have not been found; therefore indirect immunofluorescence is negative.

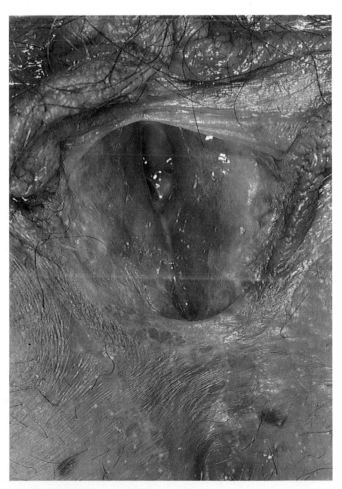

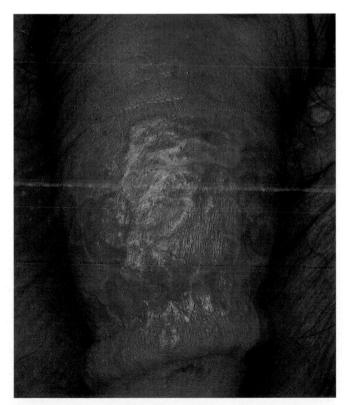

Figure 8-55 Lichen planus on the penis. A lacy, white pattern identical to that seen on the buccal mucosa.

Figure 8-56 Erosive vaginal lichen planus. The entire vaginal tract is involved in this severe case.

Treatment

THERAPY FOR CUTANEOUS LICHEN PLANUS

Topical steroids. Group I or II topical steroids (in a cream or ointment base applied two times daily) are used as initial treatment for localized disease. They relieve itching, but the lesions are slow to clear. Plastic occlusion enhances the effectiveness of topical steroids.

Intralesional steroids. Triamcinolone acetonide (Kenalog, 5 to 10 mg/mL) may reduce the hypertrophic lesions located on the wrists and lower legs. Injections may be repeated every 3 or 4 weeks.

Systemic steroids. Generalized, severely pruritic lichen planus responds to oral corticosteroids. For adults, a 2- to 4-week course of prednisone, 20 mg twice daily, is usually sufficient to clear the disease. To help prevent recurrence, gradually decrease the dosage over a 3-week period.

Acitretin. One large study showed that acitretin is an effective and acceptable therapy for severe cases of lichen planus. A significantly higher number of patients treated with 30 mg/day acitretin (64%) showed remission or marked improvement compared with placebo (13%). Furthermore, during the subsequent 8-week open phase, 83% of previously placebo-treated patients responded favorably to acitretin therapy.[164]

Azathioprine. Azathioprine can be an effective steroid sparing treatment for generalized lichen planus. Azathioprine alone is an alternative therapy, especially when there are risk factors against corticosteroid use.[164,165]

Cyclosporine. Patients with severe, chronic lichen planus were successfully treated with oral cyclosporine (6 mg/kg/day). A response was noted within 4 weeks, and complete clearing was achieved after 8 weeks of treatment. No significant adverse effect was noted. The patients remained in remission up to 10 months after therapy.[166]

Antihistamines. Antihistamines such as hydroxyzine, 10 to 25 mg every 4 hours, may provide relief from itching.

PUVA. A bilateral comparison study demonstrated that PUVA is an effective therapy for generalized, symptomatic lichen planus and suggested that maintenance therapy might not be required once complete clearance is attained.[167]

THERAPY OF MUCOUS MEMBRANE LICHEN PLANUS

The course of oral and vaginal lichen planus can extend for years. Treatment is challenging. Most treatment failures are due to improper diagnosis. Consider a biopsy to establish the diagnosis. Most patients are asymptomatic and do not need treatment. Most symptomatic forms of the disease are the erosive and atrophic types, which may need systemic therapy. The most effective treatment is short courses of systemic steroids (prednisone) and topical high-potency corticosteroids.

Tacrolimus and pimecrolimus. Topical tacrolimus (Protopic ointment 0.1, 0.03) and pimecrolimus (Elidel cream), immunomodulators approved for atopic dermatitis, have also been reported to be effective for erosive lichen planus.[168] These medications are safe and may be tried as initial therapy.

Corticosteroids. These medicines are often the initial treatment for oral lichen planus. Topical application of corticosteroids (Clobetasol propionate, fluocinonide, fluocinolone acetonide, triamcinolone acetonide [Kenalog]) in an adhesive base (orabase) is safe and effective. Fluocinolone acetonide gel 0.1% is a safe and effective alternative therapy to fluocinolone acetonide in an oral base 0.1%.[169] Clobetasol propionate in orabase was more effective than fluocinonide ointment in orabase for oral vesiculoerosive diseases.[170] The Orabase formulations are placed on the lesions, but are not rubbed in. Massaging the special cream base results in the loss of adhesiveness. Topical application of fluocinonide gel to the gingiva and buccal mucosa over a 3-week period in patients with erosive lichen planus produces no adrenal suppression.[171] Acute candidiasis may occur during treatment but responds to topical antifungal therapy (e.g., Mycelex troches).

Intralesional steroids in a single submucosal injection, 0.5 to 1.0 mL of methyl prednisolone acetate (Depo-Medrol 40 mg/mL) may be sufficient to heal erosive oral lichen planus within 1 week.[172]

Prednisone rapidly and effectively controls the disease, but recurrences may occur when the dosage is tapered.[153,173]

Dapsone (50 to 150 mg/day) may be tried if conservative medical treatment fails.[174,175]

Hydroxychloroquine sulfate (Plaquenil), 200 to 400 mg daily, is useful for oral LP. Pain relief and reduced erythema occur after 1 to 2 months; erosions required 3 to 6 months of treatment before they resolved.[176]

Azathioprine. Azathioprine is very effective for controlling oral lichen planus and may be considered for resistant, debilitating cases.[177,178]

Topical cyclosporine. In one study patients swished and expectorated 5 ml of solution (containing 100 mg of cyclosporine per milliliter) for 5 minutes three times daily. There was marked improvement after 8 weeks. There were no systemic side effects. Blood cyclosporine levels were low or undetectable.[179] Another study showed that cyclosporine was of little benefit.[180]

Griseofulvin. Griseofulvin is not effective.[181]

Lichen Sclerosus et Atrophicus

Lichen sclerosus et atrophicus (LSA) is an uncommon but distinctive chronic cutaneous disease of unknown origin. Cases in females outnumber those in males by 10:1. Although the trunk and extremities may be affected, the disease has a predilection for the vulva, perianal area, and groin. Most lesions appear spontaneously, but some may be induced by trauma or radiation (Köebner's phenomenon).[185]

At a glance, LSA may be confused with guttate morphea, lichen planus, or discoid lupus erythematosus. The difference becomes evident upon closer inspection of the surface features. Early lesions are small, smooth, pink or ivory, flat-topped, slightly raised papules. White-to-brown, horny follicular plugs appear on the surface; this feature is referred to as delling (Figures 8-57 and 8-58). Delling is not observed in lichen planus or morphea. In time, clusters of papules may coalesce to form small oval plaques with a dull or glistening, smooth, white, atrophic, wrinkled surface (Figure 8-58). Histologically, it appears that the interface area between the dermis and epidermis has dissolved. The overlying, unsupported, thin, atrophic epidermis contracts, giving the appearance of wrinkled tissue paper (Figure 8-59).

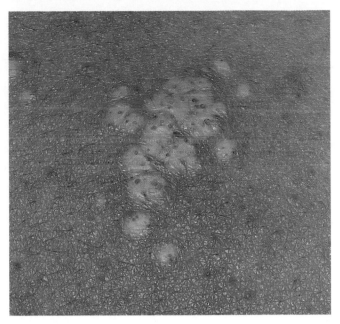

Figure 8-57 Lichen sclerosus et atrophicus. Early lesions are ivory-colored, flat-topped, slightly raised papules with follicular plugs.

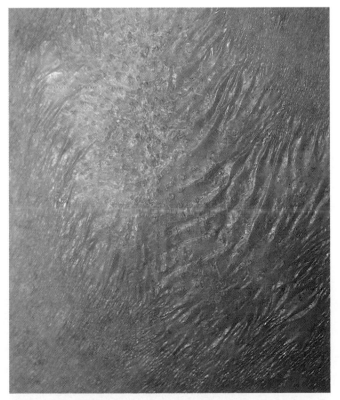

Figure 8-58 Papular lesions as illustrated in Figure 8-57 coalesce to form atrophic plaques with a wrinkled surface. White-to-brown, horny follicular plugs appear on the surface, a feature referred to as delling.

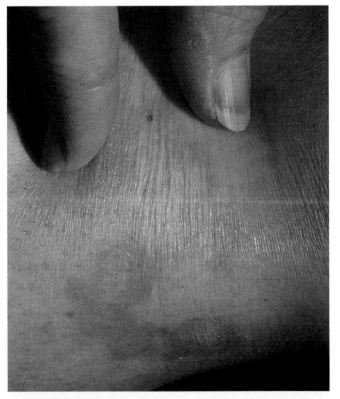

Figure 8-59 Lichen sclerosus et atrophicus. The epidermis is thin and atrophic and gives the appearance of wrinkled tissue paper when compressed.

Anogenital lesions in females

In most cases, anogenital lesions are distinctive. All of the following patterns may be present in the same individual. The first is a white atrophic plaque in the shape of an hourglass or inverted keyhole encircling the vagina and rectum (Figures 8-60 and 8-61). This distinctive pattern is seen in prepubertal females (Figure 8-62) and adults. The lesions can extend to the entire vulva, giving it a pearly white appearance, or remain localized and requiring biopsy to confirm the diagnosis. Vulvar pruritus and dyspareunia are the most common symptoms. Dysuria and pain on defecation is common.[186]

Prepubertal lichen sclerosus et atrophicus

Prepubertal LSA may occur in infants and resolves without sequelae in about two thirds of cases at or just before menarche, leaving a brown hyperpigmented area on skin that had been white and atrophic.[187] Purpura of the vulva is an occasional manifestation of pediatric LSA. It mimics sexual abuse and has led to false accusation and investigations.[188-190] The disease persists in approximately one third of patients.

Intertriginous (skin crease) lesions involve the groin and anal area and are subject to friction and maceration. The delicate, thin, white, wrinkled, compromised skin breaks down to become hemorrhagic and eroded, simulating irritant or candidal intertrigo. Bullae may precede erosions.

Adult lichen sclerosus et atrophicus

LSA of the vulva is a distressing problem. Typically, the adult form appears after menopause and has a lengthy duration. Lesions itch and may show evidence of excoriation. The disease is chronic, painful, and interferes with sexual activity. Fragile, atrophic, thin, parchmentlike tissue erodes, becomes macerated, and heals slowly. Repeated cycles of erosion and healing induce contraction and stenosis of the vaginal introitus and atrophy, and shrinkage of the clitoris and labia minora (see Figure 8-61). A watery discharge may be present. Squamous cell carcinoma, particularly of the clitoris or labia minora, has been reported in approximately 3% of patients with chronic LSA.[191] Therefore biopsy should be considered in lesions that are white and raised (leukoplakia), fissured or ulcerated, and unresponsive to medical therapy.

Lichen sclerosus et atrophicus of the penis

ADULTS. LSA of the penis in the adult (balanitis xerotica obliterans) may present as recurrent balanitis, which may be intensified by intercourse; the shaft is rarely involved. The white atrophic plaques occur on the glans and prepuce and erode and heal with contraction (Figures 8-63, 8-64, and 8-65). Most patients are uncircumcised.[192] LSA may be caused by chronic occlusion.[193] Encroachment into the urinary meatus may lead to stricture. As with vaginal LSA, degeneration into SCC is rare.[194] There does, however, appear to be an association between SCC of the penis and the presence of LSA. Fifty percent of SCC patients studied had a clinical history and/or histologic evidence of LSA. Clinical presentation of the LSA or need for circumcision may precede the SCC by many years.[195]

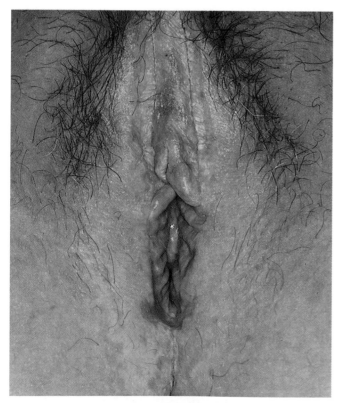

Figure 8-60 Lichen sclerosus et atrophicus. A white, atrophic plaque encircles the vagina and rectum (inverted keyhole pattern).

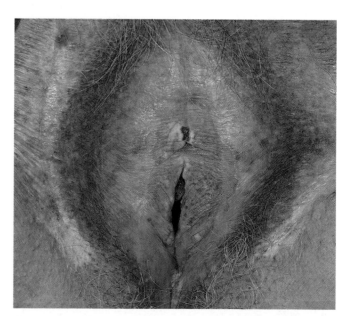

Figure 8-61 Lichen sclerosus et atrophicus of the vulva (kraurosis vulvae). The crease areas are atrophic and wrinkled, the labia is hyperpigmented, and the introitus is contracted and ulcerated.

GENITAL LICHEN SCLEROSUS ET ATROPHICUS

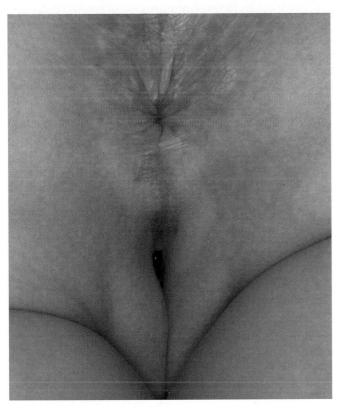

Figure 8-62 Lichen sclerosus et atrophicus. Prepubertal LSA typically involves the vulval and rectal areas. Spontaneous remission occurs in over two thirds of patients.

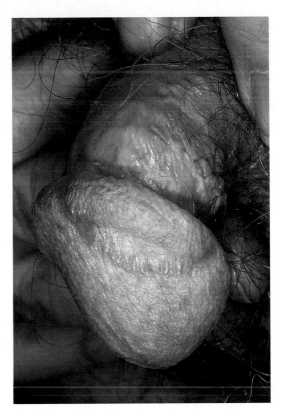

Figure 8-63 Penile shaft involvement is less common. Here an expanding sclerotic ring involves the shaft and glans.

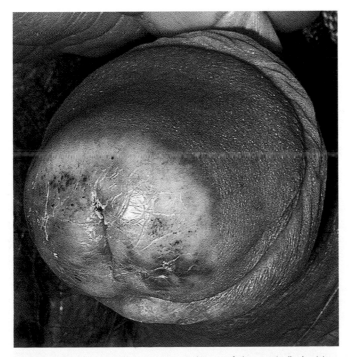

Figure 8-64 Lichen sclerosus et atrophicus of the penis (balanitis xerotica obliterans). The glans is smooth, white, and atrophic. Erosions are present on the prepuce.

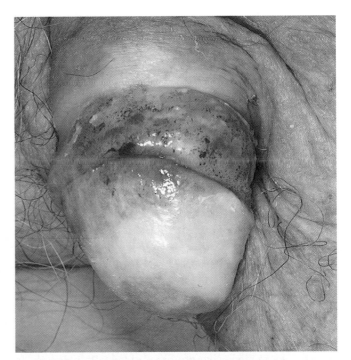

Figure 8-65 Lesions are usually confined to the glans and prepuce.

BOYS. LSA in boys was thought to be rare, but recent reports suggest that it has been overlooked in the past. Most boys are between 4 and 12 years of age at onset. Nearly all affected boys had severe phimosis in a previously retractable penis, with obvious scarring or sclerosis near the tip of the prepuce.[196] Purpura is an occasional manifestation of pediatric LSA. Genital purpura is also a sign of sexual abuse.[189]

Management

In general, the diagnosis of LSA of the skin and vulva can be made by clinical observation, but a biopsy may be necessary for confirmation. Chronically fissured, ulcerated, or hyperplastic lesions should be biopsied to rule out SCC.

TOPICAL STEROIDS. Topical steroid creams should be the initial treatment for uncomplicated vulvar and penile lesions in adults and children.[197] Vaginal and vulvar candidiasis may occur. Atrophy of the vulva may result from continual unsupervised application of topical steroids. Use should be discontinued when a favorable response is obtained, and bland lubricants can be used daily to soothe dry tissues.

CLOBETASOL. Clobetasol ointment 0.05% induces a remarkable relief of symptoms (itching, burning, pain, dyspareunia). The clinical signs of atrophy, hyperkeratosis, and sclerosis are improved and histologic alterations (atrophy of the epithelium, edema, inflammatory infiltrate, fibrosis) are reversed.[198] Treatment with topical testosterone propionate 2% is less effective.

Vulvar lichen sclerosus et atrophicus in adults. The group I topical steroid ointment, Clobetasol propionate, is reported effective for all age groups. The following regimen was reported for adults. Apply the ointment twice daily for 1 month and then once daily for 1 month, then taper down within the next month to two applications per week and remain on that regimen until a follow-up examination at 3 months after the initial visit. Treatment is then on an "as needed" basis.[199] Follow-up examinations are important when using superpotent topical steroids.

Vulvar lichen sclerosus et atrophicus in children. Premenarchal LSA patients (averaging 5.7 years) responded to clobetasol ointment 0.05% for 2 to 4 weeks. Clobetasol is then stopped and tapered to a less potent steroid.[200] Recurrences were common and required additional steroid treatment. Complications were infrequent, minor, and easily treatable. Betamethasone dipropionate 0.05% ointment applied three times each day for 3 weeks and then twice daily until the vulva appeared normal was effective. This required 1 to 6 months of treatment (average, 3 months). After this treatment course, patients received hydrocortisone 1% daily for 3 months, and then nothing. Recurrences were treated again with shorter courses. The appearance of the vulva returned to normal in most patients, leaving pigmentary changes in a few. Symptoms subsided within 6 weeks in all patients. No side effects were seen, except mild telangiectasia in three subjects. Recurrence manifested as a recurrence of symptoms.

Labial fusion is a common condition seen most frequently in infants and young children. Most cases are "physiological," but it can be the presenting feature of genital lichen sclerosus.[201] Pain and scarring develop in young women with recurrent labial and periclitoral adhesions.

Vaginal and vulvar candidiasis may occur. Atrophy of the vulva may result from continual application of topical steroids. Use should be discontinued when a favorable response is obtained, and bland lubricants can be used daily to soothe dry tissues.

Penile lichen sclerosus et atrophicus in men. Topical treatment with clobetasol propionate 0.05% is safe and effective with little risk of epidermal atrophy. Treatment significantly improves itching, burning, pain, dyspareunia, phimosis, and dysuria after 1 to 2 daily applications, for a mean of 7.1 weeks. Histologic changes are significantly reduced after treatment. There is some potential for triggering latent infections, most importantly human papillomavirus.[202]

Intralesional steroids such as triamcinolone acetonide (Kenalog, 2.5 to 5.0 mg/mL) may be useful for areas that do not respond to topical therapy.

Fissures and erosions are effectively treated with scarlet red gauze.

Surgery

The high recurrence rate of all surgical modalities makes surgical treatment suitable only for patients who failed to respond to medical treatment. Symptoms are relieved by circumcision in men and boys.[192,203] Surgical therapy of LSA of the vulva consists of: vulvectomy (with or without a skin graft), cryosurgery, and laser ablation. It is indicated when malignant transformation is present or is likely to occur. Skinning and simple vulvectomies are associated with recurrence rates as high as 50%.[204] However, better sexual function and cosmetic results have been reported in the former, especially with concomitant split skin grafting. Cryosurgery has high recurrence rates, although short-term results are favorable. Laser therapy may produce better long-term results than other treatments. Carbon dioxide laser ablation to a depth of 1 to 2 mm is acceptable treatment for patients who have LSA of the penis or vulva that is refractory to other measures.[205] The procedure may be performed under general anesthesia. Healing is complete 6 weeks postoperatively, and patients were free of symptoms for up to 3 years.[206]

Young women with recurrent labial and periclitoral adhesions respond to sharp dissection of the clitoral hood and separation of the adherent labia. Surgicel, oxidized regenerated cellulose gauze (Johnson & Johnson, Arlington, TX) is sutured to the exposed clitoral hood and labial surfaces with Vicryl suture. Complete dissolution of the Surgicel occurs between postoperative day 4 and 6 and without recurrence of adhesions. This technique has prevented the recurrence during the interval when these surfaces are at highest risk of reagglutination.[207]

ACITRETIN. Acitretin (20 to 30 mg/day for 16 weeks) is effective in treating women with severe LSA of the vulva.[208]

Pityriasis Lichenoides

Pityriasis lichenoides is a rare disease with two variants: acute (pityriasis lichenoides et varioliformis acuta [PLEVA] or Mucha-Habermann disease) and chronic (pityriasis lichenoides chronica). The terms *acute* and *chronic* refer to the characteristics of the individual lesions and not to the course of the disease. PLC and PLEVA are interrelated processes within the larger group of T-cell lymphoproliferative disorders. PLC is frequently a clonal T-cell disease. Molecular studies have shown that PLEVA is a clonal lymphoproliferative disorder.[209] Most cases occur during the first three decades of the patient's life. The diseases are more common in males. Evidence suggests that PLEVA is a hypersensitivity reaction to an infectious agent. The prognosis for both forms is good.[210] Pityriasis lichenoides chronica, PLEVA, and lymphomatoid papulosis share several clinical and immunohistologic features, suggesting that these disorders are interrelated and part of a spectrum of clonal-T-cell cutaneous lymphoproliferative disorders.[211,212] The histology of these entities is distinctive.

PLEVA

Mucha-Habermann disease, or PLEVA, is usually a benign, self-limited papulosquamous disorder. PLEVA is a clonal T cell-mediated lymphoproliferative disorder.[213] PLEVA has been documented in all age groups, with most cases occurring in the second and third decades. PLEVA begins insidiously, with few symptoms other than mild itching or a low-grade fever. Crops of round or oval, reddish-brown papules, usually 2 to 10 mm in diameter, appear, either singly or in clusters. They can occur anywhere, but they typically appear on the trunk, thighs, and upper arms (Figure 8-66). The face, scalp, palms, and soles are involved in approximately 10% of cases.

The papules may develop a violaceous center and a surrounding rim of erythema. There may be micaceous scale. Lesions can become vesicular or pustular and then undergo hemorrhagic necrosis, usually within 2 to 5 weeks, often leaving a postinflammatory hyperpigmentation and sometimes scars (Figure 8-67). Acute exacerbations are common and the disease may wax and wane for months or years. High fever is a rare complication, but it may be associated with an ulceronecrotic type of lesion.[214] Complications include a self-limited arthritis and superinfection of the skin lesions. Mucha-Habermann disease can mimic other common entities such as varicella and insect bites.

Pityriasis lichenoides chronica

Pityriasis lichenoides chronica (Juliusberg type) is a generalized eruption consisting of brownish papules with fine, micalike, adherent scale that becomes more evident when scratched. The disease may persist for years. Systemic symptoms are rare. The scale is less conspicuous than in psoriasis. Lesions clear without scarring and show only transient skin discoloration. The distribution is similar to PLEVA.

Treatment

Erythromycin produced a remission in 73% of the cases. It frequently took as long as 2 months before a significant therapeutic effect was noted. Clearing with oral erythromycin was reported in most cases at dosages of 30 to 50 mg/kg/day.[215] Erythromycin was tapered over several months, depending on the response. The disease usually recurred if erythromycin was tapered too rapidly. Psoralen ultraviolet light A (PUVA), ultraviolet light B (UVB) phototherapy,[216] tetracycline, gold, methotrexate, oral corticosteroids, and dapsone have all been used with some success.[217]

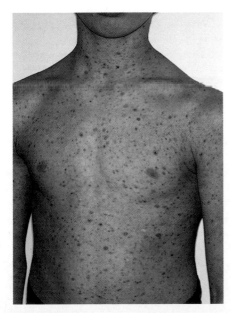

Figure 8-66 Pityriasis lichenoides et varioliformis acuta (PLEVA). A florid generalized eruption.

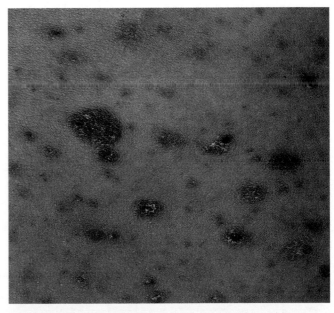

Figure 8-67 PLEVA. Scattered, discrete polymorphic red-brown papules, pustules, and erosions.

References

1. Updike J: Personal history: at war with my skin, The New Yorker 1985: Sept 2.

2. Skoven I, Thormann J: Lithium compound treatment and psoriasis,. Arch Dermatol 1979; 115:1185.

3. Gold MH, Holy AK, Roenigk HH: Beta-blocking drugs and psoriasis, J Am Acad Dermatol 1988; 19:837.

4. Slagel GA, James WD: Plaquenil-induced erythroderma, J Am Acad Dermatol 1985; 12:857.

5. Abel EA, et al: Drugs in exacerbation of psoriasis, J Am Acad Dermatol 1986; 15:1007.

6. Baker H, Ryan TJ: Generalized pustular psoriasis: a clinical and epidemiological study of 104 cases, Br J Dermatol 1968; 80:71.

7. Telfer NR, et al: The role of streptococcal infection in the initiation of guttate psoriasis, Arch Dermatol 1992; 128:39.

8. Zelickson BD, Muller SA: Generalized pustular psoriasis: a review of 63 cases, Arch Dermatol 1991; 127:1339.

9. Boyd AS, Menter A: Erythrodermic psoriasis: precipitating factors, course, and prognosis in 50 patients, J Am Acad Dermatol 1989; 21:985.

10. O'Doherty CJ, Macintyre C: Palmoplantar pustulosis and smoking, Br Med J 1985;291:861.

11. Benoldi D, et al: Reiter's disease: successful treatment of the skin manifestations with oral etretinate, Acta Derm Venereol 1984; 64:352.

12. Lesher JL, Chalker DK: Response of the cutaneous lesions of Reiter's syndrome to ketoconazole, J Am Acad Dermatol 1985; 13:161.

13. Obuch ML, et al: Psoriasis and human immunodeficiency virus infection, J Am Acad Dermatol 1992; 27:667.

14. Maurer TA, et al: The use of methotrexate for psoriasis in patients with HIV infection, J Am Acad Dermatol 1994; 3:372.

15. Ruzicka T, et al: Treatment of HIV-induced retinoid-resistant psoriasis with zidovudine, Lancet 1987; 2:1469.

16. Stern RS: The epidemiology of joint complaints in patients with psoriasis, J Rheumatol 1985; 12:315.

17. Zanolli MD, Wikle JS: Joint complaints in psoriasis patients, Int J Dermatol 1992; 31:488.

18. Ostensen M: The effect of pregnancy on ankylosing spondylitis, psoriatic arthritis, and juvenile rheumatoid arthritis, Am J Reprod Immunol 1992; 28:235.

19. Gladman DD, et al: Longitudinal study of clinical and radiological progression in psoriatic arthritis, J Rheumatol 1990; 17:809.

20. Moll JMH: The clinical spectrum of psoriatic arthritis, Clinical Orthop 1979; 143:66.

21. McHugh MJ, et al: Psoriatic arthritis: clinical subgroups and histocompatibility antigens, Ann Rheum Dis 1987; 46:184.

22. Espinoza LR, et al: Psoriatic arthritis: clinical response and side effects to methotrexate therapy, J Rheumatol 1992; 19:872.

23. Willkens R, et al: Randomized, double-blind, placebo controlled trial of low-dose pulse methotrexate in psoriatic arthritis, Arthritis Rheum 1984; 27:376.

24. Whiting-O'Keefe QE, et al: Methotrexate and histologic hepatic abnormalities: a meta-analysis, Am J Med 1991; 90:711.

25. Kammer GM, et al: Psoriatic arthritis: a clinical immunologic and HLA study of 100 patients, Semin Arthritis Rheum 1979; 9:75.

26. Gladman DD, et al: Chloroquine therapy in psoriatic arthritis, J Rheumatol 1992; 19:1724.

27. Salvarani C, et al: Low dose cyclosporine A in psoriatic arthritis: relation between soluble interleukin 2 receptors and response to therapy, J Rheumatol 1992; 19:74.

28. Wagner SA, et al: Therapeutic efficacy of oral low-dose cyclosporin A in severe psoriatic arthritis, Dermatology 1993; 186:62.

29. Chieregato GC, Leoni A: Treatment of psoriatic arthropathy with etretinate: a two-year follow-up, Acta Derm Verereol 1986; 66:321.

30. Newman ED, et al: Sulfasalazine therapy in psoriatic arthritis: clinical and immunologic response, J Rheumatol 1991; 18:1379.

31. Farr M, et al: Sulphasalazine in psoriatic arthritis. A double blind placebo-controlled study, Br J Rheumatol 1990; 26:46.

32. Gaston L, et al: Psoriasis and stress: a prospective study, J Am Acad Dermatol 1987; 17:82.

33. Gupta MA, Gupta AK, Haberman HF: Psoriasis and psychiatry: an update, Gen Hosp Psychiatry 1987; 9:157.

34. Koo J: Systemic sequential therapy of psoriasis: a new paradigm for improved therapeutic results, J Am Acad Derm 1999; 41:525.

35. Koo J, Lebwohl M: Duration of remission of psoriasis therapies, J Am Acad Dermatol 1999; 41(1):51.

36. Berth-Jones J, et al: A multicentre, parallel-group comparison of calcipotriol ointment and short-contact dithranol therapy in chronic plaque psoriasis, Br J Dermatol 1992; 127:266.

37. Lebwohl M, et al: Calcipotriene ointment and halobetasol ointment in the long-term treatment of psoriasis: effects on the duration of improvement, J Am Acad Dermatol 1998; 39(3):447.

38. Bourke JF, et al: Occlusion enhances the efficacy of topical calcipotriol in the treatment of psoriasis vulgaris, Clin Exp Dermatol 1993; 18:504.

39. Brands S, et al: No additional effect of calcipotriol ointment on low-dose narrow-band UVB phototherapy in psoriasis, J Am Acad Dermatol 1999; 41(6):991.

40. Speight E, Farr P: Calcipotriol improves the response of psoriasis to PUVA, Br J Dermatol 1994; 130(1):79.

41. Lebwohl M, et al: Interactions between calcipotriene and ultraviolet light, J Am Acad Dermatol 1997; 37(1):93.

42. Georgiou S, Tsambaos D: Hypercalcaemia and hypercalciuria after topical treatment of psoriasis with excessive amounts of calcipotriol, Acta Derm Venereol 1999; 79(1):86.

43. Lebwohl M: Strategies to optimize efficacy, duration of remission, and safety in the treatment of plaque psoriasis by using tazarotene in combination with a corticosteroid, J Am Acad Dermatol 2000; 43(2 Pt 3):S43.

44. Lebwohl M, Ali S: Treatment of psoriasis. Part 1. Topical therapy and phototherapy, J Am Acad Dermatol 2001; 45(4):487; quiz 499.

45. Hecker D, et al: Interactions between tazarotene and ultraviolet light, J Am Acad Dermatol 1999; 41(6):927.

46. Farr PM, Diffey BL, Marks JM: Phototherapy and dithranol treatment of psoriasis: new lamps for old, Br Med J 1987; 294:205.

47. Deleted in proofs.

48. Jones SK, Campbell WC, Mackie RM: Out-patient treatment of psoriasis: short contact and overnight dithranol therapy compared, Br J Dermatol 1985; 113:331.

49. Meola T, Jr, et al: Are topical corticosteroids useful adjunctive therapy for the treatment of psoriasis with ultraviolet radiation? a review of the literature, Arch Dermatol 1991; 127:1708.

50. Boer J, et al: Comparison of phototherapy (UV-B) and photochemotherapy (PUVA) for clearing and maintenance therapy of psoriasis, Arch Dermatol 1984; 120:52.

51. Marsico AR, Eaglstein WH, Weinstein GD: Ultraviolet light and tar in the Goeckerman regimen for psoriasis, Arch Dermatol 1976; 112:1249.

52. Stern RS, et al: Contribution of topical tar oil to ultraviolet B phototherapy for psoriasis, J Am Acad Dermatol 1986; 14:742.

53. Adrain RM, et al: Outpatient phototherapy of psoriasis, Arch Dermatol 1981; 117:623.

54. Stern RS, et al: Effect of continued ultraviolet B phototherapy on the duration of remission of psoriasis: a randomized study, J Am Acad Dermatol 1986; 15:546.

55. Petrozzi JW: Topical steroids and UV radiation in psoriasis, Arch Dermatol 1983; 119:207.

56. Lebwohl M, et al: Effects of topical preparations on the erythemogenicity of UVB: implications for phototherapy, J Am Acad Dermatol 1995; 32:469.

57. Perry HO, et al: The Goeckerman treatment of psoriasis, Arch Dermatol 1968; 98:178.

58. Horwitz SN, et al: Addition of a topically applied corticosteroid to a modified Goeckerman regimen for treatment of psoriasis: effect on duration of remission, J Am Acad Dermatol 1985; 13:784.

59. Paul BS, et al: Combined methotrexate—ultraviolet B therapy in the treatment of psoriasis, J Am Acad Derm 1982; 7:758.

60. Lowe N, et al: Acitretin plus UVB therapy for psoriasis. Comparisons with placebo plus UVB and acitretin alone, J Am Acad Dermatol 1991; 24(4):591.

61. Rosen K, Mobacken H, Swanbeck G: PUVA, etretinate, and PUVA-etretinate therapy for pustulosis palmoplantaris: a placebo-controlled comparative trial, Arch Dermatol 1987; 123:885.

62. Lawrence CM, et al: A comparison of PUVA-etretinate and PUVA-placebo for palmoplantar pustular psoriasis, Br J Dermatol 1984; 110:221.

63. Melski JW, Stern RS: Annual rate of psoralen and ultraviolet-A treatment of psoriasis after initial clearing, Arch Dermatol 1982; 118:404.

64. Momtaz TK, Parrish JA: Combination of psoralens and ultraviolet A and ultraviolet B in the treatment of psoriasis vulgaris: a bilateral comparison study, J Am Acad Dermatol 1984; 10:481.

65. Speight EL, Farr PM: Calcipotriol improves the response of psoriasis to PUVA, Br J Dermatol 1994; 130:79.

66. Roenigk H: Acitretin combination therapy, J Am Acad Dermatol 1999; 41(3 Pt 2):S18.

67. Morison WL, et al: Combined methotrexate-PUVA therapy in the treatment of psoriasis, J Am Acad Dermatol 1982; 6:46.

68. Stern R, Liebman E, Vakeva L: Oral psoralen and ultraviolet-A light (PUVA) treatment of psoriasis and persistent risk of non-melanoma skin cancer: PUVA Follow-up Study, J Natl Cancer Inst 1998; 90(17): 1278.

69. Studniberg HM, Weller P: PUVA, UVB, psoriasis, and non-melanoma skin cancer, J Am Acad Dermatol 1993; 29:1013.

70. Henseler T, et al: Skin tumors in the European PUVA study: eight-year follow-up of 1,643 patients treated with PUVA for psoriasis, J Am Acad Dermatol 1987;16:108.

71. Mali-Gerrits MG, et al: Psoriasis therapy and the risk of skin cancers, Clin Exp Dermatol 1991; 16:85.

72. Stern RS: Genital tumors among men with psoriasis exposed to psoralens and ultraviolet A radiation (PUVA) and ultraviolet B radiation: The Photochemotherapy Follow-up Study, N Engl J Med 1990; 322:1093.

73. Stern RS, et al: Malignant melanoma in patients treated for psoriasis with methoxsalen (psoralen) and ultraviolet A radiation (PUVA). The PUVA study, N Engl J Med 1997; 336:15.

74. Stern R, Lange R: Non-melanoma skin cancer occurring in patients treated with PUVA five to ten years after first treatment, J Invest Dermatol 1988; 91(2):120.

75. Morison W, et al: Consensus workshop on the toxic effects of long-term PUVA therapy, Arch Dermatol 1998; 134(5):595.

76. Momtaz-T K, Parrish J: Combination of psoralens and ultraviolet A and ultraviolet B in the treatment of psoriasis vulgaris: a bilateral comparison study, J Am Acad Dermatol 1984; 10(3):481.

77. Basarab T, et al: Atypical pigmented lesions following extensive PUVA therapy, Clin Exp Dermatol 2000; 25(2):135.

78. Rhodes A, Stern R, Melski J: The PUVA lentigo: an analysis of predisposing factors, J Invest Dermatol 1983; 81(5):459.

79. Stern RS, et al: Ocular lens findings in patients treated with PUVA, J Invest Dermatol 1994; 103:534.

80. Friedman SJ: Management of psoriasis vulgaris with a hydrocolloid occlusive dressing, Arch Dermatol 1987; 123:1046.

81. Shore RN: Treatment of psoriasis with prolonged application of tape, J Am Acad Dermatol 1986; 15:540.

82. Farr PM, et al: Response of scalp psoriasis to oral ketoconazole, Lancet 1985; 2:921.

83. Moy R, Kingston T, Lowe N: Isotretinoin vs etretinate therapy in generalized pustular and chronic psoriasis, Arch Dermatol 1985; 121(10):1297.

84. Weinstein GD, White GM: An approach to the treatment of moderate to severe psoriasis with rotational therapy, J Am Acad Dermatol 1993; 28:454.

85. Koo J: Systemic sequential therapy of psoriasis: a new paradigm for improved therapeutic results, J Am Acad Dermatol 1999; 41:525.

86. Collins P, Rogers S: The efficacy of methotrexate in psoriasis: a review of 40 cases, Clin Exp Dermatol 1992; 17:257.

87. V, Dooren-Greebe, et al: Methotrexate revisited: effects of long-term treatment in psoriasis, Br J Dermatol 1994; 130:204.

88. Olsen EA: The pharmacology of methotrexate, J Am Acad Dermatol 1991; 25:306.

89. Casserly CM, et al: Severe megaloblastic anemia in a patient receiving low-dose methotrexate for psoriasis, J Am Acad Dermatol 1993; 29:477.

90. Morris LF, et al: Methotrexate and reproduction in men: case report and recommendations, J Am Acad Dermatol 1993; 29:913.

91. Duhra P: Treatment of gastrointestinal symptoms associated with methotrexate therapy for psoriasis, J Am Acad Dermatol 1993; 28:466.

92. Hills RJ, Ive FA: Folinic acid rescue used routinely in psoriatic patients with known methotrexate "sensitivity," Acta Derm Venereol 1992; 72:438.

93. Roenigk HH, Jr, et al: Methotrexate in psoriasis: revised guidelines, J Am Acad Dermatol 1988; 19:145.

94. Zachariae H, Kragballe K, Sogaard H: Methotrexate-induced liver cirrhosis, Br J Dermatol 102; 07:1980.

95. Kremer JM, et al: Clinical, laboratory, radiologic, and histopathologic features of methotrexate-associated lung injury in patients with rheumatoid arthritis: a multicenter study with literature review, Arthritis Rheum 1997; 40:1829.

96. Alarcon G, et al: Risk factors for methotrexate-induced lung injury in patients with rheumatoid arthritis: a multicenter, case-control study. Methotrexate-Lung Study Group, Ann Intern Med 1997; 127(5):356.

97. Khan A, et al: Methotrexate and the photodermatitis reactivation reaction: a case report and review of the literature, Cutis 2000; 66(5):379.

98. Guzzo C, Kaidby K: Recurrent recall of sunburn by methotrexate, Photodermatol Photoimmunol Photomed 1995; 11(2):55.

99. Perry W: Methotrexate and teratogenesis, Arch Dermatol 1983; 119(11):874.

100. Mayall B, et al: Neutropenia due to low-dose methotrexate therapy for psoriasis and rheumatoid arthritis may be fatal, Med J Aust 1991; 155:480.

101. King HW, et al: Near fatal drug interactions with methotrexate given for psoriasis, Lancet 1987; 295:752.

102. Roenigk H, et al: Methotrexate in psoriasis: consensus conference, J Am Acad Dermatol 1998; 38(3):478.

103. Lebwohl M, et al: Consensus conference: acitretin in combination with UVB or PUVA in the treatment of psoriasis, J Am Acad Dermatol 2001; 45(4):544.

104. Gronhoj LF, et al: Acitretin is converted to etretinate only during concomitant alcohol intake, Br J Dermatol 2000; 143(6):1164.

105. Katz H, Waalen J, Leach E: Acitretin in psoriasis: an overview of adverse effects, J Am Acad Dermatol 1999; 41(3 Pt 2):S7.

106. Honigsmann H, Wolff K: Isotretinoin-PUVA for psoriasis, Lancet 1983; 1(8318):236.

107. Roenigk R, Gibstine C, Roenigk H: Oral isotretinoin followed by psoralens and ultraviolet A or ultraviolet B for psoriasis, J Am Acad Dermatol 1985;13(1):153.

108. Lebwohl M, et al: Cyclosporine consensus conference: with emphasis on the treatment of psoriasis, J Am Acad Dermatol 1998; 39(3):464.

109. Ho V, et al: Intermittent short courses of cyclosporine microemulsion for the long-term management of psoriasis: a 2-year cohort study, J Am Acad Dermatol 2001; 44(4):643.

110. Koo J: Systemic sequential therapy of psoriasis: a new paradigm for improved therapeutic results, J Am Acad Dermatol 1999; 41(3 Pt 2):S25.

111. Singri P, West D, Gordon K: Biologic therapy for psoriasis: the new therapeutic frontier, Arch Dermatol 2002; 138(5):657.

112. Mason C, Krueger G: Thioguanine for refractory psoriasis: a 4-year experience, J Am Acad Dermatol 2001; 44(1):67.

113. Gupta A, et al: Sulfasalazine improves psoriasis: a double-blind analysis, Arch Dermatol 1990; 126(4):487.

114. Ameen M, Smith H, Barker J: Combined mycophenolate mofetil and cyclosporin therapy for severe recalcitrant psoriasis [In Process Citation], Clin Exp Dermatol 2001; 26(6): 480.

115. Davison S, et al: Change of treatment from cyclosporin to mycophenolate mofetil in severe psoriasis, Br J Dermatol 2000; 143(2):405.

116. Paul B, et al: Combined methotrexate—ultraviolet B therapy in the treatment of psoriasis, J Am Acad Dermatol 1982; 7(6):758.

117. Zackheim H, et al: 6-Thioguanine treatment of psoriasis: experience in 81 patients, J Am Acad Dermatol 1994; 30(3):452.

118. Magro C, Crowson A: The clinical and histomorphological features of pityriasis rubra pilaris: a comparative analysis with psoriasis, J Cutan Pathol 1997; 24(7):416.

119. Griffiths WA: Pityriasis rubra pilaris: the problem of its classification, J Am Acad Dermatol 1992; 26:140.

120. Auffret N, et al: Pityriasis rubra pilaris in a patient with human immunodeficiency virus infection, J Am Acad Dermatol 1992; 27:260.

121. Blauvelt A, et al: Pityriasis rubra pilaris and HIV infection, J Am Acad Dermatol 1991; 24:703.

122. Sonnex TS, et al: The nails in adult type 1 pityriasis rubra pilaris: a comparison with Sezary syndrome and psoriasis, J Am Acad Dermatol 1986; 15:956.

123. Griffiths WAD: Pityriasis rubra pilaris: an historical approach. II. Clinical features, Clin Exp Dermatol 1976; 1:37.

124. Dicken CH: Treatment of classic pityriasis rubra pilaris, J Am Acad Dermatol 1994; 31:997.

125. Dicken CH: Isotretinoin treatment of pityriasis rubra pilaris, J Am Acad Dermatol 1987;16:297.

126. Herbst R, et al: Combined ultraviolet A1 radiation and acitretin therapy as a treatment option for pityriasis rubra pilaris, Br J Dermatol 2000; 142(3):574.

127. Kirby B, Watson R: Pityriasis rubra pilaris treated with acitretin and narrow-band ultraviolet B (Re-TL-01), Br J Dermatol 2000; 142(2):376.

128. Clayton B, et al: Adult pityriasis rubra pilaris: a 10-year case series, J Am Acad Dermatol 1997; 36(6 Pt 1):959.

129. Griffiths WAD: Vitamin A and pityriasis rubra pilaris, J Am Acad Dermatol 1982; 7:555.

130. Murry JC, Gilgor RS, Lazarus GS: Serum triglyceride elevation following high-dose vitamin A treatment for pityriasis rubra pilaris, Arch Dermatol 1983;119:675.

131. Usuki K, et al: Three cases of pityriasis rubra pilaris successfully treated with cyclosporin A, Dermatology 2000; 200(4):324.

132. Brice SL, Spencer SK: Stanozolol in the treatment of pityriasis rubra pilaris, Arch Dermatol 1985;121:1105.

133. Green CA, Farr PM, Shuster S: Treatment of seborrhoeic dermatitis with ketoconazole. II. Response of seborrhoeic dermatitis of the face, scalp and trunk to topical ketoconazole, Br J Dermatol 1987; 116:217.

134. Parsad D, et al: Topical metronidazole in seborrheic dermatitis—a double-blind study, Dermatology 2001; 202(1):35.

135. Parsons JM: Pityriasis rosea update: 1986, J Am Acad Dermatol 1986; 15:159.

136. Kempf W, et al: Pityriasis rosea is not associated with human herpesvirus 7, Arch Dermatol 1999; 135(9):1070.

137. Chuang T-Y, et al: Pityriasis rosea in Rochester, Minnesota, 1969 to 1978: a 10-year epidemiologic study, J Am Acad Dermatol 1982; 7:80.

138. Sharma P, et al: Erythromycin in pityriasis rosea: a double-blind, placebo-controlled clinical trial, J Am Acad Dermatol 2000;42(2 Pt 1):241.

139. Tay Y, Goh C: One-year review of pityriasis rosea at the National Skin Centre, Singapore, Ann Acad Med Singapore 1999; 28(6):829.

140. Kay MH, Rapini RP, Fritz KA: Oral lesions in pityriasis rosea, Arch Dermatol 1985; 121:1449.

141. Vidimos AT, Camisa C: Tongue and cheek: oral lesions in pityriasis rosea, Cutis 1992; 50:276.

142. Pierson JC, et al: Purpuric pityriasis rosea, J Am Acad Dermatol 1993; 28:1021.

143. Horn T, Kazakis A: Pityriasis rosea and the need for a serologic test for syphilis, Cutis 1987; 39:81.

144. Arndt KA, et al: Treatment of pityriasis rosea with UV radiation, Arch Dermatol 1983; 119:381.

145. Leenutaphong V, Jiamton S: UVB phototherapy for pityriasis rosea: a bilateral comparison study, J Am Acad Dermatol 1995; 33(6):996.

146. Irvine C, et al: Long-term follow-up of lichen planus, Acta Derm Venereol 1991;71:242.

147. Kofoed ML, Wantzin GL: Familial lichen planus, J Am Acad Dermatol 1985; 13:50.

148. Halevy S, Shai A: Lichenoid drug eruptions, J Am Acad Dermatol 1993; 29:249.

149. Grotty CP, Daniel SU, W.P., Winkelmann RK: Ulcerative lichen planus: follow-up of surgical excision and grafting, Arch Dermatol 1980; 116:1252.

150. Matta M, et al: Lichen planopilaris: a clinicopathologic study, J Am Acad Dermatol 1990; 22:594.

151. Mehregan DA, et al: Lichen planopilaris: clinical and pathologic study of forty-five patients, J Am Acad Dermatol 1992; 27:935.

152. Ioannides D, Bystryn JC: Immunofluorescence abnormalities in lichen planopilaris, Arch Dermatol 1992; 128:214.

153. Silverman S, Jr, Gorsky M, Lozada-Nur F: A prospective follow-up study of 570 patients with oral lichen planus: persistence, remission, and malignant association, Oral Surg Oral Med Oral Pathol 1985; 60:30.

154. Brown RS, et al: A retrospective evaluation of 193 patients with oral lichen planus, J Oral Pathol Med 1993; 22:69.

155. Vincent SD, et al: Oral lichen planus: the clinical, historical, and therapeutic features of 100 cases, Oral Surg Oral Med Oral Pathol 1990; 70:165.

156. Eisen D: The clinical features, malignant potential, and systemic associations of oral lichen planus: a study of 723 patients, J Am Acad Dermatol 2002; 46(2):207.

157. Eisen D:The vulvovaginal-gingival syndrome of lichen planus, Arch Dermatol 1994; 130:1379.

158. Romero M, et al: Clinical and pathological characteristics of oral lichen planus in hepatitis C-positive and -negative patients, Clin Otolaryngol 2002; 27(1):22.

159. Edwards L, Friedrich EG, Jr: Desquamative vaginitis: lichen planus in disguise, Obstet Gynecol 1988; 71:832.

160. Ridley CM: Chronic erosive vulval disease, Clin Exp Dermatol 1990; 15:245.

161. Eisen D: The vulvovaginal-gingival syndrome of lichen planus: the clinical characteristics of 22 patients, Arch Dermatol 1994; 130(11):1379.

162. Tosti A, et al: Nail lichen planus: clinical and pathologic study of twenty-four patients, J Am Acad Dermatol 1993; 28:724.

163. Firth NA, et al: Assessment of the value of immunofluorescence microscopy in the diagnosis of oral mucosal lichen planus, J Oral Pathol Med 1990; 19:295.

164. Laurberg G, et al: Treatment of lichen planus with acitretin: a double-blind, placebo-controlled study in 65 patients, J Am Acad Dermatol 1991; 24(3):434.

165. Lear J, English J: Erosive and generalized lichen planus responsive to azathioprine, Clin Exp Dermatol 1996; 21(1):56.

166. Ho VC, et al: Treatment of severe lichen planus with cyclosporine, J Am Acad Dermatol 1990; 22:64.

167. Gonzalez E, Momtaz TK, Freedman S. Bilateral comparison of generalized lichen planus treated with psoralens and ultraviolet A, J Am Acad Dermatol 1984; 10: 958.

168. Bergman J, Rico MJ: Tacrolimus clinical studies for atopic dermatitis and other conditions, Semin Cutan Med Surg 2001; 20:250.

169. Buajeeb W, Pobrurksa C, Kraivaphan P: Efficacy of fluocinolone acetonide gel in the treatment of oral lichen planus, Oral Surg Oral Med Oral Pathol Oral Radiol Endod 2000;89(1): 42.

170. Lozada-Nur F, Miranda C, Maliksi R: Double-blind clinical trial of 0.05% clobetasol propionate ointment in orabase and 0.05% fluocinonide ointment in orabase in the treatment of patients with oral vesiculoerosive diseases, Oral Surg Oral Med Oral Pathol 1994; 77(6):598.

171. Plemons JM, et al: Absorption of a topical steroid and evaluation of adrenal suppression in patients with erosive lichen planus, Oral Surg Oral Med Oral Pathol 1990;69:688.

172. Ferguson MM: Treatment of erosive lichen planus of the oral mucosa with depot steroids, Lancet 1977;2:771.

173. Silverman S, Lozada-Nur F, Magliorati C: Clinical efficacy of prednisone in the treatment of patients with oral inflammatory ulcerative diseases: a study of 55 patients, Oral Surg 1985; 59:360.

174. Beck H-I, Brandrup F: Treatment of erosive lichen planus with dapsone, Acta Derm Venereol (Stockh) 1986; 66:366.

175. Falk DK, Latour DL, King LE, Jr: Dapsone in the treatment of erosive lichen planus, J Am Acad Dermatol 1985; 12:567.

176. Eisen D: Hydroxychloroquine sulfate (Plaquenil) improves oral lichen planus: an open trial, J Am Acad Dermatol 1993; 28:609.

177. Silverman S, et al: A prospective study of findings and management in 214 patients with oral lichen planus, Oral Surg Oral Med Oral Pathol 1991; 72:665.

178. Lear J, English J: Erosive and generalized lichen planus responsive to azathioprine, Clin Exp Dermatol 1996; 21(1):56.

179. Eisen D, et al: Effect of topical cyclosporine rinse on oral lichen planus: a double-blind analysis, N Engl J Med 1990; 323:290.

180. Sieg P, et al: Topical cyclosporin in oral lichen planus: a controlled, randomized, prospective trial, Br J Dermatol 1995; 132(5):790.

181. Matthews RW, Scully C: Griseofulvin in the treatment of oral lichen planus: adverse drug reactions, but little beneficial effect, Ann Dent 1992; 51:10.

182. Karp DL, Cohen BA: Onychodystrophy in lichen striatus, Pediatr Dermatol 1993; 10:359.

183. Taieb A, el Y, A., et al: Lichen striatus: a Blaschko linear acquired inflammatory skin eruption, J Am Acad Dermatol 1991; 25:637.

184. Hauber K, et al: Lichen striatus: clinical features and follow-up in 12 patients, Eur J Dermatol 2000;10(7):536.

185. Yates VM, King CM, Dave VK: Lichen sclerosus et atrophicus following radiation therapy, Arch Dermatol 1985; 121:1044.

186. Berth-Jones J, et al: Lichen sclerosus et atrophicus: a review of 15 cases in young girls, Clin Exp Dermatol 1991; 16:14.

187. Helm KF, et al: Lichen sclerosus et atrophicus in children and young adults, Pediatr Dermatol 1991; 8:97.

188. Loening-Baucke V: Lichen sclerosus et atrophicus in children, Am J Dis Child 1991; 145:1058.

189. Barton PG, et al: Penile purpura as a manifestation of lichen sclerosus et atrophicus, Pediatr Dermatol 1993; 10:129.

190. Young SJ, et al: Lichen sclerosus, genital trauma and child sexual abuse, Aust Fam Physician 1993; 22:732.

191. Ridley CM: Lichen sclerosus et atrophicus, Arch Dermatol 1987 (editorial); 123:457.

192. Mallon E, et al: Circumcision and genital dermatoses, Arch Dermatol 2000; 136(3):350.

193. Weigand DA: Microscopic features of lichen sclerosus et atrophicus in acrochordons: a clue to the cause of lichen sclerosus et atrophicus? J Am Acad Dermatol 1993; 28:751.

194. Pride HB, Miller OF, Tyler QB: Penile squamous cell carcinoma arising from balanitis xerotica obliterans, J Am Acad Dermatol 1993; 29:469.

195. Powell J, et al: High incidence of lichen sclerosus in patients with squamous cell carcinoma of the penis, Br J Dermatol 2001; 145(1):85.

196. Chalmers RJG, et al: Lichen sclerosus et atrophicus: a common and distinctive cause of phimosis in boys, Arch Dermatol 1984; 120:1025.

197. Meffert JJ, Davis DM, Grimwood RE: Lichen sclerosus, J Am Acad Dermatol 1995; 32:393.

198. Cattaneo A, De M, A., et al: Clobetasol vs. testosterone in the treatment of lichen sclerosus of the vulvar region, Minerva Ginecol 1992; 44:567.

199. Bornstein J, et al: Clobetasol dipropionate 0.05% versus testosterone propionate 2% topical application for severe vulvar lichen sclerosus, Am J Obstet Gynecol 1998;178(1 Pt 1): 80.

200. Smith Y, Quint E: Clobetasol propionate in the treatment of premenarchal vulvar lichen sclerosus, Obstet Gynecol 2001; 98(4):588.

201. Gibbon K, Bewley A, Salisbury J: Labial fusion in children: a presenting feature of genital lichen sclerosus? Pediatr Dermatol 1999; 16(5):388.

202. Dahlman-Ghozlan K, Hedblad M, von KG: Penile lichen sclerosus et atrophicus treated with clobetasol dipropionate 0.05% cream: a retrospective clinical and histopathological study, J Am Acad Dermatol 1999; 40(3):451.

203. Liatsikos E, et al: Lichen sclerosus et atrophicus: findings after complete circumcision, Scand J Urol Nephrol 1997; 31(5):453.

204. Rettenmaier MA, et al: Treatment of cutaneous vulvar lesions with skinning vulvectomy, J Reproductive Med 1985; 30:478.

205. Windahl T, Hellsten S: Carbon dioxide laser treatment of lichen sclerosus et atrophicus, J Urol 1993; 150:868.

206. Stuart GC, et al: Laser therapy of vulvar lichen sclerosus et atrophicus, Can J Surg 1991; 34:469.

207. Breech L, Laufer M: Surgicel in the management of labial and clitoral hood adhesions in adolescents with lichen sclerosus, J Pediatr Adolesc Gynecol 2000; 13(1):21.

208. Bousema MT, et al: Acitretin in the treatment of severe lichen sclerosus et atrophicus of the vulva: a double-blind, placebo-controlled study, J Am Acad Dermatol 1994; 30:225.

209. Shieh S, Mikkola D, Wood G: Differentiation and clonality of lesional lymphocytes in pityriasis lichenoides chronica, Arch Dermatol 2001; 137(3):305.

210. Gelmetti C, et al: Pityriasis lichenoides in children: a long-term follow-up of eighty-nine cases, J Am Acad Dermatol 1990; 23:473.

211. Dereure O, Levi E, Kadin M: T-Cell clonality in pityriasis lichenoides et varioliformis acuta: a heteroduplex analysis of 20 cases, Arch Dermatol 2000; 136(12):1483.

212. Wood GS, et al: Immunohistology of pityriasis lichenoides et varioliformis acuta and pityriasis lichenoides chronica: evidence for their interrelationship with lymphomatoid papulosis, J Am Acad Dermatol 1987; 16:559.

213. Shieh S, Mikkola D, Wood G: Differentiation and clonality of lesional lymphocytes in pityriasis lichenoides chronica, Arch Dermatol 2001; 137(3):305.

214. Luberti AA, et al: Severe febrile Mucha-Habermann's disease in children: case report and review of the literature, Pediatr Dermatol 1991; 8:51.

215. Truhan AP, Hebert AA, Esterly NB: Pityriasis lichenoides in children: therapeutic response to erythromycin, J Am Acad Dermatol 1986; 15:66.

216. LeVine MJ: Phototherapy of pityriasis lichenoides, Arch Dermatol 1983; 119:378.

217. Powell FC, Muller SA: Psoralens and ultraviolet A therapy of pityriasis lichenoides, J Am Acad Dermatol 1984; 10:59.

Bacterial Infections

❑ **Skin infections**
Impetigo
Ecthyma
Cellulitis and erysipelas
Cellulitis of specific areas
Necrotizing fasciitis

❑ **Folliculitis**
Staphylococcal folliculitis
Keratosis pilaris
Pseudofolliculitis barbae (razor bumps)
Sycosis barbae
Acne keloidalis

❑ **Furuncles and carbuncles**
Location
Bacteria
Predisposing conditions
Recurrent furunculosis

❑ **Erysipeloid**

❑ **Blistering distal dactylitis**

❑ **Staphylococcal scalded skin syndrome**

❑ ***Pseudomonas aeruginosa* infection**
Pseudomonas folliculitis
Pseudomonas hot-foot syndrome
Pseudomonas cellulitis
External otitis
Malignant external otitis
Toe web infection
Ecthyma gangrenosum

❑ **Meningococcemia**
Transmission
Incidence
Pathophysiology

❑ **Nontuberculous mycobacteria**
M. ulcerans, M. fortuitum, M. chelonei, and
M. avium-intracellulare

Skin Infections

The two gram-positive cocci, *Staphylococcus aureus* and the group A beta-hemolytic streptococci, account for the majority of skin and soft tissue infections. The streptococci are secondary invaders of traumatic skin lesions and cause impetigo, erysipelas, cellulitis, and lymphangitis. *S. aureus* invades skin and causes impetigo, folliculitis, cellulitis, and furuncles. Elaboration of toxins by *S. aureus* causes the lesions of bullous impetigo and staphylococcal scalded skin syndrome.

Impetigo

Impetigo is a common, contagious, superficial skin infection that is produced by streptococci, staphylococci, or a combination of both bacteria. There are two different clinical presentations: bullous impetigo and nonbullous impetigo. Both begin as vesicles with a very thin, fragile roof consisting only of stratum corneum. Bullous impetigo is primarily a staphylococcal disease. Nonbullous impetigo was once thought to be primarily a streptococcal disease, but staphylococci are isolated from the majority of lesions in both bullous and nonbullous impetigo. *S. aureus* is now known to be the primary pathogen in both bullous and nonbullous impetigo.[1]

Children in close physical contact with each other have a higher rate of infection than do adults. Symptoms of itching and soreness are mild; systemic symptoms are infrequent. Impetigo may occur after a minor skin injury such as an insect bite, but it most frequently develops on apparently unimpaired skin. The disease is self-limiting, but when untreated it may last for weeks or months. Poststreptococcal glomerulonephritis may follow impetigo. Rheumatic fever has not been reported as a complication of impetigo.

Bullous impetigo

Bullous impetigo (staphylococcal impetigo) is caused by an epidermolytic toxin produced at the site of infection, most commonly by staphylococci of phage group II, and usually is not secondarily contaminated by streptococci. The toxin causes intraepidermal cleavage below or within the stratum granulosum.

CLINICAL MANIFESTATIONS. Bullous impetigo is most common in infants and children but may occur in adults. It typically occurs on the face, but it may infect any body surface. There may be a few lesions localized in one area, or the lesions may be so numerous and widely scattered that they resemble poison ivy. One or more vesicles enlarge rapidly to form bullae in which the contents turn from clear to cloudy. The center of the thin-roofed bulla collapses, but the peripheral area may retain fluid for many days in an inner tube-shaped rim. A thin, flat, honey-colored, "varnishlike" crust may appear in the center and, if removed, discloses a bright red, inflamed, moist base that oozes serum. The center may dry without forming a crust, leaving a red base with a rim of scale. In most cases, a tinea-like scaling border replaces the fluid-filled rim as the round lesions enlarge and become contiguous with the others (Figures 9-1 to 9-5). The border dries and forms a crust. The lesions have little or no surrounding erythema. In some untreated cases, lesions may extend radially and retain a narrow, bullous, inner tube rim. These individual lesions reach 2 to 8 cm and then cease to enlarge, but they may remain for months (Figure 9-5). Thick crust accumulates in these longer lasting lesions. Lesions heal with hyperpigmentation in black patients. Regional lymphadenitis is uncommon with pure staphylococcal impetigo. There is some evidence that the responsible staphylococci colonize in the nose and then spread to normal skin before infection.

Serious secondary infections (e.g., osteomyelitis, septic arthritis, and pneumonia) may follow seemingly innocuous superficial infections in infants.

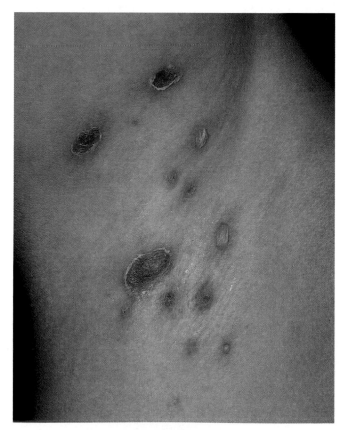

Figure 9-1 Lesions are present in all stages of development. Bullae rupture, exposing a lesion with an eroded surface and a peripheral scale.

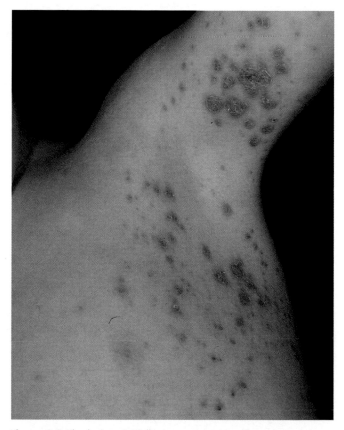

Figure 9-2 The lesions initially were present on the arm and autoinoculated the chest.

BULLOUS IMPETIGO

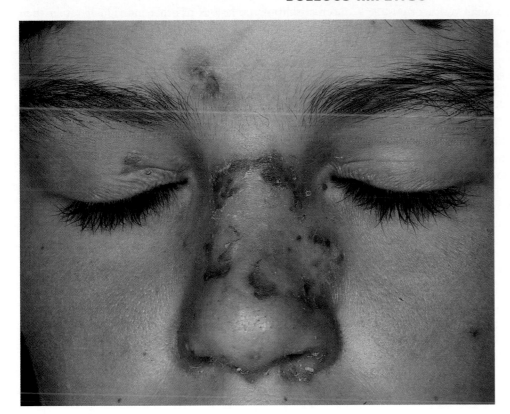

Figure 9-3 Bullae have collapsed and disappeared. The lesion is in the process of peripheral extension. Note involvement of both nares.

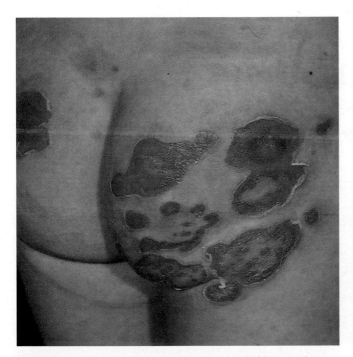

Figure 9-4 Huge lesions with a glistening, eroded base and a collarette of moist scale.

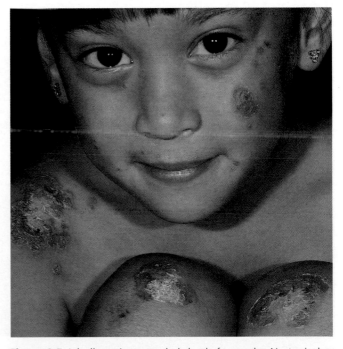

Figure 9-5 A bullous rim extended slowly for weeks. No topical or oral treatment had been attempted.

Nonbullous impetigo

Nonbullous impetigo originates as a small vesicle or pustule that ruptures to expose a red, moist base. A honey-yellow to white-brown, firmly adherent crust accumulates as the lesion extends radially (Figures 9-6 to 9-9). There is little surrounding erythema. Satellite lesions appear beyond the periphery. The lesions are generally asymptomatic. The skin around the nose and mouth and the limbs are the sites most commonly affected. The palms and soles are not affected. Untreated cases last for weeks and may extend in a continuous manner to involve a wide area (see Figure 9-7). Most lesions heal without scarring. The sequence of events leading to nonbullous impetigo is exposure to the infectious agent, carriage on exposed normal skin, and finally skin infection after a minor trauma that is aggravated by scratching. The infecting strain has been found on normal skin surfaces 2 or more weeks before the appearance of lesions.

Intact skin is resistant to colonization or infection with group A beta-hemolytic streptococci, but skin injury by insect bites, abrasions, lacerations, and burns allows the streptococci to invade. A pure culture of group A beta-hemolytic streptococci may sometimes be isolated from early lesions, but most lesions promptly become contaminated with staphylococci.[2] Regional lymphadenopathy is common. The reservoirs for streptococcus infection include the unimpaired normal skin or the lesions of other individuals rather than the respiratory tract.[3] Children ages 2 to 5 years commonly have streptococcal impetigo. Warm, moist climates and poor hygiene are predisposing factors. The antistreptolysin O (ASO) titer does not increase to a significant level following impetigo. Anti-DNAase B increases to high levels and is a much more sensitive indicator of streptococcal impetigo.

Acute nephritis

Acute nephritis tends to occur when many individuals in a family have impetigo.

Poststreptococcal glomerulonephritis (PSGN) usually develops 1 to 3 weeks following acute infection with specific nephritogenic strains of group A beta-hemolytic streptococcus. The overall incidence of acute nephritis with impetigo varies between 2% and 5%, but, in the presence of a nephritogenic strain of streptococcus, the rate varies between 10% and 25%.

PSGN occurs at any age but usually develops in children. Outbreaks in children aged 6 to 10 years are common. Infants younger than 1½ years of age are rarely affected by nephritis following impetigo. Asymptomatic episodes of PSGN exceed symptomatic episodes by a ratio of 4:1.

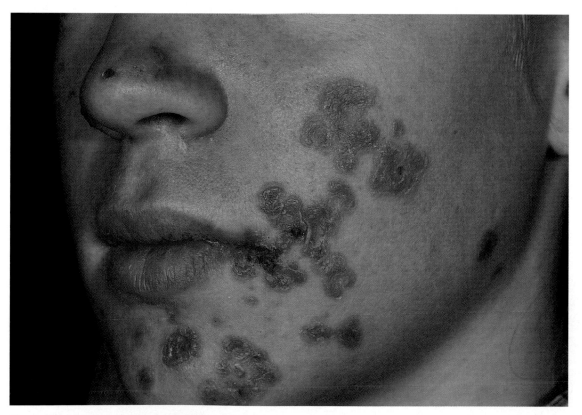

Figure 9-6 Impetigo. A thick, honey-yellow adherent crust covers the entire eroded surface.

PSGN is characterized by the onset of hematuria and proteinuria, often accompanied by decreased glomerular filtration rate and renal salt and water retention. The overall incidence and clinical features of acute nephritis[4] are as follows. Hematuria occurs in 90% of patients. Gross hematuria occurs in 25% of patients, followed by microscopic hematuria with erythrocyte casts and proteinuria that last for a variable time. Edema occurs in the majority of patients; the degree varies with the amount of dietary sodium. In the early morning, there is periorbital edema and lower extremity swelling. Hypertension occurs in 60% of patients; adults have moderate elevation of 160/100 mm Hg; in children, blood pressure readings are close to normal. The degree of hypertension varies with dietary sodium. Cerebral symptoms (headache and disturbance of consciousness), congestive heart failure, and acute renal failure are less common.

The presence of red cell casts are almost pathognomonic. Low C3 levels occur in most patients. In patients with skin infection, anti-DNase B titers increase and are more sensitive than antistreptolysin O (which remain low). Renal biopsy may be important for prognosis and therapy. Treatment for renal disease is supportive. Prognosis of acute PSGN is excellent in children. Most patients begin resolution of fluid retention and hypertension in 1 or 2 weeks. Proteinuria may persist for 6 months and microscopic hematuria for up to 1 year. Rapidly progressive renal failure develops in a few patients. Immunity to type M protein is type-specific; therefore, repeated episodes of PSGN are unusual.

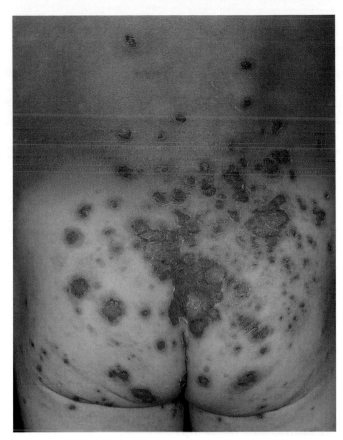

Figure 9-7 Impetigo. Widespread dissemination followed 3 weeks of treatment with a group IV topical steroid.

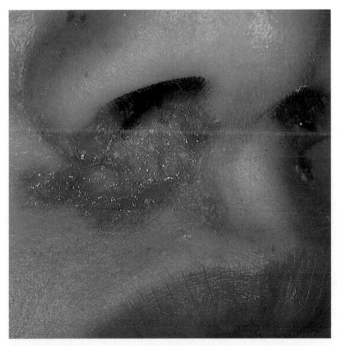

Figure 9-8 Serum and crust about the nostrils is a common presentation for impetigo.

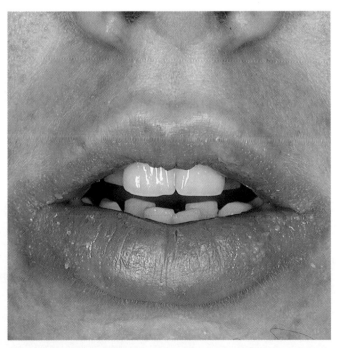

Figure 9-9 Impetigo. Serum and crust at the angle of the mouth is a common presentation for impetigo.

LABORATORY FINDINGS. Diagnosis is based on history and clinical appearance. Culture is not routinely performed. Gram-stained smears of vesicles show gram-positive cocci. Culture of exudate beneath an unroofed crust reveals group A streptococci, *S. aureus,* or a mixture of streptococci and *S. aureus.* Evidence of previous streptococcal skin infection in patients with acute glomerulonephritis is accomplished by obtaining antideoxyribonuclease B (anti-DNase B) and anti-hyaluronidase (AH) titers. More than 90% of patients with impetigo-associated acute poststreptococcal glomerulonephritis have increased anti-DNase B titers.[5]

The anti-streptolysin O titer after streptococcal impetigo is low or absent. Total serum complement activity is low during the initial stages of acute nephritis. The C3 level parallels the total serum complement. The sedimentation rate parallels the activity of the disease. C-reactive protein is usually normal. Cultures of the pharynx and any skin lesion should be made, and the serotype of the group A streptococcus that is responsible should be determined by typing with M-group and T-type antisera. M-T serotypes associated with acute nephritis are 2, 49, 55, 57, and 60.

Acute nephritis heals without therapeutic intervention. Symptoms and signs such as hypertension should be managed as they occur.

Prevention of impetigo
Mupirocin (Bactroban) or triple antibiotic ointment, containing bacitracin, Polysporin, and neomycin, applied three times daily to sites of minor skin trauma (e.g., mosquito bites and abrasions) can be efficacious as a preventative treatment.[6]

Recurrent impetigo
Patients with recurrent impetigo should be evaluated for carriage of *S. aureus.* The nares are the most common sites of carriage, but the perineum, axillae, and toe webs may also be colonized. Mupirocin ointment or cream (Bactroban) applied to the nares twice each day for 5 days significantly reduces *S. aureus* carriage in the nose and hands at 3 days and in the nasal carriage for as long as 1 year.[7]

Treatment of impetigo
Impetigo may resolve spontaneously or become chronic and widespread. Studies show that 2% mupirocin ointment is as safe and effective as oral erythromycin in the treatment of patients with impetigo.[8] Local treatment does not treat lesions that evolve in other areas. Infected children should be briefly isolated until treatment is under way.

ORAL ANTIBIOTICS. Because some cases of impetigo have a mixed infection of staphylococci and streptococci, penicillin is inadequate for treatment.[9] A 5- to 10-day course of an oral antibiotic such as dicloxacillin, or cephalosporins (e.g., cephalexin, cefadroxil) induces rapid healing.

MUPIROCIN (BACTROBAN). Mupirocin ointment or cream is the first topical antibiotic approved for the treatment of impetigo. It is active against staphylococci (including methicillin-resistant strains) and streptococci. The drug is not active against *Enterobacteriaceae, Pseudomonas aeruginosa,* or fungi. It is as effective as oral antibiotics and is associated with fewer adverse effects.[10] In superficial skin infections that are not widespread, mupirocin ointment offers several advantages. It is highly active against the most frequent skin pathogens, even those resistant to other antibiotics, and the topical route of administration allows delivery of high drug concentrations to the site of infection.[7] Mupirocin is applied three times a day until all lesions have cleared. If topical treatment is elected, then it might be worthwhile to wash the involved areas once or twice a day with an antibacterial soap such as Hibiclens or Betadine. Washing the entire body with these soaps may prevent recurrence at distant sites. Crusts should be removed because they block the penetration of antibacterial creams. To facilitate removal, soften crusts by soaking with a wet cloth compress.

Ecthyma
Ecthyma is characterized by ulcerations that are covered by adherent crusts. Poor hygiene is a predisposing factor. Ecthyma has many features similar to those of impetigo. The lesions begin as vesicles and bullae. They then rupture to form an adherent crust that covers an ulcer rather than the erosion of impetigo (see Figure 9-5). The lesion may remain fixed in size and resolve without treatment or may extend slowly, forming indolent ulcers with very thick, oyster shell-like crusts. This type of lesion occurs most commonly on the legs, where there are usually less than 10 lesions. Another more diffuse form occurs on the buttocks and legs of children who excoriate. Except for the thick crusts and underlying ulcers, the picture is approximately identical to diffuse streptococcal impetigo. Lesions heal with scarring. Ecthyma is initiated by group A beta-hemolytic streptococci but quickly becomes contaminated with staphylococci. This should be treated with a 10-day course of an oral antibiotic such as dicloxacillin or a cephalosporin such as cephalexin.

Cellulitis and erysipelas

Cellulitis and erysipelas are skin infections characterized by erythema, edema, and pain. In most instances there is fever and leukocytosis. Both may be accompanied by lymphangitis and lymphadenitis. Pathogens enter at sites of local trauma or abrasions and psoriatic, eczematous, or tinea lesions. Erysipelas involves the superficial layers of the skin and cutaneous lymphatics; cellulitis extends into the subcutaneous tissues.

Cellulitis is an infection of the dermis and subcutaneous tissue that is usually caused by a group A streptococcus and *S. aureus* in adults and *Haemophilus influenzae* type B in children younger than 3 years of age. Cellulitis is sometimes caused by other organisms. Cellulitis typically occurs near surgical wounds or a cutaneous ulcer or, like erysipelas, may develop in apparently normal skin. There is no clear distinction between infected and uninfected skin. Recurrent episodes of cellulitis occur with local anatomic abnormalities that compromise the venous or lymphatic circulation. The lymphatic system can be compromised by a previous episode of cellulitis, surgery with lymph node resection, and radiation therapy.

Erysipelas is an acute, inflammatory form of cellulitis that differs from other types of cellulitis in that lymphatic involvement ("streaking") is prominent. The area of inflammation is raised above the surrounding skin, and there is a distinct demarcation between involved and normal skin. The lower legs, face, and ears are most frequently involved.

Diagnosis of cellulitis

Recognizing the distinctive clinical features (erythema, warmth, edema, and pain) is the most reliable way of making an early diagnosis. Isolation of the etiologic agent is difficult and is usually not attempted. Fever, mild leukocytosis with a left shift, and a mildly increased sedimentation rate may be present. Patients with cellulitis of the leg often have a preexisting lesion, such as an ulcer or erosion that acts as a portal of entry for the infecting organism.[11]

ADULTS. In adults with no underlying disease, yields of cultures of aspirate specimens, biopsy specimens, and blood are low. In adults with underlying diseases (e.g., diabetes mellitus, hematologic malignancies, intravenous drug abuse, human immunodeficiency virus infection, chemotherapy) results of culture are more productive.[12] Cellulitis in these patients is often caused by organisms other than *S. aureus* or group A streptococcus, such as *Acinetobacter, Clostridium septicum, Enterobacter, Escherichia coli, H. influenzae, Pasteurella multocida, Proteus mirabilis, P. aeruginosa,* and group B streptococci. Cultures of entry sites, aspirate specimens, biopsy specimens, and blood facilitate the selection of the appropriate antibiotic for these patients.

CHILDREN. Identification of the infectious agents causing cellulitis is more successful in children. *H. influenzae* is the most common etiologic agent. Buccal infection is the most common presentation. Blood culture results were positive in 6.4%[13] to 78%[14] of reported cases. Cultures of needle aspirate specimens are more productive in children than in adults but are usually not attempted. The organism responsible for facial cellulitis can be isolated from cultures of wounds, blood, and throat or ear specimens.

CULTURE. Optimal methods for etiologic diagnosis in adults have not been delineated. Culture of the lesion is a more predictable source of information than more invasive procedures. Leading-edge and midpoint aspirates after saline injection and blood cultures are of little value in normal hosts.[11,15,16] A higher concentration of bacteria may be found at the point of maximal inflammation. Needle aspiration from the point of maximal inflammation yielded a 45% positive culture rate, compared with a 5% rate from leading-edge cultures.[17] Needle aspiration is performed by piercing the skin with a 20-gauge needle mounted on a tuberculin syringe. A 22-gauge needle is used for facial lesions. The needle is introduced into subcutaneous tissue. Suction is applied as the needle is withdrawn.

Treatment of cellulitis

ADULTS. The low yield of needle aspiration and the predictability of the organisms recovered mean that empiric treatment with antibiotics aimed at staphylococcal and streptococcal organisms is appropriate in adults. Treat with a penicillinase-resistant penicillin (dicloxacillin 500 to 1000 mg orally every 6 hours) or a cephalosporin. For more severe infections, an intravenous penicillinase-resistant penicillin such as nafcillin (500 to 1500 mg intravenously every 4 hours) or vancomycin should be used in persons allergic to penicillin. An aminoglycoside (gentamicin or tobramycin) should be considered in patients at risk for gram-negative infection. Some adults are infected with beta-lactamase–producing strains of *H. influenzae* type B (HIB) and require other appropriate antibiotics.[18] Pain can be relieved with cool Burrow's compresses. Elevation of the leg hastens recovery for lower leg infections.

CHILDREN. *H. influenzae* cellulitis therapy must be prompt. Be sure that gas formation and/or purulent collections are not present, because these lesions require aggressive surgical drainage and debridement. A decision must be made regarding the need for intubation or tracheotomy. Resistance rates to ampicillin vary from 5% to 30%. Cefotaxime and ceftriaxone are effective. Cephalosporins produce fewer drug-related side effects and provide good penetrance of cerebrospinal fluid (CSF).

H. influenzae type B can infect multiple members of a family and close contacts in day-care centers. Rifampin prophylaxis should be considered for the entire family of an index case where the household includes a child in the susceptible age group (younger than 4 years old), in a day-care classroom where a case of systemic *H. influenzae* type B disease has occurred, and in circumstances where one or more children younger than 2 years old have been exposed.[19]

Prevention of recurrent infection

Prolonged antimicrobial prophylaxis is effective and safe in preventing recurrent episodes of soft tissue infections and may be continued for months or years. An antimicrobial agent with activity against both streptococci and staphylococci is used; however, patients with recurrent disease may also respond to phenoxymethyl penicillin 250 to 500 mg twice a day. Low-dose oral clindamycin has been advocated for the prevention of recurrent staphylococcal skin infections[20] and might also be useful for the prevention of recurrent cellulitis.

Cellulitis of specific areas
Cellulitis and erysipelas of the extremities

Cellulitis of the extremities is most often caused by group A beta-hemolytic streptococci and is characterized by an expanding, red, swollen, tender-to-painful plaque with an indefinite border that may cover a small or wide area (Figures 9-10 and 9-11). Chills and fever occur as the red plaque spreads rapidly, becomes edematous, and sometimes develops bullae or suppurates. Less acute forms detected around a stasis leg ulcer spread slowly and may appear as an area of erythema with no swelling or fever. Erysipelas of the lower extremity is now more common than facial erysipelas. Group G streptococci may be a common pathogen, especially in patients older than 50 years.[21] Red, sometimes painful, streaks of lymphangitis may extend toward regional lymph nodes. Repeated attacks can cause impairment of lymphatic drainage, which predisposes the patient to more infection and permanent swelling. This series of events takes place most commonly in the lower legs of patients with venous stasis and ulceration. The end stage, which includes dermal fibrosis, lymphedema, and epidermal thickening on the lower leg, is called *elephantiasis nostras*.

TREATMENT. Treatment with oral or intravenous antibiotics should be started immediately and, if appropriate, altered according to laboratory results. The mean time for healing after treatment is initiated is 12 days, with a range of 5 to 25 days.[15] See the section on the treatment of cellulitis for more details.

TINEA PEDIS AND RECURRENT CELLULITIS OF THE LEG AFTER SAPHENOUS VENECTOMY. Tinea of the toe webs may predispose patients to cellulitis. Breaks in the dermal barrier caused by fungal infection may permit entry of bacteria through the skin. Recurrent cellulitis of the leg has been reported to occur following saphenous venectomy for coronary artery bypass grafting.[22] These patients have an acute onset of fever, erythema, and swelling of the leg arising months to years after coronary artery bypass surgery. Nongroup A beta-hemolytic streptococci (groups C, G, and B) have been implicated.[23] Tinea pedis has been observed on the foot of the infected leg. The fungal infection may be an important factor in the pathogenesis of the cellulitis. The cellulitis responds to the treatment measures outlined, and the fungal infection is treated topically or systemically as outlined in Chapter 13.

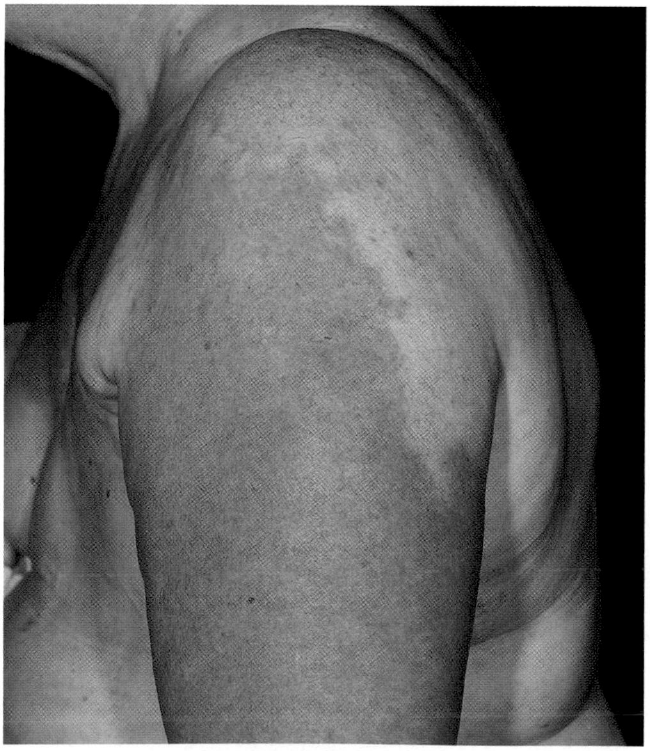

Figure 9-10 Cellulitis. Infected area is tender, deep red, and swollen.

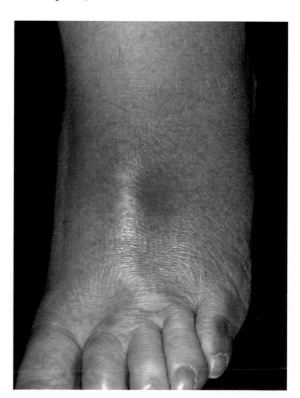

Figure 9-11 Cellulitis. There is erythema, edema, and tenderness.

Facial erysipelas and cellulitis in adults

ERYSIPELAS. The archaic term *St. Anthony's Fire* accurately describes the intensity of this eruption. Erysipelas is a superficial cellulitis with lymphatic involvement. Isolated cases are the rule; epidemic forms are rare. Facial sites have become rare but erysipelas of the legs is common. It may originate in a traumatic or surgical wound, but no portal of entry can be found in most cases. In the preantibiotic era, erysipelas was a feared disease with a significant mortality rate, particularly in infants. Most contemporary cases are of moderate intensity and have a benign course. In the majority of cases, group A streptococci are the responsible organisms. The second most frequent causative organism is group G streptococci.[21]

After prodromal symptoms that last from 4 to 48 hours and consist of malaise, chills, fever (101° to 104° F), and occasionally anorexia and vomiting, one or more red, tender, firm spots appear at the site of infection. These spots rapidly increase in size, forming a tense, red, hot, uniformly elevated, shining patch with an irregular outline and a sharply defined, raised border (Figure 9-12). As the process develops, the color becomes a dark, fiery red and vesicles appear at the advancing border and over the surface. Symptoms of itching, burning, tenderness, and pain may be moderate to severe. Without treatment, the rash reaches its height in approximately 1 week and subsides slowly over the next 1 or 2 weeks.

RECURRENCE. Recurrence after antibiotic treatment occurs in 18% to 30% of cases.[24] In particularly susceptible people, erysipelas may recur frequently for a long period and, by obstruction of the lymphatics, cause permanent thickening of the skin (lymphedema). Subsequent attacks may be initiated by the slightest trauma or may occur spontaneously to cause further irreversible skin thickening. The pinna and lower legs are particularly susceptible to this recurrent pattern (Figure 9-13).

TREATMENT. Treatment is the same as that for streptococcal cellulitis. Recurrent cases may require long-term prophylactic treatment with low-dose penicillin or erythromycin.[25] If other organisms are found on culture, a different agent is needed. See the section on the treatment of cellulitis for more details.

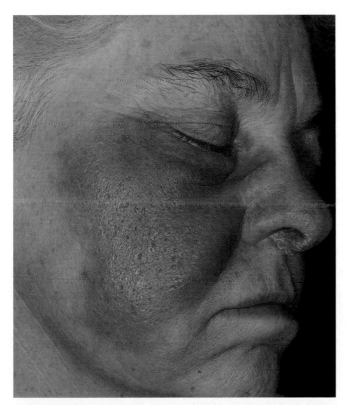

Figure 9-12 Erysipelas. Streptococcal cellulitis. The acute phase with intense erythema.

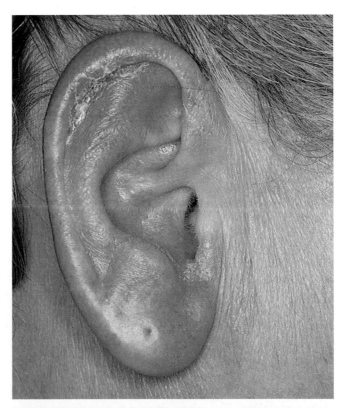

Figure 9-13 Erysipelas. Recurrent episodes of infection have resulted in lymphatic obstruction and caused permanent thickening of the skin.

Facial cellulitis in children

Facial cellulitis in children is potentially serious. Fever, irritability, and swelling and erythema of the cheek develop rapidly following 1 to 2 days of symptoms that are similar to those of an upper respiratory tract infection. Meningitis may occur.

The paramount factor in the evaluation of facial cellulitis is the presence or absence of a portal of entry. Patients older than 3 years of age who have a laceration, insect bite, eczema, dental infections, or other obvious trauma that might allow a portal of entry can be treated for staphylococcal and streptococcal infection. Children without an obvious portal of entry may be infected with *H. influenzae.*

H. INFLUENZAE TYPE B CELLULITIS.

The cellulitis is possibly caused either by local mouth trauma with subsequent soft tissue invasion or by lymphatic spread from ipsilateral otitis media. There is no obvious portal of entry. Infants are protected by maternal antibodies for the first few months of life. Children younger than 5 years of age are most susceptible. The child is typically between 6 months and 3 years of age. Symptoms usually develop after an upper respiratory infection with the rapid onset of a fever to 40° C. There is a unilateral, tender, warm, buccal discoloration, ranging from an intense erythema to a poorly demarcated violaceous hue ("bruised cheek syndrome") in approximately 50% of cases.[26] The color is not pathognomonic. Unilateral or bilateral otitis media is present in 68% of the patients. Meningitis is present in 8% of the infants, which in some cases is asymptomatic and requires lumbar puncture for demonstration. Therefore a lumbar puncture should be considered for all patients. Blood culture results are positive in 75% of the cases. Blood culture is the most sensitive test for identifying the organism. The organism may also be cultured from wounds (51%), middle ear fluid (96%), CSF (7.5%),[27] or the nasopharynx. Most cases of orbital cellulitis are associated with underlying ethmoid or maxillary sinusitis.[18] White blood counts are commonly more than 20,000 cells/mm³.

Treatment. See the section on the treatment of cellulitis on p. 273.

Cellulitis around the eye

Cellulitis around the eye is a potentially dangerous disease. Sinusitis is an important cause of these infections. Of patients who underwent radiographic evaluation, sinusitis was present in 96% of children with orbital cellulitis and 81% of patients with periorbital cellulitis.[28] Preseptal or periorbital cellulitis (infection anterior to the orbital septum) must be differentiated from infection within the orbit, which is referred to as postseptal or orbital cellulitis (behind the orbital septum). The orbital septum or palpebral fascia in the upper and lower eyelids is continuous with the periosteum of the superior and inferior margins of the orbit and inserts into the anterior surfaces of the tarsal plates. The orbital septum is the primary barrier that prevents inflammatory processes of the eyelid (preseptal) from extending posteriorly into the orbit. HIB vaccine was introduced in 1985. *H. influenzae* type B is no longer a significant pathogen in periorbital or orbital cellulitis.

Periorbital cellulitis

Periorbital cellulitis is much more common than orbital cellulitis and is limited to the eyelids in the preseptal region. It is more common in children. Sinusitis, upper respiratory infection,[29] and eye trauma are the most frequently encountered predisposing diseases. It is an acute inflammatory process associated with an increased temperature, erythema and edema of the eyelid, conjunctivitis, chemosis, normal vision, and the preservation of ocular motility (Figure 9-14). As with orbital cellulitis, staphylococci and streptococci are common pathogens in adults, and *H. influenzae* is prevalent in children. Periorbital cellulitis is rarely associated with central nervous system involvement. Routine lumbar puncture is not warranted in children 6 months of age or older unless there are clinical signs and symptoms of central nervous system involvement.[30]

TREATMENT. Adults with nonfebrile, nontoxic periorbital cellulitis can be treated with warm soaks and oral antibiotics. Young children should be treated aggressively to prevent progression to orbital cellulitis. Patients should be treated with intravenous cefuroxime, ceftriaxone or other broad-

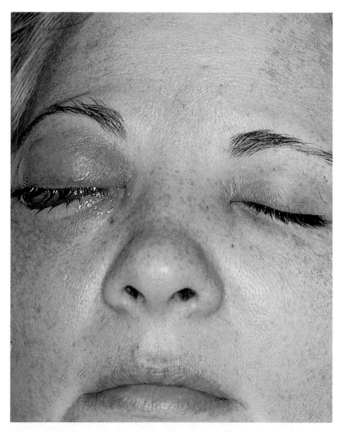

Figure 9-14 Periorbital cellulitis. An acute inflammatory process limited to the eyelids in the preseptal region. Patients are febrile. Erythema and edema of the eyelid, conjunctivitis, and chemosis occur. Sinusitis, upper respiratory infection, and eye trauma are common predisposing factors. *(Courtesy Shn R. Baker, M.D.)*

spectrum agents active against *H. influenzae* and various strains of *Streptococcus* and *Staphylococcus*. See the section on the treatment of cellulitis for more details.

Orbital cellulitis

Orbital cellulitis is an emergency. Proptosis, orbital pain, restricted movement of the eye, and chemosis occur in the majority of patients with this uncommon disease. The infection is most frequently attributed to acute sinusitis; in particular, involvement of the ethmoid and maxillary sinuses have been cited.[31] The infection spreads in two ways: direct extension and retrograde (thrombophlebitis/thromboembolism) along the valveless facial veins. Radiographic findings suggestive of sinusitis are present in 75% of patients. Visual disturbances occur in 56% of patients. *Staphylococcus* was isolated in a majority of cases in one series of adult patients.[32] *H. influenzae* is a common pathogen in children between the ages of 3 months and 4 years, and, when present, the blood culture results are positive in 10% to 60% of the cases.[33]

Complications included abscess formations, most of which are subperiosteal in location and well delineated by computed tomography (CT) scanning, persistent blindness, limitation of movement of the globe, and diplopia. Cavernous sinus thrombosis and brain abscess are rare complications.[34,35] Meningitis occurred in 1% of 214 children with periorbital and orbital cellulitis. Therefore lumbar puncture should not be a routine procedure in these patients.[36]

TREATMENT. Intravenous antibiotics are indicated for all patients. Cefuroxime is effective against all of the major etiologic agents and is especially effective against *H. influenzae*. Cefuroxime penetrates the CSF, thereby reducing the likelihood of secondary meningitis (see the section on the treatment of cellulitis for more details). The early use of CT to assess the extent of damage is important in establishing prognosis and in assessing the need for surgical therapy. CT is indicated when any degree of displacement of the globe is present or ophthalmoplegia or visual impairment is present. Serial assessment of the patient's visual acuity and ocular motility should be performed. Surgical intervention (exploration and decompression of the orbit) is indicated when there is CT evidence of intracranial involvement, a subperiosteal or orbital abscess, decreasing vision and worsening ocular motility, or the signs and symptoms do not rapidly improve over a 24- to 48-hour period in response to intravenous antibiotics.[37]

Perianal cellulitis

Cellulitis (group A beta-hemolytic streptococcus) around the anal orifice is often misdiagnosed as candidiasis. It occurs more frequently in children than adults. Bright, perianal erythema extends from the anal verge approximately 2 to 3 cm onto the surrounding perianal skin (Figure 9-15). Boys are affected more than girls. Symptoms include painful defecation (52%), tenderness, soilage from oozing, and, sometimes, blood-streaked stool and perianal itching (78%).[38,39] These children are not systemically ill. Pharyngitis may precede the infection. The differential diagnosis includes *Candida* intertrigo, psoriasis, pinworm infection, inflammatory bowel disease, a behavioral problem, and child abuse. Culture results confirm the diagnosis.

Initial treatment consists of a 10- to 14-day course of penicillin, amoxicillin-clavulanic acid, erythromycin, or other macrolides.[39] Relapses occurred in 39% of the patients.[40] After treatment, a new culture specimen should be taken to check for recurrence. The topical antibiotic mupirocin (Bactroban) may also provide rapid relief of symptoms, but systemic therapy is also required because it will treat any persistent oropharyngeal focus of streptococcal infection.

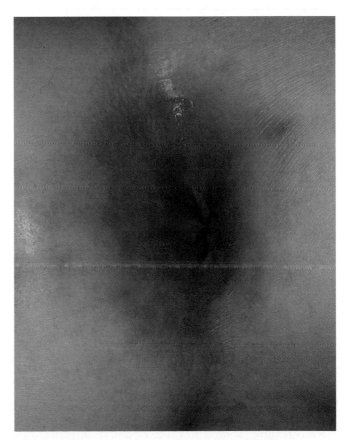

Figure 9-15 Perianal cellulitis (group A beta-hemolytic streptococcus). Bright perianal erythema extends from the anal verge approximately 2 to 3 cm onto the surrounding perianal skin. Candidiasis is usually accompanied by satellite pustules extending onto normal skin outside of the active border.

Pseudomonas *cellulitis*

Pseudomonas cellulitis is described in the section on *Pseudomonas* infection.

Necrotizing fasciitis

Necrotizing fasciitis (NF) is an infection of the subcutaneous tissue that results in the destruction of fascia and fat. The infection is most frequently polymicrobial. Ten percent of infections are caused by Group A streptococcus that can lead to toxic shock. NF most frequently occurs in the extremities, with a predilection for the lower leg. NF may mimic deep vein thrombosis. Predisposing factors include trauma (often trivial), burns, splinters, surgery, childbirth, diabetes mellitus, varicella, immunosuppression, renal failure, arteriosclerosis, odontogenic infection, malignancy, and alcoholism. Nonsteroidal antiinflammatory agents may alter the immune response, causing a minor infection to become fulminant.

Clinical manifestations

Initially there is pain, erythema, edema, cellulitis, and fever. Many patients are diagnosed with cellulitis and sent home; they return when the condition worsens. The most consistent clinical clue is unrelenting pain out of proportion to the physical findings even if there is only mild or no fever or erythema.[41] Typically there is diffuse swelling of an arm or leg and intense pain on palpation. One or 2 days after symptom onset, there are high fever, leukocytosis, edema with central patches of dusky blue discoloration, weeping blisters, and borders with cellulitis. Bullae with clear fluid rapidly turn violaceous. Septicemia may develop secondarily and should be strongly suspected in the presence of fever, anorexia, nausea, diarrhea, confusion, and hypotension. Progression to gangrene, sometimes with myonecrosis, and an extension of the inflammatory process along fascial planes are possible. Twenty-five percent will die of septic shock and organ failure.

Laboratory

Admission values of C-reactive protein and creatine kinase are higher for patients with group A beta-hemolytic streptococcal necrotizing fasciitis than for patients with cellulitis. Therefore standard laboratory tests may be useful for the early differential diagnosis of NF and cellulitis.[42]

Frozen tissue sections show massive polymorphonuclear fascial infiltrate. Most patients have a positive tissue culture result; in most cases there is more than one type of bacteria present. Streptococcal organisms are the most prevalent, but gram-negative and anaerobic bacteria are commonly found. Patients with no cutaneous evidence of infection but who have severe pain and swelling may benefit from measurements of muscle-compartment pressure. Increased compartment pressure contributes to extensive myonecrosis. Immediate fasciotomy is indicated if pressures are elevated (i.e., more than 40 mm Hg).

Imaging

CT, magnetic resonance imaging (MRI), and routine soft-tissue radiographs show soft-tissue swelling in deep tissues. CT or MRI is useful in locating the site and depth of infection. Gas may be present in clostridial and mixed aerobic/anaerobic infections. Gas is never present in group A streptococcal infections. An interpretation of soft-tissue swelling without evidence of gas may mislead the physician into thinking this is a benign process. Plain radiographs, CT, and ultrasound are useful in demonstrating the air bubbles in the soft tissues. Gas, if present, extends rapidly. When the area of abnormality on MRI is compared with the extent of infection revealed at the time of surgery, MRI generally overestimates the extent of disease presumably secondary to adjacent noninfectious edema.

Treatment

NF requires surgical debridement of necrotic tissue, antimicrobial agents, and wound and supportive care. Patients in whom the etiologic agents cannot be definitively identified should be treated with broad-spectrum antimicrobial regimens. Typical regimens include expanded-spectrum penicillins and cephalosporins, clindamycin, and aminoglycosides, in combinations suggested by the clinical manifestations and epidemiologic features of the case. Surgical exploration is indicated when the diagnosis of infection is in doubt and the patient is very ill. Surgery can establish a diagnosis by providing material for culture, Gram staining, and histopathologic examination. A diagnosis can be made at surgery with a "finger test." When the site is incised and the finger is inserted, the skin peels off easily at the subcutaneous fascia. Simple drainage, radical debridement, or amputation are the options for treatment. Intravenous immunoglobulin may be a useful adjunct in the treatment of streptococcal toxic shock syndrome associated with necrotizing fasciitis.[43]

Folliculitis

Folliculitis is inflammation of the hair follicle caused by infection, chemical irritation, or physical injury. Inflammation may be superficial or deep in the hair follicle. Folliculitis is very common and is seen as a component of a variety of inflammatory skin diseases, which are listed in Table 9-1.

In superficial folliculitis, the inflammation is confined to the upper part of the hair follicle. Clinically, it is manifested as a painless or tender pustule that eventually heals without scarring. In many instances, the hair shaft in the center of the pustule cannot be seen. Inflammation of the entire follicle or the deeper portion of the hair follicle initially appears as a swollen, red mass, which eventually may point toward the surface becoming a somewhat larger pustule than that seen in superficial folliculitis. Deeper lesions are painful and may heal with scarring.

Staphylococcal folliculitis

Staphylococcal folliculitis is the most common form of infectious folliculitis. One pustule or a group of pustules may appear, usually without fever or other systemic symptoms, on any body surface (Figure 9-16). Staphylococcal folliculitis may occur because of injury, abrasion, or nearby surgical wounds or draining abscesses. It may also be a complication of occlusive topical steroid therapy (Figure 9-17), particularly if moist lesions are occluded for many hours. Follicular pustules are cultured, not by touching the pustule with a cotton swab, but by scraping off the entire pustule with a no. 15 blade and depositing the material onto the cotton swab of a transport medium kit. Some cases can be treated with a tepid, wet Burrow's compress, but oral antibiotics are used in most cases.

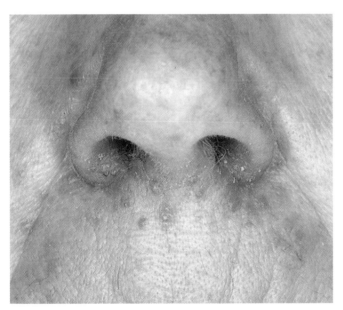

Figure 9-16 Staphylococcal folliculitis. The nares are a reservoir for *S. aureus*. Folliculitis may appear on the skin about the nose.

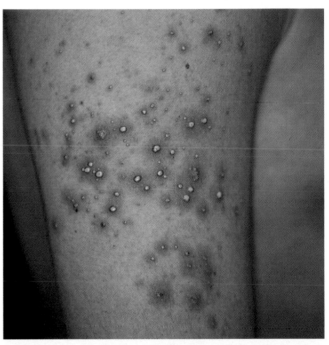

Figure 9-17 Staphylococcal folliculitis. Follicular pustules appeared after the patient's extremity had been occluded with a topical steroid and a plastic dressing for 24 hours. Gram-negative organisms may also flourish after long periods of plastic occlusion.

Table 9-1 Diseases Initially Manifesting in Folliculitis	
Superficial folliculitis	**Deep folliculitis**
Staphylococcal folliculitis	Furuncle and carbuncle
Pseudofolliculitis barbae (from shaving)	Sycosis (inflammation of the entire depth of the follicle)
Superficial fungal infections (dermatophytes)	Sycosis (beard area): sycosis barbae, bacterial or fungal
Cutaneous candidiasis (pustules also occur outside the hair follicle)	Sycosis (scalp): bacterial
Acne vulgaris	Acne vulgaris, cystic
Acne, mechanically or chemically induced	Gram-negative acne
Steroid acne after withdrawal of topical steroids	*Pseudomonas* folliculitis
Keratosis pilaris	Dermatophyte fungal infections

Keratosis pilaris

Keratosis pilaris is a common finding on the posterolateral aspects of the upper arms and anterior thighs. The eruption is probably more common in atopics (see p. 116). Clinically, a group of small, pinpoint, follicular pustules remains in the same area for years. Histologic studies show that the inflammation actually occurs outside of the hair follicle. Scratching, wearing tight-fitting clothing, or undergoing treatment with abrasives may infect these sterile pustules and cause a diffuse eruption (Figure 9-18). It is important to recognize this entity to avoid unnecessary and detrimental treatment. Many patients object to these small, sometimes unsightly bumps. Keratosis pilaris resists all types of treatment. Oral antibiotics active against *S. aureus* are used if folliculitis develops. Group V topical steroids provide temporary relief when the area becomes dry and inflamed. Urea creams (e.g., Vanamide) and lactic acid moisturizers (Lac-Hydrin, AmLactin) soften the skin.

Pseudofolliculitis barbae (razor bumps)

Pseudofolliculitis barbae (PFB) is a foreign body reaction to hair. Clinically, there is less inflammation than with staphylococcal folliculitis. The condition occurs on the cheeks and neck in individuals who are genetically inclined to have tightly curled, spiral hair, which can become ingrown (Figure 9-19). This condition is found in 50% to 75% of blacks and 3% to 5% of whites who shave. If cut below the surface by shaving, the sharp-tipped whisker may curve into the follicular wall or emerge and curve back to penetrate the skin. A tender, red papule or pustule occurs at the point of entry and remains until the hair is removed. Generally, the problem is more severe in the neck areas where hair follicles are more likely to be oriented at low angles to the skin surface, making repenetration of the skin more likely. Pseudofolliculitis can occur also in the axillae, pubic area, and legs. Normal bacterial flora may eventually be replaced by pathogenic organisms if the process becomes chronic. Pseudofolliculitis of the beard is a significant problem in the armed services (see Figure 9-19) and in professions in which individuals are required to shave.

Prevention and treatment

Programs for treatment and prevention are outlined in the Boxes 9-1 and 9-2. Wax depilation and tweezing may lead to transfollicular repenetration.[44] Electrolysis tends to be expensive, painful, and often unsuccessful. The only definitive cure is permanent removal of the hair follicle with laser-assisted hair removal.[45-47]

SHAVING TECHNIQUES. Use techniques that avoid close shaves and the production of sharply angled hair tips. Hydrating the beard before shaving by washing with soap and warm water softens the whiskers. The softened hairs are cut off directly, leaving a blunt hair and making ingrown hairs less likely. Use a highly lubricating shaving gel (e.g., Edge Gel). PFB Bumpfighter razor is a special razor that does not shave close. Shaving closely with multiple razor strokes and shaving against the grain should be avoided. Electric clippers that cut hair as stubble can be an alternative to wet shaving. Depilatories with barium sulfide (Magic Shave and Royal Crown Powders) or calcium thioglycolate (Nair lotion, Magic Shave Gold Powder, Surgex cream) are available in all pharmacies. They are an effective way of removing hair and preventing pseudofolliculitis. They are applied to the skin for 3 to 10 minutes and wiped off. The chemical reduces sulfide bonds in the cortex of the medulla of the hair shaft. The weakened hair fibers shear when the material is wiped off, leaving a soft, fluffy hair tip that is less likely to become ingrown. These products are irritating and can only be tolerated once or twice each week. If these measures fail, shaving must be discontinued indefinitely.

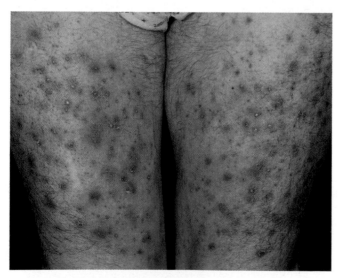

Figure 9-18 Keratosis pilaris and folliculitis. Keratosis pilaris is a common finding on the anterior thighs. A group of small, pinpoint, follicular pustules remains in the same areas for years. Scratching, wearing tight-fitting clothing, or treating with abrasives may infect these sterile pustules and cause a diffuse eruption.

PSEUDOFOLLICULITIS

A
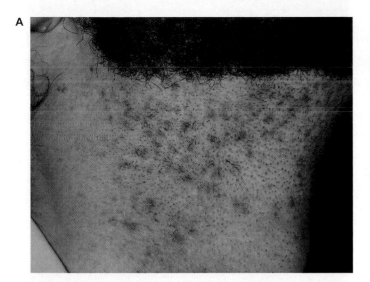

B
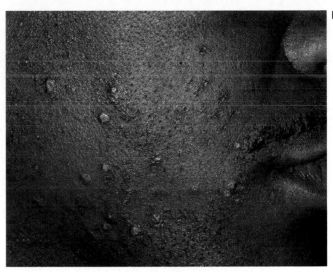

C
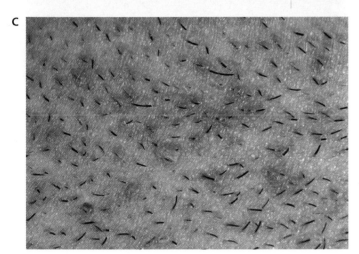

Figure 9-19 Pseudofolliculitis. **A,** Papules and pustules persist after shaving. **B,** PFB is found mostly in black males. Scarring and keloids may occur in chronic cases. **C,** Red papules occur with a hair shaft imbedded in its center.

Box 9-1 Program for Treating Pseudofolliculitis

1. Stop shaving, electrolysis, tweezing, depilatory use, and waxing. (PFB may worsen during the first week because of regrowth.)

2. Use a hair-releasing technique. Wash the beard for several minutes in a circular motion with a washcloth or toothbrush to dislodge ingrown hairs.

3. Dislodge imbedded hair shafts by inserting a firm, pointed instrument such as syringe needle under the hair loop and firmly elevating it.

4. A short course of antibiotics (e.g., tetracyclines, cephalosporins) may hasten resolution.

5. Corticosteroids (prednisone at 40 to 60 mg/day for 5 to 10 days) may be used in moderate to severe cases to reduce inflammation around the hair follicles until the hair grows and is no longer an aggravating factor.

6. Intralesional triamcinolone acetonide (2.5 to 10 mg/mL) is useful for red papules that linger.

Box 9-2 Program for Preventing Pseudofolliculitis

1. Wet beard with warm water. This hydrates the hair so that it cuts more easily and leaves a tip that is not sharp.

2. Use a soft-bristled toothbrush, in a circular motion, to dislodge hair tips that are piercing the skin. Do this before shaving and at bedtime. Use a sterile needle to dislodge stubborn tips of hair.

3. Reduce the closeness of the shave. Avoid close shaves with twin- and triple-blade razors.

4. Shave hair with electric clippers (e.g., Norelco, Braun, Remington) to a minimum length of 1 mm. Purchase at beauty supply stores or at www.electricshaver.com.

5. Shave with The Bumpfighter razor (American Safety Razor Co, Staunton, VA) (www.asrco.com), a single-edge blade with polymer coating and foil guard. This special razor cuts the hair at the correct length and prevents hair tip re-entry into the skin. Lather with a thick gel (e.g., Aveeno, Edge Gel, or Bump Fighter Shaving Gel). Avoid taut skin by not pulling it while shaving. Shave with the grain (i.e., in the direction of hair growth). Rinse blade after each shaving stroke to prevent the traction that occurs with build-up of hair between the blade and guard. Apply cool compresses after shaving.

6. Alternatively, use an electric razor, avoiding the "closest" shave setting. Razor can be ordered from Delasco, 608 13th Avenue, Council Bluffs, IA 51501-6401. 1-800-831-6273.

7. Apply a glycolic acid lotion (e.g., Nutraplus lotion) to reduce hyperkeratosis.

8. Consider use of chemical depilatories to remove hair.

*Adapted from: Crutchfield CE: Cutis 1998; 61:351, and Perry PK: J Am Acad Dermatol 2002; 46:S113.

Sycosis barbae

Sycosis implies follicular inflammation of the entire depth of the hair follicle and may be caused by infection with *S. aureus* or dermatophyte fungi. (See Chapter 13 on fungal infections for a discussion of fungal sycosis.) The disease occurs only in men who have commenced shaving. It begins with the appearance of small follicular papules or pustules and rapidly becomes more diffuse as shaving continues (Figures 9-20, 9-21, and 9-22). Reaction to the disease varies greatly among individuals. Infiltration about the follicle may be slight or extensive. The more infiltrated cases heal with scarring. In chronic cases, the pustules may remain confined to one area, such as the upper lip or neck. The hairs are epilated with difficulty in staphylococcal sycosis and with relative ease in fungal sycosis. Hairs should be removed and examined for fungi and the purulent material should be cultured. Fungal infections tend to be more severe, producing deeper and wider areas of inflammation; bacterial follicular infections usually present with discrete pustules. Pseudofolliculitis (see previous section) has a similar appearance.

Localized inflammation is treated topically with mupirocin (Bactroban ointment). Extensive disease is treated with oral antibiotics (e.g., dicloxacillin, cephalexin) for at least 2 weeks or until all signs of inflammation have cleared. Recurrences are not uncommon and require an additional course of oral antibiotics. Shaving should be performed with a clean razor.

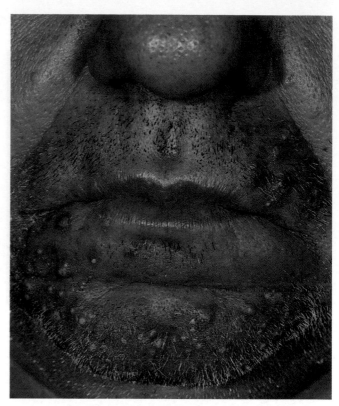

Figure 9-20 Sycosis barbae. Deep follicular pustules are concentrated in unshaved areas in this patient.

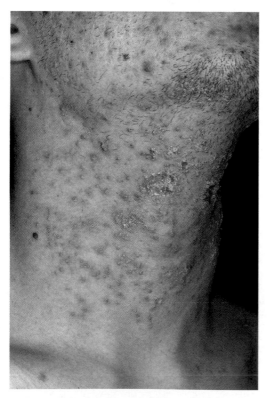

Figure 9-21 Sycosis barbae. An unusually extensive case involving the neck and face.

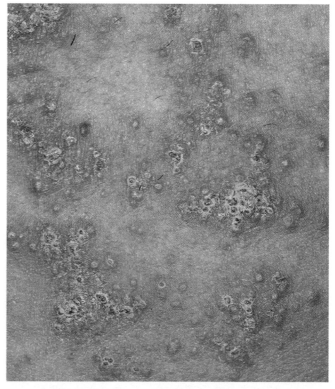

Figure 9-22 Sycosis barbae. Numerous pustules cleared rapidly with cephalexin 500 mg four times a day.

Acne keloidalis

Acne keloidalis is a primary form of scarring alopecia. The word acne is a misnomer. It is a chronic scarring folliculitis of unknown etiology located on the posterior neck that eventually results in the formation of a group of keloidal papules.[48] It occurs only in men and is more common in blacks. It may be initiated or aggravated by protective head devices.[49] Follicular papules or pustules (Figure 9-23) develop on the back of the neck. They coalesce into firm plaques and nodules. Histologically there is inflammation, fibroplasia, and disappearance of sebaceous glands.[50,51] The inflammatory stage may be asymptomatic. Extensive subclinical disease may be present and can account for some of the permanent hair loss. The patient eventually discovers a group of hard papules (Figure 9-24). The inflammatory stage lasts for months or years. The degree of inflammation varies from a group of discrete pustules to abscess formation on the entire back of the neck and scalp. Several hairs may protrude from a single follicle and look like tufted hair folliculitis.

Tufted hair folliculitis may not be a specific disease but secondary to progressive folliculitis like folliculitis decalvans, dissecting cellulitis, or acne keloidalis (p. 860).[52] Overgrowth of microorganisms does not appear to play an important role in the pathogenesis.

Treatment

A bacterial etiology has never been proven but acne keloidalis usually responds to short- or long-term courses of oral antibiotics. Different classes of antibiotics may have to be tried before control is achieved. Cephalosporins, trimethoprim-sulfamethoxazole (Bactrim, Septra), dicloxacillin, and amoxicillin-clavulanate potassium (Augmentin) have been successful in individual cases. Control with one antibiotic may diminish with time and the patient may have to be treated with a different antibiotic for continued long-term suppression. Topical steroid foams (Olux) applied bid in short courses may control inflammation and reduce the keloids. An intralesional injection of triamcinolone reduces the keloids, but this treatment should be delayed until infection has been controlled. Surgical excision may be necessary if persistent sinus tracts form. Successful surgical therapy of advanced cases can be carried out using a number of methods as long as subfollicular destruction of the process is achieved.[48] Excision with primary closure is an excellent surgical treatment for extensive and refractory cases. Extremely large lesions should be excised in multiple stages.[53,54]

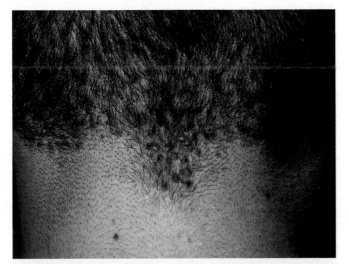

Figure 9-23 Deep folliculitis. Follicular pustules are surrounded by erythema and swelling. The entire follicular structure is inflamed. Staphylococci were isolated by culture.

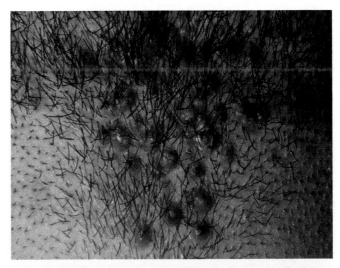

Figure 9-24 Acne keloidalis. Keloidal papules may eventually form on the back of the neck after chronic inflammation of the hair follicles.

Furuncles and Carbuncles

A furuncle (abscess or boil) is a walled-off collection of pus that is a painful, firm, or fluctuant mass. Cellulitis may precede or occur in conjunction with it. An abscess is a cavity formed by fingerlike loculations of granulation tissue and pus that extends outward along planes of least resistance. Furuncles are uncommon in children, but increase in frequency after puberty. Furunculosis occurs as a self-limited infection in which one or several lesions are present or as a chronic, recurrent disease that lasts for months or years, affecting one or several family members. Most patients with sporadic or recurrent furunculosis appear to be otherwise normal and have an intact immune system.

Location

Lesions may occur at any site but favor areas prone to friction or minor trauma, such as underneath a belt, the anterior thighs, buttocks, groin, axillae, and waist.

Bacteria

S. aureus is the most common pathogen. The infecting strain may be found during quiescent periods in the nares and perineum. There is evidence that the anterior nares are the primary site from which the staphylococcus is disseminated to the skin. Other organisms, either aerobic (*E. coli, P. aeruginosa, S. faecalis*) or anaerobic (*Bacteroides, Lactobacillus, Peptococcus, Peptostreptococcus*) may cause furuncles. In general, the microbiology of abscesses reflects the microflora of the anatomic part of the body involved. Anaerobes are found in perineal and in some head and neck abscesses. Perirectal- and perianal-region abscesses often are reflective of fecal flora. Approximately 5% of abscesses are sterile. Bacteria colonize the skin in patients with atopic dermatitis, eczema, and scabies.

Predisposing conditions

Occlusion of the groin and buttocks by clothing, especially in patients with hyperhidrosis, encourages bacterial colonization. Follicular abnormalities, evident by the presence of comedones and acneiform papules and pustules are often found on the buttocks and axillae of patients with recurrent furunculosis of those areas; these findings suggest the diagnosis of hidradenitis suppurativa (see p. 202).

Clinical manifestations

The lesion begins as a deep, tender, firm, red papule that enlarges rapidly into a tender, deep-seated nodule that remains stable and painful for days and then becomes fluctuant (Figure 9-25). The temperature is normal and there are no systemic symptoms. Pain becomes moderate to severe as purulent material accumulates. Pain is most intense in areas where expansion is restricted, such as the neck and external auditory canal. The abscess either remains deep and reabsorbs or points and ruptures through the surface. The abscess cavity contains a surprisingly large quantity of pus and white chunks of necrotic tissue. The point of rupture heals with scarring.

Carbuncles are aggregates of infected follicles. The infection originates deep in the dermis and the subcutaneous tissue, forming a broad, red, swollen, slowly evolving, deep, painful mass that points and drains through multiple openings. Malaise, chills, and fever precede or occur during the active phase. Deep extension into the subcutaneous tissue may be followed by sloughing and extensive scarring. Areas with thick dermis (i.e., the back of the neck, the back of the trunk, and the lateral aspects of the thighs) are the preferred sites. In the preantibiotic era, there were some fatalities.

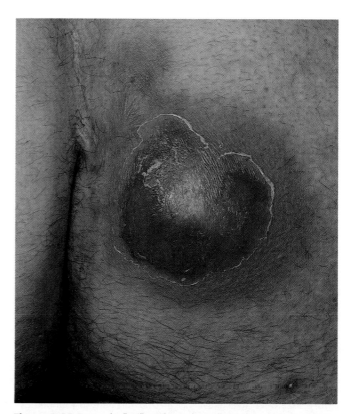

Figure 9-25 Furuncle (boil). Enlarged swollen mass with purulent material beginning to exude from several points on the surface.

Differential diagnosis

Several diseases can be manifested as a furuncle (Table 9-2). The most common structure that is misinterpreted as a furuncle is a pilar cyst of the scalp or ruptured epidermal cyst. The cyst wall ruptures spontaneously, leaking the white amorphous material into the dermis (Figure 9-26). An intense, foreign-body, inflammatory reaction occurs in hours, forming a sterile abscess. Treatment of a ruptured cyst consists of making a linear incision over the surface and evacuating the white material with manual pressure and a curette. Sometimes the cyst wall can be forced through the incision and cut out. In many cases the wall cannot be removed because it is fused to the dermis during the inflammatory process. Antibiotics are unnecessary.

Treatment of furuncles
Warm compresses

Many furuncles are self-limited and respond well to frequent applications of a moist, warm compress, which provide comfort and probably encourage localization and pointing of the abscess.

Incision, drainage, and packing

The primary management of cutaneous abscesses should be incision and drainage. In general, routine culture and antibiotic therapy are not indicated for localized abscesses in patients with presumably normal host defenses.[55] The abscess is not ready for drainage until the skin has thinned and the underlying mass becomes soft and fluctuant. The skin around the central area is anesthetized with 1% lidocaine. A pointed, lance-shaped no. 11 surgical blade is inserted and drawn parallel to skin lines through the thin, effaced skin, creating an opening from which pus may be expressed easily with light pressure. Care must be taken to avoid extending the incision into firm, noneffaced skin. A curette is inserted through the opening and carefully drawn back and forth to break adhesions and dislodge fragments of necrotic tissue. Continuous drainage may be promoted in very large abscesses by packing the cavity with a long ribbon of iodoform gauze. The end of the ribbon is inserted through a curette loop. The curette is then turned to secure the gauze, inserted deep into the cavity, twisted in the reverse direction and removed concurrently, while the gauze is held in place with a thin-tipped forceps. Next, the gauze is worked into the cavity with the forceps until resistance is met. The gauze quickly becomes saturated and should be removed hours later and replaced with a fresh packing.

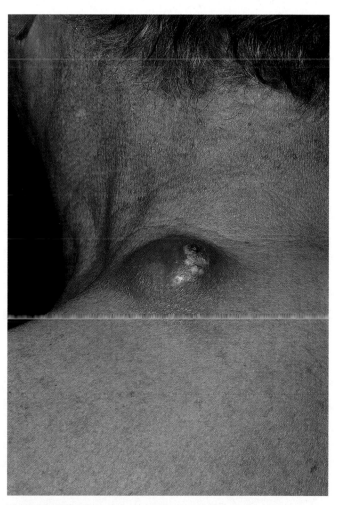

Figure 9-26 Ruptured epidermal cyst. This is commonly misinterpreted as a furuncle. A large mass of white, amorphous material and pus exudes after a linear incision is made over the surface.

Table 9-2 Disease Initially Manifesting as Furunculosis ("Boils")	
Disease	**Location**
Bacterial furunculosis	Any body surface
Recurrent furunculosis in scarred tissue	Buttock or any location
Ruptured epidermal cyst	Preauricular and postauricular areas, face, chest, back
Hidradenitis suppurativa	Axilla, groin, buttock, under breasts
Cystic acne	Face, chest, back
Primary immunodeficiency diseases*	Any body surface
Secondary immunodeficiency†	Any body surface
Others: diabetes, alcoholism, malnutrition, severe anemia, debilitation	Any body surface

*Syndrome of hyperimmunoglobulinemia E associated with staphylococcal abscesses (Job's syndrome), chronic granulomatous disease, Chédiak-Higashi syndrome, C3 deficiency, C3 hypercatabolism, transient hypogammaglobulinemia of infancy, immunodeficiency with thymoma, Wiskott-Aldrich syndrome.
†Leukemia, leukopenia, neutropenia, therapeutic immunosuppression.

Culture and Gram stain

These studies are indicated when there are recurrent abscesses, a failure to respond to conventional therapy, systemic toxicity, involvement of the central face, abscesses that contain gas or involve muscle or fascia, or when the patient is immunocompromised. Material for culture and Gram stain is collected in a sterile syringe by inserting the needle through the unbroken effaced skin over the abscess. If anaerobic organisms are suspected, the material should be rapidly transported to the laboratory in the syringe or immediately inoculated into an anaerobic tube. Culturing of an abscess usually takes 48 hours or more to determine which bacteria are present. The Gram stain provides a rapid means of diagnosis.

Antibiotics

Patients with recurrent furunculosis learn that they can sometimes stop the progression of an abscess by starting antistaphylococcal antibiotics at the first sign of the typical localized swelling and erythema. They continue to use antibiotics for 5 to 10 days. Antibiotics should be started immediately to attenuate the evolving abscess. Antibiotics have little effect once the abscess has become fluctuant.

Recurrent furunculosis

Diseases manifesting as recurrent furunculosis are listed in Table 9-2.[56] Recurrent furunculosis in otherwise healthy patients with no predisposing factors is the most common manifestation.

Management

Although recurrent infection often ceases spontaneously after 2 years, a few patients have repeated episodes of furuncles that last for years. Several members of a family may be affected. Most of these patients are normal with an intact immune system. Most people do not carry *S. aureus* in the nose, but patients with recurrent furunculosis frequently carry the pathogenic strain of *S. aureus* in their nares and perineum.[57] Therapy goals are to decrease or eliminate the pathogenic strain. The treatment program for recurrent furunculosis is described in Box 9-3.

Box 9-3 Treatment Program for Recurrent Furunculosis

ERADICATION OF *S. AUREUS* NASAL CARRIAGE

Program of first choice:

1. Instruct the patient to apply mupirocin (Bactroban) ointment to the anterior nares with a cotton swab applicator twice daily for 5 consecutive days. This treatment should be used for all verified familial carriers of the same strain.[7]
2. Culture the anterior nares every 3 months to check for the effectiveness of the above measure. Retreat with mupirocin or consider oral antibiotics for treatment failures.

Program for topical treatment failures:

Prescribe an oral semisynthetic penicillin, 0.5 to 1 gm, to be taken twice daily for 10 to 14 days; treatment for 2 months offered no benefit in preventing recurrences.[57] (Treatment with systemic antibiotics eradicates the pathogenic organisms from the nares, perineum, and furuncles*.)

OTHER MEASURES TO ERADICATE *S. AUREUS*

Instruct the patient to:

1. Wash the entire body and the fingernails with a nail brush each day for 1 to 3 weeks with Betadine, Hibiclens, or pHisoHex soap. The frequency of washing should be decreased if the skin becomes dry.
2. Change towels, washcloths, and sheets daily.
3. Change wound dressing frequently.
4. Clean shaving instruments thoroughly each day.
5. Avoid nose picking.

*The combination of 500 mg of cloxacillin every 6 hours for 7 to 10 days and 600 mg of rifampin once a day for 7 to 10 days may be more effective in eradicating coagulase-positive staphylococci from the anterior nares. When culture of the anterior nares yielded *S. aureus*, rifampin alone (given at 3-month intervals) significantly reduces the incidence of infection. A 3-month course of oral clindamycin (150 mg daily) is effective in preventing infection.[29]

Erysipeloid

Erysipeloid is an acute skin infection caused by the gram-positive, rod-shaped, nonsporulating bacillus *Erysipelothrix rhusiopathiae* (or *E. insidiosa*). It has been found to cause infection in several dozen species of mammals and other animals and fish.[58] Humans become infected through exposure to infected or contaminated animals or animal products.[59] The disease is an occupational hazard for people who handle unprocessed meat and animal products, such as fishermen (fish poisoning, crab poisoning, seal finger, whale finger), meat handlers (swine erysipelas), butchers, farmers, and veterinarians. Patients who have repeated infections know that it responds to penicillin and treat themselves.

Clinical manifestation

The most common presentation is a localized, self-limited cutaneous lesion, erysipeloid. Diffuse cutaneous and systemic infections occur rarely. Approximately 1 to 7 days (an average of 3 days) after animal contact, a dull, red erythema appears at the inoculation site and extends centrifugally for 3 to 4 days to reach a fixed size of approximately 10 cm in diameter (Figure 9-27). Central clearing often occurs. Streptococcal cellulitis (erysipelas) is bright red, painful, and spreads rapidly. Infection also occurs on the face, neck, and sole of the foot. There is burning, itching, and discomfort; lymphangitis or constitutional symptoms develop in a few patients. Arthropathy, sometimes longstanding, may develop. The disease is self-limited and may subside spontaneously. Relapse may occur from 4 days to 2 weeks after the lesions are completely resolved. Diffuse and systemic forms with extensive, red, diamond-shaped plaques, septic arthritis, and endocarditis[60] are rare.

Diagnosis

The organism may be isolated from biopsy or blood specimens on standard culture media.

Treatment

Although there are many instances of cutaneous forms of the disease running a self-limited course, all patients should receive antibiotics to prevent progression to systemic disease and the development of endocarditis.[61] The disease responds to penicillin G, cephalosporins, erythromycin, and fluoroquinolones.

Blistering Distal Dactylitis

Blistering distal dactylitis is a superficial infection of the anterior fat pad of the fingertips. It is most commonly caused by group A beta-hemolytic streptococci (Figure 9-28).[62] *S. aureus* is the cause in a few reported patients.[63,64] A large blister filled with a watery, purulent fluid forms on the volar surface of the distal portion of the fingers. The age range of most of the reported patients is 2 to 16 years but adult cases are also reported.[65] A firm diagnosis can be made with a Gram stain and culture of the blister fluid. Treatment consists of incision, drainage, and a 10-day course of antistreptococcal systemic antibiotics.

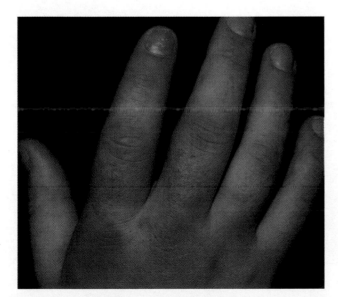

Figure 9-27 Erysipeloid. Approximately 3 days after animal or fish contact, a dull red erythema appears at the inoculation site and extends centrifugally.

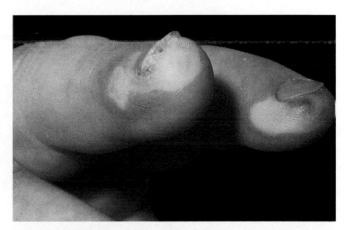

Figure 9-28 Blistering distal dactylitis. This superficial infection of the anterior fat pad of the distal portion of the fingers is caused most commonly by group A beta-hemolytic streptococci. *(Courtesy Lu'cia Martin-Moreno, M.D.)*

Staphylococcal Scalded Skin Syndrome

Staphylococcal scalded skin syndrome (SSSS), also known as Ritter's disease, is a staphylococcal epidermolytic toxin syndrome.[66] It is explained by a lack of immunity to the toxins and to renal immaturity in children that leads to poor clearance of toxins.[67] Staphylococcal scarlatiniform eruption and bullous impetigo are also diseases that are caused by an epidermolytic toxin elaborated by *S. aureus*, phage group II, including types 55, 71, 3A, and 3B.

Epidermolytic toxin

The toxin is antigenic and when elaborated elicits an antibody response. Two antigenically distinct forms: toxin A (ET A) and toxin B (ET B) have been identified. Epidermolytic toxin antibody is present in 75% of normal people older than 10 years of age, a fact that explains the rarity of SSSS in adults. It is speculated that the toxins act on an epidermal component that mediates cell-cell adhesion. This attack causes a blister just below the stratum corneum. Recent studies suggest that the toxins may have superantigen activity.[68]

Incidence

The childhood form of SSSS is most often seen in otherwise healthy children. About 62% of children are younger than 2 years old; 98% are 6 years or younger. The rare, adult type of generalized SSSS is associated with underlying diseases related to immunosuppression, abnormal immunity,[69-71] and renal insufficiency.

Clinical manifestations

SSSS begins with a localized, often inapparent, *S. aureus* infection of the conjunctivae, throat, nares, or umbilicus.[72] A diffuse, tender erythema appears; the skin has a sandpaper-like texture similar to that seen in scarlet fever. The erythema is often accentuated in flexural and periorificial areas. However, the rash of scarlet fever is not tender. The temperature rises and within 1 or 2 days the skin wrinkles, forms transient bullae, and peels off in large sheets, leaving a moist, red, glistening surface (Figures 9-29 and 9-30). Minor pressure induces skin separation (Nikolsky's sign). The area of involvement may be localized, but it is often generalized. Evaporative fluid loss from large areas is associated with increased fluid loss and dehydration. A yellow crust forms, and

Figure 9-29 Staphylococcal scalded skin syndrome. A scarlatiniform eruption appears followed by a tissue paper-like wrinkling of the epidermis. Bullae then appear around body orifices and in the axillae and groin. Sheets of epidermis then shed and reveal a moist erythematous base. Healing occurs in 5 to 7 days.

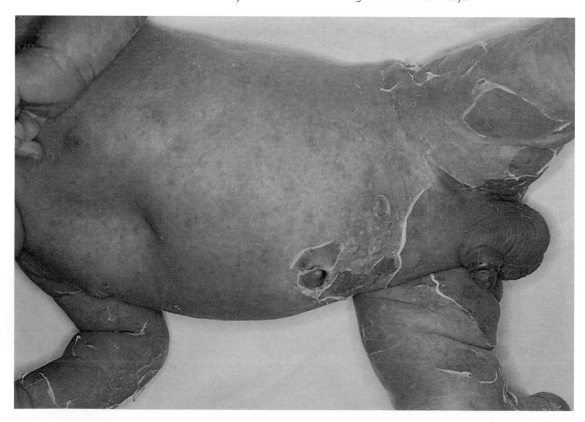

the denuded surface dries and cracks. Healing occurs in 7 to 10 days, accompanied by desquamation similar to that seen in scarlet fever. Reepithelialization is rapid because of the high level of the split in the epidermis. The distinction between the localized form of SSSS and bullous impetigo can be difficult. The criteria in favor of localized SSSS are (1) the absence of inflammatory cells in the dermis on biopsy, (2) erythematous skin with tenderness, (3) Nikolsky's phenomenon around lesions, and (4) a negative culture result from intact bullae. Staphylococcal scarlatiniform eruption is similar to SSSS, except that the skin does not blister or peel.

Pathophysiology

The epidermolytic toxin is filtered through the glomeruli and partially reabsorbed in the proximal tubule where it undergoes catabolism by the proximal tubule cells. The glomerular filtration rate of infants is less than 50% of the normal adult rate, which is reached in the second year of life. This may explain why infants, patients with chronic renal failure, and those on hemodialysis[72] may be predisposed to SSSS.

Diagnosis

With SSSS, a biopsy shows splitting of the epidermis in the stratum granulosum near the skin surface; there is scant inflammation. Thin-roofed bullae are flaccid and rupture easily. Culture specimens should be taken from the eye, nose, throat, bullae, and any obviously infected area. Skin and blood culture results are often negative in children and positive in adults. SSSS must be differentiated from toxic epidermal necrolysis, a rare, life-threatening disease in which full-thickness epidermal necrosis occurs. Histologically, toxic epidermal necrolysis shows dermal-epidermal separation, rather than the granular layer split in the epidermis seen in SSSS and an intense inflammatory infiltrate. A frozen section of peeled skin is a reliable way of rapidly establishing the diagnosis. Many of the reported adult cases had positive blood culture results; children younger than 5 years infrequently have sepsis. Cultures from bullae have also been reported to be positive, but this may have been the result of contamination. Several reported adult patients were on systemic steroids.

Treatment

Corticosteroids are contraindicated because they interfere with host defense mechanisms. Hospitalization and intravenous antibiotic therapy are desirable for extensive cases. Most of the toxin-producing *S. aureus* produce penicillinase. Nafcillin 100 to 200 mg/kg daily is used in the hospital. Patients with limited disease may be managed at home with oral antibiotics. Dicloxacillin 25 mg/kg per day, or a cephalosporin is prescribed for a minimum of 1 week. Topical antibiotics are not necessary. The patient's skin should be lubricated with bland, light lotions and washed infrequently. Wet dressings may cause further drying and cracking and should be avoided.

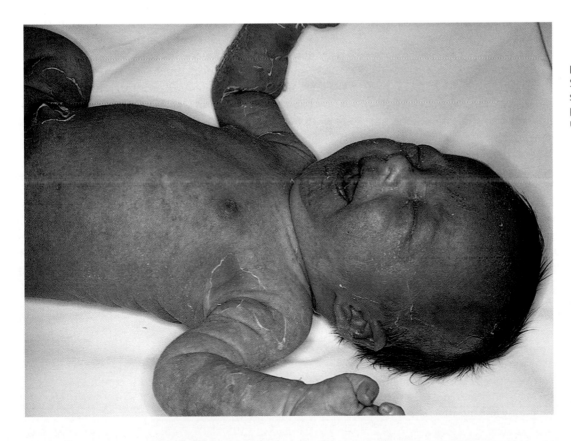

Figure 9-30
Staphylococcal scalded skin syndrome. Exfoliative phase, during which the upper epidermis is shed.

Pseudomonas aeruginosa Infection

P. aeruginosa is a saprophytic intestinal gram-negative aerobic rod with a predilection for humid environments. In normal human skin, *Pseudomonas* species are part of the transitory skin flora and are found principally in the anogenital area, axillae, and external ear canal. Gram-positive cocci exert an inhibitory effect on their growth. In immunocompromised hosts, skin fissures and erosions, venipuncture sites, nasogastric and endotracheal tubes, and urinary catheters are the usual portal of entry. The bacteria may colonize warm, moist areas such as skin folds (toe webs), ear canals, burns, ulcers, and areas beneath nails. It is also found in the moist areas of sinks and drains and in poorly preserved topical creams and ointments. It produces diffusable fluorescent pigments including pyoverdin and a soluble phenazine pigment called pyocyanin. Pyocyanin appears blue or green at neutral or alkaline pH and is the source of the name aeruginosa. An organic metabolite may impart a fruity odor to some cutaneous lesions. That same odor in culture is a specific quality of *P. aeruginosa*. *Pseudomonas* survives poorly in an acid environment. There are many serotypes.

Pseudomonas infects warm, moist areas in healthy people. Hot tub folliculitis and toe-web intertrigo occur because of a temporary change in the skin moisture content and temperature that allows pseudomonal overgrowth. Correction of the altered environment results in resolution of the infection. Severe, life-threatening infections occur in patients with impaired immunity, such as those with serious burns or acute leukemia or those receiving immunosuppressive therapy.

Oral treatment of *Pseudomonas* infections is possible with the fluoroquinolones, such as ciprofloxacin hydrochloride (Cipro).

Pseudomonas folliculitis

From 8 hours to 5 days or longer (mean incubation period is 48 hours) after using a contaminated whirlpool, home hot tub, waterslide, physiotherapy pool, or contaminated loofah sponge,[73] *Pseudomonas* folliculitis develops in 7% to 100% of exposed patients. The attack rate is significantly higher in children than in adults, possibly because they tend to spend more time in the water. Showering after using the contaminated facility offers no protection.

Clinical manifestation

The typical patient has a few to more than 50 0.5- to 3-cm, pruritic, round, urticarial plaques with a central papule or pustule located on all skin surfaces except the head. The rash may be follicular, maculopapular, vesicular, pustular, or a polymorphous eruption that includes all of these types of lesions. Women who wear one-piece bathing suits are at an increased risk. The eruption, in most cases, clears in 7 to 10 days, leaving round spots of red-brown, postinflammatory hyperpigmentation, but patients have been reported to have recurrent crops of lesions for as long as 3 months. The spread of infection from person to person is not likely. Malaise and fatigue may occur during the initial few days of the eruption. Fever is uncommon and low grade when it appears.

Pathophysiology

Under normal conditions, *P. aeruginosa* infection cannot be induced by inoculation of the microorganism onto the intact skin surface of immune-competent persons. Occlusion and superhydration of the stratum corneum favors colonization of the skin with *P. aeruginosa*. This may explain why the rash is most severe in areas occluded by a snug bathing suit (Figures 9-31 and 9-32). *P. aeruginosa* serotype 0:9 and 0:11 are most commonly isolated from skin lesions, but other serotypes[74] have been reported.[75] Three conditions are associated with folliculitis: prolonged exposure to the water, an excessive number of bathers, and inadequate pool care. The organism gains entry via the hair follicles or breaks in the skin. The increased water temperature promotes sweating, which enhances penetration of the skin by the bacteria. Also, with heavy use, there are desquamated skin cells in the water, providing a rich, organic nutrient source for the bacteria. The ubiquitous *P. aeruginosa* rapidly multiply in water at increased temperatures.

Management

The infection is self-limited, but a 5% acetic acid (white vinegar) wet compress applied for 20 minutes two to four times a day and/or silver sulfadiazine cream (Silvadene) might be of some help. Cases resistant to topical therapy can be treated orally with ciprofloxacin (Cipro) 500 or 750 mg twice each day.

Preventative measures include continuous water filtration to eliminate desquamated skin, frequent monitoring of the disinfectant levels, and frequent changing of the water, especially during heavy use. Public hot tubs and whirlpools with heavy use should be drained completely on a daily basis and the interior should be cleaned daily with an acidic solution. A heavy bather load, turbulent water, and aeration make it difficult to maintain satisfactory levels of chlorine.

Pseudomonas hot-foot syndrome

The "pseudomonas hot-foot syndrome" is described in a series of 40 children. Painful red plantar nodules developed in children within 40 hours after they had used a wading pool whose floor was coated with abrasive grit. Culture of the pustules and pool water yielded *Pseudomonas aeruginosa*. All patients recovered within 14 days. The course was benign and self-limited.[76]

PSEUDOMONAS AERUGINOSA INFECTION

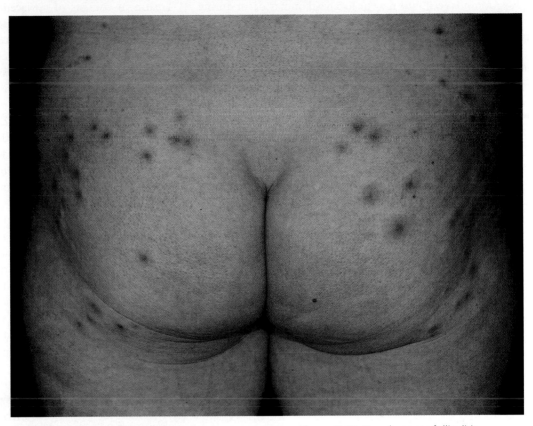

Figure 9-31 *Pseudomonas* folliculitis. Urticarial plaques surmounted by pustules located primarily in the areas covered by the bathing suit.

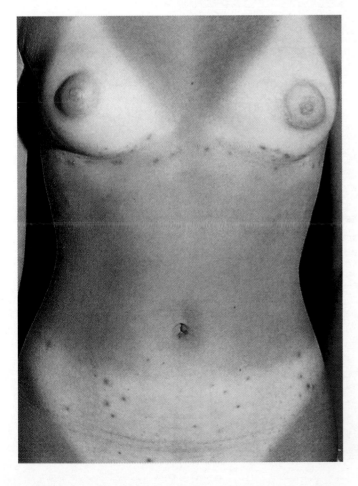

Figure 9-32 *Pseudomonas* folliculitis. Pustules form in occluded areas under the bathing suit.

Pseudomonas cellulitis

Pseudomonas cellulitis may be localized or may occur during *Pseudomonas* septicemia. The localized form occurs as a secondary infection of tinea of the toe webs or groin (Figures 9-33 and 9-34), bed sores, stasis ulcers, burns, grafted areas, under the foreskin of the penis[77,78] and following an injury[79] (Figures 9-35 and 9-36). Maceration or occlusion of these cutaneous lesions encourages secondary infection with *Pseudomonas.* Suppression of normal bacterial flora by broad-spectrum antibiotics encourages secondary infection. *Pseudomonas* infection is often unsuspected and appropriate therapy is therefore delayed. Deep erosions and tissue necrosis may occur before the correct diagnosis is made. Severe pain is highly characteristic of an evolving infection. The skin turns a dusky red (see Figure 9-34). Bluish green, purulent material with a fruity or "mousey" odor accumulates as the red, indurated area becomes macerated and then eroded. Vesicles and pustules may occur as satellite lesions. The eruption may spread to cover wide areas and be accompanied by systemic symptoms. *Pseudomonas* septicemia may produce a deep, indurated, necrotic cellulitis that resembles other forms of infectious cellulitis.

Treatment

Treatment consists of 5% acetic acid (white vinegar)[80] wet compresses applied 20 minutes four times a day. Localized infections respond to oral treatment with ciprofloxacin (Cipro) 500 or 750 mg twice each day. Severe infections may respond to clinafloxacin administered intravenously.[81]

Figure 9-33 *Pseudomonas* cellulitis. The localized form occurs as a secondary infection of tinea of the toe webs. Maceration and occlusion in moist boots predisposes to secondary infection with *Pseudomonas.* The skin becomes painful and turns a dusky red.

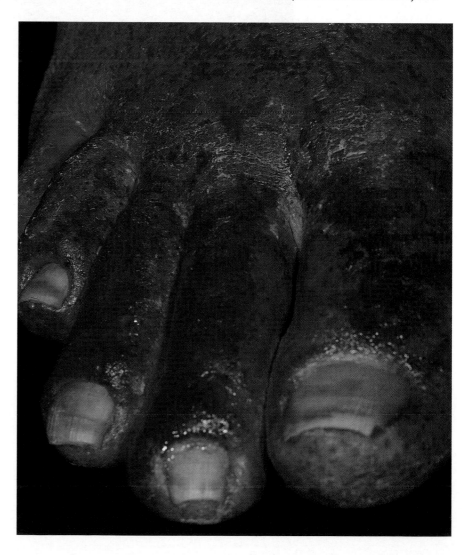

PSEUDOMONAS CELLULITIS

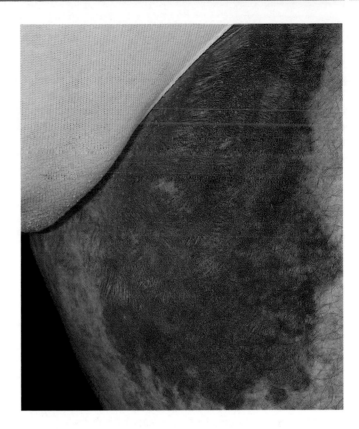

Figure 9-34 Inflamed area has a "mousey" or grape juice-like odor.

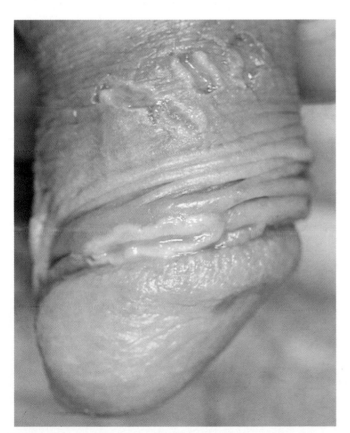

Figure 9-35 Erosions of the shaft of the penis exposed to the warmth and moisture under the foreskin may become infected with *Pseudomonas*.

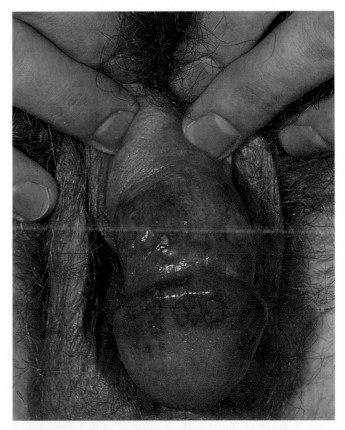

Figure 9-36 Maceration and abrasion under the foreskin can lead to secondary infection with *Pseudomonas*.

External otitis

Excessive moisture and trauma impairing the canal's natural defenses are the most common precipitants of otitis externa. Inflammation of the external auditory canal can be localized or diffuse and acute or chronic. Predisposing conditions include external trauma, loss of the canal's protective coating, maceration of the skin from water or humidity, and glandular obstruction. Acute otitis externa is generally caused by *P. aeruginosa* or *S. aureus*.[82]

External otitis is an inflammation of the external auditory canal. It occurs in a mild, self-limited form (swimmer's ear) or as an acute and chronic, recurrent, debilitating disease. The normally acidic cerumen inhibits gram-negative bacterial growth and forms a protective layer that discourages maceration. Swimming or excessive manipulation while cleaning the canal may disrupt this natural barrier. Inflammatory diseases such as psoriasis, seborrheic dermatitis, and eczematous dermatitis disrupt the normal barrier and encourage infection. *Pseudomonas* is the most common bacteria isolated from both mild and severe external otitis. Most cases, however, represent a mixed infection with other gram-negative (*Proteus mirabilis, Klebsiella pneumoniae*) and gram-positive (*S. epidermidis*, beta-hemolytic streptococci) bacteria. Fungal infection with *Candida* or *Aspergillus niger* sometimes occurs, and these organisms may be the primary pathogens.

Clinical manifestation

Discomfort, erythema, and swelling of the canal with variable discharge are the common signs and symptoms. The early stages are characterized by erythema, edema, and an accumulation of moist, cellular debris in the canal. Traction on the pinna or tragus may elicit pain. If the disease progresses, erythema radiates into the pinna and purulent material partly obstructs and exudes from the canal. Pain becomes constant and more intense. Cellulitis of the pinna and skin surrounding the ear accompanied by a dense mucopurulent exudate discharging from the canal may result from infection with *Pseudomonas* (Figures 9-37, 9-38, and 9-39). However, in most cases, this indicates a secondary infection with staphylococci and streptococci.

The lymphatics of the external ear may be permanently damaged during an attack of cellulitis, predisposing the patient to recurrent episodes of streptococcal erysipelas of the pinna. Recurrent attacks are brought on by manipulation or even the slightest trauma. Eczematous inflammation and infection of the external ear and surrounding skin may occur for a variety of reasons, such as irritation from purulent exudate, scratching and manipulation, or allergy to topical medications. Habitual manipulation may cause this disease to persist for years.

Treatment

Treatment of patients with otitis externa includes debridement, topical therapy with acidifying and antimicrobial agents and systemic antimicrobial therapy when indicated. The treatment of patients with chronic otitis externa includes cleansing and debridement accompanied by topical acidifying and drying agents.[82,83]

CLEANSING AND DEBRIDEMENT. Cleansing is essential for treatment; flushing should be avoided. Squamous debris, cerumen, and pus are removed by suction or irrigation with an ear syringe.

TOPICAL THERAPY. Acidification is accomplished with a topical solution of 2% acetic acid (Otic Domeboro). Some solutions add hydrocortisone for inflammation (VoSol Otic HC). Acidification creates an environment that is inhospitable to gram-negative bacteria and fungi. These are effective treatment in most cases and, when used after exposure to moisture, are an excellent prophylactic. Topical antibiotics should be considered for infection localized to the canal (Table 9-3). Ofloxacin given twice daily is as safe and effective as Cortisporin given four times daily for otitis externa.[84] A culture specimen of canal drainage is obtained.

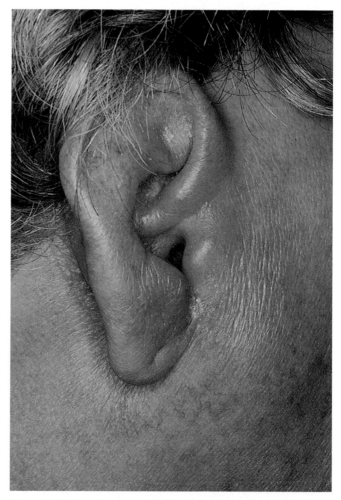

Figure 9-37 *Pseudomonas* cellulitis. The entire pinna and surrounding skin have become inflamed after an episode of external otitis.

Table 9-3 Otic Antibacterial and Anesthetic Solutions

	Active against	Dosage
FLOXIN Otic 0.3% (ofloxacin otic solution) 5 mL and 10 mL bottle	S. aureus S. pneumoniae H. influenzae Moraxella catarrhalis P. mirabilis P. aeruginosa	1-12 years old—5 drops bid—10 days 12 years and older—10 drops bid—10 days
CIPRO HC OTIC (ciprofloxacin hydrochloride and hydrocortisone otic suspension)	S. aureus P. mirabilis P. aeruginosa	3 drops bid 7 days
Otic Domeboro solution 2% acetic acid in Burrow's solution 2 fl. oz bottle	Acetic acid is antibacte- rial and antifungal	4 to 6 drops every 2 to 3 hours
Americaine otic topical (anesthetic ear drops) Benzocaine 20% in a 15 mL bottle	A local anesthetic	4 to 5 drops then insert a cotton pledget into the meatus Application may be repeated every 1 to 2 hours
VoSoL HC otic solution Hydrocortisone (1%) and acetic acid (2%) 10 mL bottle	Acetic acid is antibacte- rial and antifungal	3 to 5 drops every 4 to 6 hours
Cortisporin-TC Otic Suspension Colistin sulfate Neomycin sulfate Hydrocortisone Acetic acid	Colistin sulfate- bactericidal action against most gram- negative organisms, notably P. aerugi- nosa, E. coli, and Klebsiella aerobacter	5 drops—3 or 4 times daily 4 drops for pediatric patients
Auralgan otic solution Antipyrine Benzocaine 10 mL bottle	Topical decongestant and analgesic	Instill, permitting solution to run along the wall of the canal until it is filled. Then moisten a cotton pledget with Auralgan and insert into meatus. Repeat every 1 to 2 hours until pain and congestion are relieved. Useful for drying out the canal
PEDIOTIC Suspension Neomycin Polymyxin B sulfates Hydrocortisone 7.5 mL bottle	The combination is ac- tive against S. aureus, E. coli, H. influenzae, Klebsiella- Enterobacter species, Neisseria species, and P. aeruginosa	For adults, 4 drops 3 or 4 times daily; 3 drops for infants and children

Instructions: Lie with the affected ear upward, instill drops, maintain position for 5 minutes.

Wicks. Ear wicks are made of strands of cotton or fine cloth and are inserted into the canal to act as a conduit for application of otic solutions. If properly saturated, they will keep medication in contact with all surfaces of the canal. Solution must be added almost hourly to maintain saturation. New wicks are inserted daily. The use of a wick is usually unnecessary for mild inflammation but may be considered when the canal is partially obstructed by swelling and edema. The wick must be introduced before the canal swells, which makes insertion painful or impossible.

WICKS. Ear wicks are made of strands of cotton or fine cloth and are inserted into the canal to act as a conduit for application of otic solutions. If properly saturated, they will keep medication in contact with all surfaces of the canal. Solution must be added almost hourly to maintain saturation. New wicks are inserted daily. The use of a wick is usually unnecessary for mild inflammation but may be considered when the canal is partially obstructed by swelling and edema. The wick must be introduced before the canal swells, which makes insertion painful or impossible.

SYSTEMIC ANTIMICROBIAL THERAPY. Infections that progress beyond the canal to the pinna and surrounding tissues are treated orally with ciprofloxacin (Cipro) 500 or 750 mg twice each day.

Prevention

Prevention of recurrent external otitis is aimed at minimizing ear canal trauma and the avoidance of exposure to water. Drying the ears with a hair dryer and avoiding manipulation of the external auditory canal may help prevent recurrence.[83]

Treating eczema

Group III to IV topical steroids, wet compresses, and oral antibiotics are used when eczematous inflammation and infection occur on the external ear and surrounding skin. These can be instilled deep in the canal by connecting a syringe filled with medication to a Zollinger or disposable metal sucker tip and the ear canal can be filled under direct microscopic vision.[85] (See the section on the treatment of eczematous inflammation.)

Local injection of triamcinolone acetonide in the external auditory channel is effective in the management of chronic external otitis that may be accompanied by thickening of the skin in the external auditory channel.[86]

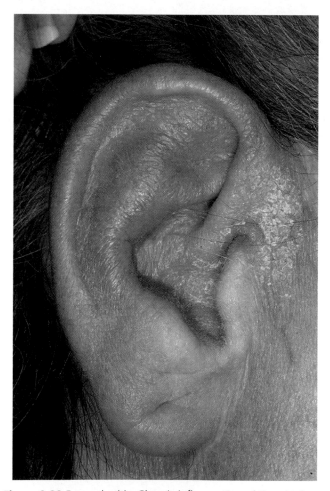

Figure 9-38 External otitis. Chronic inflammation of the canal progressed to involve the pinna. Erythema and scale (eczema) followed chronic manipulation of the pinna. Group V topical steroids were required for control

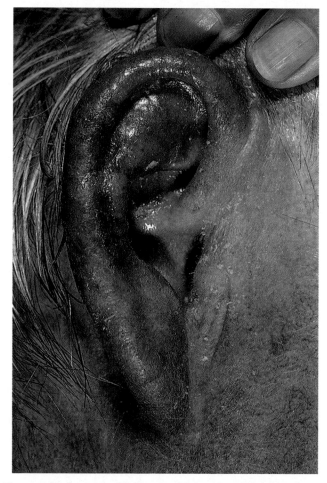

Figure 9-39 External otitis. Eczema of the pinna has become infected and painful. Culture showed staphylococcal infection and not *Pseudomonas*. Dicloxacillin 500 mg four times a day controlled the infection. Group V topical steroids were then used to treat the eczema.

Malignant external otitis

Malignant otitis externa is a life-threatening infection arising from the external auditory canal.

Patients with malignant external otitis present with a history of nonresolving otitis externa of many weeks' or months' duration (Figure 9-40). Most patients have diabetes mellitus. *Pseudomonas* infection penetrates the epithelium and invades underlying soft tissues. There is severe ear pain, which is worse at night, and purulent discharge. The external canal is edematous. Granulation tissue may be present, arising from the osseous cartilaginous junction at the floor of the canal or anteriorly. The infection then penetrates the floor of the canal at the bony cartilaginous junction and spreads to the base of the skull.[87] Malignant external otitis is an osteomyelitis of the skull base. More advanced cases demonstrate cranial nerve palsies, most frequently involving cranial nerve VII. The diagnosis is confirmed by nuclear scanning studies and CT scanning of the temporal bone and skull base. The criteria for diagnosis are listed in Box 9-4.

Treatment

The treatment of malignant external otitis has evolved from primarily surgical to one in which prolonged medical therapy of the underlying osteomyelitis with limited surgical debridement leads to a cure. Therapy consists of using a third-generation cephalosporin (ceftazidime or ceftriaxone) and a fluoroquinolone (ciprofloxacin or ofloxacin). Surgery is not indicated.

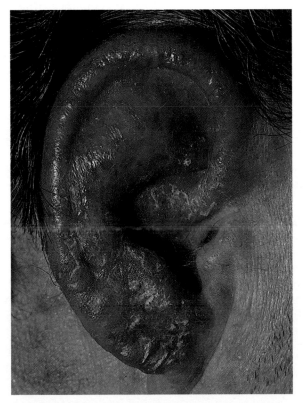

Figure 9-40 Malignant external otitis. Severe infection of the ear has occurred after months of chronic inflammation of the pinna.

Box 9-4 Criteria for Diagnosis of Malignant External Otitis
Refractory otitis externa
Severe earache, worse at night
Purulent exudate
Granulation tissue
Recovery of *P. aeruginosa*
Diabetes mellitus or other immune state compromise
Positive 99Tc bone scan of the temporal bone
From Levenson MJ, et al: Laryngoscope 1991; 101:821.

Toe web infection

Pseudomonas toe web infection is a distinctive clinical entity that is often misdiagnosed as tinea pedis.[88] A thick, white, macerated scale with a green discoloration may appear in the toe webs of people who wear heavy, wet boots. The most constant clinical feature is soggy wetness of the toe webs and immediately adjacent skin. In its mildest form, the affected tissue is damp, softened, boggy, and white. The second, third, and fourth toe webs are the most common sites of initial involvement. More severe forms may progress to denudation of affected skin and profuse, serous, or purulent discharge. In most cases, this sopping-wet denudation involves all toe webs and extends onto the plantar surface and the dorsal and plantar surfaces of the toes, and an area approximately 1 cm wide beyond the base of the toes on the plantar surface of the foot. All patients are males with broad feet, square toes, and tight interdigital spaces. Close skin-to-skin contact and friction between the toes is a constant feature. Wood's light examination may show a green-white fluorescence due to elaboration of pyoverdin, and a green stain may be found on socks, bandages, toenails, and dried exudate. The green stain is due to elaboration of bacterial pyocyanin. *Pseudomonas* or a mixed flora of *Pseudomonas* organisms and fungi may be isolated from the soggy scale.

Treatment

First, the thickened, edematous, and devitalized layers of the epidermis are debrided.[89] Repeated applications of silver nitrate (0.5%) soaks or 5% acetic acid[80] (white vinegar) to the toe webs and the dorsal and plantar surfaces promote dryness and suppress bacteria. Gentamicin cream, silver sulfadiazine cream (Silvadene), or Castellani's paint (Derma-Cas gel) are then applied until the infection has resolved. Infections that do not respond to topical therapy are treated with ciprofloxacin (Cipro) 500 or 750 mg twice each day. Some *Pseudomonas* strains have developed resistance to Cipro.

Measures to prevent reinfection include the use of gauze pledgets between toes to prevent occlusion, the use of sandals or open-weave shoes to enhance evaporation of sweat, and the use of astringents such as 20% aluminum chloride (Drysol) to promote dryness.

Ecthyma gangrenosum

Ecthyma gangrenosum (EG) is the cutaneous manifestation of *P. aeruginosa* septicemia, typically affecting immunosuppressed patients, particularly those with neutropenia. Systemic *P. aeruginosa* usually complicates debilitating conditions, such as leukemia, burns, and cystic fibrosis. It is not to be confused with pyoderma gangrenosum or streptococcal ecthyma. It is a rare but highly characteristic entity that is pathognomonic of *Pseudomonas* infection. The lesions represent either a bloodborne, metastatic seeding of *P. aeruginosa* to the skin or a primary lesion with no bacteremia. The mortality rate is high for the septicemic form and approximately 15% without bacteremia.[90] The disease is rare, occurring in only 1.3% to 6.0% of patients with *Pseudomonas* sepsis.[91] There are usually less than 10 lesions.

All patients have predisposing factors that increase their risk for infection. EG occurs in immunocompromised patients (neoplasia, leukemia, immunosuppressive treatment, graft, malnutrition, diabetes), in burn patients, and in patients who have been treated with penicillin. Many patients have a disorder that leads to severe neutropenia or pancytopenia. Most cases arise during *P. aeruginosa* septicemia, but nonsepticemic forms are described in both infants and adults.[92-94] The nonsepticemic cases occur without overt immunosuppression or neutropenia and may occur following antibiotic therapy.

Lesions consist of multiple noncontiguous ulcers or solitary ulcers. They begin as isolated, red, purpuric macules that become vesicular, indurated, and later, bullous or pustular. The pustules may be hemorrhagic. The lesions remain localized or, more typically, extend over several centimeters. The central area becomes hemorrhagic and necrotic (Figure 9-41). The lesion then sloughs to form a gangrenous ulcer with a gray-black eschar and a surrounding erythematous halo. Lesions occur mainly in the gluteal and perineal regions (57%), the extremities (30%), the trunk (6%), and the face (6%) but may occur anywhere.

Septicemic patients have high temperatures, chills, hypotension, and tachycardia or tachypnea, or both. Neutropenia is a constant finding, and the absolute neutrophil count correlates closely with the clinical outcome. Most patients died when neutrophil counts were lower than 500/mm³ during or after appropriate therapy.[95] The skin lesions are slow to heal (an average of 4 weeks).

The postulated mechanisms are a vasculitis caused by bacilli in the vessel wall, by circulating immune complexes, and/or by the effect of bacterial exotoxins or endotoxins.

Management (septicemic form)

Green et al[95] recommend the following management program:

1. Take a deep skin biopsy (4 or 5 mm) for histopathologic studies with special stains to identify bacteria in tissue.
2. Take a skin biopsy specimen for culture.
3. Perform needle aspiration of lesions to perform Gram stain for rapid diagnosis.
4. Take blood culture specimens, especially during fever spikes.
5. Start appropriate systemic antibiotics after cultures have been taken. Localized nonsepticemic disease may only require topical therapy such as silver nitrate (0.5%) or 5% acetic acid[80] (white vinegar) wet compresses or silver sulfadiazine cream.

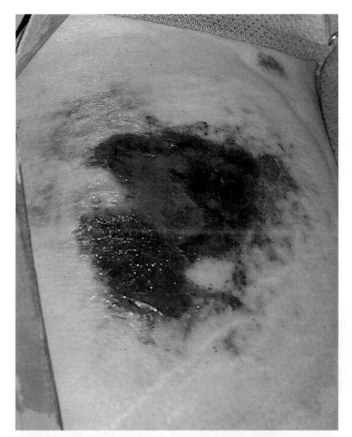

Figure 9-41 Ecthyma gangrenosum. A cutaneous manifestation of *Pseudomonas* septicemia. A large, vesicular, bullous, hemorrhagic mass is located on the thigh.

Meningococcemia

Meningococcemia is caused by the bacteria *Neisseria meningitidis*. It is transmitted by respiratory secretions. Meningitis is the most common presentation. Acute septicemia (meningococcemia) kills faster than any other infectious disease. Shock and death can occur in hours. Chronic meningococcemia is rare and resembles the arthritis-dermatitis syndrome of gonococcemia.

Transmission

Most cases are sporadic, but localized outbreaks occur.

Asymptomatic carriers are thought to be the major source of transmission. Meningococci are present in the nasopharynx of approximately 10% to 20% of healthy persons. Most cases begin with acquisition of a new organism by nasopharyngeal colonization, followed by systemic invasion and development of bacteremia. CNS invasion then occurs. Viral infection, household crowding, chronic illness, and persons who have deficiencies in the terminal common complement pathway (C3, C5-9) are at increased risk. Late complement components are required for bacteriolysis.

Incidence

Each year 2400 cases of meningococcal disease occur in the United States. Incidence is highest in infants; 32% of cases occur in persons 30 years of age or older. Serogroup C caused 35% of cases; serogroup B, 32%; and serogroup Y, 26%.[96] More than half of cases among infants younger than 1 year of age are caused by serogroup B, for which no vaccine exists.

Pathophysiology

A viral infection may facilitate the invasion of *N. meningitidis* into the bloodstream. *N. meningitidis* invades small blood vessel endothelial cells and releases bacterial endotoxin. Endotoxin causes endothelial cells, monocytes, and macrophages to release cytokines. These cause severe hypotension, lowered cardiac output, and endothelial permeability. Organ anoxia and massive disseminated intravascular coagulation can result in organ failure, shock, and death.

Decreased permeability and thrombosis lead to infarction, producing small areas of purpura with an irregular pattern.

Clinical manifestations

The incubation period varies from 2 to 10 days, but the disease typically begins 3 to 4 days after exposure. Clinical manifestations range from fever alone to fulminant septic shock with purpura fulminans. There is a sudden onset of fever, an intense headache, nausea, vomiting, a stiff neck, and a rash in more than 70% of cases.[97] Purpuric lesions (60%), erythematous papules (32%) (Figures 9-42 and 9-43),[98] faint pink macules (28%), and conjunctival petechiae (10%) are the re-

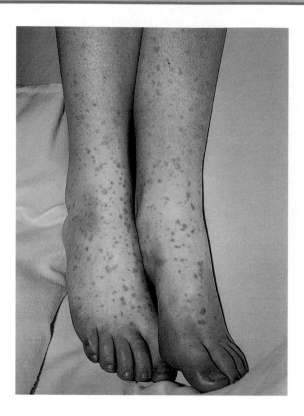

ported cutaneous signs.[99] Delirium and coma often appear. The fatality rate is 7%.[100] The highest rate occurs among infants younger than 1 year of age. Meningococcal disease causes substantial morbidity: 9% to 11% have sequelae (e.g., neurologic disability, limb loss, and hearing loss).

Purpura fulminans

With fulminating disease, accounting for approximately 3% of the cases, patients exhibit sudden prostration, ecchymoses, and shock at onset (purpura fulminans). This syndrome may lead to gangrene and autoamputation of distal extremities. It is particularly likely to complicate meningococcemia in children younger than 2 years of age. The rapidly fatal Waterhouse-Friderichsen syndrome or fulminating septicemia results in massive bleeding into the skin and hemorrhagic destruction in both adrenal glands.

Figure 9-42 Meningococcemia. A papular nonhemorrhagic rash involves the axillae, trunk, wrists, and ankles. The rash subsequently became petechial.

Figure 9-43 Meningococcemia. Petechiae may be located in the center of lighter-colored macules. Confluence of lesions may then result in hemorrhagic patches, often with central necrosis.

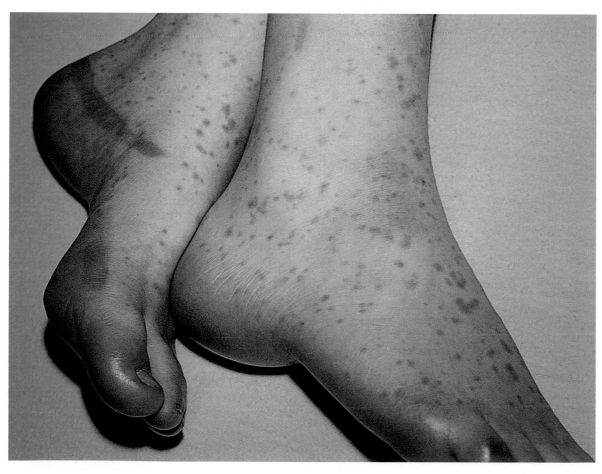

Acquired deficiencies of proteins C and S may contribute to the pathogenesis of purpura fulminans. The immaturity of the protein C system in young children may explain the increased risk.[101]

Diagnosis

Diagnosis and treatment are summarized in Box 9-5. Meningococci (*N. meningitidis*) are encapsulated gram-negative diplococci. They are separated into 13 groups on the basis of seroagglutination of capsular polysaccharides. Serogroups A, B, C, Y, and W-135 are identified in most recent cases. Serogroups B and C are responsible for most cases throughout the world.[102,103] Petechiae are the clinical sign that best discriminates patients admitted with suspected meningococcal disease.[104] Ecchymoses are specific for meningococcal disease. Reduced general condition and reduced consciousness are other valuable diagnostic signs.[105] Evaluation of the CSF remains the gold standard for the diagnosis of bacterial meningitis.[106] There is a polymorphonuclear leukocytosis in the CSF. Gram-negative diplococci are identified by Gram stain of the CSF, buffy coat, and smears taken from petechiae. A rapid diagnosis can be made with a biopsy of skin lesions. Bacteria are detected in specimens from hemorrhagic skin lesions by culture, Gram staining, or both in 63% of patients. In meningococcal sepsis, a Gram-stained skin lesion is significantly more sensitive (72%) than Gram-stained CSF (22%). The results for punch biopsy specimens are not affected by antibiotics because Gram staining gives positive results up to 45 hours after the start of treatment and culture gives positive results up to 13 hours.[107] Organisms are isolated by blood culture in almost 100% of cases, but the results are not available for 12 to 24 hours. Rule out complement deficiencies in complicated and recurrent or familial disease.

Differential diagnosis

The differential diagnosis of acute petechial eruptions includes Rocky Mountain spotted fever, echovirus and coxsackievirus infections, and toxic shock syndrome. Gonococcemia and allergic vasculitis (Henoch-Schönlein purpura, leukocytoclastic vasculitis) produce petechial and purpuric lesions that are usually elevated and palpable.

Management

Drugs effective in treating active meningococcal infection include penicillin G, chloramphenicol (for patients allergic to penicillin), and cephalosporins (i.e., cefotaxime, ceftriaxone, cefuroxime).

Meningitis and no rash

Empirical antibiotic coverage of likely meningeal pathogens is used when the etiology of meningitis is unknown. Use vancomycin and a third-generation cephalosporin. Discontinue vancomycin after the microbial diagnosis and antibiotic sensitivities are established. Empirical antibiotic therapy for meningitis based on age is as follows: neonates, ampicillin, and cefotaxime (or ampicillin and gentamicin); infants aged 1 to 3 months, ampicillin and cefotaxime with or without vancomycin; older infants, children, and adults, cefotaxime or ceftriaxone with or without vancomycin.

Box 9-5 Early Detection and Rapid Treatment of Meningococcemia	
Blood culture	Obtain before antibiotics Positive in 10%-23% Results in 12-24 hours Hold for 5 days
Lumbar puncture and culture of CSF	Polymorphonuclear leukocytosis Gram stain often negative Hold for 5 days

Gram stain
Scrapings
Lesional biopsy
Aspirate
	Positive in 50%-80%
	Diplococci in Gram-stained sections seen in purpuric skin lesions
	Histology
	  Dermal vessel thrombi
	  Vasculitis: neutrophils and nuclear dust
	  Meningococci seen thrombi and vessel walls
	  Intraepidermal, subepidermal neutrophilic pustules

Bacterial antigen test	Spinal fluid 1 mL (preferred) Urine 10 mL Identifies specific bacterial antigens in 2 hours Special labs (e.g., Mayo Clinic)
Throat culture	Obtain but unreliable Asymptomatic colonization common
Third-generation cephalosporin (e.g., cefotaxime, ceftriaxone)	Initial treatment in septic patients
Intensive supportive	
Support	Ventilatory, inotropic, intravenous fluids
DIC is present	Fresh frozen plasma
Poor tissue perfusion complications	Debridement of necrotic skin, subcutaneous tissue, and muscle + grafting MRI for diagnosis of muscle and bone involvement

DIC, Disseminated intravascular coagulation.

Septicemia and meningitis

Meningococcal infection is the most common bacterial cause of a petechial or purpuric rash and meningitis. Other organisms can cause shock and a nonblanching rash (e.g., *H. influenzae* type B and *S. pneumoniae*). A third-generation cephalosporin is appropriate until culture results are available.

Most meningococcal infections improve rapidly with antibiotics, but meningococcal disease may progress rapidly to death in a few hours.

Poor prognostic signs include:
- No meningitis
- Rapidly progressing rash
- Deteriorating consciousness
- Shock
- Coagulopathy
- Low white blood cell count

Treat with antibiotics, then manage shock and correct coagulopathy and anemia with fresh frozen plasma and blood.

Penicillin G is the treatment of choice. A third-generation cephalosporin (e.g., cefotaxime, ceftriaxone) is used initially while the diagnosis is being confirmed. Once the patient is stable, debride necrotic tissue (skin, subcutaneous tissue, muscle) and repair defects with grafts.

Acute and supportive therapy

Disseminated intravascular coagulation (DIC) is a frequent complication of meningococcal sepsis in children. Mortality is 40% in patients presenting with shock and DIC. An early assessment of the coagulation disorders in meningococcal disease can be based on few coagulation parameters.

A change of coagulation parameters occurs in the first stages of the infection. A prolongation of partial thromboplastin time and a decrease of prothrombin time help define the stage of coagulopathy. Shock is controlled by liquid substitution, compensation of metabolic acidosis, correction of clotting disorders (antithrombin III and heparin in case of pre-DIC; antithrombin III and fresh frozen plasma in case of advanced DIC), and, when necessary, catecholamine infusions.[108]

Vaccines

The quadrivalent polysaccharide meningococcal vaccine (which protects against serogroups A, C, Y, and W-135) is recommended for control of serogroup C meningococcal disease outbreaks and for use among persons in certain high-risk groups. Vaccines do not exist for serogroup B. Meningococcal C conjugate vaccine is safe and immunogenic and results in immunologic memory when given with other routinely administered vaccines to infants at 2, 3, and 4 months of age.[109] Protective levels of antibody are achieved within 7 to 10 days of vaccination. Travelers should contact the Centers for Disease Control and Prevention for information: (telephone [404] 332-4559; http://www.cdc.gov/travel/). College freshmen, especially those who live in dormitories, should be educated about meningococcal disease and the vaccine so that they can make an educated decision about vaccination.

Chemoprophylaxis

Prevention of sporadic meningococcal disease is accomplished by antimicrobial chemoprophylaxis of close contacts of infected persons (Table 9-4).[110] Individuals with at least 4 hours of close contact during the week before onset of illness have an increased risk of being infected. Close contacts include household members, daycare center contacts, and anyone directly exposed to the patient's oral secretions. Antimicrobial chemoprophylaxis should be administered as soon as possible (ideally within 24 hours after identification of the index patient). Chemoprophylaxis administered longer than 14 days after onset of illness in the index patient is probably of limited or no value. Oropharyngeal or nasopharyngeal culture specimens are not helpful in determining the need for chemoprophylaxis.

Heparin does not stop the progression of the purpuric lesions in meningococcemia. Repletion of proteins C and S with freshly frozen plasma may be important adjunctive therapy in patients with purpura fulminans complicating meningococcemia.[101]

Table 9-4 Schedule for Administering Chemoprophylaxis Against Meningococcal Disease			
Drug	**Age group**	**Dosage**	**Duration and route of administration**
Rifampin* (Rimactane)	<1 mo	5 mg/kg every 12 h	2 d, oral
Rifampin (Rimactane)	>1 mo	10 mg/kg every 12 h	2 d, oral
Rifampin (Rimactane)	Adult	600 mg every 12 h	2 d, oral
Ciprofloxacin† (Cipro)	Adult	750 mg	Single dose, oral
Ceftriaxone	<15 yr	125 mg	Single dose, IM
Ceftriaxone	Adult	250 mg	Single dose, IM
Azithromycin (Zithromax)	Adult	500 mg	Single dose, oral

Adapted from Rosenstein NE, et al: N Engl J Med 2001; 344:1378.
*Rifampin should not be used in pregnant women. Reliability of oral contraceptives may be affected by rifampin.
†Ciprofloxacin can be used for persons <18 years of age if no acceptable alternative therapy is available.

Table 9-5 Nontuberculous Mycobacteria Infection

Characteristic	M. marinum	M. ulcerans	M. fortuitum and M. chelonei	M. avium-intracellulare	M. kansasii
Source of infection	Fresh and salt water (swimming pool, wells, contaminated fish, fish tanks); immunosuppressed patients	Water; swamp areas of Australia, Uganda, and Zaire	Ocean and fresh water, dirt, dust, animal feed, sporadic postoperative infections; trauma; dialysis equipment; postinjection abscesses	Gulf coast; Pacific coast; north central U.S.; soil, house dust, water; dried plants	Unclear; has been isolated from tap water; opportunistic infection
Symptoms	Asymptomatic to painful swelling of skin	Asymptomatic to painful swelling of skin; decreased mobility of joint	Often develops in patients with preexisting lung disease Disseminated disease associated with acquired immunodeficiency syndrome	Asymptomatic fever, weight loss, bone pain	Pruritus, fever, plaques, swelling. The most common disease is a pulmonary infection in elderly men with chronic underlying pulmonary disease
Skin lesion	Lesions occur at the inoculation site. Papules; nodules; verrucous plaques; ulcers/abscesses, sporotrichoid; disseminated	Large, solitary, deep, painless ulcer on the lower extremities. Secondary necrosis occurs. Primarily affects children and young adults	Granulomatous nodules; draining abscesses; ulcers; sporotrichoid lesions; cellulitis; disseminated disease	Granulomatous synovitis; deep hand infection; panniculitis; subcutaneous nodule	Verrucous papules, sporotrichoid eruption, cellulitis, granulomatous plaques, ulcers, and necrotic papulopustules
Treatment	Minocycline or doxycycline 100 mg twice daily; trimethoprim-sulfamethoxazole 160 to 800 mg twice daily; clarithromycin, rifampin 600 mg daily and ethambutol 800 mg daily for resistant strains, sporotrichoid lesions, and disseminated infections. Treat for 1 mo to 1 yr	Wide excision with or without skin grafting is treatment of choice. Trimethoprim-sulfamethoxazole 80/400 mg twice daily followed by rifampin 600 mg daily, and minocycline, 100 mg daily, or a combination of streptomycin, dapsone, and ethambutol. Heat area with occlusive wraps because M. ulcerans is heat sensitive	Severe disease: surgical debridement; amikacin (15 mg/kg/d) plus cefoxitin (200 mg/kg/d) combined with oral administration of probenecid, followed by sulfonamide, erythromycin, or minocycline. Less severe disease: sulfonamide with erythromycin. Continue therapy for 4 to 6 wk after wound healing	Aggressive therapy with multiple drugs including INH, clofazimine, rifampin, streptomycin, ethambutol, ethionamide, cycloserine, capreomycin, or clarithromycin	Rifampin in addition to ethambutol or isoniazid. Drug resistance has been reported with isoniazid. Treatment with higher dosages of isoniazid (900 mg) has been tried. Sulfonamides and amikacin have been added when rifampin-resistant strains occur
Culture incubation temperature	30° to 33° C	30° to 33° C	Between 25° and 40° C	37° C	37° C

Adapted from Street ML, et al: J Am Acad Dermatol 1991; 24:208.

Nontuberculous Mycobacteria

Mycobacteria are rods with a waxy coating that makes them resistant to stains and to many antibiotics. Once stained, they are not easily decolored and remain "acid-fast." The most common and important mycobacteria are *M. tuberculosis* and *M. leprae.* Nontuberculous mycobacteria (previously referred to as atypical mycobacteria) usually cause systemic disease, but they may just infect the skin (Table 9-5).[111] They are widespread in nature and are found in soil, animal and human feces, and water in swimming pools and fish tanks. They differ in culture requirements, pigment production, disease manifestation, and drug susceptibility. The Runyon classification, which depends on colony pigment and growth-rate characteristics, is no longer used. The bacteria are simply referred to by genus and species. Most cutaneous disease is caused by *M. marinum*[112] and *M. marinum* (*Mycobacterium balnei*). *M. marinum* is often called swimming pool granuloma and occurs in tropical fish enthusiasts, and fisherman as a chronic granulomatous infection, often manifesting as nodular lymphangitis. Because the organism requires a temperature of 30° C to 32° C for optimal growth, infections are usually limited to the skin. The disease occurs at sites of minor trauma such as the fingers, hands; the elbows and knees follow. The incubation period is 2 to 6 weeks. A papule or nodule appears and may ulcerate and discharge a serosanguineous fluid or develop a verrucous surface. Lesions are usually solitary, but a sporotrichoid distribution, in which nodular or ulcerating lesions extend proximally along sites of lymphatic drainage may occur. Tenosynovitis is commonly present in lesions of the fingers or hand. Localized adenopathy is rare. A positive tuberculin test result is present in 50% to 80% of patients.[113] Minocycline is the treatment of choice.

M. ulcerans, M. fortuitum, M. chelonei, and M. avium-intracellulare

Mycobacterium-avium complex causes disseminated disease in as many as 15% to 40% of patients with human immunodeficiency virus infection in the United States, causing fever, night sweats, weight loss, and anemia.[114-117] The bacteria are of low pathogenicity, and transmission between persons is rare. Predisposing conditions for infection are trauma, immunosuppression, human immunodeficiency virus infection,[18] and chronic disease. Consider a nontuberculous mycobacterial infection when a lesion develops at the site of trauma and follows a chronic course.

Mycobacteria require different temperatures for culture. Instruct the laboratory to incubate the cultures at both 30° C and 37° C. Isolation of these opportunistic, widespread organisms in culture does not prove that they cause the disease. DNA probes are now available to identify the species of mycobacteria; time for identification is within 3 to 4 weeks.

References

1. Barton LL, Friedman AD: Impetigo: a reassessment of etiology and therapy, Pediatr Dermatol 1987; 4:185.
2. Dagan R, Bar-David Y: Comparison of amoxicillin and clavulanic acid (augmentin) for the treatment of nonbullous impetigo, Am J Dis Child 1989; 143:916.
3. Peter G, Smith AL: Group A streptococcal infections of the skin and pharynx, N Engl J Med 1977; 297:311.
4. Fine RN: Clinical manifestations and diagnosis of post-streptococcal acute glomerulonephritis. pp 79-82. In Nissen AR: Poststreptococcal acute glomerulonephritis: fact and controversy, Ann Intern Med 1979; 91:76.
5. Rajajee S: Post-streptococcal acute glomerulonephritis: a clinical, bacteriological and serological study, Indian J Pediatr 1990; 57:775.
6. Maddox JS, Ware JC, Dillon HC: The natural history of streptococcal skin infection: prevention with topical antibiotics, J Am Acad Dermatol 1985; 13:207.
7. Doebbeling BN, et al: Long term efficacy of intranasal mupirocin ointment: a prospective cohort study of Staphylococcus aureus carriage, Arch Intern Med 1994; 154:1505.
8. McLinn S: A bacteriologically controlled, randomized study comparing the efficacy of 2% mupirocin ointment (Bactroban) with oral erythromycin in the treatment of patients with impetigo, J Am Acad Dermatol 1990; 22:883.
9. Demidovich CW, et al: Impetigo: current etiology and comparison of penicillin, erythromycin, and cephalexin therapies, Am J Dis Child 1990; 144:1313.
10. Mertz PM, et al: Topical mupirocin treatment of impetigo is equal to oral erythromycin therapy, Arch Dermatol 1989; 125:1069.
11. Hook EW, et al: Microbiologic evaluation of cutaneous cellulitis in adults, Arch Intern Med 1986; 146:295.
12. Kielhofner MA, et al: Influence of underlying disease process on the utility of cellulitis needle aspirates, Arch Intern Med 1988; 148:451.
13. Rudoy RC, Nakashima G: Diagnostic value of needle aspiration in Haemophilus influenzae type B cellulitis, J Pediatr 1979; 94:924.
14. Goetz JP, et al: Needle aspiration in Haemophilus influenzae type B cellulitis, Pediatrics 1974; 54:504.
15. Leppard BJ, et al: The value of bacteriology and serology in the diagnosis of cellulitis and erysipelas, Br J Dermatol 1985; 112:559.
16. Epperly TD: The value of needle aspiration in the management of cellulites, J Fam Pract 1986; 23:337.
17. Howe PM, Fajardo JE, Orcutt MA: Etiologic diagnosis of cellulitis: comparison of aspirates obtained from the leading edge and the point of maximal inflammation, Pediatr Infect Dis J 1987; 6:685.
18. McDonnell WM, Roth MS, Sheagren JN: Hemophilus influenzae type B cellulitis in adults, Am J Med 1986; 81:709.
19. Broome CV, et al: Special report: use of chemoprophylaxis to prevent the spread of Hemophilus influenzae B in day-care facilities. N Engl J Med 1987; 316:1226.
20. Klemper MS, Styrt B: Prevention of recurrent staphylococcal skin infections with low dose oral clindamycin therapy, JAMA 1988; 260:2682.
21. Hugo-Persson M, Norlin K: Erysipelas and group G streptococci, Infection 1987; 15:36.
22. Baddour LM, Bisno AL: Recurrent cellulitis after saphenous venectomy for coronary bypass surgery, Ann Intern Med 1982; 97:493.

23. Baddour LM, Bisno AL: Non-group A beta-hemolytic streptococcal cellulitis: association with venous and lymphatic compromise, Am J Med 1985; 79:155.

24. Jorup-Ronstrom C: Epidemiological, bacteriological and complicating features of erysipelas, Scan J Infect Dis 1986; 18:519.

25. Bitnun S: Prophylactic antibiotics in recurrent erysipelas (letter), Lancet 1985; 9:345.

26. Charnock DR, White T: Bruised cheek syndrome: haemophilus influenzae, type B, cellulitis, Otolaryngol Head Neck Surg 1990; 103:829.

27. Ginsburg CM: Hemophilus influenzae type B buccal cellulitis, J Am Acad Dermatol 1981; 4:661.

28. Barone S, Aiuto L: Periorbital and orbital cellulitis in the Haemophilus influenzae vaccine era, J Pediatr Ophthalmol Strabismus 1997; 34(5):293.

29. Ambati B, et al: Periorbital and orbital cellulitis before and after the advent of Haemophilus influenzae type B vaccination, Ophthalmology 2000; 107(8):1450.

30. Antoine GA, Grundfast KM: Periorbital cellulitis, Int J Pediatr Otorhinolaryngol 1987; 13:273.

31. Mills RP, Kartush JM: Orbital wall thickness and the spread of infection from the paranasal sinuses, Clin Otolaryngol 1985; 10:209.

32. Jackson K, Baker SR: Clinical implications of orbital cellulitis, Laryngoscope 1986; 96:568.

33. Teele DW: Management of the child with a red and swollen eye, Pediatr Infect Dis 1983; 2:258.

34. Hodges E, Tabbara KF: Orbital cellulitis: review of 23 cases from Saudi Arabia, Br J Ophthalmol 1989; 73:205.

35. Spires JR, Smith RJH: Bacterial infection of the orbital and periorbital soft tissues in children, Laryngoscope 1986; 96:763.

36. Ciarallo LR, Rowe PC: Lumbar puncture in children with periorbital and orbital cellulitis, J Pediatr 1993; 122:355.

37. Martin-Hirsch DP, et al: Orbital cellulitis, Arch Emerg Med 1992; 9:143.

38. Marks VJ, Maksimak M: Perianal streptococcal cellulitis, J Am Acad Dermatol 1988; 18:587.

39. Rehder PA, Eliezer ET, Lane AT: Perianal cellulitis: cutaneous group A streptococcal disease, Arch Dermatol 1988; 124:702.

40. Kokx NP, Comstock JA, Facklam RR: Streptococcal perianal disease in children, Pediatrics 1987; 80:659.

41. Bisno A, Cockerill F, Bermudez C: The initial outpatient-physician encounter in group A streptococcal necrotizing fasciitis, Clin Infect Dis 2000; 31(2):607.

42. Simonart T, et al: Value of standard laboratory tests for the early recognition of group A beta-hemolytic streptococcal necrotizing fasciitis, Clin Infect Dis 2001; 32(1):E9.

43. Cawley M, et al: Intravenous immunoglobulin as adjunctive treatment for streptococcal toxic shock syndrome associated with necrotizing fasciitis: case report and review, Pharmacotherapy 1999; 19(9):1094.

44. Perry P, et al: Defining pseudofolliculitis barbae in 2001: a review of the literature and current trends, J Am Acad Dermatol 2002; 46[Suppl 2]:S113.

45. Kauvar A: Treatment of pseudofolliculitis with a pulsed infrared laser, Arch Dermatol 2000; 136(11):1343.

46. Rogers C, Glaser D: Treatment of pseudofolliculitis barbae using the Q-switched Nd:YAG laser with topical carbon suspension, Dermatol Surg 2000; 26(8):737.

47. Chui C, et al: Recalcitrant scarring follicular disorders treated by laser-assisted hair removal: a preliminary report, Dermatol Surg 1999; 25(1):34.

48. Dinehart SM, et al: Acne keloidalis: a review, J Dermatol Surg Oncol 1989; 15:642.

49. Knable A, Hanke C, Gonin R: Prevalence of acne keloidalis nuchae in football players, J Am Acad Dermatol 1997; 37(4):570.

50. Sperling L, et al: Acne keloidalis is a form of primary scarring alopecia, Arch Dermatol 2000; 136(4):479.

51. Sperling L: Scarring alopecia and the dermatopathologist, J Cutan Pathol 2001; 28(7):333.

52. Luz RM, et al: Acne keloidalis nuchae and tufted hair folliculitis, Dermatology 1997; 194(1):71.

53. Gloster H: The surgical management of extensive cases of acne keloidalis nuchae, Arch Dermatol 2000; 136(11):1376.

54. Califano J, Miller S, Frodel J: Treatment of occipital acne keloidalis by excision followed by secondary intention healing, Arch Facial Plast Surg 1999; 1(4):308.

55. Llera JL, Levy RC: Treatment of cutaneous abscess: a double-blind clinical study, Ann Emerg Med 1985; 14:15.

56. Dahl MV: Strategies for the management of recurrent furunculosis, South Med J 1987; 80:352.

57. Hedstrom SA: Recurrent staphylococcal furunculosis: bacterial findings and epidemiology in 100 cases, Scand J Infect Dis 1981; 13:115.

58. Reboli AC, Farrar WE: Erysipelothrix rhusiopathiae: an occupational pathogen, Clin Microbiol Rev 1989; 2:354.

59. Molin G, et al: Occurrence of Erysipelothrix rhusiopathiae on pork and in pig slurry, and the distribution of specific antibodies in abattoir workers, J Appl Bacteriol 1989; 67:347.

60. Gorby GL, Peacock JE: Erysipelothrix rhusiopathiae endocarditis; microbiologic, epidemiologic and clinical features of an occupational disease, Rev Infect Dis 1988; 10:317.

61. Barnett JH, et al: Erysipeloid, J Am Acad Dermatol 1983; 9:116.

62. McCray MK, Esterly NB: Blistering distal dactylitis, J Am Acad Dermatol 1981; 5:592.

63. Norcross M, Jr, Mitchell DF: Blistering distal dactylitis caused by Staphylococcus aureus, Cutis 1993; 51:353.

64. Zemtsov A, Veitschegger M: Staphylococcus aureus-induced blistering distal dactylitis in an adult immunosuppressed patient, J Am Acad Dermatol 1992; 26:784.

65. Benson PM, Solivan G: Group B streptococcal blistering distal dactylitis in an adult diabetic, J Am Acad Dermatol 1987; 17:310.

66. Lyell A: The staphylococcal scalded skin syndrome in historical perspective: emergence of dermopathic strains of Staphylococcus aureus and discovery of the epidermolytic toxin, J Am Acad Dermatol 1983; 9:285.

67. Resnick SD: Staphylococcal toxin-mediated syndromes in childhood, Semin Dermatol 1992; 11:11.

68. Amagai M, et al: Toxin in bullous impetigo and staphylococcal scalded-skin syndrome targets desmoglein 1, Nat Med 2000; 6(11):1275.

69. Goldberg NS, et al: Staphylococcal scalded skin syndrome mimicking acute graft-vs-host disease in a bone marrow transplant recipient, Arch Dermatol 1989; 125:85.

70. Herzog JL, Sexton FM: Desquamative rash in an immunocompromised adult: staphylococcal scalded skin syndrome (SSSS), Arch Dermatol 1990; 126:815.

71. Beers B, Wilson B: Adult staphylococcal scalded skin syndrome, Int J Dermatol 1990; 29:428.

72. Borchers SL, Gomez EC, Isseroff RR: Generalized staphylococcal scalded skin syndrome in an anephric boy undergoing hemodialysis, Arch Dermatol 1984; 120:912.

73. Bottone EJ, Perez A: Pseudomonas aeruginosa folliculitis acquired through use of a contaminated loofah sponge: an unrecognized potential public health problem, J Clin Microbiol 1993; 31:480.

74. Ratnam S, et al: Whirlpool-associated folliculitis caused by Pseudomonas aeruginosa: report of an outbreak and review, J Clin Microbiol 1986; 23:655.

75. Highsmith AK, et al: Characteristics of Pseudomonas aeruginosa isolated from whirlpools and bathers, Infect Control Hosp Epidemiol 1985; 6:407.

76. Fiorillo L, et al: The pseudomonas hot-foot syndrome, N Engl J Med 2001; 345(5):335.

77. Petrozzi JW, Alexander E: Pseudomonal balanitis, Arch Dermatol 1977; 113:952.

78. Manian FA, Alford RH: Nosocomial infectious balanoposthitis in neutropenic patients, South Med J 1987; 80(7):909.

79. Raz R, Miron D: Oral ciprofloxacin for treatment of infection following nail puncture wounds of the foot, Clin Infect Dis 1995; 21(1):194.

80. Milner SM: Acetic acid to treat Pseudomonas aeruginosa in superficial wounds and burns, Lancet 1992; 340:61.

81. Siami G, et al: Clinafloxacin versus piperacillin-tazobactam in treatment of patients with severe skin and soft tissue infections, Antimicrob Agents Chemother 2001; 45(2):525.

82. Brook I: Treatment of otitis externa in children, Paediatr Drugs 1999; 1(4):283-289.

83. Sander R: Otitis externa: a practical guide to treatment and prevention, Am Fam Physician 2001; 63(5):927-936, 941.

84. Jones R, Milazzo J, Seidlin M: Ofloxacin otic solution for treatment of otitis externa in children and adults, Arch Otolaryngol Head Neck Surg 1997; 123(11):1193.

85. Dekker PJ: Alternative method of application of topical preparations in otitis externa, J Laryngol Otol 1991; 105:842.

86. Stuck B, Riedel F, Hormann K: Treatment of therapy refractory chronic otitis externa by local injection of triamcinolone acetate crystalline suspension: initial experiences, HNO 2001; 49(3):199.

87. Scherbenske JM, Winton GB, James WD: Acute pseudomonas infection of the external ear (malignant external otitis), J Dermatol Surg Oncol 1988; 14:165.

88. Westmoreland TA, Ross EV, Yeager JK: Pseudomonas toe web infections, Cutis 1992; 49:185.

89. King DF, King LAC: Importance of debridement in the treatment of gram-negative bacterial toe web infection, J Am Acad Dermatol 1986; 14:278.

90. Huminer D, et al: Ecthyma gangrenosum without bacteremia: report of six cases and review of the literature, Arch Intern Med 1987; 147:299.

91. Bodey GP, Jadeja L, Elting L: Pseudomonas bacteremia: retrospective analysis of 410 episodes, Arch Intern Med 1985; 145:1621.

92. Boisseau AM, et al: Perineal ecthyma gangrenosum in infancy and early childhood: septicemic and nonsepticemic forms, J Am Acad Dermatol 1992; 27:415.

93. Fergie JE, et al: Pseudomonas aeruginosa cellulitis and ecthyma gangrenosum in immunocompromised children, Pediatr Infect Dis J 1991; 10:496.

94. el Blaze P, et al: A study of nineteen immunocompromised patients with extensive skin lesions caused by Pseudomonas aeruginosa with and without bacteremia, Acta Derm Venereol 1991; 71:411.

95. Greene SL, Daniel S, Muller SA: Ecthyma gangrenosum: report of clinical, histopathologic, and bacteriologic aspects of eight cases, J Am Acad Dermatol 1984; 11:781.

96. Rosenstein N, et al: The changing epidemiology of meningococcal disease in the United States, 1992-1996, J Infect Dis 1999; 180(6):1894.

97. Wong VK, et al: Meningococcal infections in children: a review of 100 cases, Pediatr Infect Dis J 1989; 8:224.

98. Marzouk O, Thomson AP, et al: Features and outcome in meningococcal disease presenting with maculopapular rash, Arch Dis Child 1991; 66:485.

99. Ramesh V, et al: Clinical, histopathologic & immunologic features of cutaneous lesions in acute meningococcaemia, Indian J Med Res 1990; 91:27.

100. Wang V, et al: Meningococcal disease among children who live in a large metropolitan area, 1981-1996, Clin Infect Dis 2001; 32(7):1004.

101. Powars DR, et al: Purpura fulminans in meningococcemia: association with acquired deficiencies of proteins C and S, N Engl J Med 1987; 317:571.

102. Berg S, et al: Incidence, serogroups and case-fatality rate of invasive meningococcal infections in a Swedish region 1975-1989, Scand J Infect Dis 1992; 24:333.

103. Pinner RW, et al: for the Meningococcal Disease Study Group: meningococcal disease in the United States-1986. J Infect Dis 1991; 164:368.

104. Borchsenius F, et al: Systemic meningococcal disease: the diagnosis on admission to hospital, NIPH Ann 1991; 14:11.

105. Tesoro LJ, Selbst SM: Factors affecting outcome in meningococcal infections, Am J Dis Child 1991; 145:218.

106. Pohl CA: Practical approach to bacterial meningitis in childhood, Am Fam Physician 1993; 47:1595.

107. Van DM, et al: Rapid diagnosis of acute meningococcal infections by needle aspiration or biopsy of skin lesions, BMJ 1993; 306:1229.

108. Mertens R, et al: Diagnosis and stage-related treatment of disseminated intravascular coagulation in meningococcal infections, Klin Padiatr 1999; 211(2):65.

109. MacLennan J, et al: Safety, immunogenicity, and induction of immunologic memory by a serogroup C meningococcal conjugate vaccine in infants: a randomized controlled trial, JAMA 2000; 283(21):2795.

110. Rosenstein N, et al: Meningococcal disease, N Engl J Med 2001; 344(18):1378.

111. Holland S: Nontuberculous mycobacteria, Am J Med Sci 2001; 321(1):49.

112. Hoyt RE, et al: M. marinum infections in a Chesapeake Bay community, Va Med 1989; 116:467.

113. Weitzul S, Eichhorn P, Pandya A: Nontuberculous mycobacterial infections of the skin, Dermatol Clin 2000; 18(2):359-377, xi.

114. Seevanayagam S, Hayman J: Mycobacterium ulcerans infection; is the "Bairnsdale ulcer" also a Ceylonese disease? Ceylon Med J 1992; 37:125.

115. Ingram CW, et al: Disseminated infection with rapidly growing mycobacteria, Clin Infect Dis 1993; 16:463.

116. Drabick JJ, et al: Disseminated Mycobacterium chelonae subspecies chelonae infection with cutaneous and osseous manifestations, Arch Dermatol 1990; 126:1064.

117. Wallace R, Jr: The clinical presentation, diagnosis, and therapy of cutaneous and pulmonary infections due to the rapidly growing mycobacteria: M. fortuitum and M. chelonae, Clin Chest Med 1989; 10:419.

Sexually Transmitted Bacterial Infections

❏ **Sexually transmitted disease presentations**

❏ **Genital ulcers**

❏ **Syphilis**
Incidence
Stages
Risk of transmission
T. pallidum
Primary syphilis
Secondary syphilis
Latent syphilis
Tertiary syphilis
Syphilis and human immunodeficiency virus
Congenital syphilis
Syphilis serology
Treatment of syphilis
Posttreatment evaluation of syphilis

❏ **Rare sexually transmitted diseases**
Lymphogranuloma venereum
Chancroid
Granuloma inguinale (donovanosis)

❏ **Diseases characterized by urethritis and cervicitis**
Gonorrhea
Neisseria gonorrhoeae
Nongonococcal urethritis

Sexually Transmitted Disease Presentations

Sexually transmitted diseases can present as:
- Genital ulcers
- Urethritis
- Cervicitis
- Vaginal discharge
- Papules

An overview of these diseases is presented in the diagrams on pp. 308-311. Treatment of all sexually transmitted diseases is presented in Table 10-1 (pp. 312-314).

Genital Ulcers

Genital herpes infections are discussed in Chapter 11. The differential diagnosis of genital ulcerations appears in Table 10-2 (p. 314).

In developed countries, most patients who have genital ulcers have either herpes simplex virus (HSV), syphilis, or chancroid. The frequency of each differs by geographic area and patient population. Herpes is the most prevalent. A patient may have more than one of these diseases. Not all genital ulcers are caused by sexually transmitted infections. Each disease is associated with an increased risk for human immunodeficiency virus (HIV) infection. A diagnosis-based history and physical examination is often inaccurate. All patients who have genital ulcers should have a serologic test for syphilis and diagnostic tests for herpes. Tests include:
- Rapid plasma reagin (RPR) or Venereal Disease Research Laboratories (VDRL)
- Darkfield examination for *Treponema pallidum*
- Culture and/or antigen test for HSV
- Culture for *Haemophilus ducreyi*
- Biopsy if treatment fails
- HIV testing if ulcers are caused by *T. pallidum* or *H. ducreyi*
- Consider HIV testing for patients with HSV

HIV testing should be performed in patients who have genital ulcers caused by *T. pallidum* or *H. ducreyi* and considered for those who have ulcers caused by HSV.

Treatment of genital ulcers is often desirable before test results are available. Treat for the most likely diagnosis. If the diagnosis is unclear, treat for syphilis or for both syphilis and chancroid if the patient lives in an area where *H. ducreyi* is a significant cause of genital ulcers. Even after complete diagnostic evaluation, at least 25% of patients who have genital ulcers have no laboratory-confirmed diagnosis.

Text continued on p. 315.

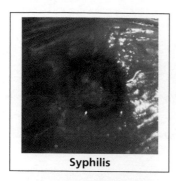

Syphilis

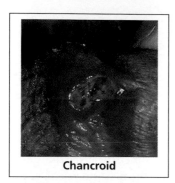

Chancroid

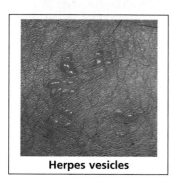

Herpes vesicles

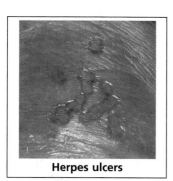

Herpes ulcers

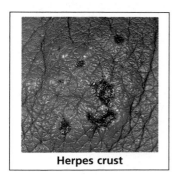

Herpes crust

SEXUALLY TRANSMITTED GENITAL DISEASES DIAGNOSIS AND MANAGEMENT

GENITAL ULCERS

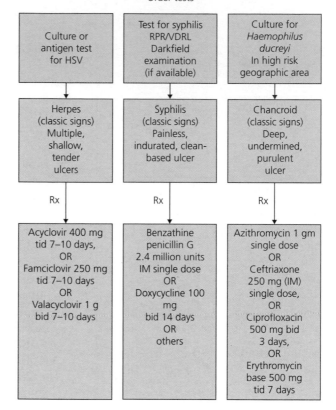

Clinical diagnosis
made in a minority of patients
Inguinal lymph node findings do not
contribute significantly to clinical
diagnostic accuracy

Order tests

Culture or antigen test for HSV	Test for syphilis RPR/VDRL Darkfield examination (if available)	Culture for *Haemophilus ducreyi* In high risk geographic area
Herpes (classic signs) Multiple, shallow, tender ulcers	Syphilis (classic signs) Painless, indurated, clean-based ulcer	Chancroid (classic signs) Deep, undermined, purulent ulcer
Rx	Rx	Rx
Acyclovir 400 mg tid 7–10 days, OR Famciclovir 250 mg tid 7–10 days OR Valacyclovir 1 g bid 7–10 days	Benzathine penicillin G 2.4 million units IM single dose OR Doxycycline 100 mg bid 14 days OR others	Azithromycin 1 gm single dose OR Ceftriaxone 250 mg (IM) single dose, OR Ciprofloxacin 500 mg bid 3 days, OR Erythromycin base 500 mg tid 7 days

Order HIV testing
1. If Dx is syphilis or chancroid
2. Consider HIV testing if Dx is HSV

If there is no laboratory-confirmed diagnosis, then consider Rx for syphilis or for both syphilis and chancroid

SEXUALLY TRANSMITTED GENITAL DISEASES
DIAGNOSIS AND MANAGEMENT

URETHRITIS AND CERVICITIS

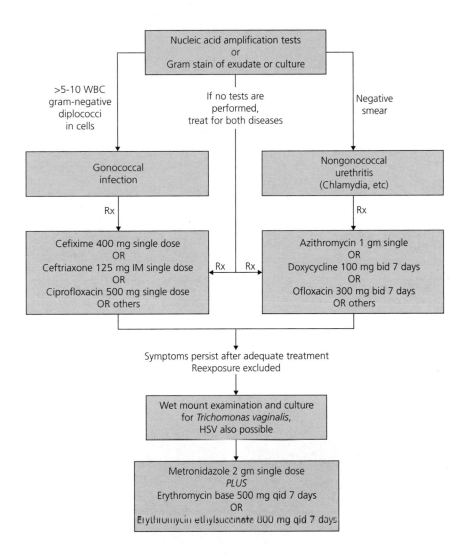

Urethritis males

1. Mucopurulent discharge
2. Burning urination or asymptomatic

Mucopurulent cervicitis

1. Exudate—canal or endocervical swab
2. Easily induced cervical bleeding
3. Vaginal discharge or bleeding

Nucleic acid amplification tests
or
Gram stain of exudate or culture

>5-10 WBC
gram-negative
diplococci
in cells

If no tests are
performed,
treat for both diseases

Negative
smear

Gonococcal
infection

Nongonococcal
urethritis
(Chlamydia, etc)

Rx

Rx

Cefixime 400 mg single dose
OR
Ceftriaxone 125 mg IM single dose
OR
Ciprofloxacin 500 mg single dose
OR others

Rx   Rx

Azithromycin 1 gm single
OR
Doxycycline 100 mg bid 7 days
OR
Ofloxacin 300 mg bid 7 days
OR others

Symptoms persist after adequate treatment
Reexposure excluded

Wet mount examination and culture
for *Trichomonas vaginalis*,
HSV also possible

Metronidazole 2 gm single dose
PLUS
Erythromycin base 500 mg qid 7 days
OR
Erythromycin ethylsuccinate 800 mg qid 7 days

SEXUALLY TRANSMITTED GENITAL DISEASES
DIAGNOSIS AND MANAGEMENT

VAGINAL DISCHARGE

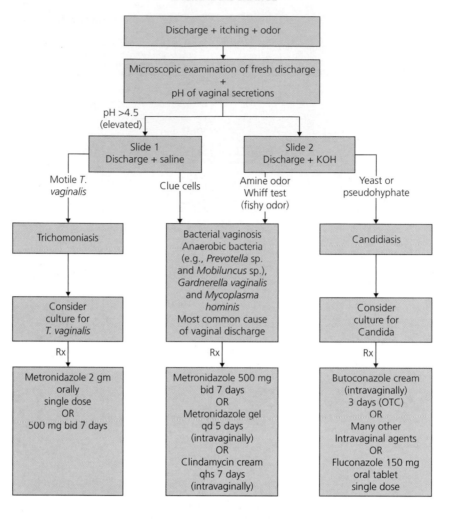

Discharge + itching + odor

↓

Microscopic examination of fresh discharge
+
pH of vaginal secretions

pH >4.5
(elevated)

| Slide 1 Discharge + saline | Slide 2 Discharge + KOH |

Motile *T. vaginalis* — Clue cells — Amine odor Whiff test (fishy odor) — Yeast or pseudohyphate

| Trichomoniasis | Bacterial vaginosis Anaerobic bacteria (e.g., *Prevotella* sp. and *Mobiluncus* sp.), *Gardnerella vaginalis* and *Mycoplasma hominis* Most common cause of vaginal discharge | Candidiasis |

| Consider culture for *T. vaginalis* | | Consider culture for Candida |

Rx — Rx — Rx

| Metronidazole 2 gm orally single dose OR 500 mg bid 7 days | Metronidazole 500 mg bid 7 days OR Metronidazole gel qd 5 days (intravaginally) OR Clindamycin cream qhs 7 days (intravaginally) | Butoconazole cream (intravaginally) 3 days (OTC) OR Many other Intravaginal agents OR Fluconazole 150 mg oral tablet single dose |

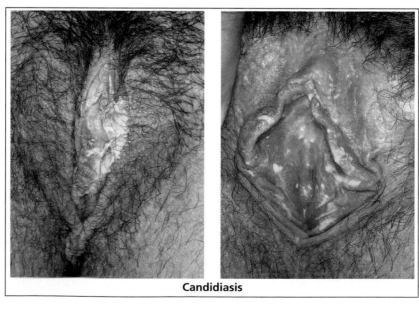

Candidiasis

SEXUALLY TRANSMITTED GENITAL DISEASES
DIAGNOSIS AND MANAGEMENT

GENITAL PAPULES

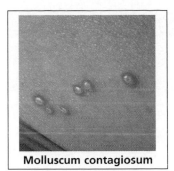

Molluscum contagiosum

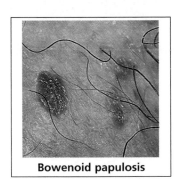

Pearly penile papules

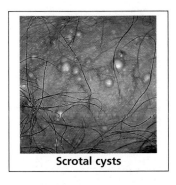

Bowenoid papulosis

Scrotal cysts

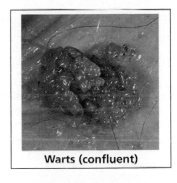

Warts (confluent)

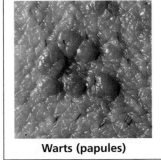

Warts (papules)

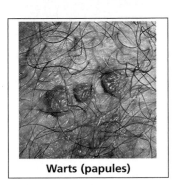

Warts (papules)

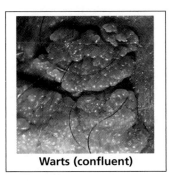

Warts (confluent)

Clinical diagnosis

Biopsy rarely needed
Acetic acid test not
recommended

Warts → Molluscum
contagiosum

Rx for
visible lesions

Rx

Cryotherapy
Aldara
Condylox
Excision
Electrocautery
TCA

Cryotherapy
Aldara
Curettage

Rx not recommended for
subclinical HPV infection
diagnosed by Pap smear,
colposcopy, biopsy, acetic acid
soaking

Differential diagnosis:

Pearly penile papules
Bowenoid papulosis
Scrotal sebaceous glands

Table 10-1 Treatment of Some Sexually Transmitted Infections (Medical Letter, 2002)

Type or stage	Drugs of choice	Dosage	Alternatives
CHLAMYDIAL INFECTION AND RELATED CLINICAL SYNDROMES[1]			
Urethritis, cervicitis, conjunctivitis, or proctitis (except lymphogranuloma venereum)			
	Azithromycin	1 gm oral once	Ofloxacin[2] 300 mg oral bid × 7 days
			Levofloxacin[3] 500 mg oral once daily × 7 days
	OR Doxycycline[2,3]	100 mg oral bid × 7 days	Erythromycin[4] 500 mg oral qid × 7 days
Infection in pregnancy			
	Amoxicillin	500 mg oral tid × 10 days	Erythromycin[4] 500 mg oral qid × 7 days
	OR Azithromycin	1 gm oral once	
Neonatal ophthalmia or pneumonia			
	Azithromycin	200 mg/kg oral once daily × 3 days	Erythromycin 12.5 mg/kg oral qid × 14 days[5]
Lymphogranuloma venereum			
	Doxycycline[2,3]	100 mg oral bid × 21 days	Erythromycin[4] 500 mg oral qid × 21 days
EPIDIDYMITIS			
	Ofloxacin	300 mg bid × 10 days	Ceftriaxone 250 mg IM once **followed by** doxycycline[3] 100 mg oral bid × 10 days
GONORRHEA[6]			
Urethral, cervical, rectal, or pharyngeal			
	Cefixime	400 mg oral once	Spectinomycin 2 g IM once[7]
	OR Ciprofloxacin[2,8]	500 mg oral once	
	OR Ofloxacin	400 mg oral once	
	OR Ceftriaxone	125 mg IM once	
PELVIC INFLAMMATORY DISEASE			
—Parenteral	Cefotetan or cefoxitin **plus**	2 g IV q12h	Ofloxacin[2] 400 mg IV q12h or levofloxacin[2]
		2 g IV q6h	500 mg IV once daily **plus** metronidazole
	doxycycline[2]	100 mg IV or oral q12h, until improved	500 mg IV q8h[9]
	followed by		Ampicillin/sulbactam 3 g IV q6h **plus**
	doxycycline[2]	100 mg oral bid to complete 14 days	doxycycline[2] 100 mg orally or IV q12h
			All continued until improved, then followed by doxycycline[2] 100 mg orally bid to complete 14 days[10]
	OR Clindamycin **plus** gentamicin	900 mg IV q8h	
		2 mg/kg IV once, then 1.5 mg/kg IV q8h[11], until improved	
	followed by doxycycline[2]	100 mg oral bid to complete 14 days[10]	
— Oral	Ofloxacin[2]	400 mg oral bid × 14 days	
	OR Levofloxacin[2] **plus** metronidazole[9]	500 mg once daily × 14 days	
		250 mg IM once	
	OR Ceftriaxone **followed by** doxycycline[2,12]		Cefoxitin 2 g once plus probenecid 1 g oral once **followed by** doxycycline[2,12]
		100 mg oral bid × 14 days	100 mg oral bid × 14 days

[1]Related clinical syndromes include nonchlamydial nongonococcal urethritis and cervicitis.
[2]Not recommended in pregnancy.
[3]Or tetracycline 500 mg oral qid.
[4]Erythromycin ethylsuccinate 800 mg may be substituted for erythromycin base 500 mg; erythromycin estolate is contraindicated in pregnancy.
[5]Pyloric stenosis has been associated with use of erythromycin in newborns.
[6]All patients should also receive a course of treatment effective for *Chlamydia*.
[7]Recommended only for use during pregnancy in patients allergic to β-lactams. Not effective for pharyngeal infection.
[8]Fluoroquinolones should not be used to treat gonorrhea acquired in Asia, Hawaii, Israel, or other areas where fluoroquinolone-resistant strains of *N. gonorrhoeae* are common.
[9]Some clinicians believe the addition of metronidazole is not required.
[10]Or clindamycin 450 mg oral qid to complete 14 days.
[11]A single daily dose of 3 mg/kg is likely to be effective but has not been studied in pelvic inflammatory disease.

Table 10-1 Treatment of Some Sexually Transmitted Infections—cont'd

Type or stage	Drugs of choice	Dosage	Alternatives
VAGINAL INFECTION			
Trichomoniasis, bacterial vaginosis			
	Metronidazole	2 gm oral once	Metronidazole 375 mg *(Flagyl 375)* or 500 mg oral bid × 7 days
	Metronidazole	500 mg oral bid × 7 days	Metronidazole 2 gm oral once[13]
	OR Metronidazole gel 0.75%[14]	5 gm intravaginally once or twice daily × 5 days	Clindamycin 300 mg orally bid × 7 days
	OR Clindamycin 2% cream[14]	5 gm intravaginally qhs × 3-7 days	Clindamycin ovules[14] 100 mg intravaginally once daily × 3 days
Vulvovaginal candidiasis			
	Intravaginal butoconazole, clotrimazole, miconazole, terconazole, or tioconazole[15]		
	OR Fluconazole	150 mg oral once	
SYPHILIS			
Early (primary, secondary, or latent less than 1 year)			
	Penicillin G benzathine	2.4 million U IM once[16]	Doxycycline[3] 100 mg oral bid × 14 days Azithromycin[17] 2 gm oral once
Late (more than 1 year's duration, cardiovascular, gumma, late-latent)			
	Penicillin G benzathine	2.4 million U IM weekly × 3 weeks	Doxycycline[2] 100 mg oral bid × 4 weeks
Neurosyphilis[18]	Penicillin G	3-4 million U IV q4h × 10-14 days	Penicillin G procaine 2.4 million U IM daily plus probenecid 500 mg qid oral, both × 10-14 days Ceftriaxone 2 gm IV once daily × 10-14 days
Congenital	Penicillin G	50,000 U/kg IV q8-12h × 10-14 days	
	OR Penicillin G procaine	50,000 U/kg IM daily × 10-14 days	
CHANCROID[19]			
	Azithromycin	1 gm oral once	Ciprofloxacin[2] 500 mg oral bid × 3 days
	OR Ceftriaxone	250 mg IM once	Erythromycin[4] 500 mg oral qid × 7 days
GENITAL WARTS[20]			
	Trichloroacetic or bichloracetic acid, or podophyllin[2] or liquid nitrogen	1-2 weeks until resolved	Surgical removal Laser surgery Intralesional interferon
	Imiquimod 5%[2]	3×/week × 16 weeks bid	
	Podofilox 0.5%[3]	bid × 3 days, 4 days rest, then repeated up to 4 times	

[12]Some experts would add metronidazole 500 mg bid.
[13]Higher relapse rate with single dose but useful for patients who may not comply with multiple-dose therapy.
[14]In pregnancy, topical preparations have not been effective in preventing premature delivery; oral metronidazole has been effective in some studies.
[15]For preparations and dosage of topical products, see Medical Letter 2001; 43:3[1].
[16]Some experts recommend repeating this regimen after 7 days, especially in patients with HIV infection.
[17]Limited experience (EW Hook III, et al: Sex Transm Dis 2002; 29, in press[2]).
[18]Patients allergic to penicillin should be desensitized and treated with penicillin.
[19]All regimens, especially single-dose ceftriaxone, are less effective in patients with human immunodeficiency virus.
[20]Recommended for external genital warts. Liquid nitrogen can also be used for vaginal, urethral, and/or oral warts. Podofilox or imiquimod can be used for urethral meatus warts. Trichloroacetic or bichloracetic acid can be used for anal warts.
[21]Antiviral therapy is variably effective for episodic treatment of recurrences; only effective if started early.
[22]Three-day regimens of acyclovir or famciclovir are probably effective, but clinical data are lacking.
[23]Preventive treatment should be discontinued for 1-2 months once a year to reassess the frequency of recurrence.
[24]Use 500 mg once daily in patients with ≥10 recurrences per year.

Continued

Table 10-1 Treatment of Some Sexually Transmitted Infections—cont'd

GENITAL HERPES

First episode	Drugs of choice	Dosage	Alternatives
	Acyclovir	400 mg oral tid × 7 -10 days	Acyclovir 200 mg oral 5×/day × 7-10 days
	OR Famciclovir	250 mg oral tid × 7-10 days	
	OR Valacyclovir	1 gm oral bid × 7-10 days	
Severe (hospitalized patients)	Acyclovir	5-10 mg/kg IV q8h × 5-7 days	
Recurrent[21]	Acyclovir	400 mg oral tid × 3-5 days[22]	
	OR Famciclovir	125 mg oral bid × 3-5 days[22]	
	OR Valacyclovir	500 mg oral bid × 3 days	
Suppression of recurrences[23]	Acyclovir	400 mg oral bid	
	OR Valacyclovir	500 mg-1 gm once daily[24]	Acyclovir 200 mg oral 2-5×/day
	OR Famciclovir	250 mg oral bid	

Table 10-2 Differential Diagnosis of Genital Ulcerations

Characteristics and treatment	Chancroid	Granuloma inguinale	Lymphogranuloma venereum (LGV)	Primary syphilis	Herpes simplex
Etiology	*Haemophilus ducreyi*	*Calymmato-bacterium (Donovania) granulomatis*	*Chlamydia*	*Treponema pallidum*	*Herpes virus hominis*
Incubation period	12 h to 3 d	3-6 wk	3 d to several weeks	3 wk	3-10 d
Initial lesion	Single or multiple, round to oval, deep ulcers with outlines, ragged and under-mined borders, and a purulent base; lesions are tender	Soft, nontender papule(s) that forms irregular ulcer with beefy-red, friable base, and raised, "rolled" border	Evanescent ulcer (rarely seen)	Nontender, eroded papule with clean base and raised, firm, indurated bor-ders; multiple lesions occa-sionally seen	Primary lesions are multiple, ede-matous, painful erosions with yellow-white membranous coating; recur-rent episodes may have grouped vesi-cles on an ery-thematous base
Duration	Undetermined (months)	Undetermined (years)	2-6 days	3-6 weeks	Primary 2-6 weeks; recurrent 7-10 days
Site	Genital or perianal	Genital, perianal, or inguinal	Genital, perianal, or rectal	Genital, perianal, or rectal	Genital or perianal
Regional adenopathy	Unilateral or bilat-eral tender, matted, fixed adenopathy that may be-come soft and fluctuant	Subcutaneous peri-lymphatic granu-lomatous lesions that produce in-guinal swellings and are not lym-phadenitis (pseudo buboes)	Unilateral or bilat-eral firm, painful inguinal adenopathy with overlying "dusky skin"; may become fluctuant and develop "grooves in the groin"	Unilateral or bi-lateral firm, movable, non-suppurative, painless in-guinal adenopathy	Bilateral, tender inguinal adenopathy, usually present with primary vulvovaginitis and may or may not be present with recurrent genital lesions
Diagnostic tests	Smear, culture, or biopsy of lesion; smear from as-pirated unrup-tured lymph node	Biopsy; touch prepa-ration from biopsy stained with Giemsa	LGV complement fixation test, culture	Dark-field exami-nation, VDRL, FTA-ABS	Tzanck smear; culture

Modified from Margolis RJ, Hood AF: J Am Acad Dermatol 1982; 6:496.

Syphilis

Syphilis is a human infectious disease caused by the bacterium *Treponema pallidum*. The disease is transmitted by direct contact with a lesion during the primary or secondary stage, in utero by the transplacental route, or during delivery as the baby passes through an infected canal. Like the gonococcus, this bacterium is fragile and dies when removed from the human environment. Unlike the gonococcus, *T. pallidum* may infect any organ, causing an infinite number of clinical presentations; thus the old adage, "he who knows syphilis knows medicine."

Incidence

The incidence of syphilis in the United States was 3.2 cases per 100,000 people in 1998 (7057 total cases), which is the lowest rate since surveillance began in 1941. Syphilis is found in the southern states, especially in African Americans[1] (Figure 10-1). Crack cocaine and the exchange of sex for drugs are contributing factors.

Stages

Untreated syphilis may pass through three stages. Syphilis begins with the infectious cutaneous primary and secondary stages that may terminate without further sequelae or may evolve into a latent stage that lasts for months or years before the now-rare tertiary stage, marked by the appearance of cardiovascular, neurologic, and deep cutaneous complications (Figure 10-2).

The Centers for Disease Control and Prevention defines the stages of syphilis as follows:

1. Infectious syphilis includes the stages of primary, secondary, and early latent syphilis of less than 1 year's duration.
2. Latent infections (i.e., those lacking clinical manifestations) are detected by serologic testing. Latent syphilis is divided into early latent disease of less than 1-year's duration and early latent disease of greater than 1 year's duration.
3. Late latent disease of 4 years' duration or longer.

Primary and Secondary Syphilis—United States, 1998*

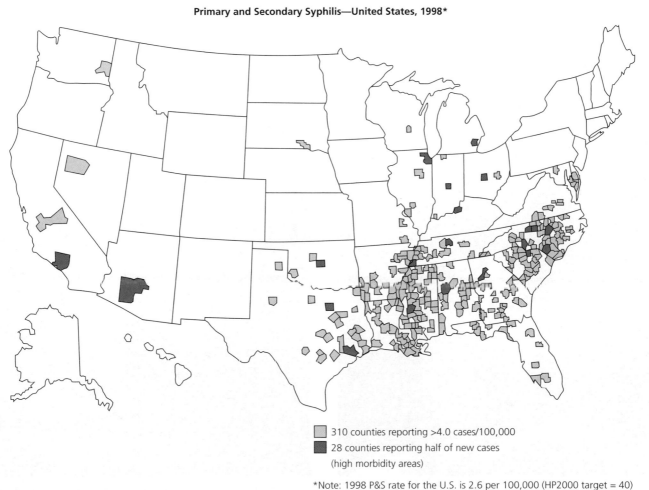

■ 310 counties reporting >4.0 cases/100,000
■ 28 counties reporting half of new cases
(high morbidity areas)

*Note: 1998 P&S rate for the U.S. is 2.6 per 100,000 (HP2000 target = 40)
Source: CDC STD Surveillance System

Figure 10-1
Incidence of primary and secondary syphilis in the United States.

Course of Disease and Blood Tests

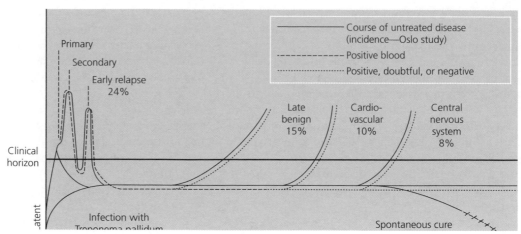

Figure legend:
——— Course of untreated disease (incidence—Oslo study)
− − − − Positive blood
· · · · · · Positive, doubtful, or negative

Primary
Secondary
Early relapse 24%
Late benign 15%
Cardio-vascular 10%
Central nervous system 8%
Clinical horizon
Latent
Infection with *Treponema pallidum*
Spontaneous cure

Figure 10-2 Natural history of untreated acquired syphilis. *(From Morgan HJ: South Med J 26:18, 1933; incidence from Clark EG, Danbolt N: J Chronic Dis 2:311, 1955.)*

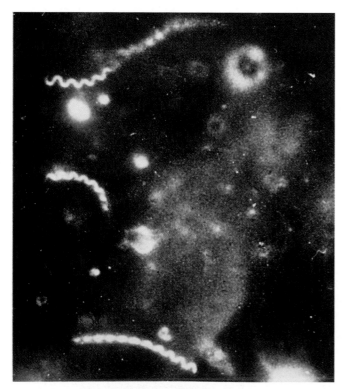

Figure 10-3 *Treponema pallidum.* Organism responsible for syphilis is seen here photographed through a dark-field microscope.

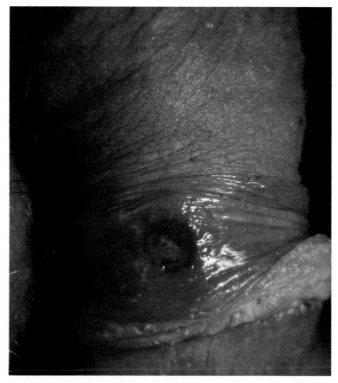

Figure 10-4 Primary syphilis. Syphilitic chancre is an ulcer with a clean, nonpurulent base and smooth, regular, sharply defined border.

Risk of transmission

The greatest risk of transmission occurs during the primary, secondary, and early latent stages of disease. The patient is most infectious during the first 1 to 2 years of infection. Patients with secondary syphilis are the most contagious because of the large number of lesions. The risk of acquiring syphilis from an infected partner is 10% to 60%. One third of persons with a single exposure to early syphilis will become infected.

T. pallidum

T. pallidum, the organism responsible for syphilis, is a very small, spiral bacterium (spirochete) whose form and corkscrew rotation motility can be observed only by dark-field microscopy (Figure 10-3). The reproductive time is estimated to be 30 to 33 hours, in contrast to most bacteria, which replicate every 30 minutes. Serum levels of antibiotics must therefore persist for at least 7 to 10 days to kill all replicating organisms. The Gram stain cannot be used, and growing the bacteria is difficult.

Primary syphilis

Primary syphilis, characterized by a cutaneous ulcer, is acquired by direct contact with an infectious lesion of the skin or the moist surface of the mouth, anus, or vagina. From 10 to 90 days (average, 21 days) after exposure, a primary lesion, the chancre, develops at the site of initial contact. Chancres are usually solitary, but multiple lesions are not uncommon. Extragenital chancres account for 6% of all chancres, and most occur on the lips and in the oral cavity and are transmitted by kissing or orogenital sex.[2] The lesion begins as a papule that undergoes ischemic necrosis and erodes, forming a 0.3- to 2.0-cm, painless to tender, hard, indurated ulcer; the base is clean, with a scant, yellow, serous discharge. Because the chancre began as a papule, the borders of the ulcer are raised, smooth, and sharply defined (Figure 10-4). The chancre of chancroid is soft and painful. Painless, hard, discrete regional lymphadenopathy occurs in 1 to 2 weeks; the lesions never coalesce or suppurate unless there is a mixed infection. Without treatment, the chancre heals with scarring in 3 to 6 weeks. Painless vaginal and anal lesions may never be detected (Figure 10-5). The differential diagnosis includes ulcerative genital lesions such as chancroid, herpes progenitalis, aphthae (Behçet's syndrome), and traumatic ulcers such as occur with biting (Table 10-2). If untreated, approximately 25% of the infections progress directly to the second stage; the other 75% enter latency.

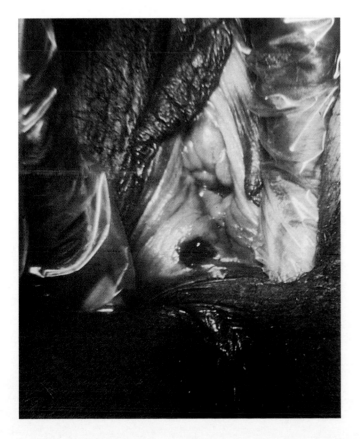

Figure 10-5 Primary syphilis. Chancre in vagina. Lesions are painless and may never be detected.

Secondary syphilis

Secondary syphilis is characterized by mucocutaneous lesions, a flulike syndrome, and generalized adenopathy. Asymptomatic dissemination of *T. pallidum* to all organs occurs as the chancre heals, and the disease then resolves in approximately 75% of cases[3] (see Figure 10-2). In the remaining 25%, the clinical signs of the secondary stage begin approximately 6 weeks (range, 2 weeks to 6 months) after the chancre appears and last for 2 to 10 weeks. Cutaneous lesions are preceded by a flulike syndrome (sore throat, headache, muscle aches, meningismus, and loss of appetite) and generalized, painless lymphadenopathy. Hepatosplenomegaly may be present. In some cases lesions of secondary syphilis appear before the chancre heals. The distribution and morphologic characteristics of the skin and mucosal lesions are varied and may be confused with numerous other skin diseases. As with most other systemic cutaneous diseases, the rash is usually bilaterally symmetric (Figures 10-6 to 10-9).

Lesions

The lesions of secondary syphilis have certain characteristics that differentiate them from other cutaneous diseases.[4] There is little or no fever at the onset. Lesions are noninflammatory, develop slowly, and may persist for weeks or months. Pain or itching is minimal or absent. There is a marked tendency to polymorphism, with various types of lesions presenting simultaneously, unlike other eruptive skin diseases in which the morphologic appearance of the lesions is uniform. The color is characteristic, resembling a "clean-cut ham" or having a coppery tint (Figure 10-10). Lesions may assume a variety of shapes, including round, elliptic, or annular. Eruptions may be limited and discrete, profuse, generalized, or more or less confluent and may vary in intensity.

The types of lesions in approximate order of frequency are maculopapular, papular, macular, annular, papulopustular, psoriasiform, and follicular. The lesions in African Americans are marked by the absence of dull-red color.[5] Lesions occur on the palms or soles in most patients with secondary syphilis (see Figure 10-10). Unlike the pigmented melanotic macules frequently seen on the palms and soles of older African Americans, lesions of secondary syphilis of the palms and soles are isolated, oval, slightly raised, erythematous, and scaly. Temporary irregular ("moth eaten") alopecia of the beard, scalp, or eyelashes may occur (Figure 10-7). Moist, anal, wartlike papules (condylomata lata) are highly infectious (Figure 10-8). Lesions may appear on any mucous membrane. All cutaneous lesions of secondary syphilis are infectious; therefore, if you don't know what it is, don't touch it. The differential diagnosis is vast. The commonly observed diseases that may be confused with secondary syphilis are pityriasis rosea (especially if the herald patch is absent), guttate psoriasis (psoriasis that appears suddenly with numerous small papules and plaques), lichen planus, tinea versicolor, and exanthematous drug and viral eruptions.

The diagnosis is based primarily on clinical and serologic grounds. Histologic studies, in the majority of cases, may confirm the disease.

Cellular immune processes are responsible for the cutaneous manifestations of secondary syphilis. Coinfection with HIV-1 has little effect on the cutaneous response to *T. pallidum.*[6]

Approximately 25% of untreated patients with secondary syphilis may experience relapse, most of them (approximately 90%) during the first year, a small percentage in the second year, and none after the fourth year.

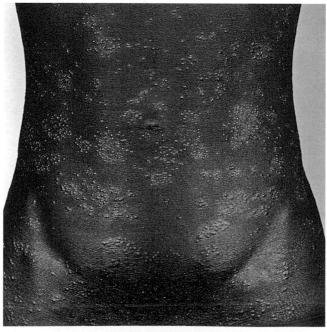

Figure 10-6 Secondary syphilis. This is the uncommon follicular secondary syphilis. *(From Hira S et al: Int J Dermatol 26:103-106, 1987.)*

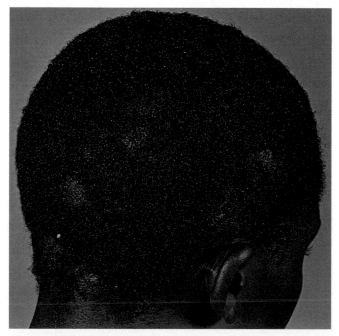

Figure 10-7 Secondary syphilis. Temporary, irregular ("moth eaten") alopecia of the scalp. *(Courtesy Subhash K. Hira, M.D.)*

SECONDARY SYPHILIS

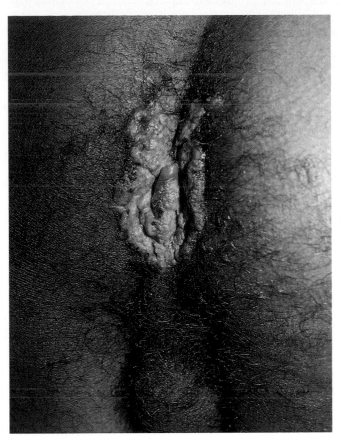

Figure 10-8 Moist, anal, wartlike papules (condylomata lata) are highly infectious.

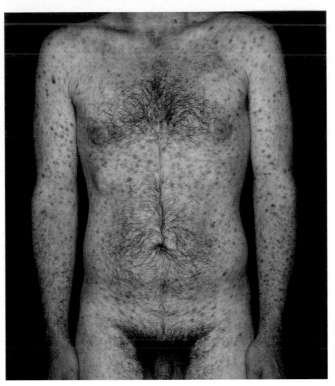

Figure 10-9 Numerous lesions are present on all body surfaces. This is a common presentation with maculopapular and psoriasiform lesions.

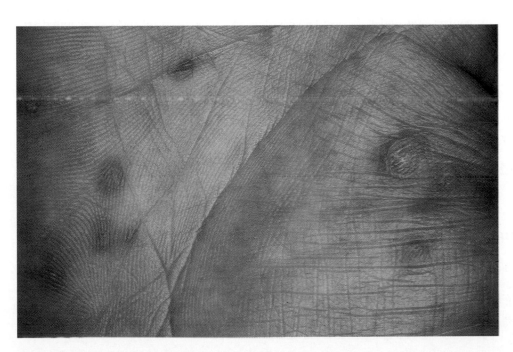

Figure 10-10 Lesions on palms and soles occur in the majority of patients with secondary syphilis. Coppery color resembling that of clean-cut ham is characteristic of secondary syphilis.

Latent syphilis

Latent syphilis is defined as syphilis characterized by seroreactivity without other evidence of disease. Patients who have latent syphilis and who acquired syphilis within the preceding year are classified as having early latent syphilis. In latent syphilis, one depends on the accuracy of the patient's history that there were characteristic signs and symptoms or that the blood test, the result of which has been discovered to be positive, was nonreactive at a specific time.

Early latent syphilis can be diagnosed if, within the year preceding the evaluation, they had:

a) A documented seroconversion (i.e., RPR, VDRL not a false-positive test result) without evidence of active disease. Often the physician is unable to confirm the specific time interval of conversion.

b) Unequivocal symptoms of primary or secondary syphilis.

c) A sex partner documented to have primary, secondary, or early latent syphilis.

By convention, early latent syphilis is of 1 year or less and late latent syphilis is more than 4 years' duration. The periods of 1 and 4 years were established to help predict a patient's chance of experiencing relapse with signs of secondary infectious syphilis. Approximately 25% of untreated patients in the secondary stage may experience a relapse, most of them (approximately 90%) during the first year, a small percentage in the second year, and none after the fourth year. The patient who experiences a relapse with secondary syphilis is infectious.

Patients who have latent syphilis of unknown duration should be treated as if they have late latent syphilis. Nontreponemal serologic titers (i.e., RPR, VDRL) usually are higher during early latent syphilis than late latent syphilis. However, early latent syphilis cannot be reliably distinguished from late latent syphilis solely on the basis of nontreponemal titers. All patients with latent syphilis should undergo careful examination of all accessible mucosal surfaces (i.e., the oral cavity, the perineum in women, and underneath the foreskin in uncircumcised men) to evaluate for internal mucosal lesions. All patients who have syphilis should be tested for HIV infection.

Tertiary syphilis

In a small number of untreated or inadequately treated patients, systemic disease develops, including cardiovascular disease, central nervous system (CNS) lesions, and systemic granulomas (gummas).[7,8]

Syphilis and human immunodeficiency virus

Syphilis (a genital ulcer disease) facilitates and is a cofactor for HIV transmission. Syphilis is associated with an increased risk of acquiring and transmitting HIV. The natural history of syphilis is altered by the human immunodeficiency virus. Reports describe an accelerated progression through the syphilitic stages in HIV patients.

Treatment of patients co-infected with syphilis and HIV is controversial; progression and relapse of neurosyphilis have been reported. Syphilis can increase the likelihood of HIV transmission and acquisition. HIV seroprevalence is high among patients with syphilis in the United States.[9] The standard recommended doses of penicillin may not be effective for HIV-infected patients with syphilis.[10] For most patients with coinfections of HIV and syphilis, laboratory tests for diagnosis and posttreatment follow-up can be interpreted as they would in an immunocompetent person.[11]

Congenital syphilis

Congenital syphilis is a problem in parts of the world where women do not receive prenatal care. *T. pallidum* can be transmitted by an infected mother to the fetus in utero. In untreated cases stillbirth occurs in 19% to 35% of reported cases, 25% of infants die shortly after birth, 12% are without symptoms at birth, and 40% will have late symptomatic congenital syphilis.[12,13] The treponeme can cross the placenta at any time during pregnancy. Adequate therapy of the infected mother before the 16th week of gestation usually prevents infection of the fetus. Treatment after 18 weeks may cure the disease but not prevent irreversible neural deafness, interstitial keratitis, and bone and joint changes in the newborn. The fetus is at greatest risk when maternal syphilis is of less than 2 years' duration. The ability of the mother to infect the fetus diminishes but never disappears in late latent stages. Condyloma lata and furuncles of Barlow can be seen toward the end of the first year of life.

The clinical manifestations occur in an early and late form.

Early congenital syphilis

Early congenital syphilis is defined as syphilis acquired in utero that becomes symptomatic during the first 2 years of life. It usually appears in the first week of life. The findings can be viewed as an exaggeration of those of acquired secondary syphilis. The fetal stigmata seen before the age of 2 years include eruptions characteristic of secondary syphilis. There are influenza-like respiratory symptoms in 20% to 50%, hepatosplenomegaly or lymphadenopathy in 50% to 75%, and mucocutaneous changes in 40% to 50%. Maculopapular rash and desquamating erythema of the palms and soles are common. Deep fissures at the angle of the mouth ("split papules") may be seen. A highly infectious hemorrhagic nasal discharge, snuffles, is a characteristic early sign. Bone and joint symptoms are common.

A vesiculobullous variant, "pemphigus syphiliticus," may occur with vesicles, bullae, and erosions. Osteochondritis with the "sawtooth" metaphysis seen on radiographs and periostitis appear with tender limbs and joints. Nontender generalized adenopathy, alopecia, iritis, and failure to thrive occur less frequently.

Late congenital syphilis

Symptoms and signs of late congenital syphilis become evident after age 5 years. The average age at first diagnosis is 30 years. It may be difficult to distinguish from acquired syphilis. The most important signs are frontal bossae (bony prominences of the forehead) (87%), saddle nose (74%), short maxilla (83%), high arched palate (76%), mulberry molars (more than four small cusps on a narrow first lower molar of the second dentition), Hutchinson's teeth (peg-shaped upper central incisors of the permanent dentition that appear after age 6 years) (63%) (Figure 10-11), Higoumenakia sign (unilateral enlargement of the sternoclavicular portion of the clavicle as an end result of periostitis) (39%), and rhagades (linear scars radiating from the angle of the eyes, nose, mouth, and anus) (8%). Hutchinson's triad (Hutchinson's teeth, interstitial keratitis, and cranial nerve VIII deafness) is considered pathognomonic of late congenital syphilis.

Syphilis serology

Culture of *T. pallidum* is not available. The diagnosis of syphilis is based on serologic findings and/or darkfield microscopic examination of the organism or direct immunofluorescent microscopy. The latter two procedures require special equipment and an experienced technician.

The interpretation[14,40] of reactive serologic tests for syphilis is shown in the diagram on p. 322. Two classes of IgM and

IgG antibodies are produced in response to infection with *T. pallidum;* these are nonspecific antibodies measured by the VDRL and RPR tests and specific antibodies measured by the fluorescent treponemal antibody absorption (FTA-ABS) test (Table 10-3). The IgM antibodies are present in the second week of infection, and they disappear 3 months after treatment for early syphilis and 12 months afterward for late syphilis. They do not pass through the placenta or blood-brain barrier. IgG antibodies reach high levels in 4 to 5 weeks and may persist for life.

Venereal Disease Research Laboratory and rapid plasma reagin tests

These tests are used for screening purposes and have a high degree of sensitivity (positive results in most patients with syphilis) but relatively low specificity (positive results in patients without syphilis). The primary chancre may be present for up to 2 weeks before serologic tests become reactive but the VDRL and RPR tests are usually reactive within 4 to 7 days of chancre development. When their results are positive, verification is by the more specific FTA-ABS test.

QUANTITATIVE TESTING. The tests give quantitative, as well as qualitative, results and can be used to monitor response to therapy. All reactive samples are titered to determine the highest reactive dilution. A rising titer indicates active disease; the titer falls in response to treatment. A fourfold change in titer, equivalent to a change of two dilutions (e.g., from 1:16 to 1:4 or from 1:8 to 1:32), is considered necessary to demonstrate a clinically significant difference between two nontreponemal test results that were obtained using the same serologic test. Nontreponemal tests usually become nonreactive with time after treatment; however, in some patients, nontreponemal antibodies can persist at a low titer for a long time, sometimes for the life of the patient. This response is referred to as the "serofast reaction."

FALSE-POSITIVE REACTIONS. Biologic false-positive reactions to nontreponemal tests (range, 3% to 20%) are defined as a positive nontreponemal antibody test result in patients for whom the FTA-ABS test result is negative (Table 10-4). False-positive test results may occur with collagen vascular disease, advancing age, narcotic drug use, chronic liver disease, several chronic infections such as HIV or tuberculosis, and several acute infections such as herpes. False-negative test results may occur if the patient has been applying topical antibiotics or ingesting systemic antibiotics.

The VDRL test result is uniformly nonreactive in Lyme disease.

PROZONE PHENOMENON. Undiluted serum containing a high titer of nonspecific antibody, as occurs in secondary syphilis, may result in a negative result on the flocculation test. This is called the prozone phenomenon and occurs because the large quantity of antibody occupies all antigen sites and prevents flocculation. The laboratory may perform flocculation tests on diluted serum in anticipation of this problem.

Table 10-3 Sensitivity of Serologic Tests in the Stages of Syphilis (Percent Positive)*					
Test	**Primary**	**Secondary**	**Latent**	**Tertiary**	**Screening**
VDRL[†]	72	100	73	77	86
FTA-ABS[‡]	91	100	97	100	99

FTA-ABS, Fluorescent treponemal antibody absorption; *VDRL,* Venereal Disease Research Laboratory.
*From Griner PF, et al: Ann Intern Med 1981; 94:585.
[†]Specificity variable by stage and proportion of population tested with chronic and autoimmune diseases. Specificity in screening general population approximately 97%.
[‡]Specificity for all stages probably 98% to 99%, including those with biologic false-positive results on nontreponemal test.

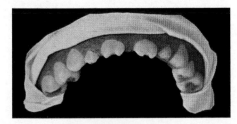

Figure 10-11 Late congenital syphilis. Hutchinson's teeth (peg-shaped upper central incisors of permanent dentition).

Interpretation of Reactive Serologic Tests for Syphilis

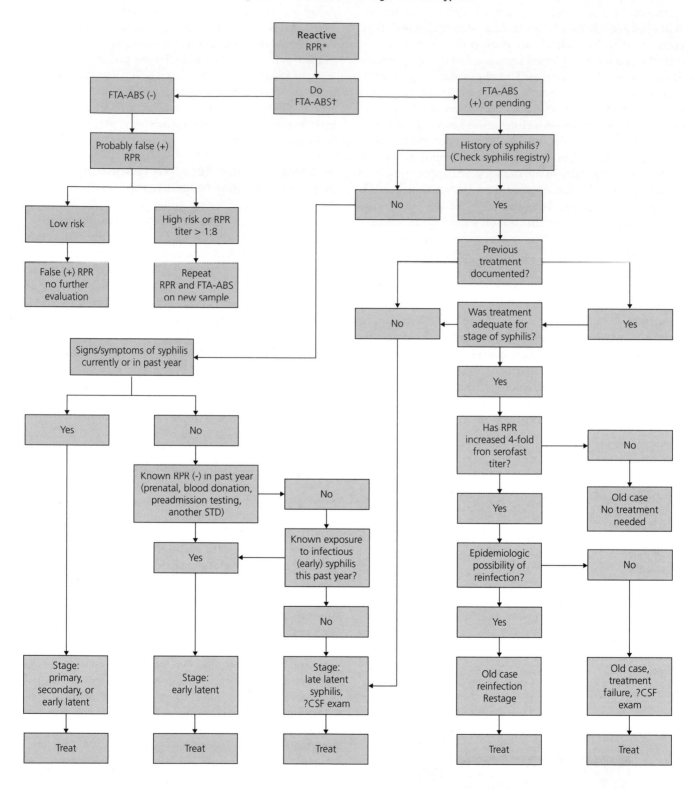

Table 10-4 Diseases That Result in Positive Reactions to Tests Although Patients Do Not Have Syphilis (False-Positive Reactions)

Nontreponemal tests		
Acute reactor (less than 6 months)	Chronic reactor (more than 6 months)	FTA-ABS
Pregnancy	Collagen vascular disease	Pregnancy
Drug-induced systemic lupus erythematosus	Senescence	Drug addiction
	Leprosy	Herpes genitalis
Acute infection	Metastasis to or cirrhosis of the liver	Lupus erythematosus, scleroderma, rheumatoid arthritis (atypical beaded fluorescence pattern)
Infectious mononucleosis		
Malaria	Hashimoto's thyroiditis	
Rubeola	Sjögren's syndrome	
Chicken pox		
Atypical pneumonia	Sarcoidosis	
	Lymphoma	Mixed connective tissue disease
Smallpox vaccine	Myeloma	
Narcotic addiction	Narcotic addiction	Alcoholic cirrhosis
	Familial false-positive findings	

Fluorescent treponemal antibody absorption and T. pallidum particle agglutination tests

Because of the decreased specificity of the nontreponemal tests, positive RPR and VDRL test results are confirmed with the more precise fluorescent treponemal antibody absorption test (FTA-ABS) or *T. pallidum* particle agglutination (TP-PA). The FTA-ABS test is also performed in patients with clinical evidence of syphilis for whom the nontreponemal test result is negative. Its main use is to rule out biologic false-positive reagin test reactions and to detect late syphilis in which the reagin test result may be nonreactive. FTA-ABS measures antibody directed against *T. pallidum* rather than from tissue (reagin), as with the RPR and VDRL tests. False-positive FTA-ABS test results occur most frequently in patients with autoantibodies. A patient who has a reactive treponemal test usually will have a reactive test for a lifetime, regardless of treatment or disease activity (15% to 25% of patients treated during the primary stage may revert to being serologically nonreactive after 2 to 3 years). Treponemal test antibody titers correlate poorly with disease activity and should not be used to assess response to treatment.

Tests for neurosyphilis

No test can be used alone to diagnose neurosyphilis. The VDRL-CSF is highly specific, but it is insensitive. Most other tests are both insensitive and nonspecific and must be interpreted in relation to other test results and the clinical assessment. Therefore the diagnosis of neurosyphilis usually depends on various combinations of reactive serologic test results, abnormalities of cerebrospinal fluid (CSF) cell count or protein, or a reactive VDRL-CSF with or without clinical manifestations. The CSF leukocyte count usually is increased (>5 white blood cells/mm^3) in patients with neurosyphilis; this count also is a sensitive measure of the effectiveness of therapy. The VDRL-CSF is the standard serologic test for CSF, and when reactive in the absence of substantial contamination of CSF with blood, it is considered diagnostic of neurosyphilis. However, the VDRL-CSF may be nonreactive when neurosyphilis is present. Some specialists recommend performing an FTA-ABS test on CSF. The CSF FTA-ABS is less specific (i.e., yields more false-positive results) for neurosyphilis than the VDRL-CSF, but the test is highly sensitive. Therefore some specialists believe that a negative CSF FTA-ABS test result excludes neurosyphilis.

Patients with human immunodeficiency virus

Some HIV-infected patients can have atypical serologic test results (i.e., unusually high, unusually low, or fluctuating titers). For such patients, when serologic tests and clinical syndromes suggestive of early syphilis do not correspond with one another, use of other tests (e.g., biopsy and direct microscopy) should be considered. However, for most HIV-infected patients, serologic tests are accurate and reliable for the diagnosis of syphilis and for following the response to treatment.

Treatment of syphilis

Patients to be treated for syphilis should have a baseline serum RPR determination. The best indication of successful therapy is a decreasing RPR titer.

The drug of choice in the treatment of syphilis is benzathine penicillin G (see Table 10-1). The latest recommendation for treatment can be found at www.cdc.gov. Conduct a search for Sexually Transmitted Diseases Treatment Guidelines.

Jarisch-Herxheimer reaction

A complex allergic response to antigens released from dead microorganisms can complicate the treatment of syphilis. A transient acute febrile reaction with headache and myalgia may develop within 24 hours of therapy. It is more prevalent with treatment of early syphilis.

Management of the patient with a history of penicillin allergy

No proven alternatives to penicillin are available for treating neurosyphilis, congenital syphilis, or syphilis in pregnant women. Penicillin is also recommended for use, whenever possible, in the treatment of HIV-infected patients. Only approximately 10% of persons who report a history of severe allergic reactions to penicillin are still allergic. Skin testing with the major and minor determinants can reliably identify persons at high risk for penicillin reactions. Those with positive

Table 10-5 Use of Nontreponemal Serologic Tests in Follow-Up After Treatment of Syphilis	
Stage	**Follow-up interval**
Early syphilis (less than 1 year)	3, 6, 12 months after treatment
Late syphilis (more than 1 year)	2 years after treatment
Neurosyphilis	Blood and CSF levels every 6 months for 3 years after Treatment
Retreatment	CSF level

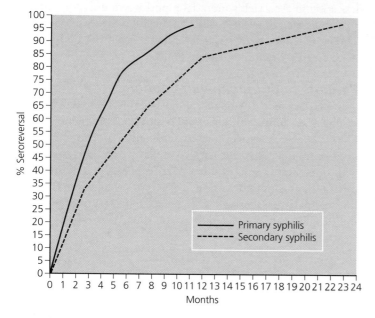

Figure 10-12 Speed of seroreversal of 500 patients with primary syphilis and 522 patients with secondary syphilis: 1977-1981. *(Graph courtesy Nicholas J. Fiumara, M.D., M.P.H.)*

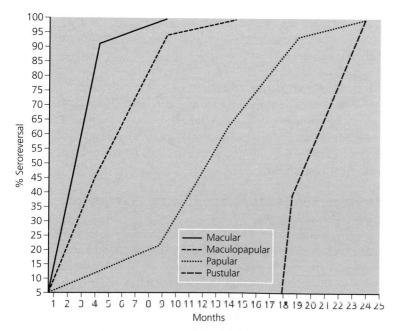

Figure 10-13 Speed of seroreversal of 522 patients with secondary syphilis by type of lesion: 1977-1981. *(Graph courtesy Nicholas J. Fiumara, M.D., M.P.H.)*

test results should be desensitized. The protocol for desensitization can be found at www.cdc.gov. Conduct a search for Sexually Transmitted Diseases Treatment Guidelines.

Posttreatment evaluation of syphilis
Serologic response to treatment
The lower the serologic titer before treatment, the quicker the blood test result will revert to normal.[15] Patients with their first attack of primary syphilis will have a nonreactive RPR result within 1 year. Patients with secondary syphilis will have a nonreactive RPR test result within 2 years (Figures 10-12 and 10-13).[16] Patients with early latent syphilis of less than 1 year will have negative serologic findings within 4 years.

Patients with a first attack of early latent syphilis of 1 to 4 years' duration treated with the schedules in Table 10-1 will have a nonreactive RPR finding in 5 years. Of patients with late latent syphilis, 45% will have negative serologic test results in 5 years, and the remainder will have reagin fast reactions. CSF examination is not performed unless the patient has neurologic or psychiatric signs and symptoms.

Persistent low-titer RPR reactivity may occur in 5% of successfully treated patients. The FTA-ABS test indicates past or present exposure and is not related to activity of the disease.

Late latent syphilis
In one study, 44% of patients with late latent syphilis had negative serologic findings within 5 years, and 56% had persistently positive reagin test results.[17] The criteria of effectiveness in the treatment of patients with late latent syphilis are reversion of the reagin blood test for syphilis from reactive to nonreactive, a fourfold or greater decrease in the reagin titer, or a fixed titer with no significant change during the period of observation.

Frequency of follow-up serologic tests
All patients treated for syphilis must be followed to assess the effectiveness of initial treatment. Quantitative nontreponemal tests (VDRL or RPR) are obtained at 3, 6, and 12 months. If antibody titers do not decrease fourfold within 6 months for patients with primary or secondary syphilis, treatment failure or reinfection should be considered, and evaluation for possible HIV infection should be initiated. Patients with secondary syphilis should be observed for possible relapse or reinfection, with monthly follow-up for the first year and quarterly visits for the second year (Table 10-5). Repeat treatment should be considered for any patient who has a sustained fourfold increase in titer or when an initially high titer does not show a fourfold decrease within a year.[18]

Reinfection in primary, secondary, and latent syphilis
The titers of reagin antibody are higher than those during the first infection, and the serologic responses to treatment are slower, taking about twice the time to become nonreactive compared with the time expected after treatment of a first episode of syphilis.

Rare Sexually Transmitted Diseases

Lymphogranuloma venereum

Lymphogranuloma venereum (LGV) is mainly a disease of lymphatic tissue that spreads to tissue surrounding lymphatics. LGV is rare in developed countries. It is more common in men (15 to 40 years).[19] Asymptomatic female carriers are probably the primary source of infection. Men present with ulcers or tender inguinal and or femoral lymphadenopathy that is usually unilateral. Women and male homosexuals might have proctocolitis or inflammatory involvement of perirectal or perianal lymphatic tissues that can result in fistulas and strictures. LGV is caused by the obligate intracellular bacteria *Chlamydia trachomatis* (serotypes L1, L2, and L3). These subtypes infect macrophages. The *C. trachomatis* serotypes that cause urethritis and cervicitis infect the squamocolumnar cells and infection is limited to mucous membranes. The diagnosis is usually made serologically and by exclusion of other causes of inguinal lymphadenopathy or genital ulcers.

Primary lesion

After an incubation period of 5 to 21 days, a small painless papule or viral (herpetiform) vesicle occurs on the penis, fourchette, posterior vaginal wall, or cervix (Figure 10-14). The lesion evolves rapidly to a small, painless erosion that heals without scarring within a week. The lesion in most cases is innocuous and most patients will not remember it. The primary lesion is rarely seen in women. A mucopurulent discharge affecting the urethra in men and the cervix in women may be present.

Figure 10-14 Lymphogranuloma venereum. Primary lesion consists of small, painless erosion that heals in a short time without scarring.

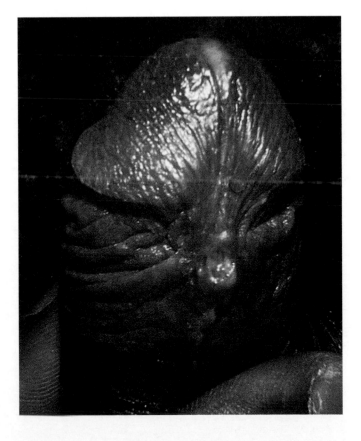

Inguinal stage

The infected macrophages drain to the regional lymph nodes. Unilateral or sometimes bilateral inguinal lymphadenopathy accompanied by headache, fever, and migratory polymyalgia and arthralgia appears from 1 to 6 weeks after the primary lesion heals (see Figure 10-14). In women, the deep pelvic nodes may also be involved. In a short time the lymph nodes become tender and fluctuant and are referred to as buboes when they ulcerate and discharge purulent material. Draining buboes may persist for months. Inflammation spreads to adjoining nodes and leads to matting. Abscesses rupture and sinus tracts eventually heal with scarring. Buboes are common in males but occur in only one third of infected females. Enlargement of inguinal nodes above and femoral nodes below Poupart's ligament creates the "groove sign" in approximately one fifth of patients, which is considered pathognomonic for LGV (Figure 10-15). Inguinal lymphadenopathy occurs in only 20% to 30% of women. They have primary involvement of the rectum, vagina, cervix, or posterior urethra, which drain to the deep iliac or perirectal nodes. This produces lower abdominal or back pain.

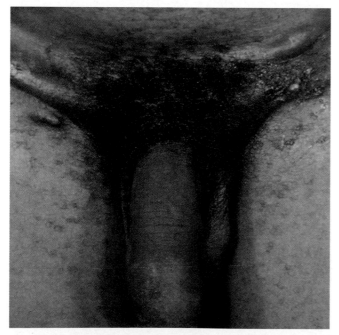

Figure 10-15 Lymphogranuloma venereum. Bilateral inguinal lymphadenopathy that discharges purulent material (buboes). Enlargement of inguinal nodes above and femoral nodes below Poupart's ligament creates the "groove sign."

Genitoanorectal syndrome

This late stage occurs more often in women who were previously asymptomatic. Proctocolitis or inflammatory involvement of perirectal or perianal lymphatic tissues may lead to perirectal abscesses, fistulas, strictures, and stenosis of the rectum and ulceration of the labia, rectal mucosa, and vagina. Chronic edema (elephantiasis) of the female external genitals is a late manifestation of lymphatic obstruction. The enlargement, thickening, and fibrosis of the labia is termed *esthiomene*. Penile and/or scrotal edema and gross distortion of the penis is called "saxophone penis."

Diagnosis

The organism is difficult to culture. The diagnosis depends mainly on serologic tests.

COMPLEMENT FIXATION TEST. The result of the LGV complement fixation test (LGV-CFT) becomes positive within 1 to 3 weeks. Cross-reaction occurs between several different serotypes that produce various chlamydial infections. CF titers greater than 1:64 are seen in most patients and are considered indicative of active LGV. Increasing titers are difficult to demonstrate because the patient is usually seen after the acute stage, when the initial lesion has healed. A four-fold rise of antibody in the course of suspected illness is diagnostic of active infection. Moderate or high serum titers may also be caused by other *C. trachomatis* infections and may persist for many years.

CULTURE. Culture of *C. trachomatis* is technically demanding and not generally available. Recovery rates are low even when specific cycloheximide-treated McCoy cells or diethylaminoethyl-treated HeLa cells were used. Material from primary ulcers may be inoculated directly onto the media. An aspirate of the involved lymph node is the best sample source. Bubo pus and tissues have to be homogenized in tissue culture medium to obtain a 10% and 20% suspension, and 10^{-1} and 10^{-2} dilutions are inoculated into tissue culture. This is necessary to reduce a toxic effect of the pus on the culture cells.

Management

DRUG REGIMEN. The drug regimen of choice is doxycycline 100 mg orally two times a day for 21 days. Erythromycin 500 mg orally four times a day for 21 days is also effective. Persons who have had sexual contact with a patient who has LGV within 30 days before the onset of the patient's symptoms should be examined, tested for urethral or cervical chlamydial infection, and treated.

LESION MANAGEMENT. Fluctuant lymph nodes should be aspirated as needed through healthy, adjacent, normal skin. Incision and drainage or excision of nodes delays healing and is contraindicated. Late sequelae such as stricture or fistula may require surgical intervention.

Chancroid

Chancroid (soft chancre) is common and endemic in many parts of the world. It occurs in discrete outbreaks in some areas of the United States (New York, California, Texas, and South Carolina). It is common in Africa, the Caribbean basin, and Southwest Asia. The overall global incidence may surpass that of syphilis. In Kenya, Gambia, and Zimbabwe, chancroid is considered to be the most common cause of genital ulceration.[19]

Bacteria

Chancroid is caused by the short gram-negative rod *H. ducreyi*. The male/female ratio is approximately 10:1. Chancroid predominantly affects heterosexual men, and most cases originate from prostitutes who are often carriers with no symptoms. Chancroid is a cofactor for HIV transmission, and high rates of HIV infection occur among patients who have chancroid. An estimated 10% of patients who have chancroid could be coinfected with *T. pallidum* or HSV.

Primary state

After an incubation period of 3 to 5 days, a painful, red papule appears at the site of contact and rapidly becomes pustular and ruptures to form an irregular-shaped, ragged ulcer with a red halo. The ulcer is deep, not shallow as in herpes; bleeds easily; and spreads laterally, burrowing under the skin and giving the lesion an undermined edge and a base covered by yellow-gray exudate (Figure 10-16). The ulcers are highly infectious, and multiple lesions appear on the genitals from autoinoculation. Unlike syphilis, the ulcers may be very painful. Untreated cases may resolve spontaneously or, more often, progress to cause deep ulceration (Figure 10-17), severe phimosis, and scarring. Systemic symptoms, including anorexia, malaise, and low-grade fever, are occasionally present. Females may have multiple, painful ulcers on the labia and fourchette and, less often, on the vaginal walls and cervix. Autoinoculation results in lesions on the thighs, buttocks, and anal areas. Female carriers may have no detectable lesions and may be without symptoms.

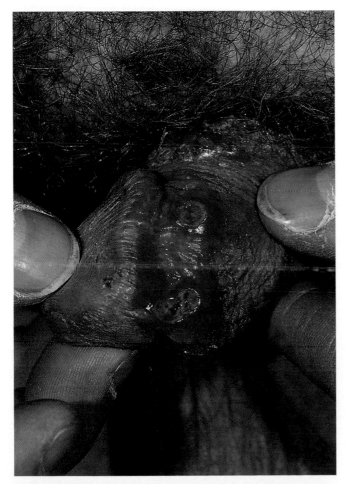

Figure 10-16 Chancroid. Several small, painful ulcers are usually present. Base is purulent, in contrast to the chancre of syphilis.

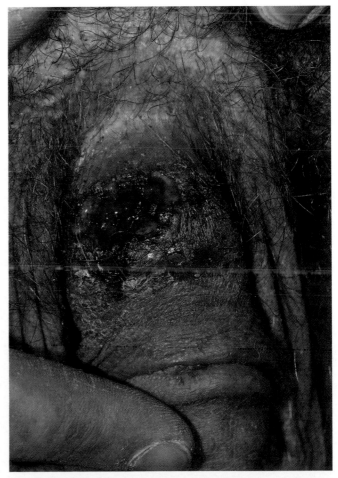

Figure 10-17 Chancroid. Ulcers have coalesced during a 4-week period without treatment.

Lymphadenopathy

Unilateral or bilateral inguinal lymphadenopathy develops in approximately 50% of untreated patients, beginning approximately 1 week after the onset of the initial lesion. The nodes then resolve spontaneously or they suppurate and break down.

Diagnosis

The combination of a painful ulcer (syphilis is not painful) with tender inguinal adenopathy is suggestive of chancroid and, when accompanied by suppurative inguinal adenopathy, is almost pathognomonic.

A probable diagnosis is made when all the following criteria are met:

- One or more painful genital ulcers
- No evidence of *T. pallidum* infection by darkfield examination of ulcer exudate or by a serologic test for syphilis performed at least 7 days after onset of ulcers
- The clinical presentation, appearance of genital ulcers and, if present, regional lymphadenopathy are typical for chancroid and
- A test result for herpes simplex virus performed on the ulcer exudate is negative. Patients should be tested for HIV infection and tested 3 months later for syphilis and HIV if initial results are negative.

Culture

Accurate diagnosis depends on the ability to culture *H. ducreyi*. The rate of isolation varies among laboratories. Most laboratories have little experience with this disease and their rates of isolation are low. A sterile swab or plastic loop is used to sample the base of the ulcers. All the newly formulated transport media maintain viability of *H. ducreyi* for more than 4 days at 4° C. More reliable results are obtained if the exudate from the ulcer is inoculated directly onto the plate, not onto transport medium. Plates are incubated at 33° C in microaerophilic conditions and examined for growth in 48 hours.

H. ducreyi cannot be cultured on routine medium. Nutritional requirements of *H. ducreyi* seem to be geographically defined. High cultural yield is obtained by using Mueller-Hinton agar base supplemented with chocolate horse blood and Isovitale X (MH-HBC).[20]

Gram stain

H. ducreyi possesses agglutination properties that account for the clumping of organisms when colonies are dispersed in saline. Agglutination may be responsible for the "school-of-fish" pattern seen on Gram staining. Smears taken from the surface areas are of little use. Material is obtained by drawing the flat surface of a toothpick under the undermined border of the ulcer. The cellular debris is then smeared on a glass slide. Exudate is obtained from the base of a new ulcer with a cotton swab. The swab is rolled in one direction over the slide to preserve the characteristic arrangement of the organisms. The slide is gently fixed with heat and stained with Gram stain. Gram-negative coccobacilli occur in parallel arrays (school-of-fish arrangement). This feature is infrequently

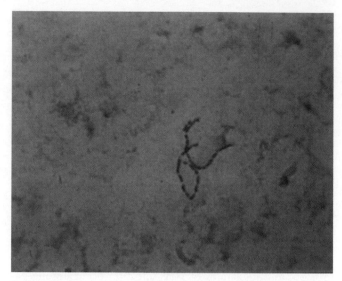

Figure 10-18 Chancroid. Wright's stain of purulent material of base of ulcer shows chain of coccobacilli.

seen and other gram-negative bacilli in the smear may result in a false-positive diagnosis (Figure 10-18). Bacteria may be intracellular. *H. ducreyi* may also be demonstrated with Wright, Giemsa, or Unna-Pappenheim stains.

Herpes simplex genital ulcers can mimic chancroid.[21] A herpes culture and Tzanck smear to look for virus-induced multinucleated giant cells help to establish the diagnosis. The histologic nature of chancroid is specific, but the biopsy procedure is so painful that other means of confirming the diagnosis should be used first.

Treatment

Drug regimens (see Table 10-1) are azithromycin 1 gm orally in a single dose, ceftriaxone 250 mg intramuscularly in a single dose, erythromycin 500 mg orally four times a day for 7 days, or ciprofloxacin 500 mg orally two times a day for 3 days. Asymptomatic carriage of *H. ducreyi* in males and females has been described[21,22]; therefore aggressive tracing and treatment of sex partners, whether or not they have symptoms, is essential for control. Test patient for HIV infection and syphilis. HIV infection slows the healing rates of chancroid ulcers despite appropriate antibiotic therapy.[23]

Fluctuant nodes can be aspirated by needle with the patient under local anesthesia; this is done superior to the abscess rather than from below to prevent continuous dripping.[24] Recent experience showed that suppurative lymphadenopathy responded to appropriate antibiotic regimens. The recommendation was to reserve surgical intervention for buboes that prove recalcitrant to antibiotic therapy.[25] Worldwide, several isolates with intermediate resistance to either ciprofloxacin or erythromycin have been reported.

Granuloma inguinale (donovanosis)

Granuloma inguinale is a predominantly tropical cause of genital ulcer occurring chiefly in small endemic foci in all continents except Europe. It is endemic in Papua, New Guinea, South-East India, the Caribbean, and adjacent areas of South America, Brazil, Durban South Africa, and among aborigines in Australia. It is a chronic, superficial, ulcerating disease of the genital, inguinal, and perianal areas. Granuloma inguinale is mildly contagious. The rates of infection between conjugal partners varies from 0.4% to 52%.[19] It is caused by *Calymmatobacterium granulomatis,* a gram-negative, facultative, obligate-intracellular, encapsulated bacillus.

Clinical presentation

The incubation period is unknown, but 14 to 50 days is suspected. The disease begins as a single or multiple papules, nodules, or ulcers on the genitals and then evolves into a painless, broad, superficial ulcer with a distinct, raised, rolled margin and a friable, beefy-red, granulation tissue-like base raised above the skin surface (Figure 10-19). The ulceration spreads contiguously causing progressive mutilation and destruction of local tissue. Autoinoculation produces lesions on adjacent skin, termed "kissing" lesions. The disease progresses to the genitocrural and inguinal folds in males and the perineal and perianal areas in females. It remains confined to areas of moist, stratified epithelium, sparing the columnar epithelium of the rectal area. Ulcers bleed to the touch and are not usually associated with inguinal lymphadenopathy as with LGV and chancroid.[26] Women present with genital ulceration (88.5%) and genital tract bleeding (19.7%). The vulva is the most frequent anatomic site involved in women. Granuloma inguinale of the cervix presents as a proliferative growth and may mimic carcinoma.[27] Systemic dissemination can occur. Most regular sexual partners of infected patients have no evidence of coexistent infection with donovanosis.[28] Delay in treatment results in significant local destruction and morbidity. Extensive and multiple perianal fistulas and abscesses may form. Granuloma inguinale does not produce constitutional symptoms. Systemic symptoms suggest hematogenous dissemination, which may cause disease at distant sites and death.[29] Extragenital sites become infected by autoinoculation (particularly the oral cavity) or extension into underlying organs, such as bone, bowel, or bladder.

Lymphatic obstruction causes genital edema. Scarring and mutilation of the anogenital region may require surgical correction.[30]

Diagnosis

Culture is very difficult on artificial culture media. The most reliable method of diagnosis involves direct visualization of the bipolar-staining intracytoplasmic inclusion bodies, called Donovan bodies. These "closed-safety-pin" appearing bodies can be seen within histiocytes of granulation tissue smears or biopsy specimens.[19] Diagnosis can be confirmed in 1 hour with the following technique.[31] The lesion is washed with

saline. EMLA ointment is applied, removed in 10 minutes, reapplied, and again removed 10 minutes later. Two scoops are taken as deeply as possible from the lesion from the advancing edge of the ulceration with a curet or chalazion spoon. The first is submitted in formalin for histopathologic study. The second is rubbed together between two glass slides to ensure a uniform spread of cells from the material. Make tissue preparations immediately while the tissue is moist. Desiccation results in rupture of the involved histiocytes. Donovan bodies are more easily recognized in smears than in tissue biopsy sections. The slides are taken to the laboratory, immediately air dried, and fixed in methyl alcohol for 5 minutes, followed by staining with 20% Giemsa for 10 minutes. Excess stain is washed off with water. Wright's or Leishman's stain is also suitable. Once dry, 100× oil-immersion, objective lens microscopic examination reveals bipolar-staining bacilli in vacuoles in the cytoplasm of large histiocytes. The intracellular organisms are called Donovan bodies and have a prominent clear capsule when mature. If slides cannot be immediately taken to the laboratory, they must be air dried and fixed with an aerosol fixative, such as that used for Papanicolaou smear tests. The RapiDiff technique is suitable for use in the diagnosis of granuloma inguinale (donovanosis) in busy sexually transmitted diseases clinics.[32]

For histopathologic study, the Warthin-Starry silver stains demonstrate the encapsulated bacilli within histiocytes.

Treatment

Trimethoprim-sulfamethoxazole, one double-strength tablet administered orally twice a day; and doxycycline, 100 mg orally twice a day, are first-line treatments. Antibiotics are administered for a minimum of 3 weeks and should be continued until all lesions have thoroughly healed. For any of the above regimens, the addition of an aminoglycoside (gentamicin 1 mg/kg IV every 8 hours) should be considered if lesions do not respond within the first few days of therapy.

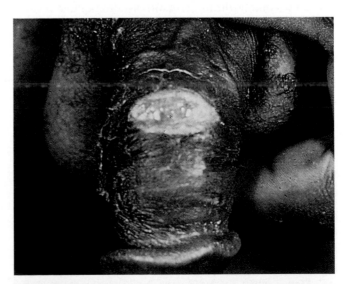

Figure 10-19 Granuloma inguinale. Painless, broad, superficial ulcer with beefy-red texture is raised above the skin surface. *(Courtesy Nicholas J. Fiumara, M.D., M.P.H.)*

Diseases Characterized by Urethritis and Cervicitis

Urethritis is characterized by (Box 10-1) urethral discharge of mucopurulent or purulent material and sometimes by dysuria or urethral pruritus. Asymptomatic infections are common. *N. gonorrhoeae* and *C. trachomatis* are the principal pathogens. Gram stain can provide an immediate diagnosis of gonorrhea. Nucleic acid amplification tests enable detection of *N. gonorrhoeae* and *C. trachomatis* on all specimens. These tests are more sensitive than culture for *C. trachomatis* and are the preferred method for the detection of this organism.

The presence of nongonococcal urethritis is demonstrated by the absence of gram-negative intracellular diplococci, a negative gonococcal culture result, and the detection of inflammatory cells (at least five polymorphonuclear leukocytes) in the urethral smear or in the urine sediment consequently for each patient with clinical symptoms of urethral inflammation.

Gonorrhea

In 1997, 324,901 cases of gonorrhea were reported in the United States. African Americans and adolescents account for the majority of cases. *N. gonorrhoeae* can survive only in a moist environment approximating body temperature. It is transmitted only by sexual contact (genital, genital-oral, or genital-rectal) with an infected person. It is not transmitted through toilet seats or the like. It most commonly infects superficial mucous membranes and initially produces discharge and dysuria. Purulent burning urethritis in males and asymptomatic endocervicitis in females are the most common forms of the disease, but gonorrhea is also found at other sites.

Gonorrhea may gain entry into the bloodstream from the primary source of infection and cause a disseminated gonococcal infection (arthritis dermatitis syndrome) that consists of fever and chills, skin lesions, and articular involvement.

From an epidemiologic point of view the disease is becoming more difficult to control because of the increasing number of asymptomatic male carriers.

"Core transmitters," or persons with repeated infections, are believed to be responsible for transmitting the majority of infections in urban areas.

Box 10-1 Urethritis Can be Documented by the Presence of Any of the Following Signs:

a. Mucopurulent or purulent discharge.

b. Gram stain of urethral secretions demonstrating >5 WBCs per oil immersion field. The Gram stain is the preferred rapid diagnostic test for evaluating urethritis.

c. Positive leukocyte esterase test on first-void urine or microscopic examination of first-void urine demonstrating >10 WBCs per high power field.

All forms of the disease previously responded to penicillin, but resistant strains have emerged.

Neisseria gonorrhoeae

N. gonorrhoeae is a gram-negative coccus that infects columnar or cuboidal epithelium. The neutrophilic response creates a purulent discharge, and stained smears show large numbers of phagocytosed gonococci in pairs (diplococci) within polymorphonuclear leukocytes. Nucleic acid amplification tests provide rapid and accurate diagnosis.

N. gonorrhoeae is a fragile organism that survives only in humans and quickly dies if all of its environmental requirements are not met. The organism can survive only in blood and on mucosal surfaces including the urethra, endocervix, rectum, pharynx, conjunctiva, and prepubertal vaginal tract. It does not survive on the stratified epithelium of the skin and postpubertal vaginal tract. The bacteria must be kept moist with isotonic body fluids and will die if not maintained at body temperature. A slightly alkaline medium is required, such as that found in the endocervix and in the vagina during the immediate premenstrual and menstrual phases. The antibodies produced during the disease offer little protection from future attacks. A fluorescent antibody test identifies the organism in tissue specimens such as in the skin in disseminated gonococcal infection (bacteremia-arthritis syndrome).

Genital infection in males

The risk of infection for a man after a single exposure to an infected woman is estimated to be 20% to 35%.

URETHRITIS. After a 3- to 5-day incubation period, most infected men have a sudden onset of burning, frequent urination, and a yellow, thick, purulent urethral discharge. In some men symptoms do not develop for 5 to 14 days. They then complain only of mild dysuria with a mucoid urethral discharge as observed in nongonococcal urethritis. Five percent to 50% of men who are infected never have symptoms and become chronic carriers for months, acting, as do women without symptoms, as major contributors to the ongoing gonorrhea epidemic. Infection may spread to the prostate gland, seminal vesicles, and epididymis, but presently these complications are uncommon because most men with symptoms are treated.

DIAGNOSIS. The diagnosis can be confirmed without culture in men with a typical history of acute urethritis by finding in urethral exudate containing gram-negative intracellular diplococci within polymorphonuclear leukocytes. Nucleic acid amplification tests (Gen-Probe, LCx Uriprobe) have high sensitivity and specificity, and they also test for *C. trachomatis*. Special transport kits provided by the laboratory are used to sample the urethra and endocervix. These tests are also performed on urine. Culture may be used for diagnostic problems.

Genital infection in females

Most cases occur in 15 to 19 year olds. The risk of infection for a woman after a single exposure to an infected man is estimated to be 50% to 90%. Female genital gonorrhea has traditionally been described as an asymptomatic disease, but symptoms of urethritis and endocervicitis may be elicited from 40% to 60% of the women. While the urethra and rectum are often involved, the locus of infection is typically the endocervix.

CERVICITIS. Endocervical infection may appear as a nonspecific, pale-yellow vaginal discharge, but in many cases this is not detected or is accepted as being a normal variation. The cervix may appear normal, or it may show marked inflammatory changes with cervical erosions and pus exuding from the os. Skene's glands, which lie on either side of the urinary meatus, exude pus if infected.

URETHRITIS. Urethritis begins with frequency and dysuria after a 3- to 5-day incubation period. These symptoms are of variable intensity. Pus may be seen exuding from the red external urinary meatus or after the urethra is "milked" with a finger in the vagina.

BARTHOLIN DUCTS. The Bartholin ducts, which open on the inner surfaces of the labia minora at the junction of their middle and posterior thirds near the vaginal opening, may, if infected, show a drop of pus at the gland orifice. After occlusion of the infected duct, the patient complains of swelling and discomfort while walking or sitting. A swollen, painful Bartholin gland may be palpated as a swollen mass deep in the posterior half of the labia majora.

DIAGNOSIS. The diagnosis of acute urethritis can be made with a high degree of certainty if gram-negative intracellular diplococci are found in the purulent exudate from the urethra. Neisseria species (e.g., *N. catarrhalis* and *N. sicca*) inhabit the female genital tract; thus the diagnosis is considered only if gram-negative diplococci are present inside polymorphonuclear leukocytes.

Nucleic acid amplification tests (Gen-Probe, LCx Uriprobe) are used on urethra and endocervix samples. These tests are also performed on urine. Culture may be used for diagnostic problems. A culture of the anal canal need be performed only if there are anal symptoms, a history of rectal sexual exposure, or follow-up of treated gonorrhea in women.

Pelvic inflammatory disease

Pelvic inflammatory disease (PID), or salpingitis, is infection of the uterus, fallopian tubes, and adjacent pelvic structures. Organisms spread to these structures from the cervix and vagina. It is present in 10% to 20% of gonococcal infections in women. Most cases are caused by *C. trachomatis* and/or *N. gonorrhoeae*. Microorganisms that can be part of the normal vaginal flora (e.g., anaerobes, *G. vaginalis*, *H. influenzae*, en-

---

Box 10-2 Criteria for Diagnosis of Pelvic Inflammatory Disease (Centers for Disease Control and Prevention)

Minimal (all present with no other cause):
- Lower abdominal tenderness
- Adnexal tenderness
- Cervical motion tenderness

Additional criteria that support a diagnosis of PID include:
- Oral temperature >101° F (38.3° C)
- Abnormal cervical or vaginal discharge
- Elevated erythrocyte sedimentation rate
- Elevated C-reactive protein
- Laboratory documentation of cervical infection with *N. gonorrhoeae* or *C. trachomatis*

Definitive criteria for diagnosing PID:
- Histopathologic evidence of endometritis on endometrial biopsy
- Laparoscopic abnormalities consistent with pelvic inflammatory disease
- Transvaginal sonography or other imaging techniques showing thickened fluid-filled tubes, with or without free pelvic fluid or tubo-ovarian complex
- Laparoscopic abnormalities consistent with PID

---

teric gram-negative rods, *Streptococcus agalactiae*) also can cause PID. In addition, *Mycoplasma hominis* and *Ureaplasma urealyticum* have been found in PID. Risk factors for ascending infection are age under 20 years, previous PID, vaginal douching, and bacterial vaginosis. Diagnostic criteria are listed in Box 10-2.

CLINICAL PRESENTATION. Symptoms range from minimal (e.g., lower abdominal tenderness) to severe pain accompanied by peritoneal signs. Pelvic inflammatory disease is an important cause of infertility. The most common presenting symptom is lower abdominal pain, usually bilateral. Gonococcal PID has an abrupt onset with fever and peritoneal irritation. The symptoms of nongonococcal disease are less dramatic. Any of these infections may be asymptomatic. Symptoms are more likely to begin during the first half of the menstrual cycle.

DIAGNOSIS. The diagnosis is usually made clinically. Lower abdominal tenderness and pain, adnexal tenderness, and pain on manipulation of the cervix are noted in most cases. Fever, leukocytosis, an increased erythrocyte sedimentation rate, elevated levels of C-reactive protein, and vaginal discharge may also occur.

Most women have either mucopurulent cervical discharge or evidence of WBCs on a microscopic evaluation of a saline preparation of vaginal fluid. If the cervical discharge appears normal and no white blood cells are found on the wet prep, the diagnosis of PID is unlikely, and alternative causes of pain should be investigated.

Endocervical specimens should be examined for *N. gonorrhoeae* and *C. trachomatis*. Direct visualization of inflamed fallopian tubes and other pelvic structures with the laparoscope is the most accurate method of diagnosis, but this procedure is usually not practical. A comprehensive microbiologic evaluation should be performed on specimens obtained through the laparoscope. The differential diagnosis includes acute appendicitis, pelvic endometriosis, hematoma of the corpus luteum, or ectopic pregnancy. Long-term complications (recurrent disease, chronic pain, ectopic pregnancy, infertility) occur from tubal damage and scarring.

MANAGEMENT. Empiric treatment of PID should be initiated in sexually active young women and others at risk for sexually transmitted diseases if all the minimum criteria in Box 10-2 are present and no other causes(s) of the illness can be identified: The recommended regimens are found in Table 10-1. Evaluate male sexual partners. Chlamydial and gonococcal infections in these men are often asymptomatic.

Rectal gonorrhea

Rectal gonorrhea is acquired by anal intercourse. Women with genital gonorrhea may also acquire rectal gonorrhea from contamination of the anorectal mucosa by infectious vaginal discharge. A history of anal intercourse is the most important clue to the diagnosis because the symptoms and signs of rectal gonorrhea are in most cases nonspecific.

Anoscopic examination of homosexual men reveals generalized exudate in 54% of culture-positive patients and 37% of culture-negative patients.[33] Many infected patients have normal-appearing rectal mucosae. These figures emphasize what is generally observed—that the specificity of the most common signs and symptoms of rectal gonorrhea is low. Some patients report pain on defecation, blood in the stools, pus on undergarments, or intense discomfort while walking.

DIAGNOSIS. Anal culture should be considered for male homosexuals with symptoms and females with symptoms who have engaged in rectal intercourse. Gonococcal proctitis does not involve segments of bowel beyond the rectum. The area of infection is approximately 2.5 cm inside the anal canal in the pectinate lining of the crypts of Morgagni. An anoscope is unnecessary to obtain culture material. A sterile cotton-tipped swab is inserted approximately 2.5 cm into the anal canal. (If the swab is inadvertently pushed into feces, another swab must be used to obtain a specimen.) The swab is moved from side to side in the anal canal to sample crypts; 10 to 30 seconds are allowed for absorption of organisms onto the swab.

Gen-Probe assays are sensitive and specific for the detection of rectal and pharyngeal gonorrhea. If non-cultural methods are used to screen for gonococcal infection, cultures should be obtained from patients with positive results so the antibiotic susceptibility and molecular epidemiology of the gonococcal population can be monitored.[34]

Gram stain is unreliable because of the presence of numerous other bacteria.

Gonococcal pharyngitis

Gonococcal pharyngitis is acquired by penile-oral exposure and rarely by cunnilingus or kissing. The possibility of infection is increased when the penis is inserted deep into the posterior pharynx as practiced by most homosexuals. Most cases are asymptomatic, and the gonococcus can be carried for months in the pharynx without being detected. In those with symptoms, complaints range from mild sore throat to severe pharyngitis with diffuse erythema and exudates.

DIAGNOSIS. Culture is most productive if exudates are present. *N. meningitidis* is a normal inhabitant of the pharynx; consequently, sugar utilization tests are necessary on *Neisseria* species isolated from the pharynx to determine accurately if infectious organisms are present.

Gram stain is useful only if exudate is present and must therefore be interpreted with caution to avoid confusion with other *Neisseria* species. Gen-Probe assays are sensitive and specific for pharyngeal gonorrhea.

Disseminated gonococcal infection (arthritis-dermatitis syndrome)

Disseminated gonococcal infection (DGI) is the most common cause of acute septic arthritis in young sexually active adults. The classic clinical triad is dermatitis, tenosynovitis, and migratory polyarthritis. It follows a genitourinary, rectal, or pharyngeal mucosal infection, which is asymptomatic in most patients. The diagnosis should be considered in any young adult or adolescent who presents with a skin rash, joint swelling, and pain.

INCIDENCE. DGI develops in approximately 1% to 3% of patients with mucosal infections and is more common in young adults. It is the most common form[35] of infectious arthritis. The male-to-female ratio is 1:4.

DISSEMINATION. Dissemination usually develops within 2 to 3 weeks of the primary infection. Hematogenous dissemination is more likely to occur within 1 week of the onset of the menstrual period. Women are more commonly affected with dissemination presumably because women more frequently have asymptomatic infection and remain untreated. Menses expose the submucosal blood vessels and increases the risk of dissemination. The risk of systemic infection increases during the second and third trimesters of pregnancy.

INITIAL PRESENTATION. Migratory polyarthralgias are the most common presenting symptoms, occurring in up to 80% of patients. Initial signs are tenosynovitis (67%), dermatitis (67%), and fever (63%). Less than 30% have symptoms or signs of localized gonorrhea, such as urethritis or pharyngitis; however, cervical culture results in women with DGI are positive in 80% to 90% of cases and men's urethral culture results are positive in 50% to 75% of cases.

JOINT DISEASE. Most patients have involvement of less than three joints. The upper extremity joints are more commonly involved, especially the wrist. The knee is the most commonly affected lower extremity joint. Tenosynovitis is present in two thirds of the patients occurring in the hands and fingers, although the tendons around the small and large joints of the lower limbs also can be affected.

TWO PRESENTATIONS. Following a genitourinary, rectal, or pharyngeal mucosal infection, which is asymptomatic in most patients, the disseminated disease can present two clinical pictures. The initial bacteremic stage, associated with fever (rarely reaching 39° C), skin rash, and tenosynovitis, is followed by localization of the infection within the joints. Approximately 60% of patients present with the bacteremic picture, and 40% present with suppurative arthritis. The features of disseminated gonococcal infection are compared with nongonococcal bacterial arthritis in Table 10-6.

ARTHRITIS-DERMATITIS SYNDROME. Chills (25%) and fever (more than 50%) are accompanied by pain, redness, and swelling of three to six small joints without effusion. This polyarthritis and tenosynovitis occur in the hands and wrists, with pain in the tendons of the wrist and fingers. Toes and ankles may also be affected. These patients are more likely to have positive results on blood culture and negative results on joint culture.

SKIN LESIONS. Dermatitis is seen in two thirds of cases. Chills and fever terminate as the rash appears on the extensor surfaces of the hands and dorsal surfaces of the ankles and toes. Lesions may develop on the trunk. The skin lesions are thought to be due to embolization of organisms to the skin with the development of microabscesses. The total number of lesions is usually less than 10. Lesions are seen in various stages of development. Many cases have only one or two lesions. The skin lesions begin as painless, nonpruritic, tiny, red papules or petechiae that either disappear or evolve

Table 10-6 Differential Features of Disseminated Gonococcal Infection and Nongonococcal Bacterial Arthritis	
Disseminated gonococcal infection	**Nongonococcal bacterial arthritis**
Generally in young, healthy adults	Often in very young, elderly, or immunocompromised persons
Initial migratory polyarthralgia (common)	Polyarthralgia rare
Tenosynovitis in majority	Tenosynovitis rare
Dermatitis in majority	Dermatitis rare
>50% polyarthritis	>85% monoarthritis
Positive blood culture result in <10%	Positive blood culture result in 50%
Positive joint fluid culture result in 25%	Positive joint fluid culture result in 85% to 95%

From Goldenberg DL, Reed JI: N Engl J Med 1985;312:767. Reprinted by permission of The New England Journal of Medicine.

through vesicular (Figure 10-20, A) and pustular stages, developing a grey necrotic and then hemorrhagic center (Figure 10-20, B). The central hemorrhagic area is the embolic focus of the gonococcus. These lesions heal in a few weeks. New lesions may appear even after antibiotic therapy has begun.

LOCALIZED SEPTIC ARTHRITIS. Usually one or two large joints are affected, most frequently the knee followed by the ankle, wrist, and elbow. The affected joint is hot, painful, and swollen, and movement is restricted. Permanent joint changes may occur. The mean leukocyte count in synovial fluid is often greater than 50,000 cells/mm^3. The joints are often sterile, possibly as a result of immunologic mechanisms. Dermatitis is usually absent.

Figure 10-20 Gonococcal septicemia.

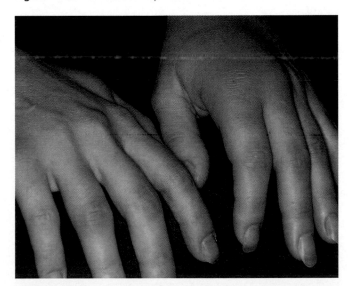

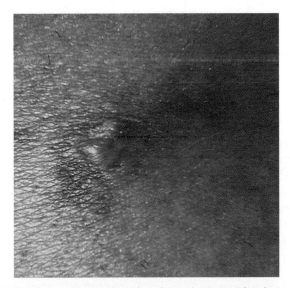

A, There is erythema and swelling of joints on the left hand. A single vesicle is present on the right hand.

B, More advanced lesion than that shown in *A.* Base has become hemorrhagic and necrotic.

Other less common complications of dissemination include endocarditis, myocarditis, and meningitis.

DIAGNOSIS. Diagnosis is based on the clinical picture and confirmed by isolation of gonococci from the primary infected mucosal site, such as the urethra, cervix, oropharynx, and rectum. Cultures of the joints, skin lesions, and blood are less apt to isolate the bacteria. Nucleic acid amplification tests allow identification of bacteria in synovial fluid even when the culture result is negative.

The most frequent laboratory findings are mild leukocytosis (10,500 to 12,500 cells/mm³) and increased ESR. A positive culture result confirms the diagnosis and allows determination of drug susceptibility.

Culture. Obtain culture specimens of blood, synovial fluid, skin lesions, endocervix, urethra, rectum, and pharynx. *N. gonorrhoeae* is cultured from synovial fluid in approximately 50% of purulent joints and from 25% to 30% of all patients with DGI. More than 80% of culture specimens obtained from primary mucosal sites or from a sexual partner show positive results. Blood culture results are positive in 20% to 30% of DGI patients, and culture specimens from skin detect infection in less than 5% of cases. Blood culture results are usually positive only during the first few days.

Gram stain. Gram stain of the skin lesions is performed on the pus obtained by unroofing the pustule. Gram-stained smears on concentrated sediment of centrifuged synovial fluid show positive results in less than 25%.

Treatment of gonococcal infection
Treatment recommendations for gonorrhea are found in Table 10-1.

Nongonococcal urethritis
Nongonococcal urethritis (NGU) and cervicitis are the most common sexually transmitted diseases in the United States. The diagnosis, as the name implies, used to be one of exclusion; however, routine diagnostic tests for identifying the various infecting organisms are now available. Epidemiologic control is difficult because many of those infected have no symptoms. Most women with cervical chlamydial infection, most homosexual men with rectal chlamydial infection, and as many as 30% of heterosexual men with chlamydial urethritis have few or no symptoms.

Organisms
Genital chlamydial infection is responsible for about half of NGU cases. *Ureaplasma urealyticum* and *Mycoplasma genitalium* may cause 10% to 30% of NGU cases. Herpes viruses, *T. vaginalis*, *Haemophilus* species, and anaerobic bacteria account for less than 10% of NGU cases. In approximately one third of cases, no infectious cause can be found.

Nongonococcal urethritis in males
In males urethritis begins with dysuria and urethral discharge. Gonococcal urethritis begins 3 to 5 days after sexual contact and produces a burning, yellow, thick to mucopurulent urethral discharge. NGU begins 7 to 28 days after sexual contact with a smarting sensation while urinating and a mucoid discharge. Table 10-7 compares the two forms of urethritis. *C. trachomatis* causes at least two thirds of the acute "idiopathic" epididymitis in sexually active men younger than 35 years.

Nongonococcal urethritis in females
The signs and symptoms in females are even more nonspecific. Nongonococcal cervicitis is asymptomatic or begins with a mucopurulent endocervical exudate or a mucoid vaginal discharge.

Diagnosis
The diagnosis is made by confirming the presence of urethritis, demonstrating the presence of *C. trachomatis*, and excluding gonococcal infection.

MOLECULAR BIOLOGIC TESTS. Molecular biologic diagnostic methods have replaced culture and antigen tests. Amplifying assays (Gen-Probe, LCx Uriprobe) are highly effective in identifying genital chlamydial and gonococcal infections by testing urethral samples and first voided urine. The results can be available in hours.

GRAM STAIN. A Gram stain is made of the urethral discharge. The presence of polymorphonuclear leukocytes confirms the diagnosis of urethritis, and the absence of gram-negative intracellular diplococci suggests urethritis is nongonococcal. Material for Gram stain is most effectively obtained at least 4 hours after urination. For those patients with urethral symptoms but without discharge, polymorphonuclear leukocytes may be seen in material obtained by a Calgiswab inserted approximately 2 cm beyond the urethral meatus.

CULTURE. Urethral discharge may be cultured for *N. gonorrhoeae*. These organisms are labile in vitro, and it is difficult to maintain viability during transport. If possible, culture

Table 10-7 Comparison of Nongonococcal and Gonococcal Urethritis		
	Nongonococcal urethritis	Gonococcal urethritis
Incubation period	7-28 days	3-5 days
Onset	Gradual	Abrupt
Dysuria	Smarting feeling	Burning
Discharge	Mucoid or purulent	Purulent
Gram stain of discharge	Polymorphonuclear leukocytes	Gram-negative intracellular diplococci

specimens should be obtained from sexual partners of men with NGU and in pregnant women who may be transmitting the organism to the fetus during birth, causing neonatal conjunctivitis.

SPECIMEN COLLECTION. The proper collection and handling of specimens are important in all the methods used to identify *Chlamydia.* Because *Chlamydiae* are obligate intracellular organisms that infect the columnar epithelium, the objective of specimen collection procedures is to obtain columnar epithelial cells from the urethra.

- Delay obtaining specimens until 2 hours after the patient has voided.
- Obtain specimens for *Chlamydia* tests after obtaining specimens for Gram-stain smear or *N. gonorrhoeae* culture.
- For nonculture *Chlamydia* tests, use the swab supplied or specified by the manufacturer.
- Gently insert the urogenital swab into the urethra (females: 1 to 2 cm, males: 2 to 4 cm). Rotate the swab in one direction for at least one revolution for 5 seconds. Withdraw the swab and place it in the appropriate transport medium or use the swab to prepare a slide for DFA testing.

C. trachomatis-*negative nongonococcal urethritis*

The most common cause of *C. trachomatis*-negative NGU is mycoplasmas, such as *U. urealyticum* and *M. genitalium. T. vaginalis,* yeasts, and anaerobic and aerobic bacteria are other possible sources of infection. Diagnosis requires cultures on specific media or detection by molecular biologic methods.

Treatment

Doxycycline or azithromycin are the drugs of choice (see Table 10-1).

References

1. Huang J, Rogers W, Bailey S: Primary and secondary syphilis in the metropolitan area of Nashville and Davidson County, Tennessee: 1996 to 1998 epidemic described, Sex Transm Dis 2000; 27(3):168.

2. Allison SD: Extragenital syphilitic chancres, J Am Acad Dermatol 1986; 14:1094.

3. Clark EG, Danbolt N: The Oslo study of the natural cause of untreated syphilis, J Chronic Dis 1955; 2:311.

4. Felman YM, Nikitas JA: Secondary syphilis, Cutis 1982; 29:322.

5. Hira SK, et al: Clinical manifestations of secondary syphilis, Int J Dermatol 1987; 26:103.

6. McBroom R, et al: Secondary syphilis in persons infected with and not infected with HIV-1: a comparative immunohistologic study, Am J Dermatopathol 1999; 21(5):432.

7. Kampmeier RH: Late and congenital syphilis. In Dermatologic Clinics. Symposium on Sexually Transmitted Diseases, 1983; 1(1):23.

8. Luxon LM: Neurosyphilis (review), Int J Dermatol 1980; 19:310.

9. Blocker M, Levine W, St. Louis M: HIV prevalence in patients with syphilis, United States, Sex Transm Dis 2000; 27(1):53.

10. Dibbern DJ, Ray S: Recrudescence of treated neurosyphilis in a patient with human immunodeficiency virus, Mayo Clin Proc 1999; 74(1):53.

11. Janier M, et al: A prospective study of the influence of HIV status on the seroreversion of serological tests for syphilis, Dermatology 1999; 198(4):362.

12. Congenital syphilis-United States, 1983-1985. MMWR 1986; 35:625.

13. Reimer CB, et al: The specificity of fetal IgM: antibody or antiantibody? Ann NY Acad Sci 1975; 254:77.

14. Griner PF, et al: Application of principles, Ann Intern Med 1981; 94(2):585.

15. Fiumara NJ: Treatment of early syphilis of less than a year's duration, Sex Transm Dis 1978; 5:85.

16. Fiumara NJ: Treatment of primary and secondary syphilis: serologic response, J Am Acad Dermatol 1986; 14:487.

17. Fiumara NJ: Serologic responses to treatment of 128 patients with late latent syphilis, Sex Transm Dis 1979; 6:243.

18. Fiumara NJ: Infectious syphilis. Dermatol Clin Symp Sexually Transmitted Dis 1983;1(1):3.

19. Brown T, Yen-Moore A, Tyring S: An overview of sexually transmitted diseases. Part I, J Am Acad Dermatol 1999; 41(4):511.

20. Pillay A, et al: Comparison of culture media for the laboratory diagnosis of chancroid, J Med Microbiol 1998; 47(11):1023.

21. Kinghorn GR, Hafiz S, McEntegart MG: Genital colonization with Haemophilus ducreyi in the absence of ulceration, Eur J Sex Transm Dis 1983; 1:89.

22. McCarley ME, Cruz PD, Jr, Sontheimer RD: Chancroid: clinical variants and other findings from an epidemic in Dallas county, 1986-1987, J Am Acad Dermatol 1988; 19:330.

23. King R, et al: Clinical and in situ cellular responses to Haemophilus ducreyi in the presence or absence of HIV infection, Int J STD AIDS 1998; 9(9):531.

24. Gollow MM, Blums M, Haverkort F: Rapid diagnosis of granuloma inguinale, Med J Aust 1986; 144:502.

25. Rosen T, et al: Granuloma inguinale, J Am Acad Dermatol 1984; 11:433.

26. O'Farrell N, et al: Genital ulcer disease: accuracy of clinical diagnosis and strategies to improve control in Durban, South Africa, Genitourin Med 1994; 70:7.

27. Hoosen AA, et al: Granuloma inguinale of the cervix: a carcinoma look-alike, Genitourin Med 1990; 66:380.

28. O'Farrell N: Clinico-epidemiological study of donovanosis in Durban, South Africa, Genitourin Med 1993; 69:108.

29. Paterson D: Disseminated donovanosis (granuloma inguinale) causing spinal cord compression. case report and review of donovanosis involving bone, Clin Infect Dis 1998; 26(2):379.

30. Bozbora A, et al: Surgical treatment of granuloma inguinale, Br J Dermatol 1998; 138(6):1079.

31. Lal S, Garg BR: Further evidence of the efficacy of cotrimoxazole in granuloma venereum, Br J Veneral Dis 1980; 56:412.

32. O'Farrell N, et al: A rapid stain for the diagnosis of granuloma inguinale, Genitourin Med 1990; 66:200.

33. Lebedeff DA, Elliott HB: Rectal gonorrhea in men: diagnosis and treatment, Ann Intern Med 1980; 92:463.

34. Young H, et al: Non-cultural detection of rectal and pharyngeal gonorrhoea by the Gen-Probe PACE 2 assay, Genitourin Med 1997; 73(1):59.

35. Cucurull E, Espinoza L: Gonococcal arthritis, Rheum Dis Clin North Am 1998; 24(2):305.

Sexually Transmitted Viral Infections

❏ **Genital warts**
Human papillomavirus

❏ **Bowenoid papulosis**

❏ **Molluscum contagiosum**

❏ **Genital herpes simplex**
Prevalence
Risk factors
Rate of transmission
Primary and recurrent infections
Prevention
Laboratory diagnosis
Serology
Psychosocial implications
Treatment of genital herpes (Centers for
Disease Control guidelines)
Genital herpes simplex during pregnancy
Neonatal herpes simplex virus infection

❏ **Acquired immunodeficiency syndrome**
Human immunodeficiency virus pathogenesis
Diagnosis
Viral burden
Assessment of immune status (CD4+ T-cells
determination)
Revised Centers for Disease Control
classification and management
Dermatologic diseases associated with
human immunodeficiency virus infection

Genital Warts

Human papillomavirus

Human papillomavirus (HPV) causes warts. HPV can reside in epithelial basal cells and lead to subclinical or latent infection. More than 80 genotypes have been identified; HPV 6, 11, and 16 are most commonly associated with genital warts. HPV 6 and 11 are rarely associated with cervical cancer. HPV 16 and 18 are more likely to be present in subclinical infection and are the types most commonly associated with genital cancer. Bowenoid papulosis is most commonly caused by HPV 16. The rare verrucous carcinoma (Buschke-Löwenstein tumor) that resembles a large wart is locally aggressive but rarely metastatic. It is associated with HPV types 6 and 11.

Incidence

The incidence of genital warts is increasing rapidly and exceeds the incidence of genital herpes. It is the most common viral sexually transmitted disease. It is estimated that 30% to 50% of sexually active adults are infected with HPV. Only 1% to 2% of that group have clinically apparent anogenital warts. Most cervical dysplasias and cancers are related to oncogenic HPV.

Transmission

Risk factors for acquisition of condyloma in women have been identified as the number of sexual partners, frequency of sexual intercourse, and presence of warts on the sexual partner. Men have been found to be at increased risk if they fail to wear a condom. Condoms reduce the transmission of HPV but they do not eliminate it. Transmission of HPV during infant delivery may rarely occur.

Clinical presentation

Genital warts (condyloma acuminata or venereal warts) are pale pink with numerous, discrete, narrow-to-wide projections on a broad base. The surface is smooth or velvety, moist, and lacks the hyperkeratosis of warts found elsewhere (Figures 11-1 to 11-5). The warts may coalesce in the rectal or perineal area to form a large, cauliflower-like mass (Figures 11-6 and 11-7). Perianal warts may be present in persons who do not practice anal sex.

Another type is seen most often in young, sexually active patients. Multifocal, often bilateral, red- or brown-pigmented, slightly raised, smooth papules have the same virus types seen in exophytic condyloma, but in some instances these papules have histologic features of Bowen's disease. (See discussion of bowenoid papulosis later in this chapter.)

Warts spread rapidly over moist areas and may therefore be symmetric on opposing surfaces of the labia or rectum (Figure 11-7). Common warts can possibly be the source of genital warts, although they are usually caused by different antigenic types of virus. Warts may extend into the vaginal tract, urethra, and anal canal or the bladder, in which case a speculum or sigmoidoscope is required for visualization and treatment. Condylomas may spontaneously regress, enlarge, or remain unchanged. Genital warts frequently recur after treatment. There are two possible reasons. Latent virus exists beyond the treatment areas in clinically normal skin.[1] Warts that are flat and inconspicuous, especially on the penile shaft and urethral meatus,[2] escape treatment.

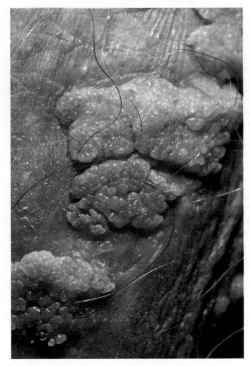

Figure 11-1 Warts on the shaft may have a papillomatous surface and a very broad base.

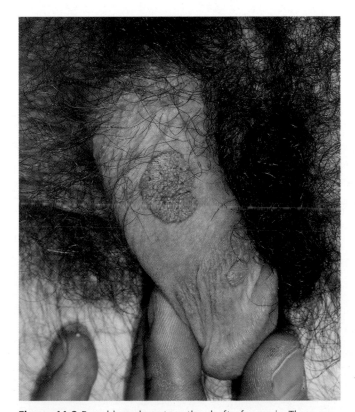

Figure 11-2 Broad-based wart on the shaft of a penis. There are numerous projections on the surface.

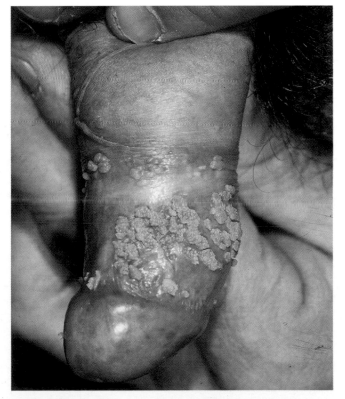

Figure 11-3 Multiple small warts under the foreskin. Multiple inoculations occur on a moist surface. Each wart is made up of many discrete, narrow projections.

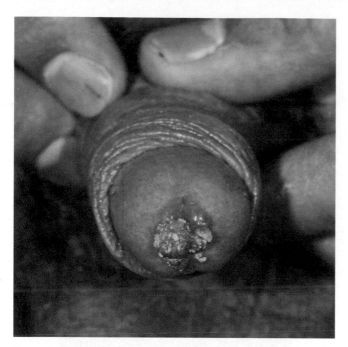

Figure 11-4 Wart at the urethral meatus.

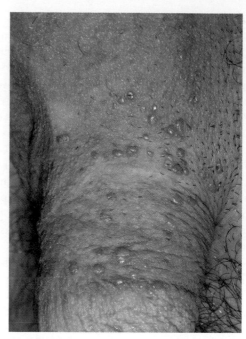

Figure 11-5 Small papular warts on the shaft of the penis. These smooth dome-shaped structures do not respond as well as broad-based papillomatous warts to topical medications. They are effectively treated with light electrodesiccation, cryosurgery, or scissor excision.

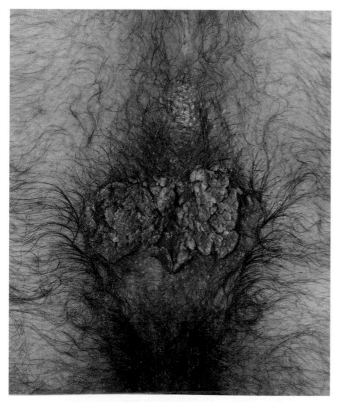

Figure 11-6 Mass of warts on opposing surfaces of the anus.

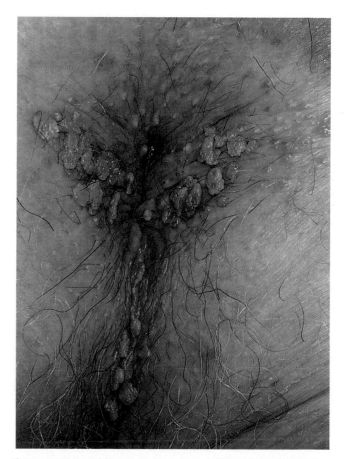

Figure 11-7 Broad-based anal warts are effectively treated with topical medications such as imiquimod cream (Aldara) or podofilox (Condylox).

Oral condyloma in patients with genital human papilloma virus infection

One study showed that 50% of patients with multiple and widespread genital HPV infection who practiced orogenital sex have oral condylomas. All lesions were asymptomatic. Magnification was necessary to detect oral lesions. The diagnosis was confirmed by biopsy. The tongue was the site most frequently affected. Oral condylomas appeared as multiple, small, white or pink papules, sessile or pedunculate, and as papillary growths with filiform characteristics. The size of oral lesions was greater than 2 mm in more than 50% of lesions, and, in 61% of cases, more than five lesions were present. HPV types 16, 18, 6, and 11 were found.[3]

Pearly penile papules

Dome-shaped or hairlike projections, called pearly penile papules, appear on the corona of the penis and sometimes on the shaft just proximal to the corona in up to 10% of male patients. These small angiofibromas are normal variants but are sometimes mistaken for warts. No treatment is required (Figure 11-8).

Genital warts in children

It has been estimated that at least 50% of the cases of condyloma acuminata in children are the result of sexual abuse.[4] In all states there are laws that in effect declare, "If child abuse is recognized or suspected, it has to be reported to the authorities."

Warts in the genital area can be acquired without sexual abuse.[5] A child with warts on the hands can transfer the warts to the mouth, genitals, and anal area.[6] A mother with hand warts can transfer warts to the child. Sexual play among children is another possible mode of transmission. It is not known whether children can acquire condyloma acuminata from adults with anogenital warts through modes of transmission other than skin-to-skin contact. The incubation period for warts is often many months; this makes it difficult to associate past events.

Figure 11-8 Pearly penile papules.

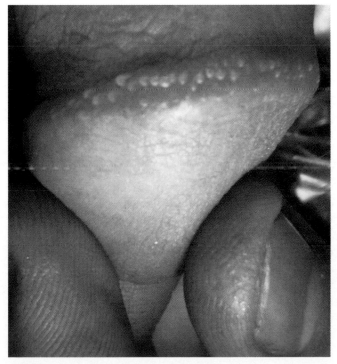

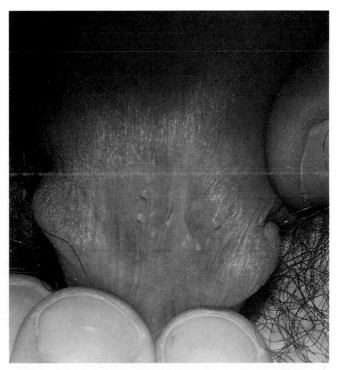

A, An anatomic variant of normal most commonly found on the corona of the penis. They are sometimes mistaken for warts. No treatment is required.

B, A group of papules found just proximal to the corona of the penis is sometimes mistaken for warts.

Genital warts and cancer

There is strong evidence that several HPV types are associated with genital cancers. Genitoanal warts are predominantly induced by HPV types 6, 11, 16, and 18.[7,8] A strong association has been established between infection by HPV-16 and HPV-18 and the subsequent development of cancer in the uterine cervix. When virus typing becomes generally available, it will be useful to identify patients harboring the high-risk HPV types. HPV-16 was demonstrated in 84% and HPV-18 in 8% of genital tumors.

Seventy-three percent of the nonmalignant, clinically and histologically normal tissue 2 to 5 cm from the tumors contained HPV-16.[9] This implies that HPV can persist latently in tissue that appears normal. Cervical carcinomas and precancerous lesions in women may be associated with genital papilloma virus infection in their male sexual partners. Forty-three percent of male sexual partners of women with genital warts had lesions that could be detected only after application of acetic acid.[10] Homosexual behavior in men is a risk factor for anal cancer. Squamous cell anal cancer is associated with a history of genital warts, which suggests that papilloma virus infection is a cause of anal cancer.[11] Male circumcision is associated with a reduced risk of penile HPV infection and, in the case of men with a history of multiple sexual partners, a reduced risk of cervical cancer in their current female partners.[12]

Diagnosis

A clinical diagnosis can be made in most cases. The differential diagnosis includes seborrheic keratoses, nevi, molluscum contagiosum, and pearly penile papules. Biopsy suspicious lesions.

Acetowhitening: acetic acid test

This test was recommended previously but is now used infrequently because it is an insensitive and nonspecific method for diagnosis. False-positive test results are common.

Treatment

HPV cannot be completely eliminated because of the surrounding subclinical HPV infection. Removal of visible lesions decreases viral transmission. All treatment methods are associated with a high rate of recurrence that is likely related to surrounding subclinical infection. Therapies with antiviral/immunomodulatory activity (e.g., imiquimod cream) may be associated with lower recurrence rates.

Management of sexual partners

Examination of sexual partners is not necessary for the management of genital warts because the role of reinfection is probably minimal. Many sexual partners have obvious warts and may desire treatment. The majority of partners are probably already subclinically infected with HPV, even if they do not have visible warts. The use of condoms may reduce transmission to partners likely to be uninfected, such as new partners. HPV infection may persist throughout a patient's lifetime in a dormant state and become infectious intermittently. Whether patients with subclinical HPV infection are as contagious as patients with exophytic warts is unknown. One study showed that the failure rate of treating women with condylomata acuminata did not decrease if their male sexual partners were also treated.[13]

Pregnancy

The use of podophyllin and podofilox is contraindicated during pregnancy. Genital papillary lesions have a tendency to proliferate and to become friable during pregnancy. Many experts advocate the removal of visible warts during pregnancy. HPV types 6 and 11 can cause laryngeal papillomatosis in infants. The route of transmission is unknown, and laryngeal papillomatosis has occurred in infants delivered by caesarean section. Caesarean delivery should not be performed solely to prevent transmission of HPV infection to the newborn. In rare instances, cesarean delivery may be indicated for women with genital warts if the pelvic outlet is obstructed or if vaginal delivery would result in excessive bleeding.

Children

Spontaneous resolution of pediatric condyloma occurs in more than half of cases in 5 years. Nonintervention is a reasonable initial approach to managing venereal warts in children.[14]

Patient-applied therapies

IMIQUIMOD. Improved efficacy and lower recurrence rates occur with imiquimod (Aldara) by inducing the body's own immunologic defenses. Imiquimod has an immunomodulatory effect and does not rely on physical destruction of the lesion. It has antiviral properties by induction of cytokines, including interferon, tumor necrosis factor, interleukin (IL)-6, IL-8, and IL-12. Imiquimod enhances cell-mediated cytolytic activity against HPV. The cream is applied at bedtime every other day, for a maximum of 16 weeks. On the morning after application, the treated area should be cleansed. Local mild-to-moderate irritation may occur. Systemic reactions have not been reported. Imiquimod has not been studied for use during pregnancy.

PODOFILOX. Podofilox, also known as podophyllotoxin, is the main cytotoxic ingredient of podophyllin. Podofilox gel (Condylox) is available for self-application and is useful for responsible, compliant patients. Patients are instructed to apply the 0.5% gel to their external genital warts twice each day for 3 consecutive days, followed by 4 days without treatment. It is recommended that no more than 10 cm² of wart tissue should be treated in a day. This cycle is repeated at weekly intervals for a maximum of 4 to 6 weeks. Approximately 15% of patients report severe local reactions to the treatment area after the first treatment cycle; this is reduced to 5% by the last treatment cycle. Local adverse effects of the drug, such as pain, burning, inflammation, and erosions have occurred in more than 50% of patients. Podofilox is not recommended for perianal, vaginal, or urethral warts and is contraindicated in pregnancy.

Provider-administered therapies

CRYOSURGERY. Liquid nitrogen delivered with a probe, as a spray, or applied with a cotton applicator is very effective for treating smaller, flatter genital warts. It is too painful for patients with extensive disease. Exophytic lesions are best treated with excision, imiquimod, or podofilox. Warts on the shaft of the penis and vulva respond very well, with little or no scarring. Cryosurgery of the rectal area is painful. A conservative technique is best. Freeze the lesion until the white border extends approximately 1 mm beyond the wart. Over-aggressive therapy causes pain, massive swelling, and scarring.

A blister appears, erodes to form an ulcer in 1 to 3 days, and the lesion heals in 1 to 2 weeks. Repeat treatment every 2 to 4 weeks as necessary. Two to three sessions may be required.

Use EMLA cream and/or 1% lidocaine injection for patients who do not tolerate the pain of cryotherapy.

Cryotherapy is effective and safe for both mother and fetus when applied in the second and third trimesters of pregnancy. An intermittent spray technique, using a small spray tip, is used to achieve a small region of cryonecrosis, limiting the run off and scattering of liquid nitrogen. Cervical involvement that requires cervical cryotherapy does not increase the risk to mother or fetus.[15]

SURGICAL REMOVAL AND ELECTROSURGERY. Scissors excision, curettage, or electrosurgery produce immediate results. They are useful for both extensive condylomas or a limited number of warts. Small isolated warts on the shaft of the penis are best treated with conservative electrosurgery or scissor excision[16] rather than subjecting the patient to repeated sessions with podophyllum. Large, unresponsive masses of warts around the rectum or vulva may be treated by scissor excision of the bulk of the mass, followed by electrocautery of the remaining tissue down to the skin surface.[17] Removal of a very large mass of warts is a painful procedure and is best performed with the patient under general or spinal anesthesia in the operating room.

TRICHLOROACETIC ACID. Application of trichloroacetic acid (TCA) and bichloracetic acid (BCA) 80% to 90% is effective and less destructive than laser surgery, electrocautery, or liquid nitrogen application. It is most effective on small, moist warts.

This is an ideal treatment for isolated lesions in pregnant women.[18] A very small amount is applied to the wart, which whitens immediately. The acid is then neutralized with water or bicarbonate of soda. The tissue slough heals in 7 to 10 days. Repeat each week or every other week as needed. Excessive application causes scars. Take great care not to treat normal surrounding skin.

PODOPHYLLUM RESIN. Podophyllin is a plant compound that causes cells to arrest in mitosis, leading to tissue necrosis. Podophyllun resin 10% to 25% in compound tincture of benzoin used to be the standard provider-administered therapy. Patient applied medications are now commonly used. The medication can be very effective especially for moist warts with a large surface area and lesions with many surface projections. Podophyllun is relatively ineffective in dry areas, such as the scrotum, penile shaft, and labia majora. It is not recommended for cervical, vaginal, or intraurethral warts. The compound is applied with a cotton-tipped applicator. The entire surface of the wart is covered with the solution, and the patient remains still until the solution dries in approximately 2 minutes. When lesions covered by the prepuce are treated, the applied solution must be allowed to dry for several minutes before the prepuce is returned to its usual position. Powdering the warts after treatment or applying petrolatum to the surrounding skin may help to avoid contamination of normal skin with the irritating resin. The medicine is removed by washing 1 hour later. The patient is treated again in 1 week. The podophyllum may then remain on the wart for 8 to 12 hours if there was little or no inflammation after the first treatment.

Overenthusiastic initial treatment can result in intense inflammation and discomfort that lasts for days. The procedure is simple and it is tempting to allow home treatment, but in most cases this should be avoided. Very frequently patients overtreat and cause excessive inflammation by applying podophyllum on normal skin. To avoid extreme discomfort, treat only part of a large warty mass in the perineal and rectal area. Warts on the shaft of the penis do not respond as successfully to podophyllum as do warts on the glans or under the foreskin; consequently, electrosurgery or cryosurgery should be used if two or three treatment sessions with podophyllum fail. Many warts disappear after a single treatment. Alternate forms of therapy should be attempted if there is no improvement after five treatment sessions.

Warning. Systemic toxicity occurs from absorption of podophyllum. Paresthesia, polyneuritis, paralytic ileus, leukopenia, thrombocytopenia, coma, and death have occurred when large quantities of podophyllum were applied to wide areas or allowed to remain in contact with the skin for an extended period.[19] Only limited areas should be treated during each session. Very small quantities should be used in the mouth, vaginal tract, or rectosigmoid. Do not use podophyllun on pregnant women.

Alteration of histopathology. Podophyllum can produce bizarre forms of squamous cells, which can be mistaken for squamous cell carcinoma. The pathologist must be informed of the patient's exposure to podophyllum when a biopsy of a previously treated wart is submitted.

5-FLUOROURACIL CREAM. Application of a 5-fluorouracil cream (Carac, Efudex) may be considered in cases of genital warts that are resistant to all other treatments. A thin layer of cream is applied one to three times per week and washed off after 3 to 10 hours, depending on the sensitivity of the location.[20,21] Treat for several weeks, as necessary. Irritation makes it intolerable for some patients.

Vaginal warts are treated by inserting an applicator (such as the one supplied by Ortho Pharmaceutical Corporation for the treatment of vaginal candida) one-third full of 5% 5-fluorouracil cream (approximately 3 mL) deeply into the vagina at bedtime, once each week for up to 10 consecutive weeks.[22,23] The vulva and urethra are protected with petrolatum. A tampon should be inserted just inside the introitus. In one study, there was no evidence of disease in 85% of patients 3 months after treatment. Resistant cases were treated twice each week. Mild irritation and vaginal discharge may develop. The vulva should be protected with zinc oxide or hydrocortisone ointments if the twice-each-week regimen is used. Application to the keratinized epithelium (vulva, anus, and penis) twice weekly on 2 consecutive days is well tolerated but less effective; such treatment should not be used for pregnant women. Patients should be warned to avoid thick coverage because the excess cream causes inflammation or ulceration in the labiocrural or anal folds. Protective gloves are not necessary, provided that the hands are carefully washed after applying the 5-fluorouracil cream. A single intravaginal dose of 1.5-gm, 5% 5-fluorouracil cream contains only 75 mg of 5-fluorouracil. This is less than 10% of the usual systemic dose and far lower than the toxicity level of the drug even if rapid and complete absorption occurs.

CARBON DIOXIDE LASER. The CO_2 laser is an ideal method for treating both primary and recurrent condyloma acuminata in men[24] and women because of its precision and the wound's rapid healing without scarring. The laser can be used with an operating microscope to find and destroy the smallest warts. For pregnant women, this is the treatment of choice for large or extensive lesions and for cases that do not respond to repeated applications of trichloroacetic acid.

ISOTRETINOIN. Oral isotretinoin (Accutane) was used in one study for the treatment of condylomata acuminata. A total of 56 males with a history of condylomata acuminata refractory to at least 1 standard therapeutic regimen were treated orally with isotretinoin (1 mg/kg daily) during a 3-month period. At the end of treatment 40% had complete response, 13 % had partial response and 47 % had no response. Immature and small condylomata acuminata respond best.[25]

INTERFERON ALFA-2B RECOMBINANT (INTRON-A). Warts that do not respond to any form of conventional treatment and patients whose disease is severe enough to impose significant social or physical limitations on their activities may be candidates for treatment with interferon.[26] Alfa interferon is approved by the U.S. Food and Drug Administration for the treatment of condyloma acuminata in patients 18 years of age or older. There are two commercially available preparations available for intralesional injection into the base of the wart. Alferon N injection (Interferon alfa-n3) is available in 1-mL vials; 0.05 mL per wart is administered twice weekly for up to 8 weeks. Intron A (Interferon alfa-2b, recombinant) is available is several size vials, but the vial of 10 million IU is the only package size specifically designed for use in treatment of condyloma acuminata. Intron-A (0.1 mL of reconstituted Intron-A) is injected into each lesion three times per week on alternate days for 3 weeks. Influenza-like symptoms usually clear within 24 hours of treatment. Total clearing occurs in approximately 40% of treated warts. The medication is very expensive.

Bowenoid Papulosis

Bowenoid papulosis is an uncommon condition seen in young, sexually active adults. It occurs on the genitals (vulva and circumcised penis) and histologically resembles Bowen's disease.[27] The mean age is 30 years for male patients and 32 years for female patients. Patients' age range is from 3 to 80 years. The duration of disease has been from 2 weeks to 11 years.[28] The natural history of the disease is unknown, but the lesions usually follow a benign clinical course and spontaneous regression is observed. Evolution of the lesions to invasive carcinoma is rare.

The papules are asymptomatic discrete, small (averaging 4 mm in diameter), flat, reddish-violaceous or brown, often coalescent, and usually have a smooth, velvety surface. They may resemble flat warts, psoriasis, or lichen planus (Figure 11-9). In women the lesions are often darkly pigmented and are not as easily confused with other entities. They are located in men on the glans, the shaft, and the foreskin of the penis and in women on the labia majora and minora, on the clitoris, in the inguinal folds, and around the anus. The lesions in women are often bilateral, hyperpigmented, and confluent. Autoinoculation probably explains the bilateral, symmetric distribution in moist areas. Many patients have a history of genital infection with viral warts or herpes simplex. Genital warts are primarily caused by HPV types 6 and 11. HPV type 16 has been found in a high percentage of women with bowenoid papulosis and in cervical and other genital neoplasias.[29] Therefore the cervix of female patients with bowenoid papulosis and other genitoanal HPV infections should be examined routinely, with careful follow-up. Female partners of patients with bowenoid papulosis should also be observed closely.

Treatment should be conservative. Individual lesions can be adequately treated by electrosurgery, carbon dioxide laser, cryosurgery, or scissor excision, much as ordinary verrucae, without the need for wide surgical margins. Alternatively, lesions may be treated for 3 to 5 weeks with 5% 5-fluorouracil cream or imiquimod cream qod until they become inflamed.

Figure 11-9 Bowenoid papulosis. Multiple brown verrucous papules on the shaft of the penis. This patient responded to imiquimod cream (Aldara) applied every other day. This is the same treatment regimen used to treat penile warts.

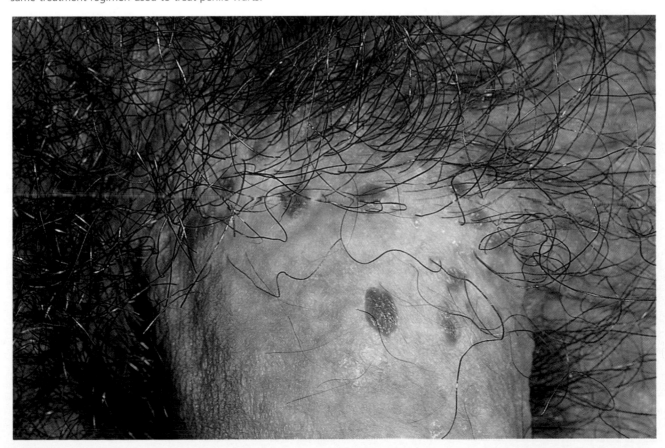

Molluscum Contagiosum

Molluscum contagiosum is a large double-stranded DNA virus that replicates entirely within the cytoplasm of keratinocytes. It is a member of the family Poxviridae and does not develop latency like the herpes virus. The virion colony is encased in a protective sac that prevents triggering of the host immune response.

Clinical manifestations

Molluscum contagiosum papules are discrete, 2 to 5 mm in diameter, slightly umbilicated, flesh colored, and dome shaped. They spread by touching, autoinoculation (particularly in atopic patients), by scratching or secondary to shaving, and may result in a linear distribution of lesions. Transmission also occurs in wrestlers, masseurs, and steam and sauna bathers. The pubic (Figure 11-10) and genital (Figure 11-11) areas are most commonly involved in adults. Molluscum lesions in other areas are described in Chapter 12. They are frequently grouped. There may be few or many covering a wide area. Erythema and scaling at the periphery of a single or several lesions may occur (Figure 11-12). This may be the result of inflammation from scratching, or it may be a hypersensitivity reaction.

Individual lesions last 6 to 8 weeks. Autoinoculation causes new lesions and the duration of infection can be up to 8 months.

The differential diagnosis includes warts and herpes simplex. Molluscum papules are dome-shaped, slightly umbilicated, firm, and white. Warts have an irregular, often velvety surface. The vesicles of herpes simplex rapidly become umbilicated.

Genital molluscum contagiosum in children may be a manifestation of sexual abuse (see Figure 11-12).

Molluscum contagiosum is a common and at times severely disfiguring eruption in patients with HIV infection (Figure 11-24). It is often a marker of late-stage disease.[30]

Diagnosis

The patient must be carefully examined because these discrete white-pink umbilicated papules are often camouflaged by pubic hair. Most patients have just a few lesions that can be easily overlooked. The focus of examination is the pubic hair, the genitals, anal area, thighs, and trunk. Lesions may appear anywhere except the palms and soles. If necessary, the diagnosis can be easily established by laboratory methods (see Chapter 12). Microscopic examination of a potassium hydroxide preparation of the soft material obtained from curette samples taken from the umbilicated part of the lesion shows inclusion bodies (molluscum bodies) within the keratinocytes.

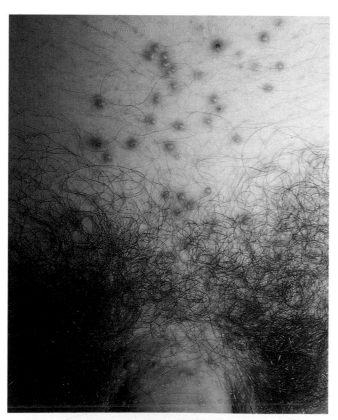

Figure 11-10 Molluscum contagiosum is a sexually transmitted disease in adults. Close observation of individual lesions is necessary to confirm the diagnosis. Lesions are often misdiagnosed as warts or herpes simplex.

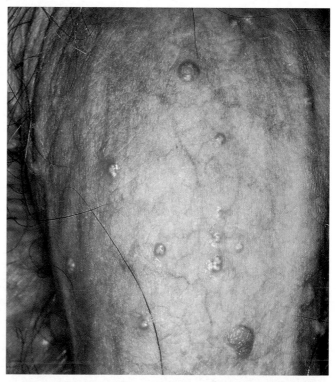

Figure 11-11 Molluscum contagiosum. Lesions are usually discrete, white, and dome shaped. They lack the many small projections found on the surface of genital warts.

Treatment

Genital lesions should be definitively treated to prevent spread through sexual contact. New lesions that were too small to be detected at the first examination may appear after treatment and require attention at a subsequent visit.

Curettage

Small papules can be quickly removed with a curette, with or without local anesthesia. Bleeding is controlled with gauze pressure or Monsel's solution. Warn the patient that Monsel's solution is painful. Curettage is useful when there are a few lesions because it provides the quickest, most reliable treatment. A small scar may form; therefore this technique should be avoided in cosmetically important areas.

Lidocaine/prilocaine (EMLA) cream applied 30 to 60 minutes before treatment helps prevent the pain of curettage for children.[31]

Cryosurgery

Cryosurgery is the treatment of choice for patients who do not object to the pain. The papule is sprayed or touched lightly with a nitrogen-bathed cotton swab until the advancing, white, frozen border has progressed down the side of the papule to form a 1-mm halo on the normal skin surrounding the lesion. This should take approximately 5 seconds. A conservative approach is necessary because excessive freezing produces hypopigmentation or hyperpigmentation.

Antiviral and immunomodulatory therapies

Males between 9 and 27 years of age with molluscum contagiosum self-administered an analog of imiquimod 5% cream (Aldara) three times daily for 5 consecutive days per week for 4 weeks. The cure rate was over 80%.[32] Children may respond with less irritation if treated once each day or every other day.[33] Children (mean age 7 years) were treated every night for 4 weeks. Adverse reactions were limited to application site reactions. There was no systemic toxicity.[34] Imiquimod is most efficacious in patients with HIV-1 disease and in the genital area in immune-competent adults.

Cantharidin

Cantharidin is a safe and effective therapy. A small drop of Cantharone (cantharidin 0.7%) is applied over the surface of the lesion, while contamination of normal skin is avoided. Temporary burning, pain, erythema, or pruritus may occur. Secondary bacterial infection does not occur. Lesions blister and may clear without scarring. New lesions occasionally appear at the site of the blister created by cantharidin. An alternate method is to apply a tiny amount of cantharidin or the more potent Verrusol (1% cantharidin, 30% salicylic acid, 5% podophyllin) and cover the area with tape for 1 day. The resulting small blister is treated with Polysporin until the reaction subsides.

Potassium hydroxide

Potassium hydroxide (KOH) 10% aqueous solution was applied twice daily, on each lesion. The therapy is continued until all lesions undergo inflammation and superficial ulceration. Thirty-two of 35 children achieved complete clinical cure after a mean treatment period of 30 days. Hypertrophic scarring occurred in 1 patient, pigmentary changes occurred in 9 others.

Oral cimetidine

Pediatric patients were treated with a 2-month course of oral cimetidine 40 mg/kg/day. All but three children who completed treatment experienced clearance of all lesions. No adverse effects were observed. Response to cimetidine may be better in atopic compared to nonatopic children.[35]

Laser therapy

The 585-nm pulsed dye laser is an effective, well-tolerated, and quick treatment for molluscum contagiosum.

Trichloroacetic acid peel

Peels performed with 25% to 50% trichloroacetic acid (average 35%) and repeated every 2 weeks as needed resulted in an average reduction in lesion counts of 40.5% (range 0% to 90%) in HIV patients with extensive molluscum contagiosum. No spread of molluscum lesions, scarring, or secondary infection developed at 2 months' follow-up.[36]

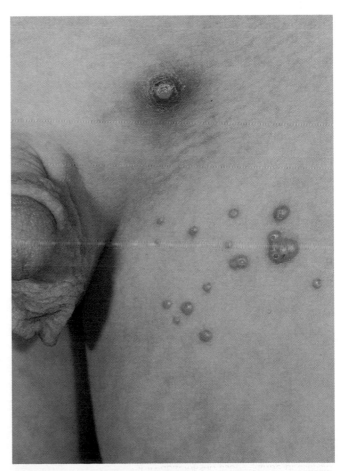

Figure 11-12 Molluscum contagiosum. A single lesion became inflamed and disappeared 10 days later.

Genital Herpes Simplex

Genital herpes simplex virus (HSV) infection is primarily a disease of young adults. It is a recurrent, life-long infection. There are two serotypes: HSV-1 and HSV-2. Most genital cases are caused by HSV-2. At least 50 million persons in the United States have genital HSV infection. Sexual encounters are often delayed or avoided for fear of acquiring or transmitting the disease. The psychologic implications are obvious. Herpes simplex virus (HSV) type 2 is not an etiologic factor in cervical cancer as was once suspected.

Most persons infected with HSV-2 have not been diagnosed. Many have mild or unrecognized infections but shed virus intermittently in the genital tract. Most genital herpes infections are transmitted by persons unaware that they have the infection or who are asymptomatic when transmission occurs. The first-episode genital infection may be severe.

Herpes simplex infection of the penis (Figures 11-13 to 11-15), vulva (Figure 11-16), and rectum is pathophysiologically identical to herpes infection in other areas.

Prevalence

From 1988 to 1994, the seroprevalence of HSV-2 in persons 12 years of age or older in the United States was 21.9%, corresponding to 45 million infected people. HSV-2 is now detectable in one of five persons 12 years of age or older nationwide.[37]

Risk factors

Risk factors for genital herpes HSV-2 are strongly related to lifetime number of sexual partners (Figure 11-17), number of years of sexual activity, male homosexuality, black race, female gender, and a history of previous sexually transmitted diseases (STD).

The seroprevalence is higher among women (25.6%) than men (17.8%) and higher among blacks (45.9%) than whites (17.6%). Less than 10% of all those who were seropositive reported a history of genital herpes infection. [37]

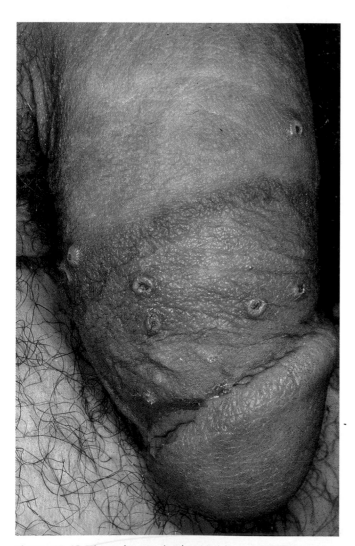

Figure 11-13 Primary herpes simplex. Vesicles are discrete and can be confused with warts and molluscum contagiosum. The primary lesion is a vesicle that rapidly becomes umbilicated.

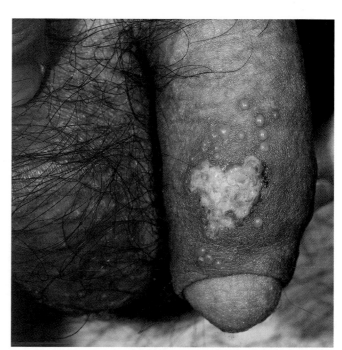

Figure 11-14 Primary herpes simplex. A group of vesicles has ruptured, leaving an erosion. Tense vesicles are at the periphery.

RECURRING GENITAL HERPES

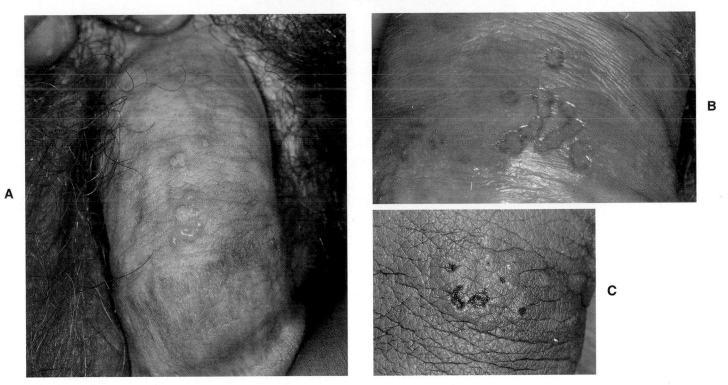

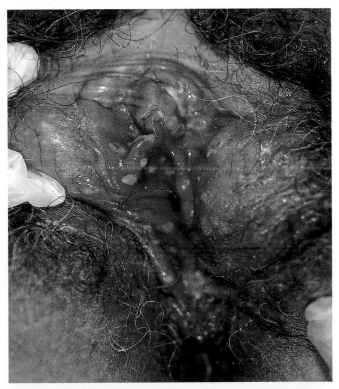

Figure 11-15 A, Grouped vesicles on a red base is the initial lesion. **B,** Vesicles do not appear under the foreskin. They are macerated away to form punched-out erosions. **C,** Crusts form and then heal with or without scarring.

Figure 11-16 Primary herpes simplex.

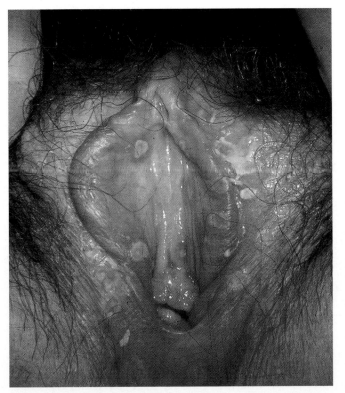

A, Scattered erosions covered with exudate.

B, Numerous erosions appeared 4 days after contact with an asymptomatic carrier.

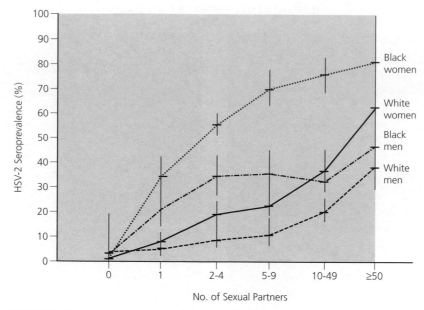

Figure 11-17 HSV-2 seroprevalence according to the lifetime number of sexual partners, adjusted for age, for black and white men and women 1988 to 1994. *(From Fleming DT, et al: N Engl J Med 1997; 337:1105.)*

Rate of transmission

Transmission of HSV occurs through both symptomatic lesions and asymptomatic viral shedding. Symptomatic lesions are more efficient transmitters of the virus because they have higher viral titers. Herpes simplex is transmitted more efficiently from males to females than from females to males. This may be due to the increased rate of recurrence, and hence infectivity, in men. Seronegative female susceptible partners have the highest risk for acquiring genital herpes infection. The 32% annual risk in seronegative women was significantly higher than the 9% risk in HSV type 1 seropositive women and than the 6% or less risk in susceptible male partners, regardless of previous HSV type 1 infection. In a large study, women acquired HSV-2 at a rate 8.9 per 10,000 episodes of sexual intercourse. Men acquired HSV-2 at a rate of 1.5 per 10,000 episodes of sexual intercourse.[38]

Previous herpes simplex virus type 1 infection

Previous infection with HSV type 1 reduces the rate of acquisition of genital HSV type 2 infection, reduces the severity of initial HSV type 2 infection, and may increase the proportion of persons acquiring HSV type 2 asymptomatically or subclinically. The presence of HSV type 1 antibody is associated with a decreased likelihood of detecting antibody to HSV type 2 in women.

Genital infections with HSV-1 are associated with less asymptomatic shedding, lower rates of clinical recurrence, and lower rates of transmission.[39-41]

Human immunodeficiency virus infection

The rates of HSV infection are increasing; the highest prevalence is in patients with the human immunodeficiency virus (HIV). Genital ulcer disease is a risk factor in the transmission of the human immunodeficiency virus-1 (HIV-1). HIV-1 virions can be detected in genital ulcers caused by HSV-2, which suggests that genital herpes infection likely increases the efficiency of the sexual transmission of HIV-1.[42]

The treatment of genital herpes decreases the rates of HIV infection. Acyclovir resistance is more common in this group, but acyclovir use may prolong survival in some HIV-seropositive patients.[43]

Primary and recurrent infections
First-episode infections

First-episode infections include true primary infection and nonprimary first-episode infections. Patients with true primary infections have seronegative test results and have never been infected with any type of herpes virus. Patients with nonprimary first-episode infections have been infected at another site with either type 1 or 2 virus (e.g., the oral area) and have serum antibody and humoral immunity.

First-episode infections are more extensive and have more systemic symptoms. Viral shedding lasts longer (15 to 16 days) in primary first-episode infections.[44] Virus infections spread easily over moist surfaces. Ten percent to 15% of patients with first-episode genital herpes have simultaneous infection in the pharynx, probably as a result of orogenital contact.[45] They have extensive genital disease and exudative or ulcerative pharyngitis.

SIGNS AND SYMPTOMS. Vesicles appear approximately 6 days after sexual contact. Vesicles become depressed in the center (umbilicated) in 2 or 3 days, then erode (see Figures 11-13 and 11-14). Crusts form and the lesion heals in the next week or two. Scars form if the inflammation has been intense. Discharge, dysuria, and inguinal lymphadenopathy are common. Systemic complaints, including fever, myalgias, lethargy, and photophobia, are present in approximately 70% of patients and are more common in women. The clinical diagnosis is insensitive and nonspecific. The typical painful multiple vesicular or ulcerative lesions are absent in many infected persons.

Women have more extensive disease and a higher incidence of constitutional symptoms probably because of the larger surface area involved. Wide areas of the female genitals may be covered with painful erosions (see Figure 11-16).

The cervix is involved in most cases, and erosive cervicitis is almost always associated with first-episode disease. The virus can be isolated from the cervix in only 10% to 15% of women with recurrent disease. Inflammation, edema, and pain may be so extreme that urination is interfered with and catheterization is required. The patient may be immobilized and require bed rest at home or in the hospital.

A similar pattern of extensive involvement, with edema and possible urinary retention, develops in males, especially if uncircumcised. Crusts do not form under the foreskin (see Figure 11-15, B). The eruption frequently extends onto the pubic area, and it is possibly spread from secretions during sexual contact. The anal area may be involved after anal intercourse.

Nearly 40% of newly acquired HSV-2 infections and nearly two thirds of new HSV-1 infections are symptomatic. Among sexually active adults, new genital HSV-1 infections are as common as new oropharyngeal HSV-1 infections.[46]

The virus ascends the peripheral sensory nerves after the primary infection and establishes latency in the nerve root ganglia. Intercourse, skin trauma, cold or heat, stress, concurrent infection, and menstruation can trigger reactivation.

Recurrent infection

CLINICAL SIGNS AND SYMPTOMS. Recurrent infection in females may be so minor or hidden from view in the vagina or cervix that it is unnoticed. This explains why some males with primary disease are not aware of the source. Recurrences cannot be predicted, but they often follow sexual intercourse. Itching or pain may precede the recurrent lesion. A small group of vesicles appears, umbilicates in 1 or 2 days, then erodes and crusts. The lesion heals in 10 to 14 days. Vesicles are not seen under the foreskin or on the moist surfaces of the vulva or vagina (see Figure 11-15).

The virus can be cultured for approximately 5 days from active genital lesions, and the lesions are almost certainly infectious during this time. Males and females who have no symptoms can transmit the disease. Infection can develop in male patients from contact with female carriers who have no obvious disease. The infection may be acquired from an active cervical infection or from cervical secretions of a female who chronically carries the virus, from vulvar ulcers, from fissures, and from anorectal infection.[47]

FREQUENCY OF RECURRENCE. A study documented the recurrence rates in patients with a symptomatic first-episode HSV-2 genital infection (Box 11-1).[48]

Approximately 80% to 90% of persons with a symptomatic first episode of HSV-2 genital infection will have a recurrent episode within the following year, compared with 50% to 60% of patients with HSV-1 infection.[49]

Reactivation decreases in frequency over time in most patients. Ninety-five percent of patients with primary HSV-2 have recurrences, with a median time to the first recurrence of approximately 50 days. The recurrence rates in patients with a symptomatic first-episode HSV-2 genital infection is documented in Box 11-1. Fifty percent of patients with primary HSV-1 have recurrent outbreaks, and the median time to the first recurrence is 1 year.

Median recurrence rates in the first year are one (HSV-1) and five (HSV-2) per year in patients with newly acquired infection. Patients infected with HSV-2 who were observed for longer than 4 years had a median decrease of two recurrences between years 1 and 5. However, 25% of these patients had an increase of at least one recurrence in year 5. Decreases among patients who never received suppressive therapy were similar to decreases during untreated periods in patients who received suppressive therapy.[39,48,50]

Box 11-1 Genital Herpes Recurrence Rates During the First Year After Symptomatic First-Episode HSV-2 Infection

89% at least 1 recurrence

38% >6 recurrences

20% >10 recurrences

NO OR 1 RECURRENCE

26% of women

8% of men

MORE THAN 10 RECURRENCES

14% of women

26% of men

Patients who had severe primary infection had recurrences nearly twice as often and had a shorter time to first recurrence compared with those who had shorter first episodes.

From Benedetti J, et al: Ann Intern Med 1994; 121:847.

ANATOMIC SITE. The frequency of recurrence varies with the anatomic site and the virus type.[39] The frequency of recurrences of genital HSV-2 herpes is higher than that of HSV-1 orolabial infection. HSV-1 oral infections recur more often than genital HSV-1 infections. HSV-2 genital infections occur six times more frequently than HSV-1 genital infections. The frequency of recurrence is lowest for orolabial HSV-2 infections.

ASYMPTOMATIC TRANSMISSION. Asymptomatic viral shedding is the primary mode of herpes virus transmission. The infected partner is almost always unaware of the herpes infection. Therefore highly motivated couples who are aware of the signs and symptoms of genital herpes and attempt to avoid sexual contact with lesions remain at substantial risk for transmission of genital herpes to the uninfected partner. Acyclovir therapy substantially decreases but does not totally eliminate symptomatic or asymptomatic viral shedding or the potential for transmission.

ASYMPTOMATIC SHEDDING. Most persons who have serologic evidence of infection with HSV-2 are asymptomatic. The site of asymptomatic shedding is unknown. Virus has not been isolated from the semen or urethra after primary infection.[51] Viral shedding can occur at any time. Asymptomatic shedding occurs most commonly in the first year after the primary episode (particularly the first 3 months), during the prodromal period, in the week after a symptomatic recurrence, and in HSV-2 infections versus HSV-1.[52]

The rate of subclinical shedding of HSV in the subjects with no reported history of genital herpes was similar to that in the subjects with such a history (3.0% vs. 2.7%).[53]

Among women with genital HSV-2 infection, subclinical shedding occurred on a mean of 2% of the days. The mean duration of viral shedding during subclinical episodes was 1.5 days, as compared with 1.8 days during symptomatic episodes. Women with frequent symptomatic recurrences also have frequent subclinical shedding and may be at high risk for transmitting HSV.[54]

Prevention

Virus can be recovered from the eroded lesions for approximately 5 days after onset, but sexual contact should be avoided until reepithelialization is complete. Male (urethra) and female (cervix) carriers who have no symptoms can conceivably transmit the infection at any time. The use of spermicidal foams and condoms should be recommended to patients who have a history of recurrent genital herpes. For sexual partners who have both had genital herpes, protective measures are probably not necessary if both carry the same virus type (one partner infected the other) and active lesions are not present. Remember that having herpes in one area is not a protection from acquiring the infection in another location. Contact should be avoided when active lesions are present.

One study showed that condom use during more than 25% of sex acts was associated with protection against HSV-2 acquisition for women but not for men. Therefore identification of heterosexual couples in which the male partner has HSV-2 infection and the female is HSV-2 negative can reduce transmission of HSV-2 for women.[38]

Laboratory diagnosis

The sensitivity of all laboratory methods depends on the stage of lesions (sensitivity is higher in vesicular than in ulcerative lesions), on whether the patient has a first or a recurrent episode of the disease (higher in first episodes), and on whether the sample is from an immunosuppressed or an immunocompetent patient (more antigen is found in immunosuppressed patients). It is crucial to document genital herpes simplex infection in pregnant women and cutaneous herpes in newborn infants. Consequently, in these instances, suspicious vesicular and eroded lesions should be cultured. In all other forms the clinical presentation is usually so characteristic that an accurate diagnosis can be made by inspection. A number of laboratory procedures are available if confirmation is desired.[55]

Culture

The most definitive method for diagnosis *in patients who present with genital ulcers or other mucocutaneous lesions* is viral culture, which can distinguish between HSV-1 and HSV-2. The culture specimen must be obtained from active lesions during viral shedding, which, on average, lasts 4 days. Fifty percent of culture results are negative in recurrent lesions. *Vesicles and wet erosions give a higher yield than dry erosions or crusts.* Vesicles are punctured and the fluid is absorbed into the swab, which is then rubbed vigorously onto the base of the lesion.

Cervical samples are taken from the endocervix with the swab. From the viewpoint of cost, the insertion of separate swabs from a number of anatomic sites (cervix, vaginal ulcers, vaginal fissures, anus) into one culture vial is the most efficient way to collect genital samples for viral culture.

Specimens are inoculated into tube cell cultures and monitored microscopically for characteristic morphologic changes (cytopathic effects for up to 5 to 7 days after inoculation for maximum sensitivity). Results may be available in 1 or 2 days.

Cytologic detection

Cytologic detection of cellular changes of herpes virus infection is insensitive and nonspecific, both in genital lesions (Tzanck preparation) (Figure 11-18) and cervical Papanicolaou smears, and should not be relied on for diagnosis of HSV infection.

Histopathologic studies

A biopsy specimen should be obtained from an intact vesicle. The histologic picture is characteristic but not unique for herpes simplex.

Polymerase chain reaction

Polymerase chain reaction assays for HSV are available in some laboratories and is the test of choice for detecting HSV in spinal fluid for diagnosis of HSV infection of the central nervous system.

Serology

Fifty percent to 90% of adults have antibody to HSV. More than 70% of the population have antibody levels ranging from 1:10 to 1:160; only 5% have titers greater than 1:160. Because of the high incidence of antibodies to herpes simplex in the population, assay of a single serum specimen is not of great value.

Subtyping

There are two serotypes of HSV. HSV-1 infections are primarily oropharyngeal; genital infections can also be caused by this serotype. HSV-2 infections are primarily genital, but are also detected in the mouth.

HERPES SIMPLEX VIRUS TYPE-1. HSV-1 seropositivity is usually associated with orolabial infection. Herpes simplex virus type-2 seropositivity is usually associated with genital infection. HSV-1 is now a significant cause of genital herpes and is implicated in 5% to 30% of all first-episode cases. The proportion of HSV-1 among initial genital herpes infections is higher among men who have sex with men (46.9%) than among women (21.4%) and is lowest among heterosexual men (14.6%). Receptive oral sex significantly increased the odds that initial infections are HSV-1 rather than HSV-2. Genital HSV-1 may often be acquired through contact with a partner's mouth.[56]

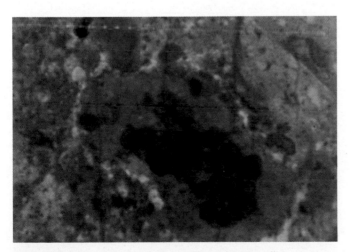

Figure 11-18 Tzanck smear. Multinucleated giant cell.

Type-specific serologic tests

Type-specific and nonspecific antibodies develop during the first several weeks following infection and persist indefinitely. Almost all HSV-2 infections are sexually acquired. Therefore HSV-2 antibody indicates anogenital infection, but the presence of HSV-1 antibody does not distinguish anogenital from orolabial infection.

The assays include POCkit HSV-2; Meridian's Premier test; HerpeSelect-1 enzyme-linked immunosorbent assay (ELISA) IgG or HerpeSelect-2 ELISA IgG; and HerpeSelect 1 and 2 Immunoblot IgG.

The POCkit HSV-2 assay is a point-of-care (performed in the office) test that provides results for HSV-2 antibodies from capillary blood or serum during a clinic visit. The other assays are laboratory-based. The sensitivities of these tests for detection of HSV-2 antibody vary from 80% to 98%, and false-negative results may occur, especially at early stages of infection. The specificities of these assays are greater than 96%. False-positive results can occur, especially in patients with low likelihood of HSV infection. Therefore repeat testing or a confirmatory test (e.g., an immunoblot assay if the initial test was an ELISA) may be indicated in some settings.

The POCkit HSV-2 Rapid Test provides rapid (6 minutes) results. It determines HSV-2 seropositivity and cannot test for HSV-1 antibodies. With Meridian's Premier test, a blood sample is sent to the laboratory. The Meridian Premier tests can detect both HSV-1 and HSV-2 type-specific HSV antibodies. With the Premier tests, seroconversion to HSV-2 can take up to 4 months, so negative results should be confirmed with Western blot analysis or a later serum sample should be tested if seroconversion is suspected.

Indications to test

Subclinical or unrecognized infections are best diagnosed with type-specific antibody tests.

PREGNANT WOMEN. Consider testing pregnant women who are at risk of acquiring herpes in the third trimester. These are women without a history of genital herpes whose partner is known to be infected or is seropositive. Infection of the neonate is most common when primary infection develops late in pregnancy. Transmission of herpes to the neonate during birth results in neonatal herpes, with devastating results.

A pregnant seronegative woman could be identified and counseled to avoid transmission during the third trimester. An HSV-2–seropositive woman can be informed that her risk of transmission to her fetus is low and that most patients can have a vaginal delivery. If a woman is entirely seronegative and her partner is HSV-1 positive, they should be instructed to avoid oral-genital and genital-genital contact in the last trimester because HSV-1 accounts for up to 30% of cases of neonatal herpes. Consider suppressive therapy for seropositive men unwilling to abstain or to use condoms.

MONOGAMOUS COUPLES. Test results can be used to counsel couples in monogamous relationships in which one partner has clinical or serologic evidence of herpes. Serologic testing can identify partners at risk. Many people are unaware of their infection. Explain the risks when one partner has antibodies and the other does not. Educate patients about the frequency of transmission, asymptomatic shedding, condoms, and suppressive therapy.

DIAGNOSIS OF RECURRENT GENITAL ERUPTIONS. Testing can be used to diagnosis or exclude the diagnosis of genital herpes as a cause of recurrent genital eruption when the diagnosis cannot be made by other means. Patients with recurrent genital eruptions frequently present after the virus can no longer be cultured. The presence of HSV-2 antibodies provides evidence of infection. The absence of seropositivity excludes genital herpes. Some patients with a clinical history of what was diagnosed as genital herpes are surprised to find that they have no serologic evidence of infection. A seropositive HSV-1 or HSV-2 result does not determine whether the infection is orolabial or genital. Viral cultures are required to confirm the diagnosis. HSV-1 recurs less frequently than HSV-2, therefore typing helps determine prognosis.

IDENTIFYING HERPES SIMPLEX VIRUS AS A RISK FACTOR FOR HUMAN IMMUNODEFICIENCY VIRUS TRANSMISSION. Testing can be used to identify HSV-2 infection in patients at high risk for HIV acquisition. Genital HSV ulcers facilitate the transmission of HIV through mucosal disruption. CD4+ lymphocytes in herpetic lesions are targets for HIV attachment and entry. Consider suppressive therapy for seropositive people at risk of HIV acquisition.

Psychosocial implications

Herpes is a benign disorder that has a tremendous psychosocial impact.[57] The sensitive physician is aware of the spectrum of symptoms that can evolve and provides emotional support, especially at initial diagnosis. The victim's response usually begins with initial shock and emotional numbing, then a frantic search for a cure. A sense of loneliness and isolation occurs after the patient becomes aware that the disease is chronic and incurable. The anxiety then generalizes to concerns about establishing relationships and that sexual gratification, marriage, and normal reproduction might not be possible. There is diminished self-esteem, social isolation, anxiety, and reluctance to initiate close relationships. Sexual drive persists, but there is a fear of initiating sexual relationships and an inhibition of sexual expression. These emotional problems appear to be worse in women than in men. A minority of patients experience deepening of depression with each recurrence, and all aspects of their lives are affected, including job performance. Recurrent disease can now be controlled by daily oral dosing with antiviral drugs such as acyclovir. This drug has significantly improved the quality of life for many herpes victims.[58]

Treatment of genital herpes (Centers for Disease Control and Prevention Guidelines)

Antiviral oral medication and counseling are the mainstays of management. Systemic antiviral drugs partially control symptoms and signs. They do not eradicate latent virus or affect the risk, frequency, or severity of recurrences after the drug is stopped. Topical antiviral drugs offer minimal benefit.

Table 11-1 Genital Herpes Simplex Virus Infection

	Acyclovir 200 mg (Zovirax)	Acyclovir 400 mg (Zovirax)	Acyclovir 800 mg (Zovirax)	Famciclovir (Famvir) 125-, 250-, 500-mg tablets	Valacyclovir (Valtrex) 500, 1000 mg caplets
First episode*	200 mg 5×/d 7-10 d	400 mg tid 7-10 d		250 mg tid 7-10 d	1g bid 7-10 d
Episodic recurrence (intermittent therapy)†	200 mg 5×/d for 5 d	400 mg tid 5 d	800 mg bid 5 d	125 mg bid 5 d	500 mg bid × 3-5 d or 1 gm qd 5 d
Chronic daily suppression		400 mg bid		250 mg bid	<10 episodes/year (500 mg qd) >10 episodes/year (1 gm qd)
Severe disease	Acyclovir 5-10 mg/kg IV every 8 h for 2-7 d or until clinical resolution				
Topical therapy is less effective than systemic drugs					

*Higher doses of medication may be needed in HIV patients.
†Treatment may be extended if healing is incomplete after 10 days of therapy.

Drugs

Three antiviral medications are effective: acyclovir, valacyclovir, and famciclovir. Valacyclovir is a valine ester of acyclovir with enhanced absorption after oral administration. Famciclovir, a prodrug of penciclovir, also has high oral bioavailability. Topical therapy with acyclovir is less effective than the systemic drug, and its use is discouraged. Acyclovir, valacyclovir, and famciclovir reduce the duration of viral shedding, the time to healing, and the development of new lesions. Dosages are listed in Table 11-1.

First clinical episode of genital herpes

Many patients with first-episode herpes present with mild clinical manifestations but severe or prolonged symptoms develop later. Therefore most patients with initial genital herpes should receive antiviral therapy. Counseling regarding the natural history of genital herpes, sexual and perinatal transmission, and methods to reduce such transmission is essential. Five percent to 30% of first-episode cases of genital herpes are caused by HSV-1, but clinical recurrences are much less frequent for HSV-1 than HSV-2 genital infection. Therefore identification of the type of the infecting strain has prognostic importance and may be useful for counseling purposes. Recommended treatment regimens are shown in Table 11-1.

Cool compresses

Extensive erosions on the vulva and penis may be treated with cool water, silver nitrate 0.5%, or Burrow's compresses applied for 20 minutes several times daily. This effective local therapy reduces edema and inflammation, macerates and debrides crust and purulent material, and relieves pain. The legs may be supported with pillows under the knees to expose the inflamed tissues and promote drying.

Counseling

Counseling is an important aspect of management. Although initial counseling can be provided at the first visit, patients benefit from learning about the chronic aspects of the disease after the acute illness subsides. Provide patients with the information in Box 11-2.

Recurrent episodes of herpes simplex virus disease

Most patients with first-episode genital HSV-2 infection will have recurrent episodes. Episodic or suppressive antiviral therapy might shorten the duration of lesions or ameliorate recurrences. Treatment is most effective when started during the prodrome or within 1 day after onset of lesions. Patient-initiated episodic treatment is more effective than provider-initiated therapy in decreasing the healing time in recurrent genital HSV infections. If episodic treatment of recurrences is chosen, the patient should be provided with antiviral therapy or a prescription for the medication, so that treatment can be initiated at the first sign of prodrome or genital lesions.

Daily suppressive therapy

The decision to initiate continuous suppressive therapy is subjective and is based on the frequency and severity of recurrences and psychosocial factors. Continuous daily suppressive therapy significantly reduces, but not completely suppresses, the amount of asymptomatic shedding and clinical outbreaks.[59] Therefore the extent to which suppressive therapy may prevent HSV transmission is unknown. Daily suppressive therapy reduces the frequency of genital herpes recurrences by 75% among patients who have frequent recurrences (i.e., six or more recurrences per year). Safety and efficacy have been documented among patients receiving daily therapy with acyclovir for as long as 6 years, and with valacyclovir and famciclovir for 1 year.

Suppressive therapy has not been associated with emergence of clinically significant acyclovir resistance among immunocompetent patients. After 1 year of continuous suppressive therapy, discontinuation of therapy should be discussed with the patient to assess the patient's psychological adjustment to genital herpes and rate of recurrent episodes, since the frequency of recurrences decreases over time in many patients. Patients with a history of less than 10 recurrences per year are effectively managed with 500 mg of valacyclovir once daily. One gram of valacyclovir once daily or 400 mg of acyclovir twice daily are more effective in patients with greater than 10 recurrences per year. Once-daily regimens offer a useful option for patients who require suppressive therapy for management of genital herpes.[60]

Box 11-2 Counseling Patients With Genital Herpes

- Explain the natural history of the disease, with emphasis on the potential for recurrent episodes, asymptomatic viral shedding, and sexual transmission.

- Abstain from sexual activity when lesions or prodromal symptoms are present and inform their sex partners that they have genital herpes. The use of condoms during all sexual exposures with new or uninfected sex partners should be encouraged.

- Sexual transmission of HSV can occur during asymptomatic periods. Asymptomatic viral shedding occurs more frequently in patients who have genital HSV-2 infection than HSV-1 infection and in patients who have had genital herpes for <12 months.

- Childbearing-aged women who have genital herpes should inform health-care providers who care for them during pregnancy about the HSV infection.

- Episodic antiviral therapy during recurrent episodes might shorten the duration of lesions.

- Suppressive antiviral therapy can ameliorate or prevent recurrent outbreaks and prevent asymptomatic transmission.

Lubrication

Occlusive ointments such as petroleum jelly should not be applied to eroded lesions. Light lubricating body lotions are soothing when inflammation subsides and tissues become dry.

Women with multiple eroded lesions on the labia experience great discomfort while urinating. Pain can be avoided by sitting in a bathtub of water and urinating while holding the labia apart.

Genital herpes simplex during pregnancy

Most mothers of infants who acquire neonatal herpes lack histories of clinically evident genital herpes. Many neonatal infections result from asymptomatic cervical shedding of virus after a primary episode of genital HSV in the third trimester. The risk for transmission to the neonate from an infected mother is high (30% to 50%) among women who acquire genital herpes near the time of delivery and is low (<1%) among women with histories of recurrent herpes at term or who acquire genital HSV during the first half of pregnancy. However, because recurrent genital herpes is much more common than initial HSV infection during pregnancy, the proportion of neonatal HSV infections acquired from mothers with recurrent herpes remains high. Prevention of neonatal herpes depends both on preventing acquisition of genital HSV infection during late pregnancy and avoiding exposure of the infant to herpetic lesions during delivery.

Pregnancy complications

The acquisition of genital herpes during pregnancy has been associated with spontaneous abortion, prematurity, and congenital and neonatal herpes.[61] Two percent or more of susceptible women acquire HSV infection during pregnancy. Acquisition of infection with seroconversion completed before labor was not associated with an increase in neonatal morbidity or with any cases of congenital herpes infection, but infection acquired shortly before labor is associated with neonatal herpes and perinatal morbidity.[62]

Prenatal screening and management

Most newborns acquire their infection by contact with infected genital secretions during delivery from an asymptomatic mother who acquired a first episode of genital herpes near the time of labor. The majority of cases of first episode genital herpes during pregnancy are unrecognized. Some experts recommend HSV serologic testing for HSV-1 and HSV-2 at the first prenatal visit.[63] This would identify patients already infected and those at risk for acquiring genital herpes. Pregnant women who are not infected with HSV-2 are advised to avoid intercourse during the third trimester with men who have genital herpes. Pregnant women who are not infected with HSV-1 should be counseled to avoid genital exposure to HSV-1 during the third trimester (e.g., cunnilingus with a partner with oral herpes and vaginal intercourse with a partner with genital HSV-1 infection). Antiviral prophylaxis with acyclovir may be considered in late pregnancy for women with a known history of genital herpes.[64]

Prevention

Prevention of neonatal herpes should emphasize prevention of acquisition of genital HSV infection during late pregnancy. Susceptible women whose partners have oral or genital HSV infection, or those whose sex partners' infection status is unknown, should be counseled to avoid unprotected genital and oral sexual contact during late pregnancy or take suppressive therapy with an oral antiviral (see Box 11-2).

Antiviral therapy

The safety of systemic acyclovir and valacyclovir therapy in pregnant women has not been established. Current findings do not indicate an increased risk for major birth defects after acyclovir treatment. The first clinical episode of genital herpes during pregnancy may be treated with oral acyclovir. Acyclovir treatment near term might reduce the rate of abdominal deliveries among women who have frequently recurring or newly acquired genital herpes by decreasing the incidence of active lesions. Routine administration of acyclovir to pregnant women who have a history of recurrent genital herpes is not recommended by most clinicians.

Viral cultures

The results of viral cultures during pregnancy do not predict viral shedding at the time of delivery, and such cultures are not indicated routinely.

Management at labor

At the onset of labor, all women should be examined and carefully questioned regarding whether they have symptoms of genital herpes. Infants of women who do not have symptoms or signs of genital herpes infection or its prodrome may be delivered vaginally. A study does not support the policy of cesarean section in case of maternal recurrent herpes simplex infection at delivery.[65] If a woman experiences her first attack of genital HSV infection around the time of delivery, the risk that her neonate will acquire an HSV infection is high. In this circumstance a cesarean delivery is probably prudent. Cesarean section, where the amniotic membranes are intact or have been ruptured for less than 4 hours, is recommended for those women who have clinical evidence of active herpes lesions on the cervix or vulva at the time of labor.[66]

Abdominal delivery does not completely eliminate the risk for HSV infection in the neonate. Infants exposed to HSV during birth, as proven by virus isolation or presumed by observation of lesions, should be observed carefully. Some authorities recommend that such infants undergo surveillance cultures of mucosal surfaces to detect HSV infection before development of clinical signs. Available data do not support the routine use of acyclovir for asymptomatic infants exposed during birth through an infected birth canal, because the risk for infection in most infants is low. However, infants born to women who acquired genital herpes near term are at high risk for neonatal herpes, and some experts recommend acyclovir therapy for these infants. Such pregnancies and newborns should be managed in consultation with an expert. All infants who have evidence of neonatal herpes should be promptly evaluated and treated with systemic acyclovir.

Neonatal herpes simplex virus infection

Neonatal infection is serious but rare. Approximately half the infected babies are born prematurely, which raises the question of whether reactivation can trigger early onset of labor. The mortality rate is approximately 50% in the absence of therapy, and many survivors have ocular or neurologic complications. Most infected neonates are exposed to the virus during vaginal delivery, but infection may occur in utero, by transplacental or ascending infection, or postnatally from relatives or attendants. Many of the infections result from asymptomatic cervical shedding of virus after a primary episode of genital HSV in the third trimester. Herpes simplex virus–positive papules may be present on the skin at birth. Infants born to women who have an active primary HSV infection have a risk of approximately 50% of acquiring an infection.[67]

Clinical signs

The diagnosis of neonatal HSV should be suspected in any newborn with irritability, lethargy, fever, or poor feeding at 1 week of age. Clinical signs of infection in the neonate are usually present between 1 and 7 days of life. Neonatal infections are clinically categorized according to the extent of the disease. They are: (1) skin, eye and mouth (17%) (SEM) infections; (2) CNS infection (32%) (encephalitis)—neonatal encephalitis can include SEM infections; and (3) disseminated infection (39%) involving several organs, causing hepatitis, pneumonitis, intravascular coagulopathy, or encephalitis. The CNS may also be involved in disseminated infections.[66,68] A significant minority of patients do not have skin vesicles at presentation, and vesicles do not develop during the acute HSV disease.

Progression to systemic infection from isolated skin vesicles can occur in a matter of days. The mean age at diagnosis is 12.8 days, but at the time of diagnosis these infants have had symptoms for an average of 5 days. This delay in diagnosis puts the infant at great risk of internal disease, which is preventable with antiviral therapy if treatment is started when only skin disease is present. The infection can be limited to the skin, eyes, or mouth, or can affect the CNS or visceral organs.

Diagnosis

Diagnosis is made by culturing the blood; cerebrospinal fluid; urine; and fluid from eyes, nose, and mucous membranes. Herpes simplex virus was detected most early and frequently in pharyngeal swabs (in one third on postnatal days 2 to 5).

Prognosis

A large collaborative study showed no deaths among infants with localized HSV infection. The mortality rate was 57% in neonates with disseminated infection and 15% in neonates with encephalitis. Therefore the most important predictor of death is visceral involvement. The risk of death was increased in neonates who were in or near coma, had disseminated intravascular coagulopathy, or were premature. In babies with disseminated disease, HSV pneumonitis was associated with greater mortality. In the survivors, morbidity was most frequent in infants with encephalitis, disseminated infection, seizures, or infection with HSV type 2. With HSV infection limited to the skin, eyes, or mouth, the presence of three or more recurrences of vesicles was associated with an increased risk of neurologic impairment as compared with two or fewer recurrences.[69] Death is unusual when disease is limited to the skin but occurs in 15% to 50% of cases of brain and disseminated disease, even with antiviral therapy. Despite antiviral therapy, there is evidence of impairment in approximately 10% of children and debility in more than 50% with CNS and visceral disease.

Treatment

Early institution of antiviral therapy is crucial to the outcome of the disease.[68]

The early identification of skin lesions is critical for the outcome of infections that originate in the skin. Ninety percent of infants with initial herpetic skin lesions treated with acyclovir 30 mg/kg/day had no sequelae.[70]

All infants who have evidence of neonatal herpes should be promptly treated with systemic acyclovir. The recommended regimen for infants treated for known or suspected neonatal herpes is acyclovir 20 mg/kg body weight intravenously every 8 hours for 21 days for disseminated and CNS disease, or 14 days for disease limited to the skin and mucous membranes.[71]

Acquired Immunodeficiency Syndrome

Acquired immunodeficiency syndrome (AIDS) is the end stage of HIV infection. The infection causes a profound defect in cell-mediated immunity, which causes complicating opportunistic infections and neoplastic processes. The initial event is a symptomatic or an asymptomatic HIV infection. The infection may then not be apparent for months or years. In an undetermined number of patients, symptoms emerge and the disease progresses to AIDS. Internal infections are the major cause of death. Infections can be controlled but are rarely curable. Most result from reactivation of previously acquired organisms. Concurrent or consecutive infections with a different organism are common. Infections are severe and commonly disseminated.

Human immunodeficiency virus pathogenesis

HIV is a retrovirus. Retroviruses carry a positive-stranded ribonucleic acid (RNA) and use a dexoyribonucleic acid (DNA) polymerase enzyme called reverse transcriptase to convert viral RNA to DNA. This reverses the usual process of transcription whereby DNA is converted to RNA, thus the term *retrovirus*. HIV attaches to a protein receptor site (CD4) on the surface of CD4+ lymphocytes, penetrates the cell, and exposes its RNA core; then reverse transcriptase converts viral RNA to DNA, which becomes part of the host genome. New viral particles are then produced during normal cellular division and CD4+ lymphocytes are destroyed. A repetitive cycle of immune activation, and partial clearing of the virus, and reinfection of immune cells by replicating virus occurs. Every component of the immune system attempts to stop the disease but fails. Components of the immune system wear down or are destroyed, leading to severe immunosuppression and progression of HIV disease to AIDS and death. The immune system produces cytokines that have an inflammatory effect that promotes spread of HIV infection and penetrance of HIV into several types of cells.

CD4+ T-lymphocyte destruction leads to infection

HIV selectively attacks helper/inducer CD4+ T lymphocytes, decreases their number, and interferes with their function. CD4+ T lymphocytes are responsible for modulation of essentially the entire immune response. Lymphopenia occurs because of the reduced numbers of CD4+ T lymphocytes. Infections normally controlled by cellular immunity occur with markedly increased frequency.

The initial human immunodeficiency virus infection

The incubation period is unknown but has been estimated to be 3 to 6 weeks. An acute mononucleosis-like syndrome develops in 50% to 70% of patients approximately 3 to 6 weeks after initial infection. There is fever, myalgia-arthralgias, pharyngitis, and a diffuse red eruption[72] consisting of macules 0.5 to 2.0 cm in diameter.[73] The symptoms resolve spontaneously within 8 to 12 days. Seroconversion may take place within 1 week to 3 months, and then there is a dramatic decline in viremia. The CD4+ cells remain at a normal level of more than 500/mm³, and the patient is without symptoms. After the initial infection viremia may persist for life.

The evolution of disease

After primary infection, viral dissemination, and the appearance of HIV-specific immunity, most patients have a period of "clinical latency" that lasts for years (Figure 11-19). The clinical presentation of patients with HIV infections ranges from asymptomatic, through chronic generalized lymphadenopathy, to subclinical and clinical T-cell deficiency. There is strong association between the development of life-threatening opportunistic illnesses and the absolute number of CD4+ T lymphocytes. As the number of CD4+ T lymphocytes decreases, the risk and severity of opportunistic illnesses increase. The revised Centers for Disease Control and Prevention classification system for HIV infection categorizes persons on the basis of clinical conditions associated with HIV infection and CD4+ T-lymphocyte counts. Measures of CD4+ T lymphocytes are used to guide clinical and therapeutic management.

Progression to acquired immunodeficiency syndrome

Patients have a number of symptoms during disease progression. They exhibit prolonged constitutional symptoms such as chronic fatigue, night sweats, fever, weight loss, and diarrhea. They frequently have clinical manifestations of T-cell dysfunction such as mucous membrane disease (oral candidiasis, hairy leukoplakia) and dermatologic diseases (herpes simplex/zoster, fungal infections).

AIDS is the end stage of HIV infection. It is characterized by a variety of unusual tumors and opportunistic infections. There appears to be a spectrum of disease, and long-term survival with new drug regimens may be possible.

Diagnosis

In adults, the diagnosis is made with serologic tests (ELISA) and confirmed with the Western blot antibody test. These tests are then repeated to confirm the diagnosis. Virologic tests (p24 antigen, DNA tests, HIV cultures) may be ordered to confirm the diagnosis. HIV RNA polymerase chain reaction (PCR) test is used to measure viral burden.

Viral burden

The onset of infection, the initial immune response, and the long-term prognosis of the disease can be monitored by determining the viral burden. This is measured with PCR tests for HIV RNA. HIV RNA increases soon after infection in adults, declines within 3 weeks because of an immune response, and adjusts to a viral set point, which is predictive of outcome. Patients with a high viral set point experience early onset of AIDS and death, those with a low viral set point live longer with relatively asymptomatic disease.

Assessment of immune status (CD4+ T-cell determinations)

The pathogenesis of AIDS is attributable to the decrease in T lymphocytes that bear the CD4 receptor. The degree of immunosuppression is indicated by the T-helper (CD4+) lymphocyte count. Measures of CD4+ T lymphocytes (CD4+ T-cells) are essential to the assessment of the immune system of HIV-infected persons. Progressive depletion of CD4+ T lymphocytes is associated with an increased likelihood of clinical complications.[74] CD4+ T-cell levels are monitored every 3 to 6 months in all HIV-infected persons.

The measurement of CD4+ T-cell levels is used to establish decision points for initiating antiviral therapy, determining prophylaxis for opportunistic infections, and monitoring the efficacy of treatment.

Revised Centers for Disease Control and Prevention classification and management

The revised Centers for Disease Control and Prevention classification system (1993) for HIV-infected adolescents and adults is primarily intended for use in public health practice. It categorizes persons on the basis of clinical conditions associated with HIV infection and CD4+ T-lymphocyte counts. The system is based on three ranges of CD4+ T-lymphocyte counts and three clinical categories of conditions associated with HIV infection and is represented by a matrix of nine mutually exclusive categories. The three CD4+ T-lymphocyte categories are defined as follows:

- Category 1: greater than 500 cells/mL
- Category 2: 200 to 499 cells/mL
- Category 3: less than 200 cells/mL

Antimicrobial prophylaxis and antiretroviral therapies have been shown to be most effective within certain levels of immune dysfunction. Therefore CD4+ T-lymphocyte determinations are an integral part of medical management of HIV-infected persons.

Figure 11-19
AIDS. Evolution of the disease.

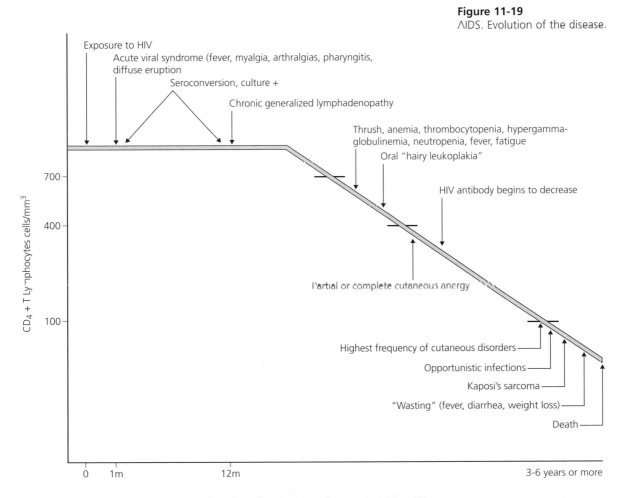

Note: The natural history of HIV infection is highly variable.
This chart shows approximate relationships of signs and symptoms.

Table 11-2 Frequency and Percentage of Patients Presenting with Specific Skin Disorders in a Population of 528 Patients Infected with HIV		
Presenting diagnosis	**No.**	**%**
Pruritic papular eruption	60	11.4
Herpes simplex	57	10.8
Kaposi's sarcoma	45	8.5
Molluscum contagiosum	43	8.1
Condyloma acuminatum	42	8.0
Seborrheic dermatitis	39	7.4
Drug eruption	33	6.3
Xerosis	28	5.3
Eosinophilic folliculitis	21	4.0
Tinea	19	3.6
Verruca vulgaris	18	3.4
Scabies	17	3.2
Bacterial cellulitis	15	2.8
Syphilis	12	2.3
Psoriasis	12	2.3
Zoster	11	2.1
Nonmelanoma skin cancer	10	1.9

Adapted from Goldstein B, Berman B, Sukenik E, Frankel SJ: J Am Acad Dermatol 1997; 36:262.

Incidence

The incidence, severity and number[82] of skin disorders increase as immune function deteriorates (Tables 11-2 and 11-3). The number of mucocutaneous diseases, like the CD4+ count, is an indicator of the status of the immune system and the prognosis. Cutaneous disorders found to correlate with CD4 cell counts are shown in the Figure 11-20. Herpes zoster and drug reactions correlated with a higher CD4 cell count (424/mm³ and 301/mm³, respectively), whereas the other seven disorders correlated with a more advanced degree of immunosuppression with CD4 counts less than 75/mm³. Therefore, in the majority of patients infected with HIV, cutaneous manifestations may reflect the underlying degree of immunosuppression.

Dermatologic diseases associated with human immunodeficiency virus infection

Disorders of the skin and mucous membranes occur throughout the course of HIV infection, affecting more than 90% of patients at some time.[75-80] Cutaneous disease may be the initial or only problem for much of the course of the HIV infection and may be the most debilitating element of the patient's condition. Serious opportunistic infections may present for the first time in the skin. Skin disorders in patients with HIV may look unusual and may not be accurately diagnosed. Response to treatment may be poorer than expected.[81]

Complete lists of diseases and treatments are found in Tables 11-2 and 11-3. Illustrations of these diseases are found in Figures 11-21 to 11-36. The most common skin disorders in HIV disease are caused by infections.

The frequency and percentage of patients presenting with specific skin disorders in a population of 528 patients infected with HIV is shown in Table 11-2.

Figure 11-20 Correlation of mean CD4 cells/mm³ and incidence of specific skin disorders in 528 patients with HIV infection and a CD4 cell count within 3 weeks of presentation. *(From Goldstein B, Berman B, Sukenik E, Frankel SJ: J Am Acad Dermatol 1997; 36:262.)*

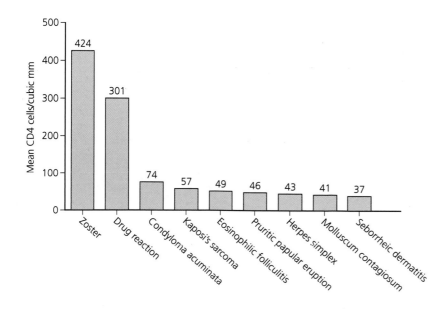

Table 11-3 HIV Infection—Cutaneous Manifestations

Disease	Clinical manifestations	Diagnosis	Treatment
VIRAL INFECTIONS			
Acute HIV exanthema (HIV primary infection)	Fever, myalgias, urticaria Truncal maculopapular eruption Mononucleosis-like syndrome Generalized lymphadenopathy follows later	Time to seroconversion unknown Antibodies found 3 wk to 6 mo after initial infection Low white blood cell count, thrombocytopenia, hyper-gammaglobulinemia	Antiretroviral drugs
Herpes simplex (common)	Persistent erosions and ulcerations Widely disseminated Resembles other infections Intractable perirectal ulcerations Regional lymphadenopathy	HSV culture Tzanck smear for multinucle-ated giant cells HSV-2 infection is risk factor for subsequent or concur-rent HIV infection[79]	Acyclovir, valacyclovir or famciclovir Acyclovir or penciclovir (Denavir) ointment Foscarnet
Herpes zoster Shingles (common sign of AIDS)	Shingles may be severe, re-sulting in deep scarring Persistent disseminated lesions Intractable herpetic pain	Herpes virus culture Tzanck smear for multinucle-ated giant cells	Acyclovir, valacyclovir or famciclovir
Chicken pox (uncommon)	Chicken pox with numerous lesions and pneumonia		Same treatment as for herpes zoster
Molluscum contagiosum	Clusters of white umbili-cated papules Persistent on face, groin Cutaneous cryptococcus[83,84] can mimic molluscum contagiosum	KOH preparations of soft ma-terial in center of lesion show large viral inclusions Biopsy—large viral inclusions	Cryosurgery, curettage Scissor excision with blunt-tipped scissors Trichloroacetic acid peels for ex-tensive cases[36] Imiquimod cream (Aldara)
Warts/condyloma (common) Human papillomavirus (HPV)	Common warts—extensive[82] and persistent Condylomas—increased prevalence, number, size Cervical, anal squamous cell carcinoma (HPV-16,18)	Biopsy or clinical appearance Profound reduction in CD4+ cells	Cryosurgery, blunt dissection, ex-cision, surgery Imiquimod cream (Aldara) Podophyllotoxin (Condylox)
Hairy leukoplakia (Epstein-Barr virus) (common)	Whitish, nonremovable ver-rucous hairy plaques on sides of tongue May resemble fungal tongue infections	Biopsy—acanthosis and parak-eratosis with large pale-staining cells with pyknotic nuclei	Treating oral *Candida* improves appearance Podophyllin resin 25% in ethanol and acetone
FUNGAL INFECTIONS			
Candida albicans (very common)	White plaques on cheeks, tongue Sore throat, dysphagia Deep tongue erosions, thick plaques back of throat Esophageal infection Intractable vaginal infection *Candida* nail infection	Culture Obtain specimen for KOH slide preparation with cotton swab	Nystatin oral suspension Clotrimazole (Mycelex Troche) 10 mg 5×/daily Ketoconazole (200 mg PO qd) Fluconazole 100-200 mg PO qd Amphotericin B (severe cases) 0.3 mg/kg IV qd
Tinea versicolor (common)	Common early and late in HIV infection Thick, scaly hypopigmented or light-brown plaques on trunk	KOH slide preparation shows numerous short hyphae and spores Wood's light accentuates lesions	Oral: fluconazole, itraconazole, ketoconazole (various dosages)

Continued

Table 11-3 HIV Infection—Cutaneous Manifestations—cont'd

Disease	Clinical manifestations	Diagnosis	Treatment
FUNGAL INFECTIONS—cont'd			

Dermatophytes
  Tinea corporis
  Tinea pedis
  Tinea cruris
  Onychomycoses
    (common)
	Extensive involvement, especially groin and feet
	Thick keratoderma—blennorrhagic-like lesions on feet
	Proximal subungual onychomycosis
		KOH slide preparation shows branched, septated hyphae	Dosage schedules
			  See Table 13-2, page 437

Cryptococcus neoformans (rare)	White papules that resemble molluscum contagiosum	Assays for antigen in serum or cerebrospinal fluid India ink or Wright stain Culture Biopsy	Amphotericin B 0.5-0.6 mg/kg IV qd or add flucytosine Itraconazole 200 mg PO bid Fluconazole 200-400 mg PO qd
Histoplasma capsulatum (rare)	Multiple papules, nodules, macules and oral and skin ulcers on arms, face, trunk Travel history (South America)	Biopsy—PAS stain Crushed tissue preparation—rapid diagnosis Culture—several weeks required	Amphotericin B 0.5-0.6 mg/kg IV qd Itraconazole 200 mg PO bid
Penicillium marneffei (Southeast Asia)	Fever, anemia, weight loss, molluscum-like papules, cough, lymphadenopathy, Hepatomegaly	Culture—skin, blood, bone marrow Skin touch prep Yeast forms with central septae	Amphotericin B, oral imidazoles, lifelong prophylaxis to prevent recurrence
BACTERIAL INFECTIONS			
Staphylococcus aureus (common)	Bullous impetigo—axillae or groin Facial or truncal folliculitis (resembling acne) Impetigo of beard and body	Culture	Dicloxacillin Cefadroxil (many others)
Syphilis (uncommon)	Generalized papulosquamous papules and plaques Can mimic almost any inflammatory cutaneous disorder Incubation period for neurosyphilis may be very brief (months)	VDRL titer may be very high or negative; obtain sequential tests or skin biopsy with special stains	Standard recommended treatment may not be sufficient to prevent central nervous system disease. See Chapter 10
ARTHROPOD			
Scabies (uncommon)	Generalized crusted papules Norwegian scabies—generalized hyperkeratotic eruption	KOH or oil preparation shows mites	Lindane (Kwell) Premethrin (Elimite)
PROLIFERATIVE DISORDERS			
Seborrheic dermatitis (common)	Red scaling plaques with yellowish, greasy scales and crust Distinct margins, hypopigmentation of scalp, face; sometimes groin, extremities Severity correlates with degree of clinical deterioration	Biopsy differs from ordinary seborrheic dermatitis Parakeratosis is widespread Necrotic keratinocytes Dermoepidermal obliteration by lymphocytes Sparse spongiosis Thick-walled vessels Do KOH to rule out tinea	Ketoconazole cream Loprox gel
Psoriasis (uncommon)	Activation of previous disease or no history	Biopsy	Treatment-resistant cases may respond to acitretin or antiretroviral drugs Calcipotriol ointment (Dovonex)

Table 11-3 HIV Infection—Cutaneous Manifestations—cont'd

Disease	Clinical manifestations	Diagnosis	Treatment
PROLIFERATIVE DISORDERS—cont'd			
Xeroderma (common) Ichthyosis (uncommon)	Severe dry skin may be associated with erythroderma, seborrheic dermatitis, and dementia Ichthyosiform scaling of legs, keratoderma of palms and soles	Clinical presentation	Lactic acid emollients (Lac-Hydrin)
Pruritic papular eruption (common)	2-5 mm skin-colored papules on head, neck, upper trunk Pruritus and number of papules may wax and wane with time	Biopsy—lymphocytic perivascular infiltrate with numerous eosinophils Follicular damage	Ultraviolet B phototherapy[85,86] Often resistant to topical steroids and oral antihistamines Antipruritic lotions (Sarna) Dapsone 100 mg qd possibly effective
Eosinophilic pustular folliculitis (rare)	Groups of small vesicles and pustules becoming confluent to form irregular pustular lakes and erosions Polycyclic plaques with central hyperpigmentation Severe, intractable pruritus Chronic and persistent Many nonfollicular lesions	Biopsy is diagnostic Eosinophils that invade sebaceous glands and outer root sheaths of hair follicles Moderate eosinophilia and leukocytosis (50%) CD4 counts <250-300 cells/mm³	Permethrin cream (Elimite) qd until lesions clear Ultraviolet B phototherapy Antihistamines Group I topical steroids Itraconazole 100-400 mg/day Dapsone 100 mg qd possibly effective Metronidazole[87] Acitretin[88]
VASCULAR DISORDERS			
Telangiectasias of anterior chest wall (uncommon)	Linear telangiectasia in broad, crescent distribution across the chest[89] Associated with erythema in the same distribution	Biopsy shows dilated blood vessels with perivascular small cell infiltrate No endothelial proliferation	None
Bacillary (epithelioid) angiomatosis (rare)	Solitary or multiple dome-shaped friable, bright-red granulation tissue-like papules and subcutaneous nodules (1 mm-2 cm)[90] of face, trunk, extremities Visceral angiomatosis Cat bite or scratch[91]	Biopsy—proliferation of small blood vessels lined with plump endothelial cells projecting into lumen *Rochalimaea* bacilli seen with Warthin-Starry silver stain	Ciprofloxacin, trimethoprim-sulfamethoxazole, doxycycline, azithromycin, erythromycin, rifampin and gentamycin
Thrombocytopenic purpura (common)	Petechia	Complete blood count	
NEOPLASTIC DISORDERS			
Kaposi's sarcoma	Pale to deep violaceous, thin, oval plaques Long axis of lesions aligned with skin tension lines Many unusual presentations Numbers vary from few to numerous lesions Any skin surface and mouth, usually palate Visceral lesions Lesions induced by trauma	Biopsy Proliferation of small vessels Proliferation of bundles of interweaving plump spindle cells Slitlike intercellular spaces with extravasated red blood cells	Radiation for individual lesions Intralesional vinblastine (0.1 to 0.5 mg/mL every 4 wks) Liquid nitrogen cryotherapy (keep blister covered to prevent exposure of others to HIV) Many others
MISCELLANEOUS			
Cutaneous drug reactions	Morbilliform eruptions predominate Urticaria Much greater incidence than general population	Trimethoprim-sulfamethoxazole Dapsone Aminopenicillins	Stop drug if possible

Continued

Table 11-3 HIV Infection—Cutaneous Manifestations—cont'd

Disease	Clinical manifestations	Diagnosis	Treatment
MISCELLANEOUS—cont'd			
Pruritus (uncommon)	Intractable pruritus without internal malignancy May be presenting symptom of AIDS	Numerous excoriations Rule out other causes of pruritus (e.g., renal, thyroid, hepatic dysfunction; drugs; malignancy; diabetes; iron deficiency anemia)	Emollients, topical steroids, and prednisone are not effective
Yellow nails	Yellow discoloration of nail plate Many associated with *Pneumocystis carinii* pneumonia	Differentiate from yellow nail syndrome: yellow nail plate + absent cuticles + diminished growth rate + transverse overcurvature of nail plate + subungual hyperkeratosis	Treat possible aggravating conditions (e.g., *P. carinii* pneumonia)
Dark-blue nails	Darkened bluish appearance at bases of fingernails (black patients > white patients)	Recent history of zidovudine treatment	None
Vitiligo (uncommon) Premature graying of hair (common)	Loss of pigmentation of hair and skin usually follows other AIDS signs and symptoms	Physical examination	None

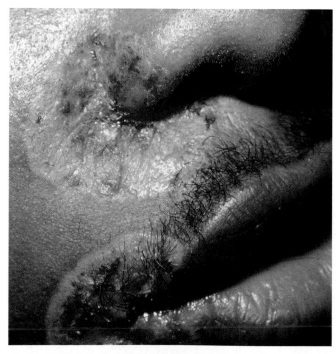

Figure 11-21 Herpes simplex. Erosive. *(Courtesy Neal S. Penneys, M.D., Ph.D.)*

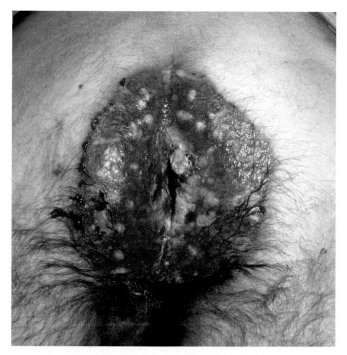

Figure 11-22 Herpes simplex. Erosive. *(Courtesy Benjamin K. Fisher, M.D.)*

CUTANEOUS MANIFESTATIONS OF HIV

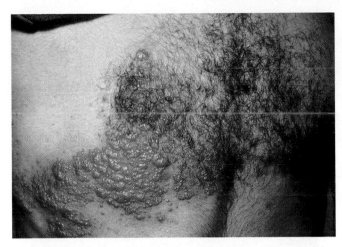

Figure 11-23 Herpes zoster. *(Courtesy Benjamin K. Fisher, M.D.)*

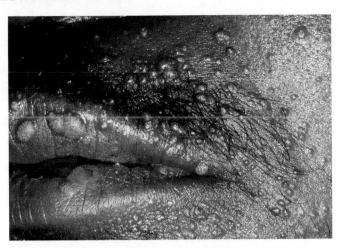

Figure 11-24 Molluscum contagiosum. *(From Redfield RR, James WD, Wright DC: J Am Acad Dermatol 13:821, 1985.)*

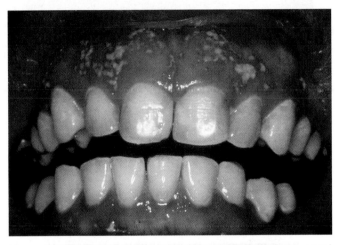

Figure 11-25 Candida albicans. *(Courtesy William D. James, M.D.)*

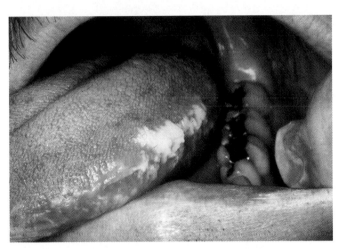

Figure 11-26 Hairy leukoplakia. *(Courtesy Deborah S. Greenspan.)*

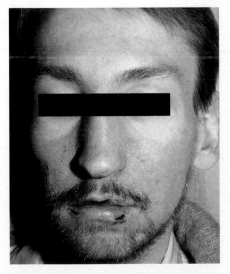

Figure 11-27 Seborrheic dermatitis. *(Courtesy Benjamin K. Fisher, M.D.)*

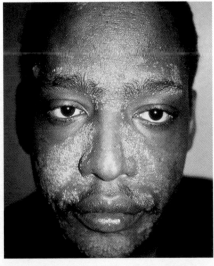

Figure 11-28 Seborrheic dermatitis. *(Courtesy William D. James, M.D.)*

CUTANEOUS MANIFESTATIONS OF HIV

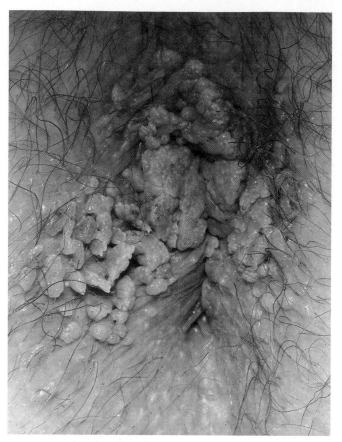

Figure 11-29 Anal warts.

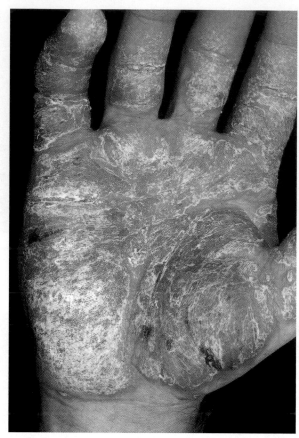

Figure 11-30 Psoriasis. *(Courtesy William D. James, M.D.)*

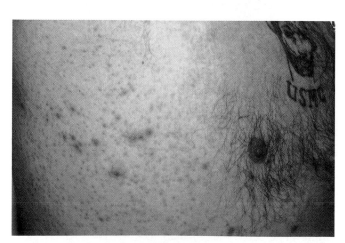

Figure 11-31 Papular eruption. *(Courtesy David Goodman, M.D.)*

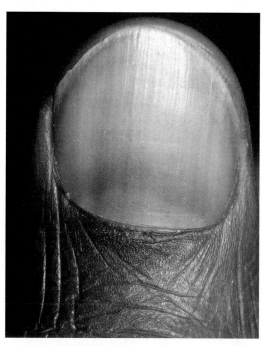

Figure 11-32 Dark-blue nails (after treatment with zidovudine). *(Courtesy William D. James, M.D.)*

KAPOSI'S SARCOMA IN HIV PATIENTS

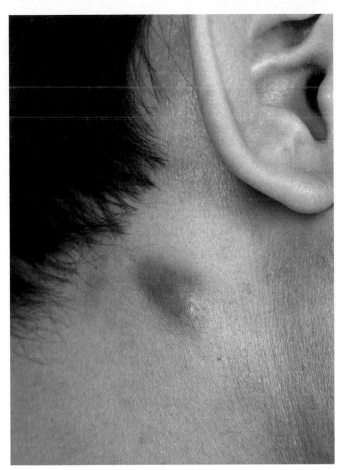

Figure 11-33 Kaposi's sarcoma. *(Courtesy H.J. Hulsebosch, M.D.)*

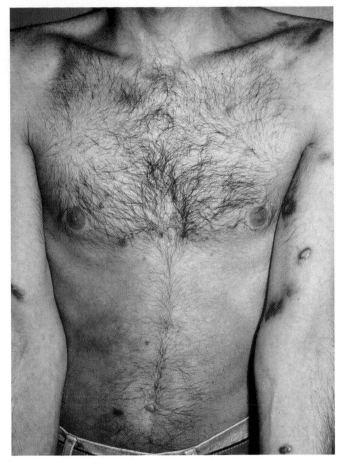

Figure 11-34 Kaposi's sarcoma. *(Courtesy Benjamin K. Fisher, M.D.)*

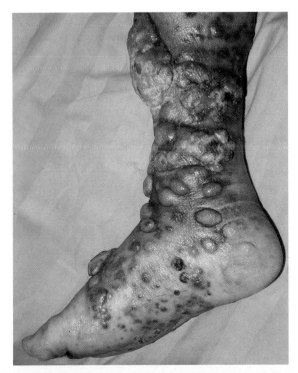

Figure 11-35 Kaposi's sarcoma. *(Courtesy Benjamin K. Fisher, M.D.)*

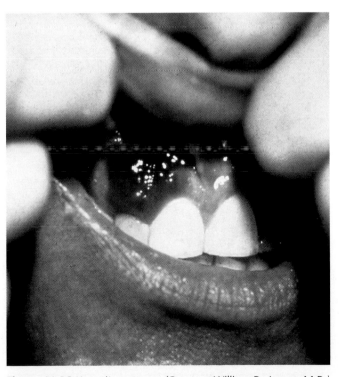

Figure 11-36 Kaposi's sarcoma. *(Courtesy William D. James, M.D.)*

References

1. Ferenczy A, et al: Latent papillomavirus and recurring genital warts, N Engl J Med 1985; 313:784.

2. Rosenberg SK: Subclinical papilloma viral infection of male genitalia, Urology 1985; 26:554.

3. Panici PB, et al: Oral condyloma lesions in patients with extensive genital human papillomavirus infection, Am J Obstet Gynecol 1992; 167:451.

4. American Academy of Dermatology Task Force on Pediatric Dermatology: Genital warts and sexual abuse in children, J Am Acad Dermatol 1984; 11:529.

5. Cohen BA, Honing P, Androphy E: Anogenital warts in children, Arch Dermatol 1990; 126:1575.

6. Obalek S, et al: Condylomata acuminata in children: frequent association with human papillomaviruses responsible for cutaneous warts, J Am Acad Dermatol 1990; 23:205.

7. Reeves WC, et al: Human papillomavirus infection and cervical cancer in Latin America, N Engl J Med 1989; 320:1437.

8. Von K, G. Syrjanen SM, Syrjanen KJ: Advantage of human papillomavirus typing in the clinical evaluation of genitoanal warts, J Am Acad Dermatol 1988; 18:495.

9. Macnab JCM, et al: Human papillomavirus in clinically and histologically normal tissue of patients with genital cancer, N Engl J Med 1986; 315:1052.

10. Barrasso R, et al: High prevalence of papillomavirus-associated penile intraepithelial neoplasia in sexual partners of women with cervical intraepithelial neoplasia, N Engl J Med 1987; 317:916.

11. Daling JR, et al: Sexual practices, sexually transmitted diseases, and the incidence of anal cancer, N Engl J Med 1987; 317:973.

12. Castellsague X, et al: Male circumcision, penile human papillomavirus infection, and cervical cancer in female partners, N Engl J Med 2002; 346(15):1105.

13. Krebs H-B, Helmkamp BF: Treatment failure of genital condylomata acuminata in women: role of the male sexual partner, Am J Obstet Gynecol 1991; 165:337.

14. Allen A, Siegfried E: The natural history of condyloma in children, J Am Acad Dermatol 1998; 39(6):951.

15. Matsunaga J, Bergman A, Bhatia NN: Genital condylomata acuminata in pregnancy: effectiveness, safety and pregnancy outcome following cryotherapy, Br J Obstet Gynaecol 1987; 94:168.

16. Bonnez W, et al: Therapeutic efficacy and complications of excisional biopsy of condyloma acuminatum, Sex Transm Dis 1996; 23(4):273.

17. Robinson JK: Extirpation by electrocautery of massive lesions of condyloma acuminatum in genito-perineo-anal region, J Dermatol Surg Oncol 1980; 6:733.

18. Schwartz DB, et al: The management of genital condylomas in pregnant women, Obstet Gynecol Clin North Am 1987; 14:589.

19. Fisher AA: Severe systemic and local reactions to topical podophyllum resin, Cutis 1981; 28:233.

20. Beutner K, Ferenczy A: Therapeutic approaches to genital warts, Am J Med 1997; 102(5A):28.

21. Beutner K, et al: Genital warts and their treatment, Clin Infect Dis 1999; 28(1):S37.

22. Krebs H-B: Treatment of vaginal condylomata acuminata by weekly topical application of 5-fluorouracil, Obstet Gynecol 1987; 70:68.

23. Krebs H-B: Treatment of genital condylomata with topical 5-fluorouracil, Dermatol Clin 1991; 9:333.

24. Bar-Am A, et al: Treatment of male genital condylomatous lesions by carbon dioxide laser after failure of previous nonlaser methods, J Am Acad Dermatol 1991; 24:87.

25. Tsambaos D, et al: Treatment of condylomata acuminata with oral isotretinoin, J Urol 1997; 158(5):1810.

26. Browder JF, et al: The interferons and their use in condyloma acuminata, Ann Pharmacother 1992; 26:42.

27. Schwartz RA, Janniger CK: Bowenoid papulosis, J Am Acad Dermatol 1991; 24:261.

28. Obalek S, et al: Bowenoid papulosis of the male and female genitalia: risk of cervical neoplasia, J Am Acad Dermatol 1986; 14:433.

29. Rudlinger R: Bowenoid papulosis of the male and female genital tracts: risk of cervical neoplasia, J Am Acad Dermatol 1987; 16:625.

30. Schwartz JJ, Myskowski PL: Molluscum contagiosum in patients with human immunodeficiency virus infection: a review of twenty-seven patients, J Am Acad Dermatol 1992; 27:583.

31. de W-v, der, et al: Treatment of molluscum contagiosum using a lidocaine/prilocaine cream (EMLA) for analgesia, J Am Acad Dermatol 1990; 23:685.

32. Syed T, et al: Treatment of molluscum contagiosum in males with an analog of imiquimod 1% in cream: a placebo-controlled, double-blind study, J Dermatol 1998; 25(5):309.

33. Liota E, et al: Imiquimod therapy for molluscum contagiosum, J Cutan Med Surg 2000; 4(2):76.

34. Barba A, Kapoor S, Berman B: An open label safety study of topical imiquimod 5% cream in the treatment of Molluscum contagiosum in children, Dermatol Online J 2001; 7(1):20.

35. Cunningham B, Paller A, Garzon M: Inefficacy of oral cimetidine for nonatopic children with molluscum contagiosum, Pediatr Dermatol 1998; 15(1):71.

36. Garrett SJ, et al: Trichloroacetic acid peel of molluscum contagiosum in immunocompromised patients, J Dermatol Surg Oncol 1992; 18:855.

37. Fleming D, et al: Herpes simplex virus type 2 in the United States, 1976 to 1994 [see comments], N Engl J Med 1997; 337(16):1105.

38. A W, AG L, K L, et al: Effect of condoms on reducing the transmission of herpes simplex virus type 2 from men to women, JAMA 2001; 285(24):3100.

39. Lafferty WE, et al: Recurrences after oral and genital herpes simplex virus infection: influence of site of infection and viral type, N Engl J Med 1987; 316:1444.

40. Kinghorn G: Limiting the spread of genital herpes, Scand J Infect Dis Suppl 1996; 100:20.

41. Koelle D, et al: Asymptomatic reactivation of herpes simplex virus in women after the first episode of genital herpes, Ann Intern Med 1992; 116(6):433.

42. Schacker T, et al: Frequent recovery of HIV-1 from genital herpes simplex virus lesions in HIV-1-infected men, JAMA 1998; 280(1):61.

43. Severson J, Tyring S: Relation between herpes simplex viruses and human immunodeficiency virus infections, Arch Dermatol 1999; 135(11):1393.

44. Corey L: First-episode, recurrent, and asymptomatic herpes simplex infections, J Am Acad Dermatol 1988; 18:169.

45. Miller RG, et al: Acquisition of concomitant oral and genital infection with herpes simplex virus type 2, Sex Transm Dis 1987; 14:41.

46. Langenberg A, et al: For the Chiron HSV Vaccine Study Group: a prospective study of new infections with herpes simplex virus type 1 and type 2, N Engl J Med 1999; 341(19):1432.

47. Koutsky LA, et al: Underdiagnosis of genital herpes by current clinical and viral-isolation procedures, N Engl J Med 1992; 326:1533.

48. Benedetti J, et al: Recurrence rates in genital herpes after symptomatic first-episode infection, Ann Intern Med 1994; 121:847.

49. Pereira F: Herpes simplex: Evolving concepts [see comments], J Am Acad Dermatol 1996; 35(4):503-520; 521.

50. Benedetti J, Zeh J, Corey L: Clinical reactivation of genital herpes simplex virus infection decreases in frequency over time, Ann Intern Med 1999; 131(1):14.

51. McGowan MP, et al: Prevalence of cytomegalovirus and herpes simplex virus in human semen, Int J Androl 1983; 6:331.

52. Mertz G: Epidemiology of genital herpes infections, Infect Dis Clin North Am 1993; 7(4):825.

53. Wald A, et al: Reactivation of genital herpes simplex virus type 2 infection in asymptomatic seropositive persons, N Engl J Med 2000; 342(12):844.

54. Wald A, et al: Virologic characteristics of subclinical and symptomatic genital herpes infections, N Engl J Med 1995; 333(12):770.

55. Solomon AR: New diagnostic tests for herpes simplex and varicella zoster infections, J Am Acad Dermatol 1988; 18:218.

56. Lafferty W, et al: Herpes simplex virus type 1 as a cause of genital herpes: Impact on surveillance and prevention, J Infect Dis 2000; 181(4):1454.

57. Luby ED, Klinge V: Genital herpes: a pervasive psychosocial disorder, Arch Dermatol 1985; 121:494.

58. Mindel A: Psychological and psychosexual implications of herpes simplex virus infections, Scand J Infect Dis Suppl 1996; 100:27.

59. Wald A, et al: Suppression of subclinical shedding of herpes simplex virus type 2 with acyclovir, Ann Intern Med 1996; 124(1 Pt 1):8.

60. Reitano M, et al., for the International Valacyclovir HSV Study Group: valaciclovir for the suppression of recurrent genital herpes simplex virus infection: a large-scale dose range-finding study, J Infect Dis 1998; 178(3):603.

61. Monif GRG, Kellner KR, Donnelly W, Jr: Congenital herpes simplex type II infection, Am J Obstet Gynecol 1985; 152:1000.

62. Brown Z, et al: The acquisition of herpes simplex virus during pregnancy, N Engl J Med 1997; 337(8):509.

63. Brown Z: HSV-2 specific serology should be offered routinely to antenatal patients, Rev Med Virol 2000; 10(3):141.

64. Braig S, et al: Acyclovir prophylaxis in late pregnancy prevents recurrent genital herpes and viral shedding, Eur J Obstet Gynecol Reprod Biol 2001; 96(1):55.

65. Fonnest G, de IFFI, Weber T: Neonatal herpes in Denmark 1977-1991, Acta Obstet Gynecol Scand 1997; 76(4):355.

66. Kesson A: Management of neonatal herpes simplex virus infection, Paediatr Drugs 2001; 3(2):81.

67. Whitley RJ, et al: Changing presentation of herpes simplex virus infection in neonates, J Infect Dis 1988; 158:109.

68. Kimberlin D, et al: Natural history of neonatal herpes simplex virus infections in the acyclovir era, Pediatrics 2001; 108(2):223.

69. Whitley R, et al: For The National Institute of Allergy and Infectious Diseases Collaborative Antiviral Study Group: predictors of morbidity and mortality in neonates with herpes simplex virus infections, N Engl J Med 1991; 324:450.

70. Arvin AM: Antiviral treatment of herpes simplex infection in neonates and pregnant women, J Am Acad Dermatol 1988; 18:200.

71. Kimberlin D, et al: Safety and efficacy of high-dose intravenous acyclovir in the management of neonatal herpes simplex virus infections, Pediatrics 2001; 108(2):230.

72. Kessler HA, et al: Diagnosis of human immunodeficiency virus infection in seronegative homosexuals presenting with an acute viral syndrome, JAMA 1987; 258:1196.

73. Rustin MHA, et al: The acute exanthem associated with seroconversion to human T-cell lymphotrophic virus III in a homosexual man, J Infect 1986; 12:161.

74. Uthayakumar S, et al: The prevalence of skin disease in HIV infection and its relationship to the degree of immunosuppression [see comments], Br J Dermatol 1997; 137(4):595.

75. Kaplan MH, et al: Dermatologic findings and manifestations of acquired immunodeficiency syndrome (AIDS), J Am Acad Dermatol 1987; 16:485.

76. Coopman SA, et al: Cutaneous disease and drug reactions in HIV infection, N Engl J Med 1993; 328:1670.

77. Matis WL, Triana A, Shapiro R: Dermatologic findings associated with human immunodeficiency virus infection, J Am Acad Dermatol 1987; 17:746.

78. Valle S-L: Dermatologic findings related to human immunodeficiency virus infection in high-risk individuals, J Am Acad Dermatol 1987; 17:951.

79. Penneys NS, Hicks B: Unusual cutaneous lesions associated with acquired immunodeficiency syndrome, J Am Acad Dermatol 1985; 13:845.

80. Samet J, et al: Dermatologic manifestations in HIV-infected patients: a primary care perspective, Mayo Clin Proc 1999; 74(7):658.

81. Porras B, et al: Update on cutaneous manifestations of HIV infection, Med Clin North Am 1998; 82(5):1033.

82. Jensen B, et al: Incidence and prognostic significance of skin disease in patients with HIV/AIDS: a 5-year observational study [In Process Citation], Acta Derm Venereol 2000; 80(2):140.

83. Rico MJ, Penneys NS: Cutaneous cryptococcus resembling molluscum contagiosum in a patient with AIDS, Arch Dermatol 1985; 121:901.

84. Miller SJ: Cutaneous cryptococcus resembling molluscum contagiosum in a patient with acquired immunodeficiency syndrome, Cutis 1988; 41:411.

85. Pardp RJ, et al: UVB phototherapy of the pruritic papular eruption of the acquired immunodeficiency syndrome, J Am Acad Dermatol 1992; 26:423.

86. Meola T, et al: The safety of UVB phototherapy in patients with HIV infection, J Am Acad Dermatol 1993; 29:216.

87. Inaoka M, Hayakawa J, Shiohara T: HIV seronegative eosinophilic pustular folliculitis successfully treated with metronidazole, J Am Acad Dermatol 2002; 46(5 Suppl):S153.

88. Dubost-Brama A, et al: Ofuji's eosinophilic pustular folliculitis: efficacy of acitretin, Ann Dermatol Venereol 1997; 124(8):540.

89. Fallon T, Jr, et al: Telangiectasias of the anterior chest in homosexual men, Ann Intern Med 1986; 105:679.

90. Cockerell CJ, et al: Epithelioid angiomatosis: a distinct vascular disorder in patients with the acquired immunodeficiency syndrome or AIDS-related complex, Lancet 1987; 2:654.

91. Tappero JW, et al: The epidemiology of bacillary angiomatosis and bacillary peliosis, JAMA 1993; 269:770.

Warts, Herpes Simplex, and Other Viral Infections

❏ **Warts**
  Common warts
  Filiform and digitate warts
  Flat warts
  Plantar warts
  Subungual and periungual warts
  Genital warts

❏ **Molluscum contagiosum**

❏ **Herpes simplex**
  Oral-labial herpes simplex
  Cutaneous herpes simplex
  Eczema herpeticum

❏ **Varicella**
  Chickenpox in the immunocompromised
    patient
  Chickenpox and HIV infection
  Chickenpox during pregnancy
  Congenital and neonatal chickenpox

❏ **Herpes zoster**
  Herpes zoster after varicella immunization
  Herpes zoster and HIV infection
  Herpes zoster during pregnancy
  Syndromes
  Prevention of postherpetic neuralgia: early
    combined antiviral drugs and antidepres-
    sants
  Treatment of postherpetic neuralgia

Warts

Warts are benign epidermal neoplasms that are caused by human papilloma viruses (HPVs), which are small DNA viruses. There are more than 100 different types of HPVs, and new types are discovered each year. HPVs infect epithelial cells of the skin, mouth, esophagus, larynx, trachea, and conjunctiva and cause both benign and malignant lesions.[1] They induce a variety of infections (Table 12-1).

Clinical infection

Warts commonly occur in children and young adults, but they may appear at any age. Warts are transmitted simply by touch; it is not unusual to see warts on adjacent toes ("kissing lesions"). Warts commonly appear at sites of trauma, on the hands, in periungual regions as a result of nail biting, and on plantar surfaces. Plantar warts may be acquired from moist surfaces in communal swimming areas. Their course is highly variable; most resolve spontaneously in weeks or months, and others may last years or a lifetime. Infection with HPV can be latent, subclinical, or clinical. Latent infections are detected with molecular biologic techniques. Subclinical infections are found with a colposcope or microscope. HPVs induce hyperplasia and hyperkeratosis.

Table 12-1 Different Types of HPV and Their Clinical Manifestations

Clinical manifestation	HPV types
Plantar warts	1
Common warts	2, 4, 29
Flat warts	3, 10, 28, 49
Epidermodysplasia verruciformis	5, 8, 9, 12, 14, 15, 17, 19-25, 36, 47, 50
Genital warts, laryngeal papillomas	6, 11
Butcher's warts	7
Oral focal epithelial hypoplasia	13, 32
Anogenital dysplasias and neoplasms (rarely laryngeal carcinomas)	16, 18, 26, 27, 30, 31, 33-35, 39, 40, 42-45, 51-59, 61, 62, 64, 66-69, 71-74
Keratoacanthoma	37
Cutaneous squamous cell carcinoma	38, 41, 48
Oral papillomas, inverted nasal and papillomas	57
Buschke Loewenstein tumors	6, 11
Bowenoid papulosis	16, 18, 33, 39
Epidermal cysts	60
Pigmented wart	65
Vulvar papilloma	70
Oral papillomas (in HIV-infected patients)	72, 73
Common wart in renal allograft recipient	75-77
Cutaneous wart	78

From Tyring S: J Am Acad Dermatol 2000; 43(1 Pt 2):pS18.

Immunologic response

The regression of virus-infected cells involves a multifactorial response that includes cell-mediated immunity and induction of interferons. Individual variations in cell-mediated immunity may account for differences in severity and duration. Warts develop on many immunosuppressed patients. Warts occur more frequently, last longer, and appear in greater numbers in patients with AIDS or lymphomas and those taking immunosuppressive drugs. Patients with atopic eczema may not be at increased risk for viral warts, as was once suspected.

Treatment

Some types of warts respond quickly to routine therapy, whereas others are resistant. It should be explained to patients that warts often require several treatment sessions before a cure is realized. Because warts are confined to the epidermis, they can be removed with little, if any, scarring. To avoid scarring, treatment should be conservative. Treatment that results in a hand with many scars is not worthwhile for lesions that undergo spontaneous resolution (Figure 12-1).

Warts obscure normal skin lines; this is an important diagnostic feature. When skin lines are reestablished, the warts are gone. Warts vary in shape and location and are managed in several different ways.

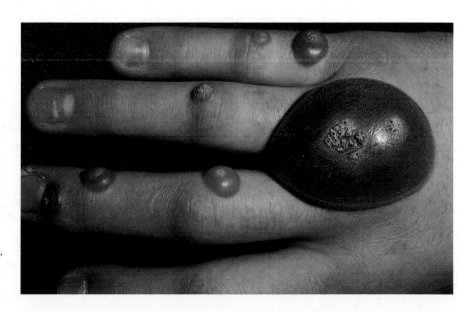

Figure 12-1 Cryosurgery for warts. Excessive, prolonged freezing with liquid nitrogen resulted in a huge blister that healed with scarring.

WARTS: THE PRIMARY LESION

Viral warts are tumors initiated by a viral infection of keratinocytes. The cells proliferate to form a mass but the mass remains confined to the epidermis. There are no "roots" that penetrate the dermis. Several types of warts form cylindrical projections. These projections are clearly seen in digitate warts that occur on the face (Figure 12-2). The projections become fused together in common warts on thicker skin (Figure 12-3); this produces a highly organized mosaic pattern on the surface. This pattern is unique to warts and is a useful diagnostic sign (Figure 12-4). Thrombosed black vessels become trapped in these projections and are seen as black dots on the surface of some warts (Figure 12-5). Although warts remain confined to the epidermis, the growing mass can protrude down and displace the dermis. Blunt dissection of a wart shows that the undersurface is smooth (Figure 12-6).

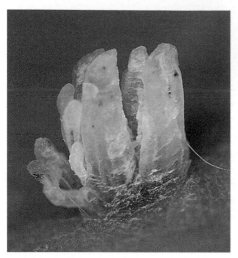

Figure 12-2 Warts form cylindrical projections. They diverge when the wart grows in thin skin.

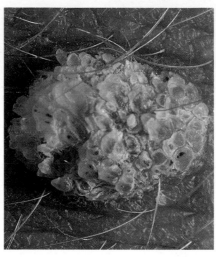

Figure 12-3 The cylindrical projections are partially fused together in this larger wart.

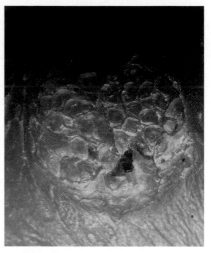

Figure 12-4 The cylindrical projections are tightly packed together, confined by the surrounding skin. This uniform mosaic surface pattern is unique to warts and is a useful diagnostic sign. The pattern can be easily seen with a hand lens.

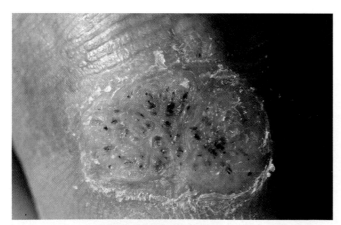

Figure 12-5 Thrombosed black vessels are trapped in the cylindrical projections. They appear as black dots when only the surface of the projections can be seen.

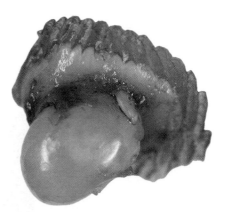

Figure 12-6 The undersurface of a wart. Contrary to popular belief, warts do not have roots. The undersurface is round and smooth. The wart is confined to the epidermis, but it expands and displaces the dermis, giving the impression that it extends into the dermis or subcutaneous tissue.

Common warts

Common warts (Verruca vulgaris) begin as smooth, flesh-colored papules and evolve into dome-shaped, gray-brown, hyperkeratotic growths with black dots on the surface (Figures 12-7 and 12-8). The black dots, which are thrombosed capillaries, are a useful diagnostic sign and may be exposed by paring the hyperkeratotic surface with a #15 surgical blade. The hands are the most commonly involved areas, but warts may be found on any skin surface. In general, the warts are few in number, but it is not unusual for common warts to become so numerous that they become confluent and obscure large areas of normal skin.

TREATMENT. Topical salicylic acid preparations, liquid nitrogen (Figures 12-9 and 12-10), and very light electrocautery are the best methods of initial therapy. Blunt dissection is used for resistant or very large lesions. (See Chapter 27 for surgical techniques.) The technique for the application of salicylic acid is described in the treatment section for plantar warts.

CRYOTHERAPY. The hyperkeratotic surface should be pared. Liquid nitrogen is then applied with either spray or cotton applicator application so that a 1- to 2-mm zone of frozen tissue is created and maintained around lesional skin for about 5 seconds. The area is allowed to thaw. A second or third freeze during the same treatment secession may increase the cure rate.[2] A small blister, sometimes hemorrhagic, is expected. Excessive freezing causes massive swelling, hemorrhagic blisters (see Figure 12-1), hypopigmentation or hyperpigmentation, and scarring. Sharp pain lasts for minutes and sometimes hours; some children tolerate the pain. Freezing may be repeated in 2 to 4 weeks.

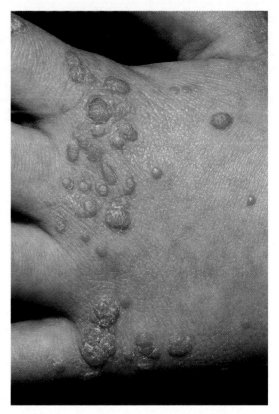

Figure 12-7 Common warts on the back of the hand.

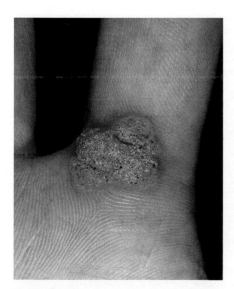

Figure 12-8 A common wart with black dots on the surface.

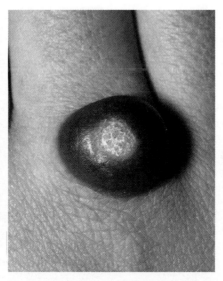

Figure 12-9 Cryosurgery produced the expected hemorrhagic blister.

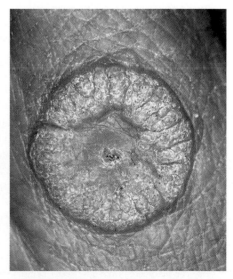

Figure 12-10 A side effect of cryosurgery. The wart spreads to the blister edge.

Treatment of recalcitrant warts

IMIQUIMOD. Nightly application of the immunomodulatory drug imiquimod (Aldara cream) may be effective. The patient is instructed to soak the wart to soften the keratin surface. Removal of the keratin with an abrasive material, such as a pumice stone and application of tape to cover the area, facilitates penetration of the imiquimod cream.

CANDIDA ALBICANS SKIN TEST ANTIGEN INJECTION. *C. albicans* skin test antigen injection is safe and well accepted. There is minimal pain and no scarring. A 1:1 mixture of *C. albicans* skin test antigen (Candin; Allermed Laboratories, San Diego, California; Candida, Bayer, Spokane, Washington; or Candid, ALK-Abelló, Round Rock, Texas) solution and 1% lidocaine is prepared. The mixture (0.1 ml) is injected into and intradermally at the margins of each wart (genital and facial warts excluded) up to a total of 1.0 ml. Injections are repeated every 4 weeks for a total of three injection visits or until there was no evidence of warts, whichever occurs first. Seventy-two percent of patients were completely cured within 8 weeks of the last injection, without subsequent recurrence.[3-5]

CONTACT IMMUNOTHERAPY. The use of squaric acid dibutylester (SADBE) may be considered for recalcitrant warts, especially in patients who do not tolerate painful procedures. Contact immunotherapy is believed to work by inducing a cell-mediated response. SADBE requires refrigeration and is not mutagenic. Sensitization is achieved by applying 1% or 2% SADBE in acetone with or without occlusion to a 2-cm² area of normal skin on the upper arm overnight, after which the patient is instructed to wash the area thoroughly with soap and water. Ninety percent of patients were successfully sensitized after one application of SADBE.*

Sensitization was determined to have occurred when a second or third dose was applied to a different area, inducing erythema and pruritus in the new area of application. A maximum of six attempts were made at sensitization. After sensitization occurred, 0.5% to 1% SADBE was applied directly to the warts during office visits scheduled every 2 to 4 weeks. A concentration of 0.5% SADBE was used on warts in sensitive areas such as the perianal region and on warts of patients who experienced an exuberant contact dermatitis. SADBE is not usually used on the face. The applied concentration of SADBE was increased to 2% and occasionally to 5% if no change in the warts appeared after several treatments, especially on the palms or soles. Clearing of all warts was achieved in 69% of patients. The cured patients had a mean duration of therapy of 4.4 months and achieved complete regression within 12 months with a mean of 5.9 treatments.[6,7]

*SADBE can be ordered from Spectrum Chemical Mfg. Corp., 14422 S. San Pedro St, Gardena, CA 90248. (310) 516-8000, Fax: (310) 516-9843. A pharmacist can compound the various concentrations in acetone.

Filiform and digitate warts

These growths consist of a few or several fingerlike, flesh-colored projections emanating from a narrow or broad base. They are most commonly observed about the mouth (Figure 12-11), beard (Figure 12-12), eyes, and ala nasi.

TREATMENT. These are the easiest warts to treat. Those with a very narrow base do not require anesthesia. A firm base is created by retracting the skin on either side of the wart with the index finger and thumb. A curette is then firmly drawn across the base, removing the wart with one stroke. Bleeding is controlled with gauze pressure rather than by using Monsel's solution, which is painful. This technique is particularly useful for young children who refuse local anesthesia with a needle. Light electrocautery is an alternative.

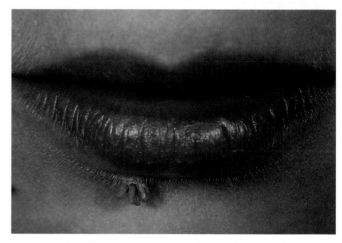

Figure 12-11 Filiform wart with fingerlike projections. These are most commonly observed on the face.

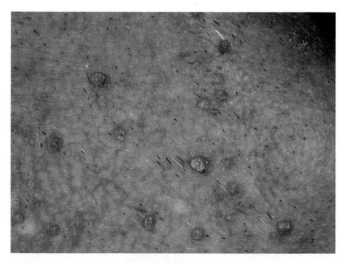

Figure 12-12 Small digitate and filiform warts in the beard area. Shaving spreads the virus over wide areas of the beard. Recurrences are common after cryotherapy or curettage. The infection may last for years.

Flat warts

Flat warts (Verruca plana) are pink, light brown, or light yellow and are slightly elevated, flat-topped papules that vary in size from 0.1 to 0.5 cm. There may be only a few, but in general they are numerous. Typical sites of involvement are the forehead (Figures 12-13, A and 12-14), about the mouth (Figure 12-13, B), the backs of the hands, and shaved areas such as the beard area in men and the lower legs in women. A line of flat warts may appear as a result of scratching these sites.

TREATMENT. Flat warts present a special therapeutic problem. Their duration may be lengthy, and they may be very resistant to treatment. In addition, they are usually located in cosmetically important areas where aggressive, scarring procedures are to be avoided. Imiquimod 5% cream (Aldara) applied every day or every other day may be effective.[8] Freezing of individual lesions with liquid nitrogen or exercising a very light touch with the electrocautery needle may be performed for patients who are concerned with cosmetic appearance and desire quick results. Treatment with 5-fluorouracil cream (carac) applied once or twice a day for 3 to 5 weeks may produce dramatic clearing of flat warts; it is worth the attempt if other measures fail.[9,10] Persistent hyperpigmentation may occur following 5-fluorouracil use. This result may be minimized by applying the ointment to individual lesions with a cotton-tipped applicator. Warts may reappear in skin inflamed by 5-fluorouracil.

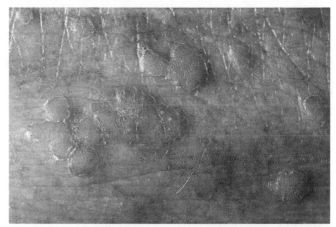

A

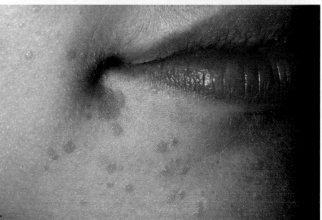

B

Figure 12-13 Flat warts. **A,** Lesions are slightly elevated, flesh-colored papules that often appear grouped. **B,** The face, back of the hands and shins are the most common areas. Flatter lesions are brown.

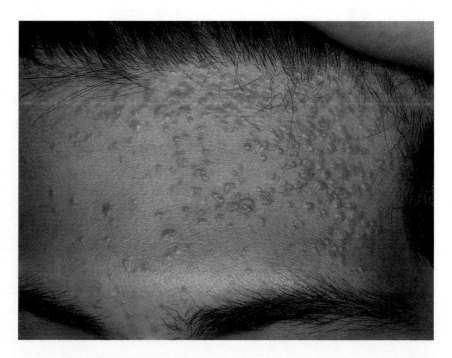

Figure 12-14 Lesions may be numerous and often appear in a linear distribution as a result of scratching.

Plantar warts

Warts of the soles are called plantar warts. Patients may, incorrectly, refer to warts on any surface as plantar warts. Plantar warts frequently occur at points of maximum pressure, such as over the heads of the metatarsal bones or on the heels (Figure 12-15). A thick, painful callus forms in response to pressure and the foot is repositioned while walking. This may result in distortion of posture and pain in other parts of the foot, leg, or back. A little wart can cause a lot of trouble.

Warts may appear anywhere on the plantar surface. A cluster of many warts that appears to fuse is referred to as a mosaic wart (Figure 12-16).

DIFFERENTIAL DIAGNOSIS

Corns. Corns are a mechanically induced lesion that forms over or under a weight-bearing surface or structure. Corns (clavi) over the metatarsal heads are frequently mistaken for warts. The two entities can be easily distinguished by paring the callus with a #15 surgical blade. Warts lack skin lines that cross their surface and have centrally located black dots that bleed with additional paring. Examination with a hand lens shows a highly organized mosaic pattern on the surface (see Figure 12-4). Clavi or corns also lack skin lines crossing the surface, but they have a hard, painful, well-demarcated, translucent central core (Figure 12-17, A). The core or kernel can be removed easily by inserting the point of a #15 surgical blade into the cleavage plane between normal skin and the core, holding the scalpel vertically, and smoothly drawing the blade circumferentially. The hard kernel is freed by drawing the blade horizontally through the base to reveal a deep depression (Figure 12-17, B). Pain is greatly relieved by this simple procedure. Lateral pressure on a wart causes pain, but pinching a plantar corn is painless.

The treatment of corns is targeted at reducing the friction or pressure at a specific location. This can be accomplished with orthotic therapy and/or surgical correction of the osseus deformity creating the mechanical pressure point. Podiatric or orthopedic surgeons familiar with biomechanics and reconstructive surgery perform these corrective procedures.

Black heel. Horizontally arranged clusters of blue-black dots (ruptured capillaries-petechiae) may appear on the upper edge of the heel or anywhere on the plantar surface following the shearing trauma of sports that involve sudden stops or position changes (Figure 12-18, A). It is caused by the shearing force of the epidermis sliding over the rete pegs of the papillary dermis. At first glance, this may be confused with a wart or acral lentiginous melanoma, but closer examination reveals normal skin lines, and paring does not cause additional bleeding (Figure 12-18, B). The condition resolves spontaneously in a few weeks.

Black warts. Warts in the process of undergoing spontaneous resolution, particularly on the plantar surface, may turn black (Figure 12-19) and feel soft when pared with a blade. Cell-mediated immunity against virus-infected keratinocytes may take place in the process of regression of some warts.

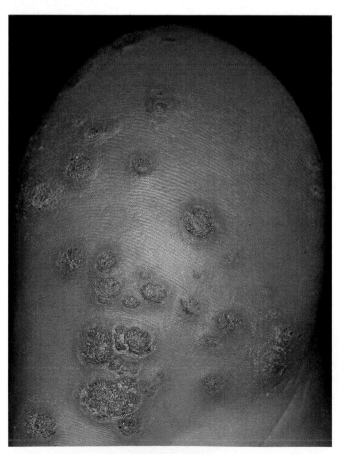

Figure 12-15 Plantar warts. Warts on weight-bearing surfaces accumulate callus and may become painful.

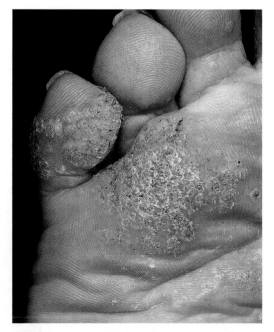

Figure 12-16 Plantar wart. Fusion of numerous small warts to form a mosaic wart. Examination with a hand lens shows a highly organized mosaic pattern on the surface (see Figure 12-3).

PLANTAR WARTS

A

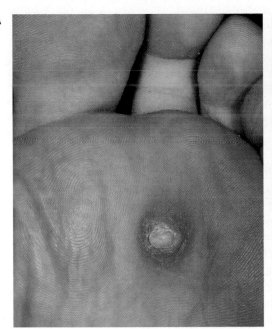

B

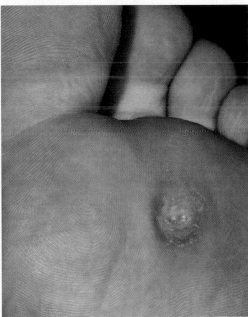

Figure 12-17 A, Corns (clavi) on the plantar surface are frequently mistaken for warts. **B,** Plantar surface depicted in *A* with soft and hard callus removed from the corn to reveal a deep depression. Examination with a hand lens shows no organized surface pattern as is seen in a plantar wart.

A

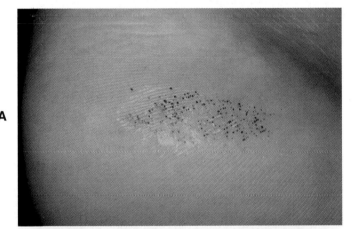

B

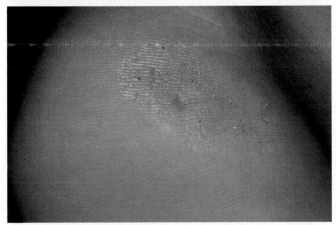

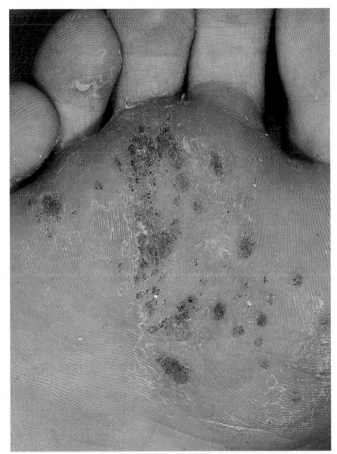

Figure 12-18 A, Black heel. Trauma causes capillaries to shear, resulting in a group of black dots; appearance may be confused with warts. **B,** Paring the skin over the black dots in *A* reveals normal skin lines, proving that a wart is not present.

Figure 12-19 Spontaneous resolution. Warts in the process of resolving may be painful and turn black. They are easily removed without anesthesia with a curette.

TREATMENT. Plantar warts do not require therapy as long as they are painless. Although their number may increase, it is sometimes best to explain the natural history of the virus infection and wait for resolution rather than subject the patient to a long treatment program. Minimal discomfort can be relieved by periodically removing the callus with a blade or pumice stone.

Painful warts must be treated (Figures 12-20 and 12-21). A technique that does not cause scarring should be used; scars on the soles of the feet may be painful for years.

DEBRIDEMENT. It is very important to debride the hyperkeratotic tissue over and around plantar warts to ensure that the medication can penetrate. This may require seeing the patient every 2 to 3 weeks.

COMBINATION THERAPY. Multiple simultaneous techniques are often required to successfully treat plantar warts and may include the following regimens.

Keratolytic therapy (salicylic acid liquid). Keratolytic therapy with salicylic acid (DuoPlant gel [salicylic acid in flexible collodion], Occlusal-HP liquid [salicylic acid in polyacrylic vehicle], and many others that are now available over-the-counter) is conservative initial therapy for plantar warts. The treatment is nonscarring and relatively effective but requires persistent application of medication once each day for many weeks.

The wart is pared with a blade, pumice stone, or sandpaper (emery board). The affected area is soaked in warm water to hydrate the keratin surface; this facilitates penetration of the medicine. A drop of solution is applied with the applicator and allowed to dry. Solution may be added as needed to cover the entire surface of the wart. Penetration of the acid mixture is enhanced if the treated wart is covered with a piece of adhesive tape. Inflammation and soreness may follow tape occlusion, necessitating periodic interruption of treatment; consequently, the patient may be satisfied with the longer, more comfortable process of simply applying the solution at bedtime. White, pliable keratin forms in a few days and should be pared with a blade or worn away with abrasives such as sandpaper or a pumice stone. Ideally, the white keratin should be removed to expose pink skin; to accomplish this, an occasional visit to the office may be necessary.

Keratolytic therapy (40% salicylic acid plasters). This is a safe, nonscarring treatment similar to keratolytic therapy with salicylic acid liquid except the salicylic acid has been incorporated into a pad. Salicylic acid 40% plasters (Mediplast and many others) are particularly useful in treating mosaic warts that cover a large area.

The plaster is cut to the size of the wart. The backing of the plaster is removed and the sticky surface is applied to the wart and secured with tape. The plaster is removed in 24 to 48 hours, the pliable white keratin is reduced in the manner previously described, and another plaster is applied. The treatment requires many weeks, but it is effective and less irritating than salicylic acid and lactic acid liquid. Pain is relieved because a large amount of keratin is removed during the first few days of treatment.

Blunt dissection. Blunt dissection is a surgical alternative that is fast, effective (90% cure rate), and usually nonscarring. It is superior to both electrodesiccation-curettage and excision because normal tissue is not disturbed.[11] (See Chapter 27 for surgical techniques.)

Imiquimod. The immunomodulating drug imiquimod (Aldara cream) is more effective on thicker keratinized (nongenital) skin when occluded and used in combination with cryotherapy or a keratolytic agent.[12] It is essential to debride the thick scale before applying imiquimod. The patient applies the cream daily and covers with tape (for ≥12 hours) to enhance penetration. Response to the use of imiquimod on the plantar surface is usually not preceded by an inflammatory reaction.

Suggestive therapy. Suggestive therapy generally works through the age of 10 years. A banana peel, potato eye, or a penny applied to the skin and covered with tape for a 1- to 2-week period has been effective in young children. Another technique is to draw the body part on a piece of paper and then draw a picture of the wart on the diagram. Crumble the pictures and throw them in the wastebasket.

Vitamin A. Some physicians have had success by treating children with vitamin A 10,000 U for 4 to 6 weeks.

Cantharidin. Cantharidin mixtures are very effective for plantar warts. Apply Canthacur PS (cantharone plus podophyllin 5% plus salicylic acid 30%) in the office and allow to dry. Avoid touching normal skin. Cover with occlusive tape (e.g., Blenderm) or Moleskin and remove in 24 hours or earlier for significant discomfort. A blister usually appears. Patients can relieve pain by breaking the blister. Patients may apply moleskin or felt padding around but not over the lesion to reduce pressure. In 2 to 3 days, remove the blister under local anesthesia by scissors excision or curette. Retreat weekly if necessary.

Laser. Various lasers are available for treating resistant warts. The procedure is expensive and at times painful.

Chemotherapy. For years a variety of acids has been successfully used to treat plantar warts. This technique is occasionally used to treat warts that have recurred after treatment with other techniques and occasionally used as initial therapy. Like keratolytic therapy, repeated application is required. Home application of acids is too dangerous; therefore, weekly or biweekly visits to the office are required. A number of acids may be used (bichloracetic acid is commercially available).

Treatment is as follows. The excess callus is pared. The surrounding area is protected with petrolatum. The entire lesion is coated with acid and the acid is worked into the wart with a sharp toothpick. This procedure is repeated every 7 to 10 days.

Formalin. This may be considered for resistant cases. Mosaic warts or other large involved areas may be treated with daily soaking for 30 minutes in 4% formalin solution. The firm, fixed tissue is pared before subsequent soaking.

Lazerformaldehyde solution (10% formaldehyde) is commercially available for direct application to warts. There is a risk of inducing sensitization to formalin.

Cryosurgery. Cryosurgery on the sole may produce a deep, painful blister and interfere with mobility. Repeated light applications of liquid nitrogen are preferred to aggressive treatment. Cryotherapy is equally effective when applied with a cotton wool bud or by means of a spray.[13] A surgical blade is used to debulk the wart before freezing. Liquid nitrogen is applied until ice-ball formation has spread from the center to include a margin of 2 mm around each wart. A double or triple freeze-thaw cycle may be more effective than a single freeze. Treatment is given every 2 to 4 weeks for up to 3 months.

Contact immunotherapy. See the section on common warts.

Intralesional bleomycin sulfate. Intralesional bleomycin may be considered when all other treatments fail. The drug is expensive. Three milliliters of bacteriostatic saline is added to a 15-U vial of bleomycin sulfate (Blenoxane; Bristol-Myers). The solution is transferred into an empty 20-ml vial, to which an additional 12 ml of saline is added to produce a total of 15 ml of solution of 1U/ml. This vial now becomes a storage container. A 3-ml syringe is filled, capped, and refrigerated. The solution will remain stable for 4 weeks. After the induction of local anesthesia with topical EMLA cream (lidocaine and prilocaine), one or two drops of the bleomycin solution is dropped onto the wart and 'pricked' into the wart using a Monolet or 25-gauge needle until bleeding points appear. The site is covered with a plastic bandage strip, which is removed that evening or the next day. The patient returns in 2 weeks for additional treatment. The responsive warts show hemorrhagic eschars that heal without scarring. Blackened or macerated tissue is removed with a blade, and the bleomycin is readministered. A 92% success rate was achieved.[14,15] The use of bleomycin for the treatment of warts results in significant systemic drug exposure; therefore, it is prudent to exclude pregnancy before treating women of child-bearing age.[16] The patient can be given a prescription for the drug and bring the medication to the office; insurance companies will often pay for the medication if it is obtained at a pharmacy.

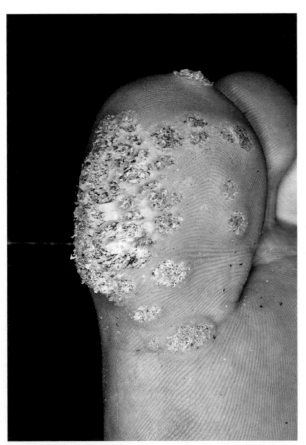

Figure 12-20 Plantar wart. This large mosaic wart is not on a pressure area. It has very long projections. Cryosurgery combined with other treatments would be appropriate.

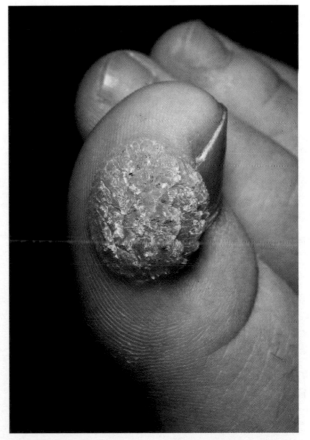

Figure 12-21 Plantar wart. Warts off the plantar surface are elevated and exophytic like common warts in other locations and could be treated with cryosurgery and other techniques.

Subungual and periungual warts

Subungual and periungual warts (Figure 12-22) are more resistant to both chemical and surgical methods of treatment than are warts located in other areas. A wart next to the nail may simply be the tip of the iceberg; much more of the wart may be submerged under the nail.

TREATMENT. The tips of the fingers and toes are a confined area. Therapeutic measures that cause inflammation and swelling, such as cryosurgery, may produce considerable pain.

Cryosurgery. Small periungual warts respond to conservative cryosurgery; warts that extend under the nail do not respond. The use of aggressive cryosurgery over superficial nerves on the volar or lateral aspects of the proximal phalanges of the fingers has caused neuropathy. Permanent nail changes may occur if the nail matrix is frozen.

Cantharidin. Cantharidin (Cantharone) causes blister formation at the dermoepidermal junction but does not cause scarring. Adverse effects are postinflammatory hyperpigmentation, painful blistering, and dissemination of warts to the area of blistering.

In treatment, the solution is applied to the surface and allowed to dry. The patient is seen 1 week later for evaluation. Blisters are opened and the remaining wart is retreated. If blistering does not occur, then cantharidin is applied in one to three layers and covered with tape for 48 hours. Each layer should be dry before the next application of cantharidin. The treatment is very effective for some patients, but there are some warts that do not respond to repeated applications.

Keratolytic preparations. The same procedures described for treating plantar warts with salicylic acid and lactic acid paint and salicylic acid plasters are useful for periungual warts.[17]

Blunt dissection. When conventional measures fail, blunt dissection offers an excellent surgical alternative[18] (see Chapter 27). Local anesthesia is induced with 2% lidocaine without epinephrine around and under small warts. A digital block is required for larger warts. Hemostasis during the procedure is maintained by firm pressure over the digital arteries or with a rubber-band tourniquet. The nail should be removed only if the wart is very large and imbedded. The procedure is exactly the same as that described for blunt dissection of plantar warts.

Duct tape occlusion. Duct tape occlusion therapy may be more effective than cryotherapy for common warts.[19] To completely cover the wart, the tip of the finger is wrapped with duct tape. The tape remains in place for 6 days, is removed at home, is then reapplied in a similar manner 12 hours later, and remains in place for an additional 6 days. This procedure is repeated for up to 2 months.

Genital warts

Genital warts are discussed in Chapter 11.

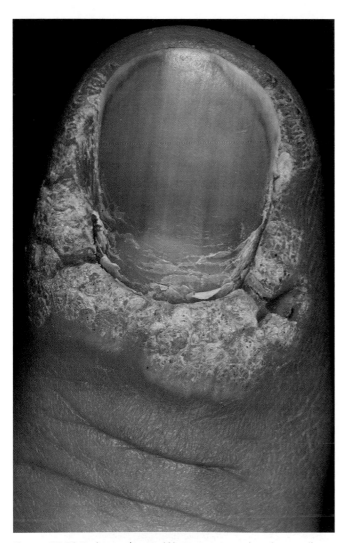

Figure 12-22 Periungual wart. Warts may extend under a nail. Cuticle biting may spread warts.

Molluscum Contagiosum

CLINICAL MANIFESTATIONS. Molluscum contagiosum is a double-stranded DNA poxvirus infection of the skin characterized by discrete, 2- to 5-mm, slightly umbilicated, flesh-colored, dome-shaped papules (Figure 12-23). It spreads via autoinoculation, scratching, or touching a lesion and fomites. The areas most commonly involved are the face (Figure 12-24), trunk, axillae, extremities in children, and the pubic and genital areas in adults (see Figures 11-10 and 11-11). Lesions are frequently grouped; there may be few or many covering a wide area. Unlike warts, the palms and soles are not involved. It is not uncommon to see erythema and scaling at the periphery of a single or several lesions (see Figure 11-12). This may be the result of inflammation from scratching or may be a hypersensitivity reaction. Lesions spread to inflamed skin, such as areas of atopic dermatitis (Figure 12-25). The individual lesion begins as a smooth, dome-shaped, white- to flesh-colored papule. With time, the center becomes soft and umbilicated. Most lesions are self-limiting and clear spontaneously in 6 to 9 months; however, they may last 2 to 4 years or longer. Genital molluscum contagiosum may be a manifestation of sexual abuse in children.

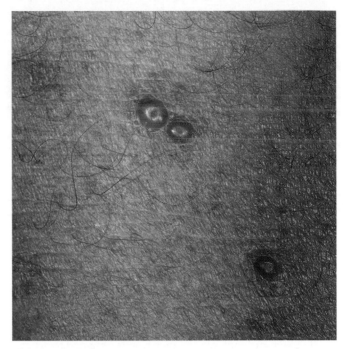

Figure 12-23 Molluscum contagiosum. Individual lesions are 2- to 5-mm, flesh-colored, dome-shaped umbilicated papules.

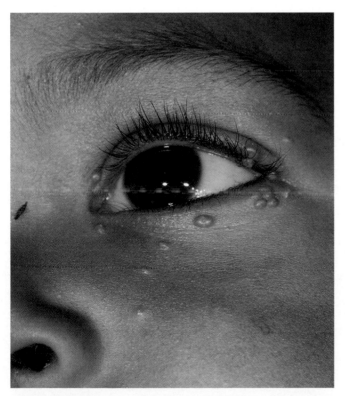

Figure 12-24 Molluscum contagiosum. Inoculation around the eye, a typical presentation for children.

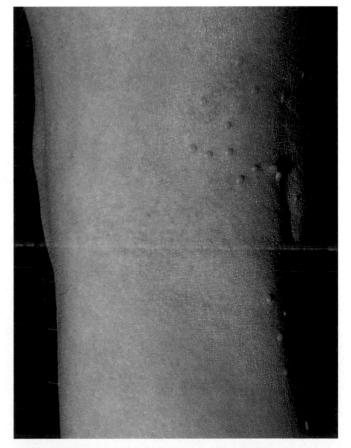

Figure 12-25 Molluscum contagiosum spreads rapidly in eczematous skin. This patient has atopic dermatitis of the popliteal fossa.

MOLLUSCUM CONTAGIOSUM IN HIV-INFECTED PATIENTS. Molluscum contagiosum is a common and at times severely disfiguring cutaneous viral infection in patients with HIV. Atypical facial lesions occur with either multiple small papules or giant nodular tumors. Cutaneous cryptococcosis may resemble molluscum contagiosum in AIDS patients. Cytologic examination of skin brushing reveals encapsulated budding yeasts. An inverse relation between $CD4^+$ count and the number of molluscum contagiosum lesions is observed.

DIAGNOSIS. If necessary the diagnosis can be established easily with laboratory methods. The virus infects epithelial cells, creating very large intracytoplasmic inclusion bodies and disrupting cell bonds by which epithelial cells are generally held together. This lack of adhesion causes the central core of the lesion to be soft. Rapid confirmation can be made by removing a small lesion with a curette and placing it with a drop of potassium hydroxide between two microscope slides. The preparation is gently heated and then crushed with firm twisting pressure. Larger umbilicated papules have a soft center, the contents of which can be obtained by scooping with a needle. This material contains only infected cells and can be examined directly in a heated potassium hydroxide preparation. The infected cells are dark and round and disperse easily with slight pressure, whereas normal epithelial cells are flat and rectangular and tend to remain stuck together in sheets. Virions streaming out of the amorphous mass can be seen if Sedi-Stain, a supravital stain used to stain urine sediments, is used.[20] Toluidine blue gives the same results. Viral inclusions (large, eosinophilic, round, intracytoplasmic bodies) are easily seen in a fixed and stained biopsy specimen.

TREATMENT. Treatment must be individualized. Conservative nonscarring methods should be used for children who have many lesions. Genital lesions in adults should be definitively treated to prevent spread by sexual contact (see Chapter 11). New lesions that are too small to be detected may appear after treatment and may require additional attention. Topical corticosteroids are used to treat dermatitis near or involving the lesions.

Curettage. Small papules can be quickly removed with a curette and without local anesthesia in adults. Children might tolerate curettage after using a lidocaine/prilocaine cream (EMLA) for analgesia. The cream is applied 30 to 60 minutes before treatment. Bleeding is controlled with gauze pressure. Monsel's solution is painful to use in an unanesthetized area in children. Curettage is useful when there are a few lesions because it provides the quickest, most reliable treatment. A small scar may form; therefore this technique should be avoided in cosmetically important areas.

Cryosurgery. Cryosurgery is the treatment of choice for patients who do not object to the pain. Most children will not tolerate cryosurgery. The papule is touched lightly with a nitrogen-bathed cotton swab or spray until the advancing, white, frozen border has progressed to form a 1-mm halo on the normal skin surrounding the lesion. This should take approximately 5 seconds. This conservative method destroys most lesions in one to three treatment sessions at 1- or 2-week intervals and rarely produces a scar.

Cantharidin. Cantharidin, a chemovesicant extract from the blister beetle, is very effective, well tolerated, and safe in children.[21] It penetrates the epidermis and induces vesiculation through acantholysis. Cantharidin is sparingly applied to each nonfacial lesion with the blunt wooden end of a cotton-tipped applicator. Contact with surrounding skin is avoided, and a maximum of 20 lesions are treated per visit. The treated areas are washed with soap and water after 4 to 6 hours, or sooner if burning, discomfort, or vesiculation occurs; therapy is repeated at 2- to 4-week intervals. Lesions blister and may clear without scarring. Occasionally, new lesions appear at the site of the blister created with cantharidin. Blistering and pain are mild to moderate. Pitted shallow depressions sometimes occur.

Imiquimod. Nightly application of the immunomodulatory drug Imiquimod (Aldara cream) has been reported to be effective in both immunocompromised and immunocompetent children and adults.[22] The cream is applied for several weeks.[23]

Potassium hydroxide 5%. Parents are instructed to apply the pharmacist prepared solution twice daily with a cotton swab. A brief stinging may occur shortly after the application. Most lesions clear in 4 weeks.[24]

Podophyllotoxin 0.5%. The daily application of podophyllotoxin 0.5% (Condylox) may be tried for cases resistant to other therapies.[25]

Hypoallergenic surgical adhesive tape. Tape is applied once each day after showering and is used each day until the lesion ruptures and the core is discharged. The average time to clearance is 16 weeks.

Tretinoin. Tretinoin (Retin-A) cream (0.025%, 0.05%, or 0.1%) or gel (0.01% or 0.025%) should be applied once or twice daily to individual lesions. Weeks or months of treatment may be required. This method is useful for children whose parents are anxious for some type of treatment, but it is not very effective.

Salicylic acid. Salicylic acid (Occlusal) applied each day without tape occlusion may cause irritation and encourage resolution.

Laser therapy. Lesions on the genital area may be treated with the carbon dioxide laser.

Trichloroacetic acid peel in immunocompromised patients. Patients with HIV infection who have extensive facial molluscum contagiosum infection were treated with trichloroacetic acid peels. Peels were performed with 25% to 50% trichloroacetic acid (average, 35%) and were repeated every 2 weeks as needed. A total of 15 peels were performed with an average reduction in lesion counts of 40.5% (range, 0% to 90%).[26]

Herpes Simplex

Genital herpes simplex virus (HSV) infections are discussed in Chapter 11.

HSV infections are caused by two different virus types (HSV-1 and HSV-2), which can be distinguished by laboratory and office tests. HSV-1 is generally associated with oral infections, and HSV-2 is associated with genital infections. HSV-1 genital infections and HSV-2 oral infections are becoming more common, possibly as a result of oral-genital sexual contact. Both types seem to produce identical patterns of infection. Many infections are asymptomatic, and evidence of previous infection can be detected only by an elevated IgG antibody titer. HSV infections have two phases: the primary infection, after which the virus becomes established in a nerve ganglion; and the secondary phase, characterized by recurrent disease at the same site. The rate of recurrence varies with virus type and anatomic site. Genital recurrences are nearly 6 times more frequent than oral-labial recurrences; genital HSV-2 infections recur more often than genital HSV-1 infections; and oral-labial HSV-1 infections recur more often than oral HSV-2 infections.[27] Infections can occur anywhere on the skin. Infection in one area does not protect the patient from subsequent infection at a different site. Lesions are intraepidermal and usually heal without scarring.

Primary infection

Many primary infections are asymptomatic and can be detected only by an elevated IgG antibody titer. Like most virus infections, the severity of disease increases with age. The virus may be spread via respiratory droplets, direct contact with an active lesion, or contact with virus-containing fluid such as saliva or cervical secretions in patients with no evidence of active disease. Symptoms occur from 3 to 7 or more days after contact. Tenderness, pain, mild paresthesias, or burning occurs before the onset of lesions at the site of inoculation. Localized pain, tender lymphadenopathy, headache, generalized aching, and fever are characteristic prodromal symptoms. Some patients have no prodromal symptoms.

LESIONS. Grouped vesicles on an erythematous base appear and subsequently umbilicate (Figure 12-26). The vesicles in primary herpes simplex (Figures 12-27 and 12-28) are more numerous and scattered than those in the recurrent infection (Figures 12-29 and 12-30). The vesicles of herpes simplex are uniform in size in contrast to the vesicles seen in herpes zoster, which vary in size. Mucous membrane lesions accumulate exudate, whereas skin lesions form a crust. Lesions last for 2 to 4 weeks unless secondarily infected and heal without scarring.

The virus replicates at the site of primary infection. Virons are then transported by neurons via retrograde axonal flow to the dorsal root ganglia, and latency is established in the ganglion.

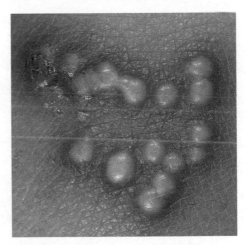

A, Vesicles appear on a red base.

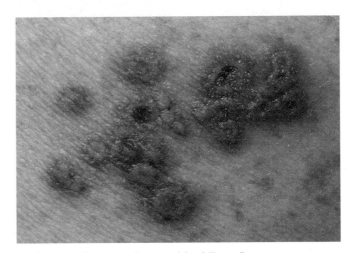

B, The center becomes depressed (umbilicated).

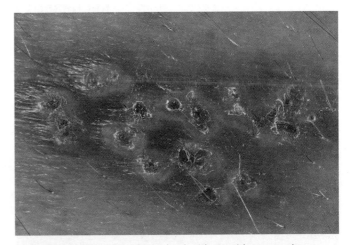

C, Crusts form and the lesions heal with or without scarring.

Figure 12-26 Herpes simplex—the evolution of lesions.

PRIMARY HERPES SIMPLEX

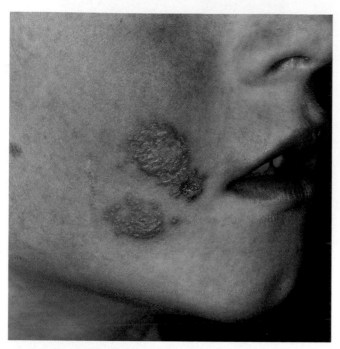

Figure 12-27 Primary infections in children typically begin in or about the oral cavity. Blisters are numerous and confluent.

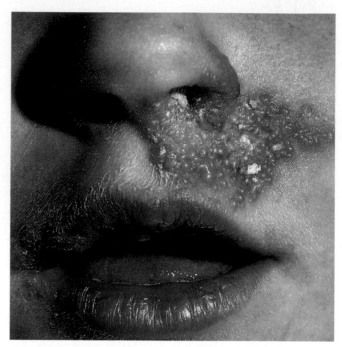

Figure 12-28 A particularly extensive eruption involving the mouth, lips, and nasal orifice.

RECURRENT HERPES SIMPLEX

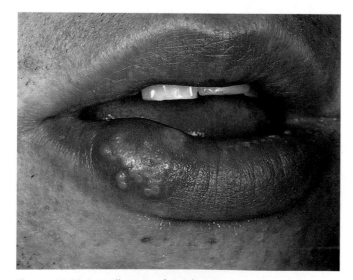

Figure 12-29 A small group of vesicles on an erythematous base are the primary lesion.

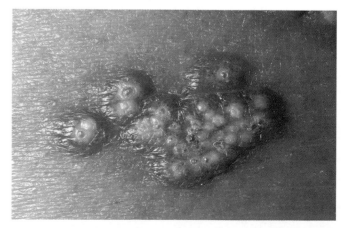

Figure 12-30 Vesicles evolve to pustules and become umbilicated.

Table 12-2 Herpes Simplex Virus Infection (Systemic Medication)

	Acyclovir (Zovirax)			Famciclovir (Famvir) (125-, 250-, and 500-mg tablets)	Valacyclovir (Valtrex) 500-, 1000-mg caplets
	200 mg	400 mg	800 mg		
First episode*	200 mg 5 times/day × 7-10 days	400 mg tid × 7-10 days		250 mg tid × 7-10 days	1 gm bid 7-10 days
Episodic recurrence Intermittent therapy	200 mg 5 times/day × 5 days	400 mg tid × 5 days	800 mg bid × 5 days	125 mg bid × 5 days	500 mg qd or bid × 3 days 2 gm bid 1 day (herpes labialis)
Chronic daily suppression		400 mg bid		250 mg bid	<10 episodes/year (500 mg qd) >10 episodes/year (1 gm qd)
Severe disease	Acyclovir 5-10 mg/kg IV every 8 hours for 5-7 days or until clinical resolution				
Topical therapy is less effective than systemic drugs.					
*Treatment may be extended if healing is incomplete after 10 days of therapy; higher doses of medication may be needed in HIV patients.					

Recurrent infection

Local skin trauma (e.g., ultraviolet light exposure, chapping, abrasion) or systemic changes (e.g., menses, fatigue, fever) reactivate the virus, which then travels down the peripheral nerves to the site of initial infection and causes the characteristic focal, recurrent infection. Recurrent infection is not inevitable. Many individuals have a rise in antibody titer and never experience recurrence. The prodromal symptoms of itching or burning, lasting 2 to 24 hours, resemble those of the primary infection. Within 12 hours, a group of lesions evolves rapidly from an erythematous base to form papules and then vesicles. The dome-shaped, tense vesicles rapidly umbilicate. In 2 to 4 days, they rupture, forming aphthaelike erosions in the mouth and vaginal area or erosions covered by crusts on the lips and skin. Crusts are shed in approximately 8 days to reveal a pink, reepithelialized surface. In contrast to the primary infection, systemic symptoms and lymphadenopathy are rare unless there is secondary infection.

The frequency of recurrence varies with anatomic site and virus type.[27] HSV-1 oral infections recur more often than genital HSV-1 infections; HSV-2 genital infections recur 6 times more frequently than HSV-1 genital infections; and the frequency of recurrence is lowest for oral-labial HSV-2 infections.

LABORATORY DIAGNOSIS. The laboratory diagnosis of herpes simplex is covered in Chapter 11, which discusses sexually transmitted viral infections.

TREATMENT. A number of measures can be taken to relieve discomfort and promote healing; these are described in the following sections. The appropriate use of topical, oral, and intravenous antiviral agents is outlined (Table 12-2 and Box 12-1). Oral drugs decrease the duration of viral excretion, new lesion formation, and vesicles and promote rapid healing. The subsequent recurrence rate is not influenced by acyclovir. Acyclovir-resistant HSV infections are becoming a problem in patients with AIDS. L-Lysine is not effective.

Box 12-1 Recurrent Herpes Simplex Infection (Topical Medication)

Apply the creams frequently (e.g., every 2 hours)
Acyclovir cream
Penciclovir cream (Denavir)
n-Docosanol cream (Abreva) over-the-counter
Topical corticosteroids plus oral antiviral drug
Famciclovir (500 mg tid × 5 days) + topical fluocinonide (0.05% tid × 5 days)

Oral-labial herpes simplex
Primary infection

Transmission is dependent on intimate, personal contact with someone excreting HSV. Gingivostomatitis and pharyngitis are the most frequent manifestations of first-episode HSV-1 infection. Infection occurs most commonly in children between ages 1 and 5 years. The incubation period is 3 to 12 days. Although most cases are mild, some are severe. Sore throat and fever may precede the onset of painful vesicles occurring anywhere in the oral cavity or on the face (see Figures 12-27 and 12-28). The vesicles rapidly coalesce and erode with a white, then yellow, superficial, purulent exudate. Children are unable to swallow liquids because of the edema, ulcerations, and pain. Tender cervical lymphadenopathy develops. Fever subsides in 3 to 5 days, and oral pain and erosions are usually gone in 2 weeks; in severe cases, they may last for 3 weeks.

Recurrent infection

Recurrences average two or three each year but may occur as often as 12 times a year. Oral HSV-1 infections recur more often than oral HSV-2 infections.[27] Recurrent oral herpes simplex can appear as a localized cluster of small ulcers in the oral cavity, but the most common manifestation consists of eruptions on the vermilion border of the lip (recurrent herpes labialis) (Figures 12-29, 12-31, 12-33, and 12-34). Fever (fever blisters), upper respiratory infections (cold sores), and exposure to ultraviolet light (Figure 12-31), among other things, may precede the onset. The course of the disease in the oral-labial area is the same as it is in other areas. Immunosuppressed patients are at greater risk of developing lesions on the lips, in the oral cavity, and on surrounding skin (Figure 12-32). Lesions may also appear on the upper lip and chin (Figure 12-35). The recurrence rate and long-term natural history are not well defined. Many people experience a decrease in the frequency of recurrences, but others experience an increase. A history of recurrent herpes labialis is present in 38% of college students. The prevalence of asymptomatic excretion of HSV following recurrence varies from 1% to 5% in adults.

TREATMENT. A number of treatment modalities have been used for herpes on the vermilion border. Oral acyclovir, famciclovir, and valacyclovir can be used to treat the primary infection and episodic recurrences and for suppression (see Table 12-2 and Box 12-1). Oral antiviral drugs have a modest clinical benefit only if initiated very early after recurrence. They may be of value in patients whose recurrences are associated with protracted clinical illness. Oral antiviral drugs can alter the severity of sun-induced reactivation. Short-term prophylactic treatment may help patients who anticipate high-risk activity (e.g., intense sunlight exposure). Intermittent administration does not alter the frequency of subsequent recurrences.

COMBINATION TREATMENT. Corticosteroids in combination with an oral antiviral agent may be beneficial for episodic treatment of herpes labialis. Famciclovir (500 mg tid for 5 days) and topical fluocinonide (0.05% tid for 5 days) significantly reduced lesion size and pain.[28]

TOPICAL TREATMENT. Topical treatments include penciclovir cream (Denavir), *n*-docosanol cream (Abreva), and acyclovir cream. Abreva is an over-the-counter drug. The cream is applied frequently (e.g., every 2 hours while awake) at the first sign of prodromal symptoms or erythema. These creams may shorten an episode of herpes labialis by a few hours or a day and may not be worth the high cost. Many patients believe that these creams are effective and prefer them to oral medication.

The lips should be protected from sun exposure with an opaque cream such as zinc oxide or with sun-blocking agents incorporated into a lip balm (Chap Stick). A cool water or Burrow's solution compress decreases erythema and debrides crusts to promote healing.

Lubricating creams may be applied if the lips become too dry.

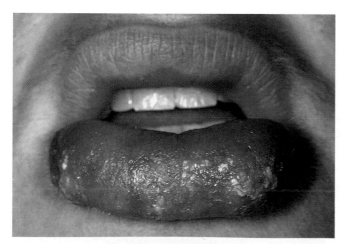

Figure 12-31 Sun exposure triggered this extensive recurrence.

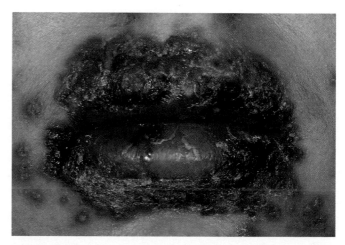

Figure 12-32 Recurrent herpes in an HIV patient.

RECURRENT ORAL-LABIAL HERPES SIMPLEX

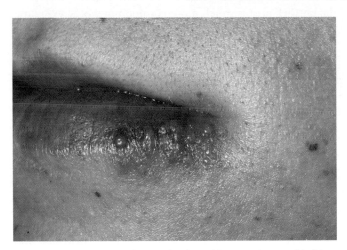

Figure 12-33 Recurrent herpes begins with a prodrome of itching or burning. A group of vesicles appears on an erythematous base. Previous episodes in the same area are typical.

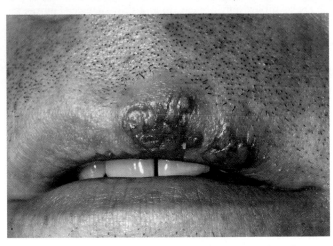

Figure 12-34 Vesicles of recurrent herpes evolve in a few days to form crusts. The diagnosis is suspected because crusts are small, round, and grouped. Previous episodes support the diagnosis.

Figure 12-35 Recurrent oral labial herpes can appear on the lips or surrounding skin. Patients unaware of this do not understand that lesions on the chin, nose, or cheeks can be "cold sores." The typical grouped crusts support the diagnosis. Impetigo is often suspected. Impetigo does not present as a group of highly uniform small crusts.

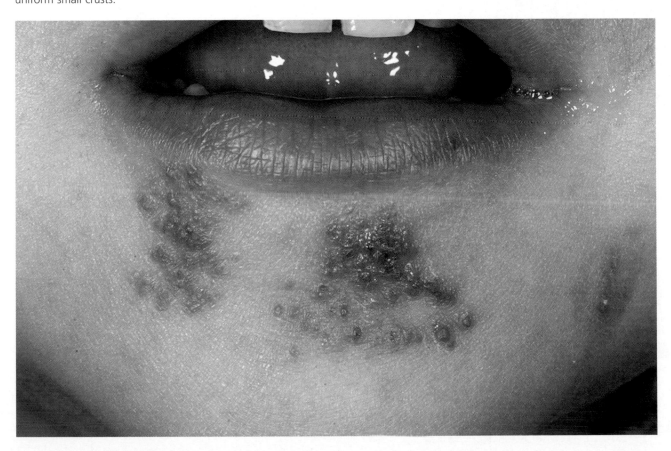

Cutaneous herpes simplex

Herpes simplex may appear on any skin surface (Figures 12-36 and 12-37). It is important to identify all of the characteristic features when attempting to differentiate cutaneous herpes from other vesicular eruptions.

HERPETIC WHITLOW. Herpes simplex of the fingertip (herpetic whitlow) (Figure 12-38) can resemble a group of warts or a bacterial infection. Health care professionals who had frequent contact with oral secretions used to be the most commonly affected group; the incidence has decreased, probably as a result of heightened awareness of the condition and stricter infection-control precautions. Herpetic whitlow is most often reported in pediatric patients with gingivostomatitis and in women with genital herpes.[29]

HERPES GLADIATORUM. Cutaneous herpes in athletes involved in contact sports is transmitted via direct skin-to-skin contact. This is a recognized health risk for wrestlers.[30] Prompt identification and exclusion of wrestlers with skin lesions may reduce transmission.

HERPES SIMPLEX OF THE BUTTOCK. Herpes simplex of the buttock area is much more common in women (Figures 12-39 and 12-40). The cause of infection in this area has not been identified.

HERPES SIMPLEX OF THE TRUNK. Herpes simplex of the lumbosacral region or trunk may be very difficult to differentiate from herpes zoster; the diagnosis becomes apparent only at the time of recurrence.

TREATMENT. Oral antiviral drugs are useful for suppressive therapy, particularly for recurrent fingertip and buttock infections.[31]

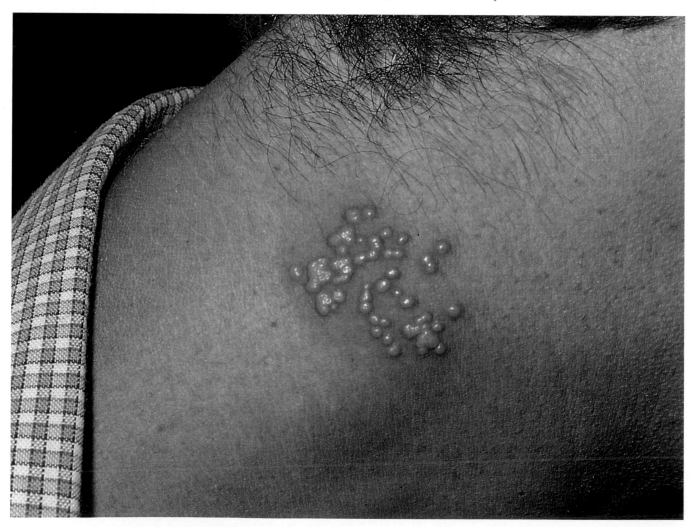

Figure 12-36 Herpes simplex of the skin: vesicular stage. The uniform size of the vesicles helps differentiate this from herpes zoster, in which vesicles vary in size.

CUTANEOUS HERPES SIMPLEX

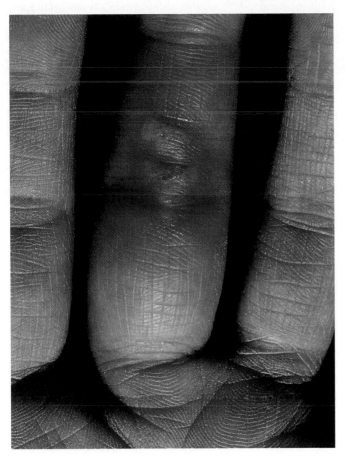

Figure 12-37 Infections in this area are unusual and mimic other blistering eruptions such as poison ivy or bites.

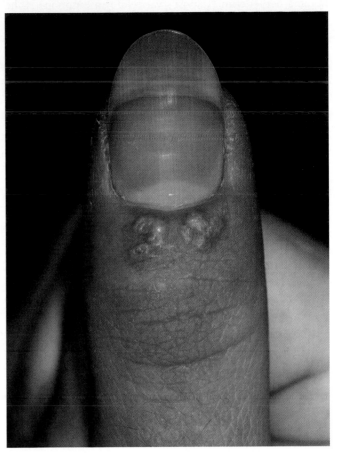

Figure 12-38 Herpetic whitlow. Inoculation followed examination of a patient's mouth.

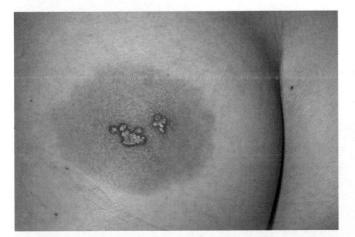

Figure 12-39 Herpes of the buttock. The diagnosis is suspected because of the classic presentation of recurrent disease with highly characteristic grouped vesicles of uniform size on an erythematous base. This presentation is seen almost exclusively in women. Recurrences may be frequent and very annoying; suppressive therapy can greatly improve the quality of life.

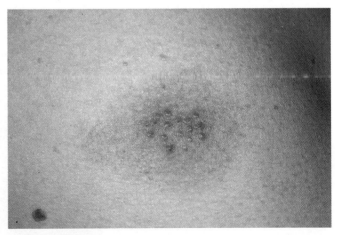

Figure 12-40 Recurrent herpes of the buttock. Recurrent lesions in the same area that progress from vesicles to crusts make the clinical diagnosis. Patients with herpes of the buttock may have recurrences in several different areas of the buttock. Groups of small round scars may be the only evidence of past recurrences.

Eczema herpeticum

Eczema herpeticum (Kaposi's varicelliform eruption) is the association of two common conditions: atopic dermatitis and HSV infection. Certain atopic infants and adults may develop the rapid onset of diffuse cutaneous herpes simplex. The severity of infection ranges from mild and transient to fatal. The disease is most common in areas of active or recently healed atopic dermatitis, particularly the face, but normal skin can be involved. The disease in most cases is a primary HSV infection. In one third of the patients in a particular study, there was a history of herpes labialis in a parent in the previous week.[32] Recurrences are uncommon and usually limited. Approximately 10 days after exposure, numerous vesicles develop, become pustular, and umbilicate markedly (Figure 12-41). Secondary staphylococcal infection commonly occurs. New crops of vesicles may appear during the following weeks. The most intense viral dissemination is located in the areas of dermatitis, but normal appearing skin may ultimately be involved. High fever and adenopathy occur 2 to 3 days after the onset of vesiculation. The fever subsides in 4 to 5 days in uncomplicated cases, and the lesions evolve in the typical manner (Figure 12-42). Viremia with infection of internal organs can be fatal. Recurrent disease is milder and usually without constitutional symptoms.

TREATMENT. Eczema herpeticum of the young infant is a medical emergency; early treatment with acyclovir can be life saving.[33,34] Eczema herpeticum is managed with cool, wet compresses, similar to the management of diffuse genital herpes simplex. Oral dosages of acyclovir 25 to 30 mg/kg/day have been effective.[35] Infants were successfully treated with intravenous acyclovir, 1500 mg/m²/day administered over a 1-hour period tid.[36,37] Oral antistaphylococcal antibiotics are an important part of treatment. Minor relapses do not require a second course of acyclovir. Adults respond to the standard intravenous acyclovir dosage of 250 mg tid. Oral antiviral drugs (see Table 12-2) are expected to be equally effective.

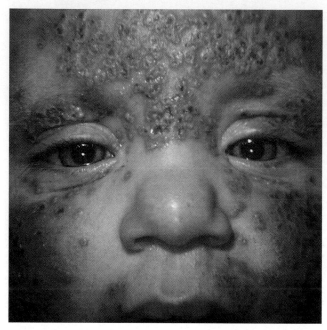

Figure 12-41 Eczema herpeticum. Numerous umbilicated vesicles of the face.

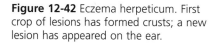

Figure 12-42 Eczema herpeticum. First crop of lesions has formed crusts; a new lesion has appeared on the ear.

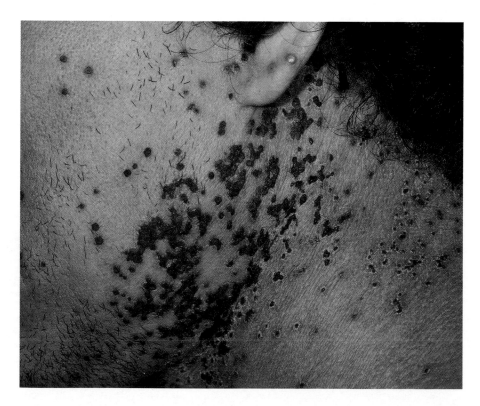

Varicella

Varicella, or chickenpox, is a highly contagious viral infection that, during epidemics, affects the majority of urban children before puberty. The incidence peaks sharply in March, April, and May in temperate climates. Transmission occurs via airborne droplets or vesicular fluid. Patients are contagious from 2 days before onset of the rash until all lesions have crusted. The systemic symptoms, extent of eruption, and complications are greater in adults; thus some parents intentionally expose their young children. Patients with defective, cell-mediated immunity or those using immunosuppressive drugs, especially systemic corticosteroids, have a prolonged course with more extensive eruptions and a greater incidence of complications. An attack of chickenpox usually confers lifelong immunity. After it has produced chickenpox, varicella-zoster virus (VZV) becomes latent in ganglia along the entire neuraxis. Unlike HSV, however, VZV cannot be cultured from human ganglia. Varicella vaccine is effective and approved for use in children and adults.

CLINICAL COURSE. The incubation period averages 14 days, with a range of 9 to 21 days; in the immunosuppressed host, the incubation period can be shorter. The prodromal symptoms in children are absent or consist of low fever, headache, and malaise, which appear directly before or with the onset of the eruption. Symptoms are more severe in adults. Fever, chills, malaise, and backache occur 2 to 3 days before the eruption.

ERUPTIVE PHASE. Lesions of different stages are present at the same time in any given body area. New lesion formation ceases by day 4 and most crusting occurs by day 6; the process lasts longer in the immunosuppressed patient. The lesion starts as a 2- to 4-mm red papule that develops an irregular outline (rose petal) as a thin-walled clear vesicle appears on the surface (dewdrop) (Figure 12-43). This lesion, "dewdrop on a rose petal," is highly characteristic. The vesicle becomes umbilicated and cloudy and breaks in 8 to 12 hours to form a crust as the red base disappears. Fresh crops of additional lesions undergoing the same process occur in all areas at irregular intervals during the following 3 to 5 days, giving the characteristic picture of intermingled papules, vesicles, pustules, and crusts (see Figures 12-44 and 45). Moderate to intense pruritus is usually present during the vesicular stage. The degree of temperature elevation parallels the extent and severity of the eruption and varies from 101° to 105° F. The temperature returns to normal when the vesicles have disappeared. Crusts fall off in 7 days (with a range of 5 to 20 days) and heal without scarring. Secondary infection or excoriation extends the process into the dermis, producing a craterlike, pockmark scar. Vesicles often form in the oral cavity and vagina and rupture quickly to form multiple, aphthaelike ulcers.

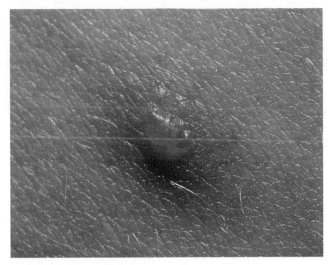

A, "Dewdrop on a rose petal": a thin-walled vesicle with clear fluid forms on a red base.

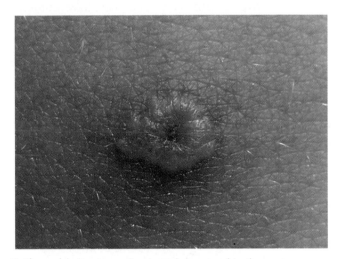

B, The vesicle becomes cloudy and depressed in the center (umbilicated), the border is irregular (scalloped).

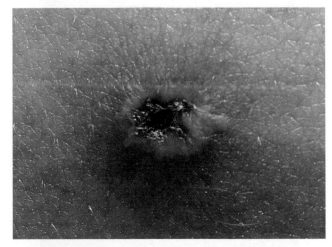

C, A crust forms in the center and eventually replaces the remaining portion of the vesicle at the periphery.

Figure 12-43 Chickenpox—the evolution of lesions.

The rash begins on the trunk (centripetal distribution) (Figure 12-44) and spreads to the face (Figure 12-45) and extremities (centrifugal spread). The extent of involvement varies considerably. Some children have so few lesions that the disease goes unnoticed. Older children and adults have a more extensive eruption involving all areas, sometimes with lesions too numerous to count.

DIFFERENTIAL DIAGNOSIS. The differential diagnosis includes drug eruptions, smallpox, other viral exanthemas, scabies, erythema multiforme, and insect bites.

COMPLICATIONS

Skin infection. The most common complication in children is bacterial skin infection. Secondary infection should be suspected when the vesiculopustules develop large, moist, denuded areas, and particularly when the lesions become painful.

Neurologic complications. The most common extracutaneous complication is central nervous system involvement. Encephalitis and Reye's syndrome are complications of chickenpox.[38] There are two forms of encephalitis. The cerebellar form seen in children is self-limited and complete recovery occurs. There is ataxia with nystagmus, headache, nausea, vomiting, and nuchal rigidity. Adult patients with encephalitis have altered sensorium, seizures, and focal neurologic signs with a mortality rate of up to 35%.[39] Reye's syndrome is an acute, noninflammatory encephalopathy associated with hepatitis or fatty metamorphosis of the liver; 20% to 30% of Reye's syndrome cases are preceded by varicella. The fatality rate is 20%. Salicylates used during the varicella infection may increase the risk of the development of Reye's syndrome.

Pneumonia. Varicella pneumonia occurs in 1:400 cases. Pneumonia is rare in normal children, but it is the most common serious complication in normal adults. Viral pneumonia develops 1 to 6 days after onset of the rash. In most cases it is asymptomatic and can be detected only with a chest x-ray examination. Cough, dyspnea, fever, and chest pain can occur. The mortality rate for adult varicella pneumonia is 10% of immunocompetent patients and 30% of immunocompromised patients.

Other. Hepatitis is the most common complication in immunosuppressed patients. Mild degrees of thrombocytopenia can accompany routine cases.

CHICKENPOX

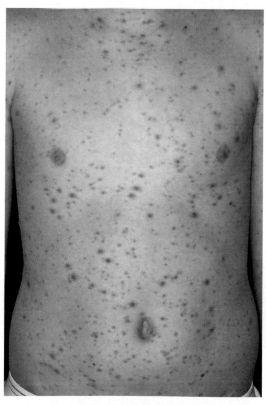

Figure 12-44 Numerous lesions on the trunk (centripetal distribution).

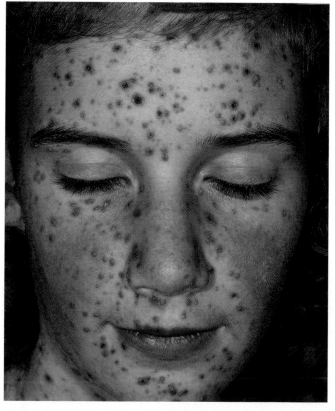

Figure 12-45 Lesions present in all stages of development.

Chickenpox in the immunocompromised patient

Patients with cancer or patients who are taking immunosuppressive drugs, particularly systemic and intranasal corticosteroids, have extensive eruptions and more complications. The mortality rate for immunosuppressed children or children with leukemia is 7% to 14%. Adults with malignancy and varicella have a mortality rate as high as 50% (Figure 12-46). Hemorrhagic chickenpox, also called malignant chickenpox, is a serious complication, in which the lesions are numerous and often bullous and bleeding occurs in the skin at the base of the lesion.[40] The bullae turn dark brown and then black as blood accumulates in the blister fluid. Patients are usually toxic, have high fever and delirium, and may develop convulsions and coma. They frequently bleed from the gastrointestinal tract and mucous membranes. Pneumonia with hemoptysis commonly occurs. The mortality rate was 71% in one series.[41]

Chickenpox and HIV infection

Many children with HIV infection who acquire varicella have an uncomplicated clinical course and have a significant antibody response to VZV.[42] Some, however, have chronic, recurrent, or persistent varicella.[43,44] Varicella in adult HIV-infected patients is a potentially severe infection, but these patients respond well to acyclovir therapy. Immune status to varicella does not correlate with the declining CD4+ counts and is well preserved, even in patients with fewer than 200 CD4+ cells/mm³.[45]

Chickenpox during pregnancy

Varicella during pregnancy poses a risk for both the mother and the unborn child. In a study of 43 pregnant women, 4 developed symptomatic pneumonia and 1 died of the infection.[46] Smoking is a possible risk factor. Pregnant women with pneumonitis, who received high-dose intravenous acyclovir, ranging from 10 to 18 mg/kg every 8 hours, showed rapid improvement. Lower dosages may not be effective.[47]

Figure 12-46 Hemorrhagic chickenpox. Numerous vesicular and bullous lesions with hemorrhage at the base.

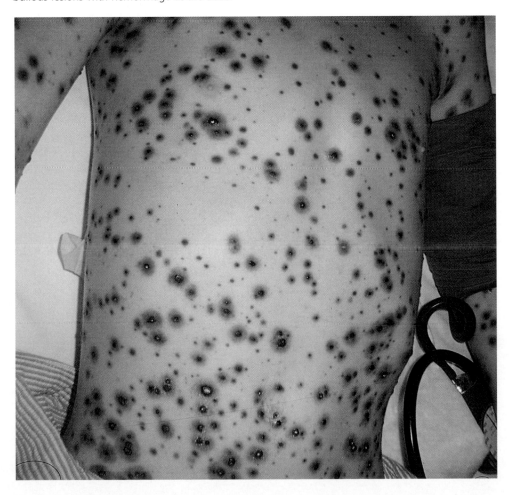

Congenital and neonatal chickenpox
Maternal varicella

FIRST TRIMESTER. Infection with the VZV during pregnancy can produce an embryopathy characterized by limb hypoplasia, chorioretinitis, cortical atrophy, and cutaneous scars (congenital varicella syndrome).[46] The risk is greatest when infection occurs during the first 20 weeks of pregnancy. The absolute risk of embryopathy after maternal varicella infection in the first 20 weeks of pregnancy is approximately 2%.[48, 49]

SECOND TRIMESTER. Maternal varicella in the middle months of pregnancy may result in undetected fetal chickenpox. The newborn child who has already had chickenpox is at risk for developing herpes zoster (shingles). This may explain why some infants and children develop herpes zoster without the expected history of chickenpox.

NEAR BIRTH. The time of onset of maternal lesions correlates directly with the frequency and severity of neonatal disease (Figure 12-47). If the mother has varicella 2 to 3 weeks before delivery, the fetus may be infected in utero and be born with or develop lesions 1 to 4 days after birth. Transplacental maternal antibody protects the infant and the course is usually benign. The risk of infection and complications is greatest when the maternal onset of varicella is from 5 days before to 2 days after delivery. When maternal infection appears more than 5 days before delivery, maternal antibody can develop and transfer via the placenta. Maternal infection that develops more than 2 days after delivery is associated with onset of disease in a newborn approximately 2 weeks later, at which point the immune system is better able to respond to the infection.

There is a high incidence of disseminated varicella in the infant when the mother's eruption appears 1 to 4 days before delivery or the child's eruption appears 5 to 10 days after birth. When the maternal rash appears within 5 days before delivery, approximately one third of infants become infected. After 5 days, transmission occurs in approximately 18%.[50] When the rash appears in infants between 5 and 10 days old, the mortality rate may be as high as 20%.[51] In this situation, the virus is either acquired transplacentally or from contact with maternal lesions during birth; there is insufficient time to receive adequate maternal antibody. The infant is immunologically incapable of controlling the infection and is at great risk of developing a disseminated disease. These infants should be given zoster immune globulin (ZIG), varicella-zoster immune globulin (VZIG), or gamma globulin if ZIG or VZIG is not available.

LABORATORY DIAGNOSIS

Culture. In questionable cases, virus can be cultured from vesicular fluid. Culture is not easily obtained because VZV is a labile virus that is cultured much less readily than HSV.

Serologic testing. The main value of serologic testing is the assessment of the immune status of immunocompromised patients, such as children with neoplastic diseases, who are at risk of developing severe disease with VZV infection. There are qualitative and quantitative tests that measure IgG and IgM antibodies. The presence of IgM antibodies or a fourfold or greater rise in paired sera IgG titer indicates recent infection. The presence of IgG indicates past exposure and immunity.

Tzanck smear. Cytologic smear (Tzanck smear), as described for the diagnosis of herpes simplex (Figure 11-18), is a valuable tool for rapid diagnosis. The test does not differentiate herpes simplex from varicella. Scrape the base of an early lesion and stain with hematoxylin-and-eosin, Giemsa, Wright's, toluidine blue, or Papanicolaou. Multinucleated giant cells and epithelial cells containing eosinophilic intranuclear inclusions are seen.

A chest x-ray examination should be obtained if respiratory symptoms develop. The white blood cell count is variably elevated, but it is necessary to obtain a count only if the disease progresses.

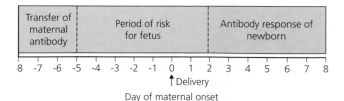

Figure 12-47 Varicella in newborns. For neonates, the risk of varicella infection and its associated complications is greatest when maternal onset of disease occurs in a 7-day period from 5 days before delivery to 2 days after delivery.

Varicella vaccine

The live attenuated varicella vaccine was approved for use in the United States in 1995 and is recommended for all susceptible persons 12 months of age or older. One dose is given for healthy children 12 to 18 months of age, and two doses, in a 4- to 8-week interval, is given to susceptible persons older than 13 years. The vaccine is highly effective; it prevented chickenpox in 85% of immunized children, with 97% protection against moderately severe and severe disease. A documented history of vaccination is sufficient to predict a level of immunity to VZV that will prevent severe cases of chickenpox in healthy children.[52]

Studies show that protection against varicella seems to last at least 6 years.[53] The incidence of zoster in children with leukemia is no greater than that in children who have had natural varicella infection.[54] The live attenuated vaccine should not be given to patients with HIV infection or to other immunosuppressed patients.

Treatment

Bland antipruritic lotions (e.g., Sarna Anti-Itch [camphor and menthol over-the-counter]), cool wet compresses, tepid baths, and antipyretics (excluding aspirin because of its association with Reye's syndrome) provide symptomatic relief. Antihistamines (e.g., hydroxyzine) may help control excoriation. Oral antibiotics active against *Streptococcus* and *Staphylococcus* are indicated for secondarily infected lesions.

ACYCLOVIR AND VIDARABINE

Children and adolescents. Oral acyclovir therapy initiated within 24 hours of illness for otherwise healthy children with varicella typically results in a 1-day reduction in fever and an approximately 15% to 30% reduction in the severity of cutaneous and systemic signs and symptoms. Therapy has not been shown to reduce the rate of acute complications, pruritus, spread of infection, or duration of absence from school.

The American Academy of Pediatrics Committee on Infectious Diseases published recommendations for the use of oral acyclovir in otherwise healthy children with varicella. Recommendations are that (1) oral acyclovir therapy is not routinely recommended for the treatment of uncomplicated varicella in otherwise healthy children and that (2) for certain groups at increased risk of severe varicella or its complications, oral acyclovir therapy for varicella should be considered if it can be initiated within the first 24 hours after the onset of rash. These groups include otherwise healthy, nonpregnant individuals 13 years of age or older,[55] children older than 12 months with a chronic cutaneous or pulmonary disorder, and those receiving long-term salicylate therapy, although in the latter instance a reduced risk for Reye's syndrome has not been shown to result from oral acyclovir therapy or from milder illness with varicella.

Adults. Early therapy with oral acyclovir (800 mg 5 times per day for 7 d) decreases the time to cutaneous healing of adult varicella, decreases the duration of fever, and lessens symptoms. Initiation of therapy after the first day of illness is of no value in uncomplicated cases of adult varicella.[56]

Immunocompromised patients. Studies show that immunosuppressed patients treated with acyclovir had decreased morbidity from visceral dissemination; there was a modest effect on the cutaneous disease (see Table 12-2).[57,58] Acyclovir (500 mg/m² intravenous every 8 hours for 7 to 10 days) is the drug of choice for treatment of varicella in immunocompromised patients.

A continuous infusion of acyclovir may be beneficial for severe, life-threatening VZV infections that are resistant to treatment with the conventional regimen, and perhaps even acyclovir-resistant herpesvirus infections. A continuous infusion of acyclovir at a rate of 2 mg/kg body weight/hr (2250 mg/day) was effective in one report.[59]

The recommended dose for vidarabine is 10 mg/kg/day intravenously for 5 to 10 days, the risk of neurotoxicity limits its use.

Acyclovir-resistant strains of VZV have been reported in AIDS patients. Foscarnet is a potentially effective with acyclovir-resistant VZV strains.

VARICELLA-ZOSTER IMMUNE GLOBULIN. VZIG, a more readily available preparation than ZIG, has been used to modify the course of varicella. It is indicated for immunosuppressed patients and certain nonimmunosuppressed patients. VZIG must be administered as early as possible after the presumed exposure but may be effective when given as late as 96 hours after exposure. VZIG is not known to be useful in treating clinical varicella or zoster or in preventing disseminated zoster. The duration of protection is estimated to be 3 weeks. Patients exposed again more than 3 weeks after a dose of VZIG should receive another full dose. VZIG is given intramuscularly.[60]

GAMMAGLOBULIN. Intravenous gammaglobulin may be an acceptable substitute if VZIG is not available.[61]

Herpes Zoster

Herpes zoster, or shingles, a cutaneous viral infection generally involving the skin of a single dermatome (Figure 12-48), occurs during the lifetime of 10% to 20% of all persons. People of all ages are afflicted; it occurs regularly in young individuals, but the incidence increases with age as T-cell immunity to the virus wanes. Patients who have T-cell immunosuppression are at greater risk. There is an increased incidence of zoster in normal children who acquire chickenpox when younger than 2 months.[62] Patients with zoster are not more likely to have an underlying malignancy.[63,64] Zoster may be the earliest clinical sign of the development of AIDS in high-risk individuals.

Zoster results from reactivation of varicella virus that entered the cutaneous nerves during an earlier episode of chickenpox, traveled to the dorsal root ganglia, and remained in a latent form. Age, immunosuppressive drugs, lymphoma, fatigue, emotional upsets, and radiation therapy have been implicated in reactivating the virus, which subsequently travels back down the sensory nerve, infecting the skin. Some patients, particularly children with zoster, have no history of chickenpox. They may have acquired chickenpox via the transplacental route. Although reported, herpes zoster acquired through direct contact with a patient with active varicella or zoster is rare. After contact with such patients, infections are more inclined to result from reactivation of latent infection. Virus reactivation usually occurs once in a lifetime; the incidence of a second attack is less than 5%.

Varicella zoster virus can be cultured from vesicles during an eruption. It may also cause chickenpox in those not previously infected.

The elderly are at greater risk to develop segmental pain, which can continue for months after the skin lesions have healed.

CLINICAL PRESENTATION. Preeruptive pain (preherpetic neuralgia), itching, or burning, generally localized to the dermatome, precedes the eruption by 4 to 5 days. An extended period of pain (7 to 100 days) has been reported.[65] The pain may simulate pleurisy, myocardial infarction, abdominal disease, or migraine headache and may present a difficult diagnostic problem until the charactcristic eruption provides the answer. Preeruptive tenderness or hyperesthesia throughout the dermatome is a useful predictive sign. *Zoster sine herpete* refers to segmental neuralgia without a cutaneous eruption and is rare. Constitutional symptoms of fever, headache, and malaise may precede the eruption by several days. Regional lymphadenopathy may be present. Segmental pain and constitutional symptoms gradually subside as the eruption appears and then evolves (Figures 12-49 to 12-52). Prodromal symptoms may be absent, particularly in children.

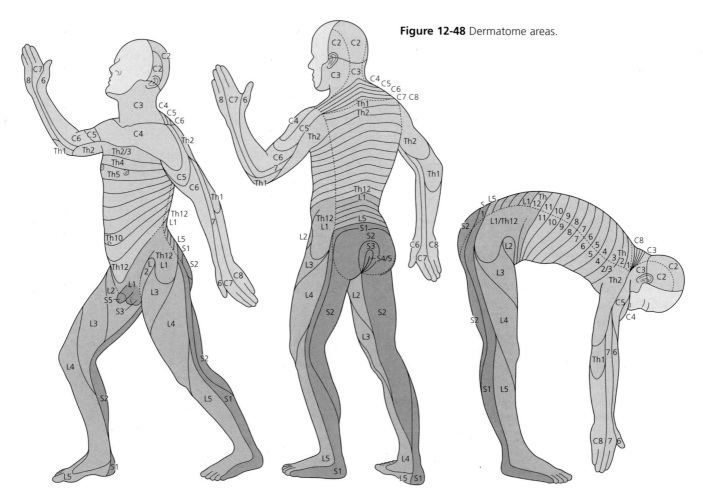

Figure 12-48 Dermatome areas.

HERPES ZOSTER—THE EVOLUTION OF LESIONS

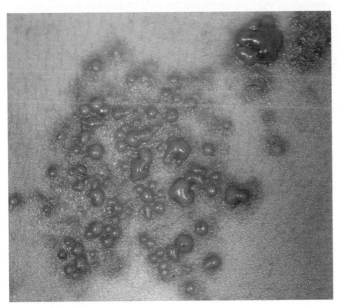

Figure 12-49 A group of vesicles that vary in size. Vesicles of herpes simplex are of uniform size.

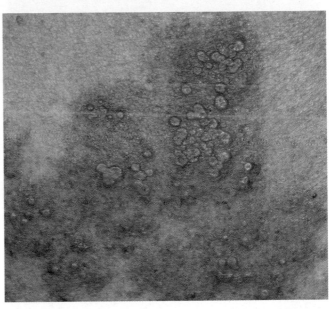

Figure 12-50 Vesicles become umbilicated and then form crusts.

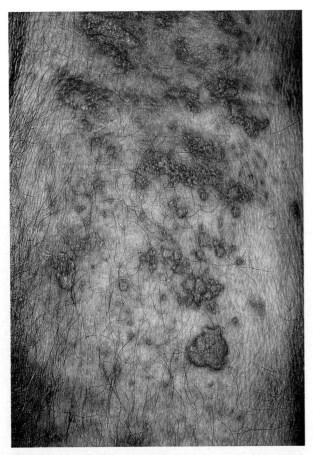

Figure 12-51 Confluent groups of vesicles in a highly inflamed case.

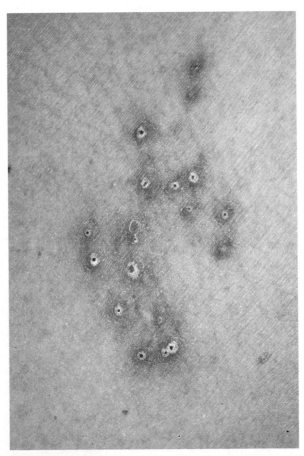

Figure 12-52 Vesicles evolve to crusts and may eventually scar if inflammation is intense.

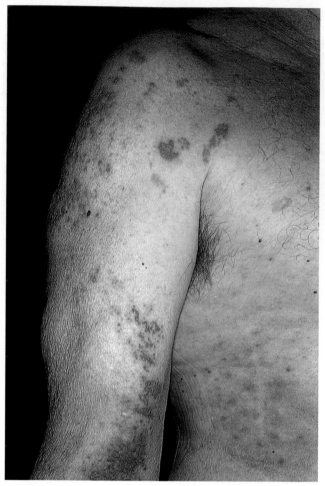

Figure 12-53 Herpes zoster may involve any dermatome. Patients are confused by this presentation. They think that "shingles" can appear only on the trunk.

ERUPTIVE PHASE. The eruption begins with red, swollen plaques of varying sizes and spreads to involve part or all of a dermatome (Figures 12-49 through 12-56). The vesicles arise in clusters from the erythematous base and become cloudy with purulent fluid by day 3 or 4. In some cases vesicles do not form or are so small that they are difficult to see. The vesicles vary in size, in contrast to the cluster of uniformly sized vesicles noted in herpes simplex (Figure 12-49). Successive crops continue to appear for 7 days. Vesicles either umbilicate (Figure 12-50) or rupture before forming a crust, which falls off in 2 to 3 weeks. The elderly or debilitated patients may have a prolonged and difficult course. For them, the eruption is typically more extensive and inflammatory, occasionally resulting in hemorrhagic blisters, skin necrosis, secondary bacterial infection, or extensive scarring (Figure 12-57), which is sometimes hypertrophic or keloidal (Figure 12-58).

Although generally limited to the skin of a single dermatome (Figures 12-55 and 12-56), the eruption may involve one or two adjacent dermatomes (Figure 12-54). Occasionally, a few vesicles appear across the midline. Eruption is rare in bilaterally symmetric or asymmetric dermatomes. Approximately 50% of patients with uncomplicated zoster have a viremia, with the appearance of 20 to 30 vesicles scattered over the skin surface outside the affected dermatome. Possibly because chickenpox is centripetal (located on the trunk), the thoracic region is affected in two thirds of herpes zoster cases. An attack of herpes zoster does not confer lasting immunity, and it is possible, although very unusual, to have two or three episodes in a lifetime.

Figure 12-54 Herpes zoster may involve one, two, or three adjacent dermatomes.

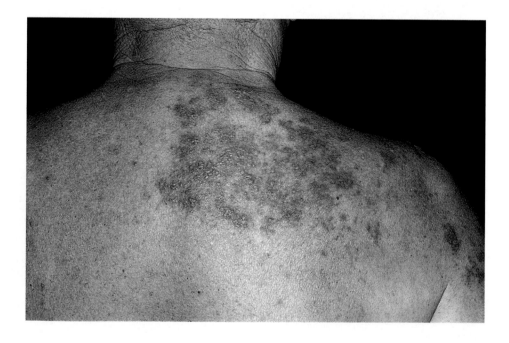

HERPES ZOSTER

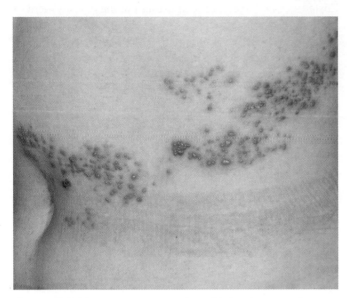

Figure 12-55 A common presentation with involvement of a single thoracic dermatome.

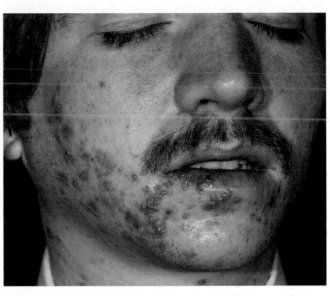

Figure 12-56 Unilateral single-dermatome distribution involving the mandibular branch of the fifth nerve.

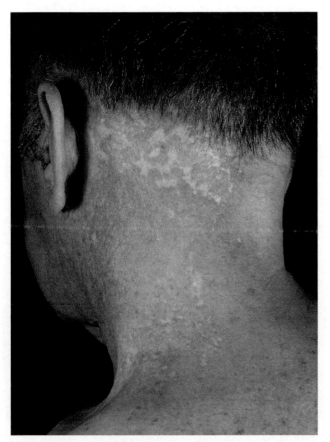

Figure 12-57 Several scars localized to a dermatome.

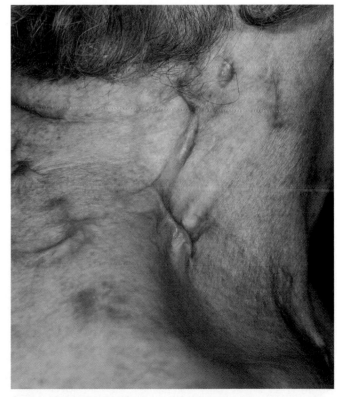

Figure 12-58 Hypertrophic scars. Plastic surgery was required to improve mobility of the neck.

PAIN. The pain associated with acute zoster and postherpetic neuralgia (PHN) is neuropathic and results from injury of the peripheral nerves and altered central nervous system signal processing. After the injury, peripheral neurons discharge spontaneously, have lower activation thresholds, and display exaggerated responses to stimuli. Axonal regrowth after the injury produces nerve sprouts that are also prone to unprovoked discharge. The excessive peripheral activity is thought to lead to hyperexcitability of the dorsal horn, resulting in exaggerated central nervous system responses to all input. These changes may be so complex that no single therapeutic approach will ameliorate all the abnormalities.[66]

Herpes zoster after varicella immunization

Herpes zoster may be less common after immunization than after natural infection. The incidence of zoster in children with leukemia who receive the vaccine is lower than that in leukemic children who have natural varicella infection.

Herpes zoster and HIV infection

Zoster may be the earliest clinical sign of the development of AIDS in high-risk individuals. The incidence of herpes zoster is significantly higher among HIV-seropositive patients. The risk of herpes zoster is not associated with duration of HIV infection and is not predictive of faster progression to AIDS.[67]

Herpes zoster during pregnancy

Herpes zoster during pregnancy, whether it occurs early or late in the pregnancy, appears to have no deleterious effects on either the mother or infant.[68]

Syndromes

OPHTHALMIC ZOSTER. Herpes zoster ophthalmicus presents with vesicular and erythematous involvement of the cranial nerve V1 dermatome, ipsilateral forehead, and upper eyelid. The fifth cranial, or trigeminal, nerve has three divisions: the ophthalmic, maxillary, and mandibular. The oph-

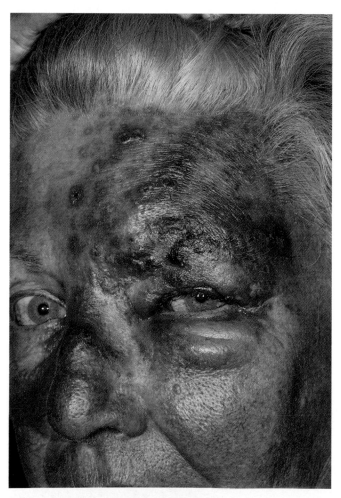

Figure 12-59 Herpes zoster (ophthalmic zoster). Involvement of the first branch of the fifth nerve. Vesicles on the side of the nose are associated with the most serious ocular complications.

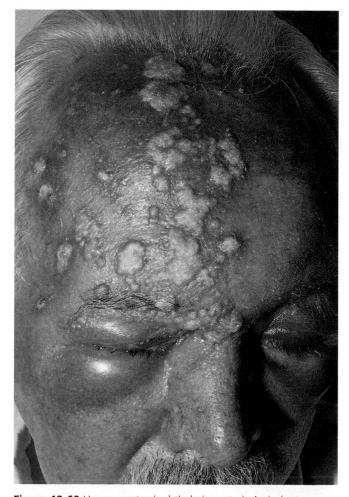

Figure 12-60 Herpes zoster (ophthalmic zoster). A virulent infection of the skin and eye.

thalmic division further divides into three main branches: the frontal, lacrimal, and nasociliary nerves. Involvement of any branch of the ophthalmic nerve is called herpes zoster ophthalmicus. It constitutes 10% to 15% of all zoster cases. Involvement of the ophthalmic branch of the fifth cranial nerve is 5 times as common as involvement of the maxillary or mandibular branches.

CLINICAL PRESENTATION. Headaches, nausea, and vomiting are prodrome symptoms. Ipsilateral preauricular and, sometimes, submaxillary nodal involvement is a common prodromal event. Reactive lymphadenopathy can occur later with secondary infection of vesicles. The ophthalmic branch of the fifth cranial nerve sends branches to the tentorium and to the third and sixth cranial nerves, which may explain the meningeal signs and, occasionally, the third and sixth cranial palsies associated with herpes zoster ophthalmicus. The rash extends from eye level to the vertex of the skull but does not cross the midline (Figures 12-59 and 12-60). Herpes zoster ophthalmicus may be confined to certain branches of the trigeminal nerve. The tip and side of the nose and eye are innervated by the nasociliary branch of the trigeminal nerve. Vesicles on the side or tip of the nose (Hutchinson's sign) that occur during an episode of zoster are associated with the most serious ocular complications, including conjunctival, corneal, scleral, and other ocular diseases, although this is not invariable. Involvement of the other sensory branches of the trigeminal nerve is most likely to yield periocular involvement but spare the eyeball. Acute pain occurs in 93% of patients and remains in 31% at 6 months. Of patients aged 60 and older, pain persists in 30% for 6 months or longer, and this rises to 71% in those aged 80 and older.

Eye involvement. Between 20% and 72% develop ocular complications. Anterior uveitis and the various varieties of keratitis are most common, affecting 92% and 52% of patients with ocular involvement, respectively. Sight-threatening complications include neuropathic keratitis, perforation, secondary glaucoma, posterior scleritis/orbital apex syndrome, optic neuritis, and acute retinal necrosis (Table 12-3). Twenty-eight percent of initially involved eyes develop long-term ocular disease (6 months), with chronic uveitis, keratitis, and neuropathic ulceration being the most common.

Prompt treatment with oral antiviral drugs (see Table 12-4) reduces the severity of the skin eruption, the incidence and the severity of late ocular manifestations, and the intensity of PHN. At 6 months, late ocular inflammatory complications are seen in 29.1% of acyclovir-treated patients versus 50% to 71% of untreated patients. Ophthalmic 3% acyclovir ointment may be used for established ocular complications.[69]

Ramsay Hunt syndrome. The strict definition of the Ramsay Hunt syndrome (geniculate ganglion zoster) is peripheral facial nerve palsy accompanied by a vesicular rash on the ear (zoster oticus) or in the mouth. It is caused by zoster of the geniculate ganglion. Other frequent signs and symptoms include tinnitus, hearing loss, nausea, vomiting, vertigo, and nystagmus. These eighth nerve features are caused by the close proximity of the geniculate ganglion to

the vestibulocochlear nerve within the bony facial canal. Bell's palsy (facial paralysis without rash) is significantly associated with herpes simplex virus infection.

There is involvement of the sensory portion and motor portion of the seventh cranial nerve. There may be unilateral loss of taste on the anterior two thirds of the tongue and vesicles on the tympanic membrane, external auditory meatus, concha, and pinna. Involvement of the motor division of the seventh cranial nerve causes unilateral facial paralysis. Auditory nerve involvement occurs in 37.2% of patients, resulting in hearing deficits and vertigo.[70] Recovery from the motor paralysis is generally complete, but residual weakness is possible. Sweeney discusses and diagrams the complex neuroanatomy of this syndrome.[71]

The syndrome also may result from zoster of ninth or tenth cranial nerves since the external ear has complex innervation by branches of several cranial nerves.

Compared with Bell's palsy (facial paralysis without rash), patients with Ramsay Hunt syndrome often have more severe paralysis at onset and are less likely to recover completely. About 14% developed vesicles after the onset of facial weakness. Thus Ramsay Hunt syndrome may initially be indistinguishable from Bell's palsy.

Some patients develop peripheral facial paralysis without ear or mouth rash, associated with a fourfold rise in antibody to VZV. This indicates that a proportion of patients with "Bell's palsy" have Ramsay Hunt syndrome zoster sine herpete (zoster without the rash). Treatment of these patients with acyclovir and prednisone within 7 days of onset has been shown to improve the outcome of recovery from facial palsy.[71]

Table 12-3 Ocular Complications in 86 Patients with Herpes Zoster Ophthalmicus*	
Complication	**No. of patients**
Lid involvement	11
Corneal involvement	66
Scleral involvement	4
Canalicular scarring	2
Uveitis	37
Glaucoma (secondary)	10
Glaucoma persistent	2
Cataract	7
Neuroophthalmic involvement	7
Postherpetic neuralgia	15

Modified from Womack LW, Liesegang T J: Arch Ophthalmol 101:44, 1983. By permission of Mayo Foundation.

*Some patients had more than one manifestation of involvement.

Sacral zoster (S2, S3, or S4 dermatomes). A neurogenic bladder with urinary hesitancy or urinary retention has reportedly been associated with zoster of the sacral dermatome S2, S3, or S4 (Figures 12-61 and 12-62). Migration of virus to the adjacent autonomic nerves is responsible for these symptoms.[72]

COMPLICATIONS

Pain and postherpetic neuralgia. Pain persisting after herpes zoster is called *postherpetic neuralgia*. It is the most common and most feared complication and the major cause of morbidity. The risk of PHN increases with age (especially in patients older than 50 years) and increases in patients who have severe pain or severe rash during the acute episode or who have a prodrome of dermatomal pain before the rash appears. The pain is often severe, intractable, and exhausting. The patient protects areas of hyperesthesia to avoid the slightest pressure, which activates another wave of pain. There is a yearning for a few hours of sleep, but sharp paroxysms of lancinating pain invade the mind and the patient is again awakened. "The pain is sometimes so severe as to make the patient weary of existence." These words were written more than 100 years ago. Despair and sometimes suicide occur if hope and encouragement are not provided.

Duration of pain. Pain can persist in a dermatome for months or years after the lesions have disappeared. The probability of longstanding pain in patients not treated with antiviral drugs is low. One large study provided the following data. Regardless of age, the prevalence of pain was 19.2% at 1 month, 7.2% at 3 months, and 3.4% at 1 year. Among pa-

tients younger than 60 years, the risk of PHN 3 months after the start of the zoster rash was 2% and pain was mild in all cases. After the age of 60, both the frequency and severity of pain increased, although moderate pain was rare after 3 months and severe pain was uncommon at all times (Figure 12-63). The probability of having severe PHN after 3 months in this age group was less than 7%, and it was less than 3% at 12 months.[73]

Once present, neuralgia can persist for years, but spontaneous remission may occur after several years.

Pathophysiology of pain. Postherpetic neuralgia is associated with scarring of the dorsal root ganglion and atrophy of the dorsal horn on the affected side. These changes are caused by the extensive inflammation that occurs during the active infection.

Dissemination. A few vesicles may be found remote from the affected dermatome in immunocompetent patients and is probably a result of hematogenous spread of the virus. Cutaneous dissemination is defined as more than 20 vesicles outside the primary and immediately adjacent dermatomes. Visceral dissemination (lungs, liver, brain) occurs in 10% of immunocompromised patients. In addition, patients with

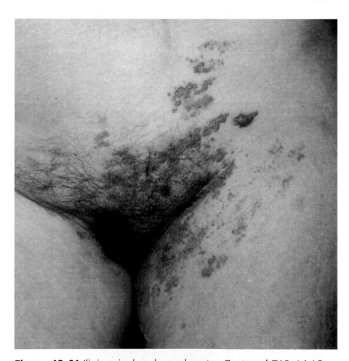

Figure 12-61 Ilioinguinal and sacral zoster. Zoster of T12, L1-L2, and S2-S4 dermatomes can occasionally cause a neurogenic bladder. Acute urinary retention and polyuria are the most common symptoms.

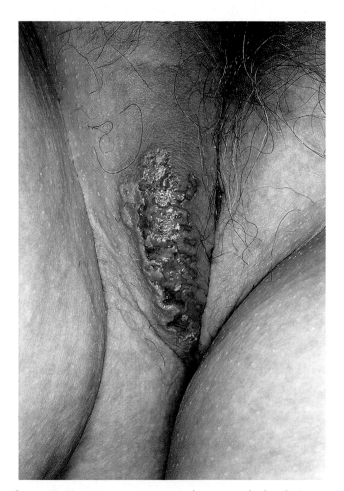

Figure 12-62 Herpes zoster may not be expected when lesions appear in unusual areas. The prodrome of pain and sudden appearance of grouped vesicles, crusts, or erosions support the diagnosis. Vesicles are macerated to form erosions in intertriginous areas.

**Plot of Duration of Any Pain from Start of
Herpes Zoster Among Patients in Two Age Groups**

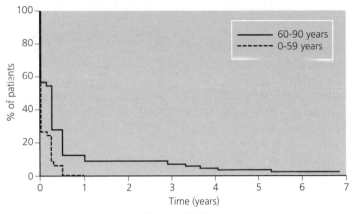

Figure 12-63

Hodgkin's disease are uniquely susceptible to herpes zoster. Furthermore, 15% to 50% of zoster patients with active Hodgkin's disease have disseminated disease involving the skin, lungs, and brain; 10% to 25% of those patients die.[74] In patients with other types of cancer, death from zoster is unusual. HIV-infected patients with zoster have increased neurologic (e.g., aseptic meningitis, radiculitis, and myelitis) and ophthalmologic complications.

Motor paresis. Muscle weakness in the muscle group associated with the infected dermatome may be observed before, during, or after an episode of herpes zoster. The paralysis usually occurs in the first 2 to 3 weeks after rash onset and can persist for several weeks. The weakness results from the spread of the virus from the dorsal root ganglia to the anterior root horn. Patients in the sixth to eighth decade of life are most commonly involved. Motor neuropathies are usually transient and approximately 75% of patients recover. They occur in approximately 5% of all cases of zoster but in up to 12% of patients with cephalic zoster. Ramsay Hunt syndrome accounts for more than half of the cephalic motor neuropathies.

Encephalitis. Neurologic symptoms characteristically appear within the first 2 weeks of onset of the skin lesions. It is possible that encephalitis is immune mediated rather than a result of viral invasion. Patients at greatest risk are those with trigeminal and disseminated zoster, as well as the immunosuppressed. The mortality rate is 10% to 20%; most survivors recover completely. The diagnosis is hampered by the fact that the virus is rarely isolated from the spinal fluid. Cell counts and protein concentration of the spinal fluid are elevated in encephalitis and in approximately 40% of typical zoster patients.

Necrosis, infection, and scarring. Elderly, malnourished, debilitated, or immunosuppressed patients tend to have a more virulent and extensive course of disease. The entire skin area of a dermatome may be lost after diffuse vesiculation. Large adherent crusts promote infection and increase the depth of involvement (Figure 12-64). Scarring, sometimes hypertrophic or keloidal (see Figures 12-57 and 12-58), follows.

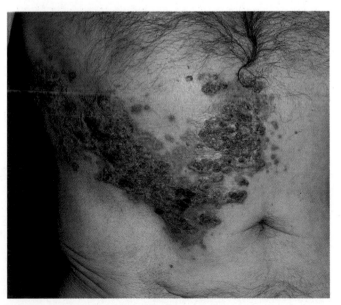

Figure 12-64 Herpes zoster. Massive involvement of a dermatome: numerous vesicles have been replaced by large crusts.

Pregnancy

Herpes zoster during pregnancy is not associated with maternal or fetal morbidity.

DIFFERENTIAL DIAGNOSIS

Herpes simplex. The diagnosis of herpes zoster is usually obvious. Herpes simplex can be extensive, particularly on the trunk. It may be confined to a dermatome and possess many of the same features as zoster (zosteriform herpes simplex). The vesicles of zoster vary in size, whereas those of simplex are uniform within a cluster. A later recurrence proves the diagnosis.

Poison ivy. A group of vesicles on a red, inflamed base may be mistaken for poison ivy (Figure 12-65).

"Zoster sine herpete." Neuralgia within a dermatome without the typical rash can be confusing. A concurrent rise in varicella zoster complement–fixation titers has been demonstrated in a number of such cases.

Cellulitis. The eruption of zoster may never evolve to the vesicular stage. The red, inflamed, edematous, or urticarial-like plaques may appear infected, but they usually have a fine, cobblestone surface indicative of a cluster of minute vesicles. A skin biopsy shows characteristic changes.

Laboratory diagnosis

A clinical diagnosis is made in most cases; laboratory confirmation is usually unnecessary. The laboratory methods for identification are the same as for herpes simplex. Tzanck smears, skin biopsy (Figures 12-66 and 12-67), antibody titers, vesicular fluid immunofluorescent antibody stains, electron microscopy, and culture of vesicle fluid are some of the studies to consider. The initial test of choice is a cytologic smear (Tzanck smear). The test does not differentiate herpes simplex from varicella. The base of an early lesion is scraped and stained with hematoxylin-and-eosin, Giemsa, Wright's, toluidine blue, or Papanicolaou. Multinucleated giant cells and epithelial cells containing acidophilic intranuclear inclusions are seen. Zoster is seen about 7 times more frequently in HIV patients. An HIV test should be ordered if indicated.

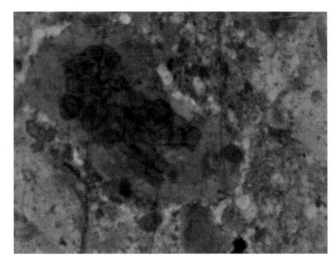

Figure 12-66 Tzanck smear. A cytologic smear of the base of a herpetic blister. The multinucleated giant cells are characteristic of herpes simplex and herpes zoster.

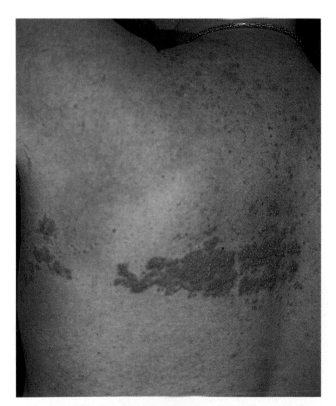

Figure 12-65 Herpes zoster mimicking poison ivy. A group of blisters on a broad base is often mistaken for an acute eczematous eruption.

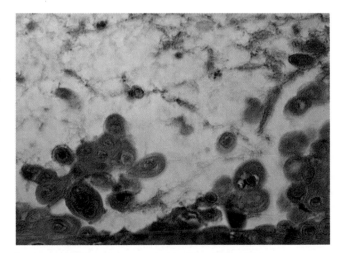

Figure 12-67 Herpes zoster. A skin biopsy showing multinucleated giant cells at the base of a vesicle.

Treatment

The aim of treatment is the suppression of inflammation, pain, and infection.

TREATMENT STRATEGY. Acute herpes zoster causes mixed somatic and neuropathic pain (pain from nerve injury) of varying intensity. Pain must be controlled. Antiviral therapy within the first 72 hours from the onset of rash or radicular pain and the use of analgesics, including opioids (if necessary), nerve blocks, and early antidepressant therapy, are treatment options. The dose and drug should be selected according to the needs of the individual patient. If less potent analgesic medications are ineffective, stronger agents should be prescribed until pain is relieved or dose-limiting side effects occur. It is possible that early, aggressive treatment may prevent PHN. Treatment with amitriptyline and related drugs, nerve blocks, and/or opioids soon after the development of acute pain may help prevent the sensitization of the central nervous system that may lead to persistence of the pain.[75] It has been suggested that vaccination of older adults may prevent PHN.[76] Varicella vaccination of older persons can boost immunity to herpes zoster.

Topical therapy. Burrow's solution or cool tap water can be used in a wet compress. The compresses, applied for 20 minutes several times a day, macerate the vesicles, remove serum and crust, and suppress bacterial growth. A whirlpool with Betadine (povidone-iodine) solution is particularly helpful in removing the crust and serum that occur with extensive eruptions in the elderly.

Antiviral drugs. Antiviral drugs reduce the severity, duration, and prevalence of PHN by as much as 50%, but 20% of patients over 50 years of age treated with famciclovir or valacyclovir report pain at 6 months (Table 12-4).[77]

Topical acyclovir. Topical acyclovir ointment applied 4 times a day for 10 days to immunocompromised patients significantly shortened complete-healing time.

Valacyclovir (Valtrex). Valacyclovir is available only as an oral formulation. After ingestion, the drug is converted to acyclovir in the gastrointestinal tract and liver. Its oral bioavailability is 3 to 5 times that of acyclovir. Studies demonstrate a significant advantage of Valtrex compared with Zovirax on decreasing the duration and incidence of pain, including both acute pain and PHN. Valacyclovir reduced the median duration of pain from 60 days after healing (with acyclovir) to 40 days. Six months after healing, only 19% of patients taking valacyclovir had pain compared with 26% of patients taking acyclovir. Patients who may have trouble complying with 5-times-daily dosing of oral Zovirax, and patients at highest risk for PHN (e.g., older patients and those with prodromal pain) may benefit from valacyclovir.

Famciclovir (Famvir). Famciclovir is an analogue of penciclovir. It is well absorbed after oral administration and is rapidly metabolized to penciclovir in the gastrointestinal tract, blood, and liver. The intracellular half-life of the active drug, penciclovir triphosphate, is very long. Famciclovir is available for oral treatment of acute uncomplicated herpes zoster. The benefits appear to be similar to those of acyclovir. It was found to decrease the duration of PHN among elderly patients compared with placebo.

Oral and intravenous acyclovir. Acyclovir decreases acute pain, inflammation, vesicle formation, and viral shedding. The median duration of pain in acyclovir recipients is 20 days vs. 62 days for their placebo counterparts. Several studies show no effect on the subsequent development of PHN, even in patients who experience immediate pain relief. A study showed a possible reduction in the incidence of PHN if treatment began within 4 days of the onset of pain or within 48 hours of the onset of rash.[78] Acyclovir appears to change the nature of PHN. Its use should be considered for immunosuppressed, debilitated patients who appear to be developing extensive cutaneous disease and for patients with ophthalmic zoster who are at increased risk of ocular complications. Treatment is most effective when started within the first 72 hours of infection. If lesions are not completely crusted and the patient is older than 50 years, immunocompromised, and/or has trigeminal zoster, treatment after 72 hours of the onset of vesicles should be considered. The recommended oral dosage is shown in Table 12-4. Proper hydration and urine flow must be maintained.

Table 12-4 Drugs for Varicella-Zoster Infections*			
	Acyclovir (Zovirax) (200-, 400-, and 800-mg capsules)	Famciclovir (Famvir) (125-, 250-, and 500-mg tablets)	Valacyclovir (Valtrex) (500- and 1000-mg caplets)
Varicella-zoster	800 mg qid daily × 7 days	500 mg q8h × 7 days	1 gm tid × 7 days
Varicella chickenpox	20 mg/kg per dose (800 mg maximum) qid × 5 days		
Varicella or zoster in immunocompromised patients	10 mg/kg IV q8h × 10 days (adult dose)		
Acyclovir-resistant infections: foscarnet (Foscavir) 40 mg/kg IV q8h × 10 days			
*Higher doses of medication may be needed in HIV-infected patients.			

Acyclovir-resistant infection. Persons with AIDS who have CD4$^+$ counts of less than 100 cells/mm^3 and transplant recipients, especially bone marrow allograft recipients, may experience infections with acyclovir-resistant VZV. Patients who have received prior repeated acyclovir treatment appear to be at the highest risk of harboring acyclovir-resistant strains. Treatment with foscarnet (40 mg/kg intravenously every 8 hours) should be initiated within 7 to 10 days in patients suspected to have acyclovir-resistant VZV infections. Foscarnet therapy should be continued for at least 10 days or until lesions are completely healed.[79]

Disseminated herpes zoster in the immunocompromised host. Acyclovir (30 mg/kg/day at 8-hour intervals) and vidarabine (continuous 12-hour infusion at 10 mg/kg/day) for 7 days (longer if resolution of cutaneous or visceral disease is incomplete) are equally effective for the treatment of disseminated herpes zoster. The resultant mortality rate is low.[80]

Oral steroids. The use of systemic steroids during the early acute phases of herpes zoster to prevent PHN has been controversial. A double-blind, controlled trial showed that prednisolone therapy initiated at a dose of 40 mg/day and tapered over a 3-week period does not reduce the frequency of PHN. Pain reduction is, however, greater during the acute phase of disease and a quicker rash resolution.[81]

There are no significant differences between steroid-treated and non–steroid-treated patients in the time to a first or a complete cessation of pain. Steroid recipients report more complications.[81]

In another controlled study, patients were treated with acyclovir and prednisone (60 mg/day for the first 7 days, 30 mg/day for days 8 to 14, and 15 mg/day for days 15 to 21). Time to total crusting and healing was accelerated. There was accelerated time to cessation of acute neuritis, time to return to uninterrupted sleep, time to return to usual daily activity, and time to cessation of analgesic therapy. Resolution of pain during the 6 months after disease onset did not statistically differ from that of patients with no treatment. No important clinical or laboratory adverse events occurred in any group. The authors concluded that in relatively healthy persons older than 50 years who have localized herpes zoster, combined acyclovir and prednisone therapy can improve quality of life.[82]

Intradermal steroids, xylocaine, and epinephrine. Attenuation or elimination of pain in the eruptive stage and for PHN may be accomplished with the following technique.[83] Lidocaine (Xylocaine) 0.5% to a total of 4 to 5 ml is injected into the subcutaneous tissue at the most painful sites. For patients with intolerable pain and/or necrotic herpes zoster, 2 ml of 1% lidocaine is injected deep into the proximal area, innervating the herpes zoster lesions. Injections are repeated every 4 to 5 days as needed. Others have claimed substantial relief with a similar schedule using subcutaneous injections through the affected skin with a combination of lidocaine and triamcinolone acetonide (Kenalog).[84] The mixture is prepared by diluting triamci-

nolone acetonide (10 mg/5 ml) with equal parts 1% lidocaine. Tumescent infiltration of corticosteroids, lidocaine, and epinephrine into dermatomes of acute herpetic pain or PHN provided immediate and sustained relief in several patients in a pilot study.[85]

Nerve blocks. Sympathetic blocks (stellate ganglion or epidural) with 0.25% bupivacaine terminates the pain of acute herpes zoster[86] and possibly prevents or relieves PHN in patients treated within 2 months of onset of the acute phase of the disease. Three injections are made on alternate days. When thoracic dermatomes are involved, an epidural catheter is left in place for the 5 days of therapy to avoid having to replace the needle each time. Epidural injections are made at or just above the highest dermatome of the rash. There is prompt relief of pain and all symptoms are usually gone after the second injection.[87] Sympathetic blockade applied within the first 2 months after the onset of acute herpes zoster terminates[88] the acute phase of the disease, probably by restoring intraneural blood flow and thus preventing the death of the large fibers and avoiding the development of PHN. After 2 months, the damage to the large fibers is irreversible.

Prevention of postherpetic neuralgia: early combined antiviral drugs and antidepressants

It is possible that very early treatment with an antiviral and an antidepressant would greatly shorten the duration of pain in herpes zoster and thereby reduce the likelihood of PHN. Patients were given amitriptyline 25 mg, starting within 48 hours of onset of the rash and continuing for 90 days. The results of this study strongly suggest that early treatment of older patients with acute herpes zoster with low-dose amitriptyline reduces the long-term prevalence of PHN.[89]

Treatment of postherpetic neuralgia

The nature of the pain. PHN has many characteristics. There is frequently a steady, burning pain; a paroxysmal pain like that of an electric shock; and exquisite sensitivity of the skin, often with allodynia (pain from an ordinarily nonpainful stimulus). Allodynic pain from light tactile stimulation, such as that from clothing, hair, or even a breeze, can be one of the most debilitating problems faced by patients with PHN. There may be deterioration in the quality of life; patients may become reclusive, unable to bear the lightest contact of clothing against the affected skin.[90]

POSTHERPETIC NEURALGIA TREATMENT OPTIONS. An algorithm for the treatment of herpes zoster and PHN appears on p. 405. First-line therapy for neuropathic pain may be either an older-generation antidepressant such as amitriptyline or nortriptyline or the anticonvulsant gabapentin. For refractory cases, chronic opioid therapy may be the only avenue of relief, and evidence is accumulating that this approach is safe if proper guidelines are observed.[75]

TREATMENT OF HERPES ZOSTER AND POSTHERPETIC NEURALGIA

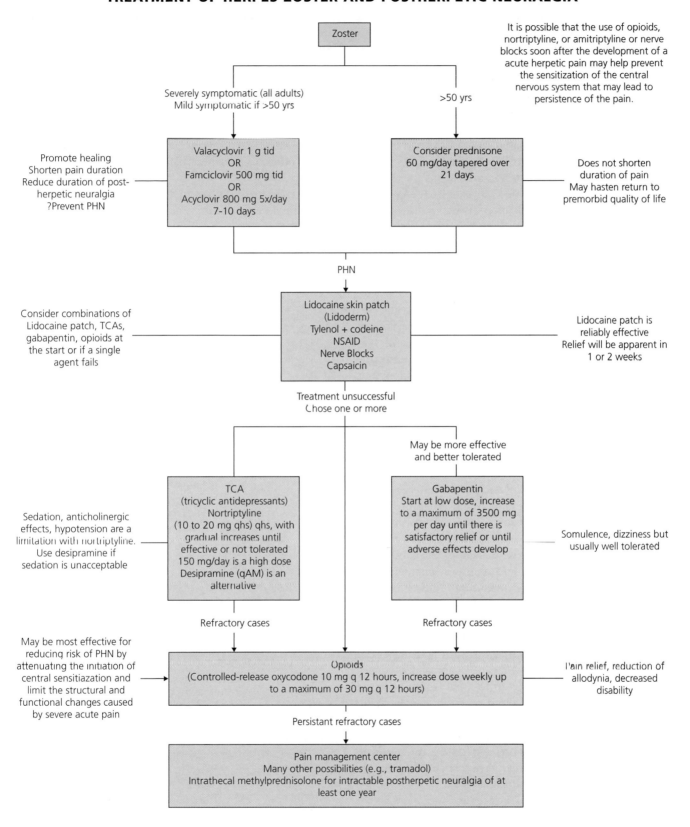

Zoster

It is possible that the use of opioids, nortriptyline, or amitriptyline or nerve blocks soon after the development of a acute herpetic pain may help prevent the sensitization of the central nervous system that may lead to persistence of the pain.

Severely symptomatic (all adults)
Mild symptomatic if >50 yrs

>50 yrs

Promote healing
Shorten pain duration
Reduce duration of post-
herpetic neuralgia
?Prevent PHN

Valacyclovir 1 g tid
OR
Famciclovir 500 mg tid
OR
Acyclovir 800 mg 5x/day
7-10 days

Consider prednisone
60 mg/day tapered over
21 days

Does not shorten
duration of pain
May hasten return to
premorbid quality of life

PHN

Consider combinations of
Lidocaine patch, TCAs,
gabapentin, opioids at
the start or if a single
agent fails

Lidocaine skin patch
(Lidoderm)
Tylenol + codeine
NSAID
Nerve Blocks
Capsaicin

Lidocaine patch is
reliably effective
Relief will be apparent in
1 or 2 weeks

Treatment unsuccessful
Chose one or more

May be more effective
and better tolerated

Sedation, anticholinergic
effects, hypotension are a
limitation with nortriptyline.
Use desipramine if
sedation is unacceptable

TCA
(tricyclic antidepressants)
Nortriptyline
(10 to 20 mg qhs) qhs, with
gradual increases until
effective or not tolerated
150 mg/day is a high dose
Desipramine (qAM) is an
alternative

Gabapentin
Start at low dose, increase
to a maximum of 3500 mg
per day until there is
satisfactory relief or until
adverse effects develop

Somulence, dizziness but
usually well tolerated

Refractory cases

Refractory cases

May be most effective for
reducing risk of PHN by
attenuating the initiation of
central sensitiazation and
limit the structural and
functional changes caused
by severe acute pain

Opioids
(Controlled-release oxycodone 10 mg q 12 hours, increase dose weekly up
to a maximum of 30 mg q 12 hours)

Pain relief, reduction of
allodynia, decreased
disability

Persistant refractory cases

Pain management center
Many other possibilities (e.g., tramadol)
Intrathecal methylprednisolone for intractable postherpetic neuralgia of at
least one year

Topical lidocaine patch (Lidoderm). The topical lidocaine patch is the first Food and Drug Administration–approved drug for PHN. It has no systemic side effects and is easy to use.

Analgesics. Oral analgesics (e.g., Tylenol [acetaminophen] with codeine, Percodan [oxycodone HCl], Percocet [oxycodone HCl and acetaminophen]) should be used as needed. Aspirin and other mild analgesic drugs are commonly used in patients with PHN, but their value is limited. Ibuprofen is ineffective.

Tricyclic antidepressants. Antidepressants such as amitriptyline, nortriptyline, desipramine, and maprotiline, given in low doses, have been used for years. They are thought to act independent of their antidepressant actions (because relief of PHN occurs at less than antidepressant dosages). Amitriptyline is a standard therapy for PHN. Start amitriptyline at low doses (10 to 25 mg) and gradually increase this to doses of 50 to 75 mg over 2 to 3 weeks in all patients older than 60 years as soon as shingles is diagnosed. Nortriptyline is a noradrenergic metabolite of amitriptyline. Amitriptyline and nortriptyline have a similar analgesic action. Pain relief occurs without an antidepressant effect with nortriptyline, and there are fewer side effects with nortriptyline.[91] Therefore nortriptyline is the preferred antidepressant, although desipramine may be used if the patient experiences unacceptable sedation from nortriptyline. Desipramine has a low incidence of anticholinergic and sedative effects. As many as half the patients do not have a response to these drugs or have intolerable side effects. These drugs have only a moderate effect.

Gabapentin. The anticonvulsant drug gabapentin is effective in the treatment of pain and sleep interference associated with PHN. Mood and quality of life also improve with gabapentin therapy. In one study the dosage was increased over a 4-week period to a maximum dosage of 3600 mg/day. Dosage is increased until there is satisfactory relief or until serious adverse effects develop. Treatment was maintained for an additional 4 weeks at the maximum tolerated dose.[92] Somnolence, dizziness, ataxia, and peripheral edema are side effects.

Oxycodone. Controlled-release oxycodone (10 mg every 12 hours) is an effective analgesic for the management of steady pain, paroxysmal spontaneous pain, and allodynia. The dose was increased weekly up to a maximum of 30 mg every 12 hours.[93] Others have found narcotics ineffective for the long-term control of pain from PHN and to be associated with unacceptable side effects.[94]

Intrathecal methylprednisolone. Patients with intractable PHN for at least 1 year were treated with intrathecal methylprednisolone and lidocaine (3 ml of 3% lidocaine with 60 mg of methylprednisolone acetate) once per week for up to 4 weeks. Each dose was injected into the lumbar intrathecal space. The treatment provided good or excellent analgesia for the burning and lancinating pain and allodynia of PHN in nearly all of the patients who received it. The pain relief lasted throughout the 2 years of follow-up.[95] This procedure is performed only by anesthesiologists, with appropriate monitoring and equipment.

Capsaicin. Capsaicin is a chemical that depletes the pain impulse transmitter substance P and prevents its resynthesis within the neuron. Substantial relief of pain follows the application (3 to 5 times daily) of this chemical in the form of a white cream (Zostrix and Zostrix-HP).[96] Substantial pain relief occurs in 4 weeks in most patients. Maximum benefit occurs when capsaicin cream is applied for many weeks. The application of EMLA or topical lidocaine before capsaicin may prevent burning. Do not apply capsaicin to the unhealed skin lesions of acute zoster. Capsaicin is available without prescription. Some experts believe that this medication is not effective.

Emotional support. Patients with PHN can be miserable for several months. Emotional support is as important as other therapeutic measures.

References

1. Tyring S: Human papillomavirus infections: epidemiology, pathogenesis, and host immune response, J Am Acad Dermatol 2000; 43(1 Pt 2):S18.

2. Berth-Jones J, et al: Value of a second freeze-thaw cycle in cryotherapy of common warts, Br J Dermatol 1994; 131:883.

3. Phillips RC, et al: Treatment of warts with Candida antigen injection, Arch Dermatol 2000; 136:1274.

4. Johnson SM, Roberson PK, Horn TD: Intralesional injection of mumps or Candida skin test antigens: a novel immunotherapy for warts, Arch Dermatol 2001; 137:451.

5. Signore RJ: Candida immunotherapy of warts, Arch Dermatol 2001; 137:1250.

6. Silverberg NB, et al: Squaric acid immunotherapy for warts in children, J Am Acad Dermatol 2000; 42(5 Pt 1):803.

7. Micali G, et al: Treatment of cutaneous warts with squaric acid dibutylester: a decade of experience, Arch Dermatol 2000; 136:557.

8. Schwab R, Elston D: Topical imiquimod for recalcitrant facial flat warts, Cutis 2000; 65:160.

9. Lockshin NA: Flat facial warts treated with fluorouracil, Arch Dermatol 1979; 115:929.

10. Lee S, Kim J-G, Chun SI: Treatment of verruca plana with 5% 5-fluorouracil ointment, Dermatologica 1980; 160:383.

11. Pringle WM, Helms BC: Treatment of plantar warts by blunt dissection, Arch Dermatol 1973; 108:79.

12. Sparling J, Checketts S, Chapman M: Imiquimod for plantar and periungual warts, Cutis 2001; 68:397.

13. Ahmed I, et al: Liquid nitrogen cryotherapy of common warts: cryo-spray vs. cotton wool bud, Br J Dermatol 2001; 144:1006.

14. Munn S, et al: A new method of intralesional bleomycin therapy in the treatment of recalcitrant warts, Br J Dermatol 1996; 135:969.

15. Sollitto R, Pizzano D: Bleomycin sulfate in the treatment of mosaic plantar verrucae: a follow-up study, J Foot Ankle Surg 1996; 35:169.

16. James MP, et al: Histologic, pharmacologic, and immunocytochemical effects of injection of bleomycin into viral warts, J Am Acad Dermatol 1993; 28:933.

17. Tosti A, Piraccini B: Warts of the nail unit: surgical and nonsurgical approaches, Dermatol Surg 2001; 27:235.

18. Habif TP, Graf FA: Extirpation of subungual and periungual warts by blunt dissection, J Dermatol Surg Oncol 1981; 7:553.

19. Focht DR, et al: The efficacy of duct tape vs cryotherapy in the treatment of verruca vulgaris (the common wart), Arch Pediatr Adolesc Med 2002; 156(10):971.

20. Shelley WB, Burmeister V: Office diagnosis of molluscum contagiosum by light microscopic demonstration of virions, Cutis 1985:465.

21. Silverberg N, Sidbury R, Mancini A: Childhood molluscum contagiosum: experience with cantharidin therapy in 300 patients, J Am Acad Dermatol 2000; 43:503.

22. Strauss R, et al: Successful treatment of molluscum contagiosum with topical imiquimod in a severely immunocompromised HIV-positive patient, Int J STD AIDS 2001; 12:264.

23. Barba A, Kapoor S, Berman B: An open label safety study of topical imiquimod 5% cream in the treatment of Molluscum contagiosum in children, Dermatol Online J 2001; 7:20.

24. Romiti R, Ribeiro A, Romiti N: Evaluation of the effectiveness of 5% potassium hydroxide for the treatment of molluscum contagiosum, Pediatr Dermatol 2000; 17:495.

25. Markos A: The successful treatment of molluscum contagiosum with podophyllotoxin (0.5%) self-application, Int J STD AIDS 2001; 12:833.

26. Garrett SJ, Robinson JK, Roenigk RR Jr: Trichloroacetic acid peel of molluscum contagiosum in immunocompromised patients, J Dermatol Surg Oncol 1992; 18:855.

27. Lafferty WE, et al: Recurrences after oral and genital herpes simplex virus infection: influence of site of infection and viral type, N Engl J Med 1987; 316:1444.

28. Spruance S, McKeough M: Combination treatment with famciclovir and a topical corticosteroid gel versus famciclovir alone for experimental ultraviolet radiation-induced herpes simplex labialis: a pilot study, J Infect Dis 2000; 181:1906.

29. Gill MJ, Arlette J, Buchan K: Herpes simplex virus infection of the hand: a profile of 79 cases, Am J Med 1988; 84:89.

30. Belongia EA, et al: An outbreak of herpes gladiatorum at a high-school wrestling camp, N Engl J Med 1991; 325:906.

31. Laskin OL: Acyclovir and suppression of frequently recurring herpetic whitlow, Ann Intern Med 1985; 102:494.

32. Novelli VM, Atherton DJ, Marshall WC: Eczema herpeticum: clinical and laboratory features, Clin Pediatr 1988; 27:231.

33. Ingrand D, et al: Eczema herpeticum of the child, Clin Pediatr 1985; 24:660.

34. Sanderson IR, et al: Eczema herpeticum: a potentially fatal disease, Br Med J 1987; 294:693.

35. Muelleman PJ, Doyle JA, House RF Jr: Eczema herpeticum treated with oral acyclovir, J Am Acad Dermatol 1986; 15:716.

36. Jawitz JC, Hines HC, Moshell AN: Treatment of eczema herpeticum with systemic acyclovir, Arch Dermatol 1985; 121:274.

37. Taieb A, Fontan I, Maleville J: Acyclovir therapy for eczema herpeticum in infants, Arch Dermatol 1985; 121:1380.

38. Jackson MA, Burry VF, Olson LC: Complications of varicella requiring hospitalization in previously healthy children, Pediatr Infect Dis J 1992; 11:441.

39. Preblud SR: Varicella: complications and costs, Pediatrics 1986; 78:728.

40. Miller HC, Stephan M. Hemorrhagic varicella: a case report and review of the complications of varicella in children, Am J Emerg Med 1993; 11:633.

41. Feldman S, Hughes WT, Daniel CB: Varicella in children with cancer: seventy-seven cases, Pediatrics 1975; 56:388.

42. Kelley R, et al: Varicella in children with perinatally acquired human immunodeficiency virus infection, J Pediatr 1994; 124:271.

43. Leibovitz E, et al: Varicella-zoster virus infection in Romanian children infected with the human immunodeficiency virus, Pediatrics 1993; 92:838.

44. Srugo I, et al: Clinical manifestations of varicella-zoster virus infections in human immunodeficiency virus-infected children, Am J Dis Child 1993; 147:742.

45. Wallace MR, et al: Varicella immunity and clinical disease in HIV-infected adults, South Med J 1994; 87:74.

46. Paryani SG, Arvin AM: Intrauterine infection with varicella-zoster virus after maternal varicella, N Engl J Med 1986; 314:1542.

47. Boyd K, Walker E: Use of acyclovir to treat chicken pox in pregnancy, Br Med J 1988; 296:393.

48. Pastuszak AL, et al: Outcome after maternal varicella infection in the first 20 weeks of pregnancy, N Engl J Med 1994; 330:901.

49. Balducci J, et al: Pregnancy outcome following first-trimester varicella infection, Obstet Gynecol 1992; 79:5.

50. Meyers JD: Congenital varicella in term infants: risk reconsidered, J Infect Dis 1974; 129:215.

51. Stagno S, Whitley RJ: Herpesvirus infections of pregnancy. Part II. Herpes simplex virus and varicella-zoster virus infections, N Engl J Med 1985; 313:1327.

52. Vazquez M, et al: The effectiveness of the varicella vaccine in clinical practice, N Engl J Med 2001; 344:955.

53. Watson B, et al: Persistence of cell-mediated and humoral immune responses in healthy children immunized with live attenuated varicella vaccine, J Infect Dis 1994; 169:197.

54. Lawrence R, et al: The risk of zoster after varicella vaccination in children with leukemia, N Engl J Med 1988; 318:543.

55. Balfour H Jr, et al: Acyclovir treatment of varicella in otherwise healthy adolescents: the Collaborative Acyclovir Varicella Study Group, J Pediatr 1992; 120:627.

56. Wallace MR, et al: Treatment of adult varicella with oral acyclovir: a randomized, placebo-controlled trial, Ann Intern Med 1992; 117:358.

57. Whitley R, et al: Vidarabine therapy of varicella in immunosuppressed patients, J Pediatr 1982; 101:125.

58. Prober CG, Kirk LE, Keeney RE: Acyclovir therapy of chicken pox in immunosuppressed children: a collaborative study, J Pediatr 1982; 101:622.

59. Kakinuma H, Itoh E: A continuous infusion of acyclovir for severe hemorrhagic varicella, N Engl J Med 1997; 336:732.

60. Varicella-zoster immune globulin for the prevention of chicken pox: recommendations of the Immunization Practices Advisory Committee, Centers for Disease Control, Department of Health and Human Services, Atlanta, Ga, Ann Intern Med 1984; 100:859.

61. Paryani SG, et al: Varicella zoster antibody titers after the administration of intravenous immune serum globulin or varicella zoster immune globulin, Am J Med 1984; 76:124.

62. Baba K, et al: Increased incidence of herpes zoster in normal children infected with varicella zoster virus during infancy: community-based follow-up study, J Pediatr 1986; 108:372.

63. Ragozzino MW, et al: Risk of cancer after herpes zoster: a population-based study, N Engl J Med 1982; 307:393.

64. Fueyo MA, Lookingbill DP: Herpes zoster and occult malignancy, J Am Acad Dermatol 1984; 11:480.

65. Gilden DH, et al: Preherpetic neuralgia, Neurology 1991; 41:1215.

66. Kost R, Straus S. Postherpetic neuralgia: predicting and preventing risk, Arch Intern Med 1997; 157:1166.

67. Buchbinder SP, et al: Herpes zoster and human immunodeficiency virus infection, J Infect Dis 1992; 166:1153.

68. McKinlay WJD: Herpes zoster in pregnancy, Br Med J 1980; 280:561.

69. Harding SP: Management of ophthalmic zoster, J Med Virol 1993; 1:97.

70. Scott MJ Sr, Scott MJ Jr: Ipsilateral deafness and herpes zoster ophthalmicus, Arch Dermatol 1983; 119:235.

71. Sweeney C, Gilden D: Ramsay Hunt syndrome, J Neurol Neurosurg Psychiatry 2001; 71:149.

72. Yamanishi T, et al: Urinary retention due to herpes virus infections, Neurourol Urodyn 1998; 17:613.

73. Helgason S, et al: Prevalence of postherpetic neuralgia after a first episode of herpes zoster: prospective study with long term follow up, BMJ 2000; 321:794.

74. Mazur MH, Dolin R: Herpes zoster at the NIH: a 20-year experience, Am J Med 1978; 65:738.

75. Watson C: The treatment of neuropathic pain: antidepressants and opioids, Clin J Pain 2000; 16(2 suppl):S49.

76. Watson C, et al: Nortriptyline versus amitriptyline in postherpetic neuralgia: a randomized trial, Neurology 1998; 51:1166.

77. Dworkin R: Prevention of postherpetic neuralgia, Lancet 1999; 353:1636.

78. Klenerman P, et al: Antiviral treatment and postherpetic neuralgia, Br Med J 1989; 298:832.

79. Balfour H Jr, et al: Management of acyclovir-resistant herpes simplex and varicella-zoster virus infections, J Acquir Immune Defic Syndr 1994; 7:254.

80. Whitley RJ, Gnann J Jr: Disseminated herpes zoster in the immunocompromised host: a comparative trial of acyclovir and vidarabine. The NIAID Collaborative Antiviral Study Group, J Infect Dis 1992; 165:450.

81. Wood MJ, et al: A randomized trial of acyclovir for 7 days or 21 days with and without prednisolone for treatment of acute herpes zoster, N Engl J Med 1994; 330:896.

82. Whitley R, et al: Acyclovir with and without prednisone for the treatment of herpes zoster: a randomized, placebo-controlled trial. The National Institute of Allergy and Infectious Diseases Collaborative Antiviral Study Group, Ann Intern Med 1996; 125:376.

83. Ogata A, et al: Local anesthesia for herpes zoster, J Dermatol 1980; 7:161.

84. Epstein E: Treatment of herpes zoster and postzoster neuralgia by subcutaneous injection of triamcinolone, Int J Dermatol 1981; 20:65.

85. Chiarello S: Tumescent infiltration of corticosteroids, lidocaine, and epinephrine into dermatomes of acute herpetic pain or postherpetic neuralgia, Arch Dermatol 1998; 134:279.

86. Riopelle JM, Naraghi M, Grush KP: Chronic neuralgia incidence following local anesthetic therapy for herpes zoster, Arch Dermatol 1984; 120:747.

87. Burney RG, Peeters-Asdourian C: Herpetic neuralgia, Semin Anesth 1985; 4:275.

88. Winnie AP, Hartwell PW: Relationship between time of treatment of acute herpes zoster with sympathetic blockade and prevention of postherpetic neuralgia: clinical support for a new theory of the mechanism by which sympathetic blockade provides therapeutic benefit, Reg Anesth 1993; 18:277.

89. Bowsher D: The effects of pre-emptive treatment of postherpetic neuralgia with amitriptyline: a randomized, double-blind, placebo-controlled trial, J Pain Symptom Manage 1997; 13:327.

90. Watson C: A new treatment for postherpetic neuralgia, N Engl J Med 2000; 343:1563.

91. Watson C, Babul N: Efficacy of oxycodone in neuropathic pain: a randomized trial in postherpetic neuralgia, Neurology 1998; 50:1837.

92. Rowbotham M, et al: Gabapentin for the treatment of postherpetic neuralgia: a randomized controlled trial, JAMA 1998; 280:1837.

93. Watson C: Postherpetic neuralgia: the importance of preventing this intractable end-stage disorder, J Infect Dis 1998; 178(suppl 1):S91.

94. Gilden D, et al: Neurologic complications of the reactivation of varicella-zoster virus, N Engl J Med 2000; 342:635.

95. Kotani N, et al: Intrathecal methylprednisolone for intractable postherpetic neuralgia, N Engl J Med 2000; 343:1514.

96. Bernstein JE, et al: Treatment of chronic postherpetic neuralgia with topical capsaicin, J Am Acad Dermatol 1987; 17:93.

❑ **Dermatophyte fungal infections**
  Tinea
  Tinea of the foot
  Pitted keratolysis
  Tinea of the groin
  Tinea of the body and face
  Tinea of the hand
  Tinea incognito
  Tinea of the scalp
  Tinea of the beard
  Treatment of fungal infections

❑ **Candidiasis (moniliasis)**
  Candidiasis of normally moist areas
  Candidiasis of large skin folds
  Candidiasis of small skin folds
  Chronic mucocutaneous candidiasis

❑ **Tinea versicolor**
  Pityrosporum folliculitis

Dermatophyte Fungal Infections

The dermatophytes include a group of fungi (ringworm) that under most conditions have the ability to infect and survive only on dead keratin; that is, the top layer of the skin (stratum corneum or keratin layer), the hair, and the nails. They cannot survive on mucosal surfaces such as the mouth or vagina where the keratin layer does not form. Very rarely, dermatophytes undergo deep local invasion and multivisceral dissemination in the immunosuppressed host. Dermatophytes are responsible for the vast majority of skin, nail, and hair fungal infections. Lesions vary in presentation and closely resemble other diseases; therefore laboratory confirmation is often required. There is evidence that genetic susceptibility may predispose a patient to dermatophyte infection. Studies show that although several blood-related members of a family may share similar manifestations of disease;[1] spouses, despite prolonged exposure, do not become infected. Patients with chronic dermatophytosis have a relatively specific defect in

delayed hypersensitivity to *Trichophyton*, but their cell-mediated responses to other antigens are somewhat depressed. There also is a greater frequency of atopy in chronically infected patients.[1]

CLASSIFICATION. Dermatophytes are classified in several ways. The ringworm fungi belong to three genera: *Microsporum, Trichophyton,* and *Epidermophyton.* There are several species of *Microsporum* and *Trichophyton* and one species of *Epidermophyton.*

Place of origin. The anthropophilic dermatophytes grow only on human skin, hair, or nails. The zoophilic varieties originate from animals but may infect humans. Geophilic dermatophytes live in soil but may infect humans.

Type of inflammation. The inflammatory response to dermatophytes varies. In general, zoophilic and geophilic dermatophytes elicit a brisk inflammatory response on skin and in hair follicles. The inflammatory response to anthropophilic fungi is usually mild.

Type of hair invasion. Some species are able to infect the hair shaft. Microscopic examination of infected hairs shows fungal spores and hyphae either inside the hair shaft or both inside and on the surface. The endothrix pattern consists of fungal hyphae inside the hair shaft, whereas the ectothrix pattern consists of fungal hyphae inside and on the surface of the hair shaft.

Spores of fungi are either large or small. The type of hair invasion is further classified as large- or small-spored ectothrix or large-spored endothrix.

CLINICAL CLASSIFICATION. *Tinea* means fungal infection. Clinically, dermatophyte infections are classified by body region. The dermatophytes, or ringworm fungi, produce a variety of disease patterns that vary with the location and species. Learning the numerous patterns of disease produced by each species is complicated and unnecessary because all dermatophytes respond to the same topical and oral agents. It is important to be familiar with the general patterns of inflammation in different body regions and to be able to interpret accurately a potassium hydroxide wet mount preparation of scale, hair, or nails. Species identification by culture is necessary only for scalp infections, inflammatory skin infections, and some nail infections.

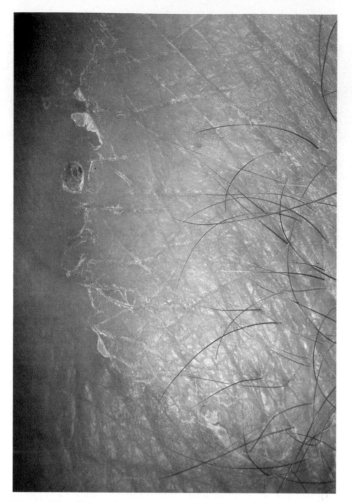

Figure 13-1 Tinea infection. Active border (classic presentation). The border is red, scaly, and slightly raised. The central area is often lighter than the surrounding normal skin.

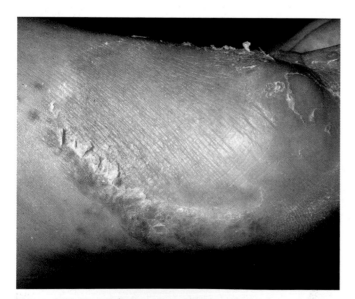

Figure 13-2 Tinea infection. Active border, which contains vesicles that indicate acute inflammation.

The active border. One very characteristic pattern of inflammation is the active border of infection. The highest numbers of hyphae are located in the active border, and this is the best area to obtain a sample for a potassium hydroxide examination. Typically the active border is scaly, red, and slightly elevated (Figure 13-1). Vesicles appear at the active border when inflammation is intense (Figure 13-2). This pattern is present in all locations except the palms and soles.

DIAGNOSIS

Potassium hydroxide wet mount preparation. The single most important test for the diagnosis of dermatophyte infection is direct visualization under the microscope of the branching hyphae in keratinized material.

Sampling scale. Scale is obtained by holding a #15 surgical blade perpendicular to the skin surface and smoothly but firmly drawing the blade with several short strokes against the scale. If an active border is present, the blade is drawn along the border at right angles to the fringe of the scale. If the blade is drawn from the center of the lesion out and parallel to the active border, some normal scale may also be included.

WET MOUNT PREPARATION. The small fragments of scale are placed on a microscope slide and gently separated, and a coverslip is applied. Potassium hydroxide (10% or 20% solution) is applied with a toothpick or eye dropper to the edge of the coverslip and allowed to run under via capillary action. The preparation is gently heated under a low flame and then pressed to facilitate separation of the epithelial cells and fungal hyphae. Potassium hydroxide dissolves material that binds together cells but does not distort the epithelial cells or fungi. Lowering the condenser of the microscope and dimming the light enhance contrast, makes hyphae easier to identify.

Nail plate keratin is thick and difficult to digest. The nail plate can be adequately softened by leaving the fragments along with several drops of potassium hydroxide in a watch glass covered with a Petri dish for 24 hours. Hair specimens require no special preparation or digestion and can be examined immediately.

MICROSCOPY. The preparation is studied carefully by scanning the entire area under the coverslip at low power. The presence of hyphae should be confirmed by examination with the ×40 objective. Slight back-and-forth rotation of the focusing knob aids visualization of the entire segment of the hyphae, which may be at different depths. It is not uncommon to find one small fragment of scale containing many hyphae and the rest of the preparation free of hyphae. The entire preparation should be studied carefully.

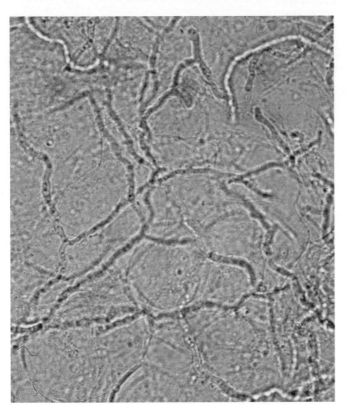

Figure 13-3 Fungal hyphae in a potassium hydroxide wet mount. The identifying characteristic is the branching, filamentous structure that is uniform in width.

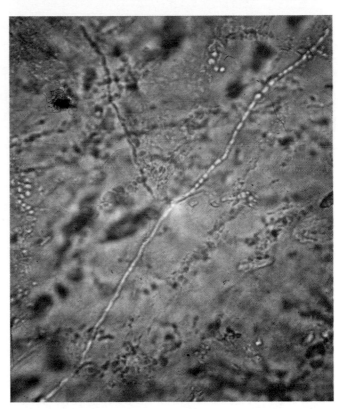

Figure 13-4 A drop of ink added to the potassium hydroxide wet mount accentuates hyphae. *(Courtesy Dr. Leanor Haley, Centers for Disease Control and Prevention.)*

INTERPRETATION. The interpretation of potassium hydroxide wet mounts takes experience. Dermatophytes appear as translucent, branching, rod-shaped filaments (hyphae) of uniform width, with lines of separation (septa) spanning the width and appearing at irregular intervals (Figures 13-3 and 13-4). The uniform width and characteristic bending and branching distinguish hyphae from hair and other debris. Hair tapers at the tip. Lines that intersect across cell walls at different planes of the scale are viewed using the fine adjustment knob of the microscope. Some hyphae contain a single-file line of bubbles in their cytoplasm. Hyphae may fragment into round or polygonal fragments that look like spores. Hyphae may be seen in combination with scale or floating free in the potassium hydroxide.

ARTIFACT. Confusion may arise with the so-called mosaic artifact produced by lipid droplets appearing in a single-file line between cells, especially from specimens taken from the palms and soles (Figure 13-5). These disappear when the cells are separated further by additional heating and pressure. Although spores and branching and short, nonbranching hyphae are seen in superficial *Candida* infections and tinea versicolor, only branching hyphae are seen in dermatophyte infections. Longitudinal, rod-shaped potassium hydroxide crystals that simulate hyphae may appear if the wet mount is heated excessively.

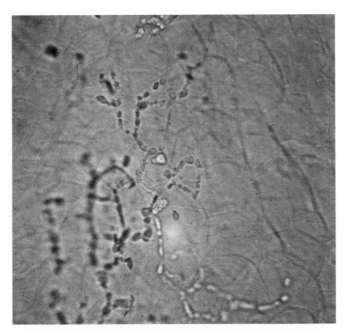

Figure 13-5 Mosaic artifact. Lipid droplets appearing in a single-file line between epithelial cells simulate fungal hyphae in potassium hydroxide wet mounts. Heat encourages cell separation and the artifact disappears. *(Courtesy Dr. Leanor Haley, Centers for Disease Control and Prevention.)*

Special stains. Hyphae may be difficult to find in a potassium hydroxide wet mount. Chlorazol Fungal Stain,[2] Swartz Lamkins Fungal Stain, or Parker's blue ink[3] clearly stains hyphae, rendering them visible under low power. The specialized stains are available from Dermatologic Lab and Supply, Inc. (www.delasco.com).

Culture. It is usually not necessary to know the species of dermatophyte infecting skin in most cases because the same oral and topical agents are active against all of them. Fungal culture is necessary for hair and nail fungal infections. Scalp hair infections in children may originate from an animal that carries a typical species of dermatophyte. The animal can then be traced and treated or destroyed to prevent further infection of other humans. Nail plate, especially of the toenails, may be infected with nondermatophytes, such as the saprophytic mold Scopulariopsis, which do not respond to treatment. Identification of the genus of fungus responsible for nail plate infection is therefore necessary before embarking on a long course of treatment.

COTTON SWAB TECHNIQUE FOR CULTURE. A sterile cotton swab that is moistened with sterile water or agar from an agar plate and rubbed vigorously over the lesion produces results comparable to those obtained by scraping with a scalpel blade.[4] A light sweep over the lesion does not collect sufficient material; therefore the swab must be rubbed vigorously over the active part of the lesion and then over the surface of the agar. The swab is useful in areas that are difficult to scrape, such as the scalp, eyelids, ears, nose, and between the toes. The sterile swab is less threatening than a blade, and it is safer in situations in which the sudden movement of a child could lead to a painful stab or cut.

CULTURE MEDIA FOR TINEA. Dermatophytes are aerobic and grow on the surface of media. The three types of culture media used most often for isolation and identification are Dermatophyte Test Medium (DTM), Mycosel agar, and Sabouraud's dextrose agar. Many hospital laboratories lack the experience to interpret fungal cultures and instead send them to outside laboratories for analysis. Material to be cultured can be sent directly to a laboratory because, unlike many bacteria, fungi remain viable for days in scale and hair without being inoculated onto media. Alternatively, many hospitals and individual practitioners now rely on DTM for faster but slightly less accurate results.

DTM is a commercially available medium supplied in vials that are ready for direct inoculation. The yellow medium, which contains the indicator phenol red, turns pink in the presence of the alkaline metabolic products of dermatophytes in approximately 6 or 7 days but remains yellow in the presence of the acid metabolic products of nonpathogenic fungi. It must be discarded after 2 weeks because saprophytes can induce a similar color change from this time on. Species identification is possible with DTM but is more accurately determined with Mycosel agar and Sabouraud's agar because the dye in DTM may interfere with interpretation.

Mycosel agar is a modification of Sabouraud's medium that contains cycloheximide and chloramphenicol to prevent the growth of bacteria and saprophytic fungi; the dextrose content of Mycosel agar has been lowered and the pH has been raised to allow for better growth of dermatophytes.

Sabouraud's agar, which does not contain antibiotics, allows the growth of most fungi, including nondermatophytes. This may be useful for nail infections because the detection of nondermatophytes is desirable in nail infections; but the more selective Mycosel agar is best for evaluation of hair tinea because only dermatophytes cause hair tinea. Cultures usually become positive in 1 to 2 weeks.

CULTURE MEDIA FOR YEAST. Yeast may be isolated on plates obtained from the hospital laboratory. Acu-Nickerson is a commercially available medium in a slant for use in the isolation and identification of *Candida* species.

Wood's light examination. Light rays with a wavelength above 365 nm are produced when ultraviolet light is projected through a Wood's filter. Hair, but not the skin of the scalp, fluoresces with a blue-green color if infected with *Microsporum canis* or *Microsporum audouinii*. The rarer *Trichophyton schoenleinii* produces a paler green fluorescence of infected hair; no other dermatophytes that infect hair produce fluorescence. Fungal infections of the skin do not fluoresce, except for tinea versicolor, which produces a pale white-yellow fluorescence. Erythrasma, a noninflammatory, pale brown, scaly eruption of the toe webs, groin, and axillae caused by the bacteria *Corynebacterium minutissimum,* shows a brilliant coral-red fluorescence with the Wood's light. Wood's light examination should be performed in a dark room with a high-intensity instrument. The fluorescence of hair may be caused by tryptophan metabolites.

Tinea

Clinically, dermatophyte infections have traditionally been classified by body region. *Tinea* means fungus infection. The term *tinea capitis,* for example, indicates "dermatophyte infection of the scalp."

Tinea of the foot

The feet are the most common area infected by dermatophytes (*tinea pedis,* or "athlete's foot"). Shoes promote warmth and sweating, which encourage fungal growth. Fungal infections of the feet are common in men and uncommon in women; although uncommon, tinea pedis does occur in prepubertal children. Tinea should be considered in the differential diagnosis of children with foot dermatitis.[5,6] The occurrence of tinea pedis seems to be inevitable in immunologically predisposed individuals regardless of elaborate precautions taken to avoid the infecting organism. Locker-room floors contain fungal elements, and the use of communal baths may create an ideal condition for repeated exposure to infected material.[7] White socks do nothing to prevent tinea pedis. Once established, the individual becomes a carrier and is more susceptible to recurrences. There are many different clinical presentations of tinea pedis.

CLINICAL PRESENTATIONS. Tinea of the feet may present with the classic "ringworm" pattern (Figure 13-6), but most infections are found in the toe webs or on the soles.

Interdigital tinea pedis (toe web infection). Tight-fitting shoes compress the toes, creating a warm, moist environment in the toe webs; this environment is suited to fungal growth. The web between the fourth and fifth toes is most commonly involved, but all webs may be infected. The web can become dry, scaly, and fissured (Figure 13-7) or white, macerated, and soggy (Figure 13-7). Itching is most intense when the shoes and socks are removed. The bacterial flora is unchanged when the tinea-infected webs demonstrate scale and peeling without maceration. Overgrowth of the resident bacterial population determines the severity of interdigital toe web infection. The macerated pattern of infection occurs from an interaction of bacteria and fungus.[8] Dermatophytes initiate the damage to the stratum corneum and, by the production of antibiotics, influence the selection of a more antibiotic-resistant bacterial population.[9] The prevalence of *Staphylococcus aureus,* gram-negative bacteria, *Corynebacterium minutissimum, Staphylococcus epidermidis,* and *Micrococcus sedentarius* increases. Extension out of the web space onto the plantar surface or the dorsum of the foot is common and occurs with the typical, chronic, ringworm type of scaly, advancing border or with an acute, vesicular eruption (Figures 13-8 and 13-9). Identification of fungal hyphae in the macerated skin of the toe webs may be difficult.

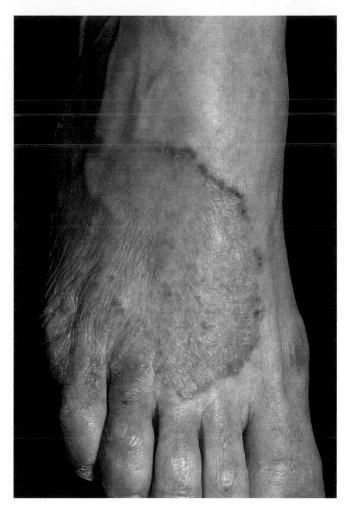

Figure 13-6 Tinea pedis. The classic "ringworm" pattern of tinea can appear on any body surface.

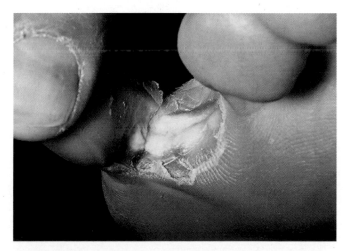

Figure 13-7 Tinea pedis (toe web infection). The toe web space contains macerated scale. The fourth web is the most commonly involved web space.

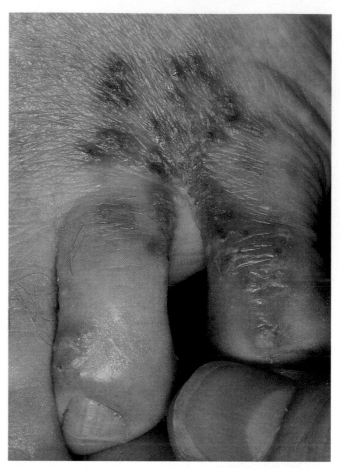

Figure 13-8 Tinea pedis. The infection has spread out of the toe web.

Chronic scaly infection of the plantar surface. Plantar hyperkeratotic or moccasin-type tinea pedis is a particularly chronic form of tinea that is resistant to treatment. The entire sole is usually infected and covered with a fine, silvery white scale (Figures 13-10 to 13-12). The skin is pink, tender, and/or pruritic. The hands may be similarly infected. It is rare to see both palms and soles infected simultaneously; rather, the pattern is infection of two feet and one hand or of two hands and one foot. *T. rubrum* is the usual pathogen. This pattern of infection is difficult to eradicate. *Trichophyton rubrum* produce substances that diminish the immune response and inhibit stratum corneum turnover.

Acute vesicular tinea pedis. A highly inflammatory fungal infection may occur, particularly in people who wear occlusive shoes. This acute form of infection often originates from a more chronic web infection. A few or many vesicles evolve rapidly on the sole or on the dorsum of the foot. The vesicles may fuse into bullae or remain as collections of fluid under the thick scale of the sole and never rupture through the surface. Secondary bacterial infection occurs commonly in eroded areas after bullae rupture. Fungal hyphae are difficult to identify in severely inflamed skin. Specimens for potassium hydroxide examination should be taken from the roof of the vesicle. A second wave of vesicles may follow shortly in the same areas or at distant sites such as the arms, chest, and along the sides of the fingers. These itchy sterile vesicles represent an allergic response to the fungus and are termed a *dermatophytid,* or *id, reaction.*[9] They subside when the infection is controlled. At times the id reaction is the only clinical manifestation of a fungus infection. Careful examination of these patients may show an asymptomatic fissure or area of maceration in the toe webs.

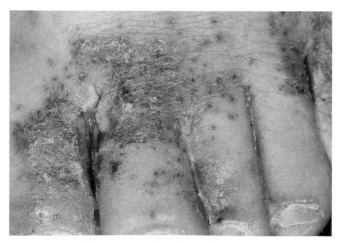

Figure 13-9 Tinea pedis. A chronic toe web and dorsal foot fungal infection have become secondarily infected with staphylococci.

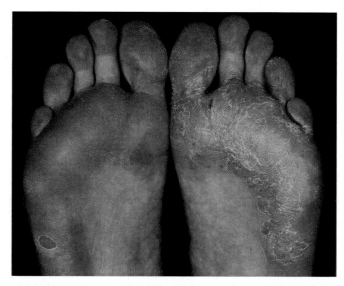

Figure 13-10 Tinea pedis. Web spaces and plantar surfaces of one foot have been inflamed for years; the other foot remains clear.

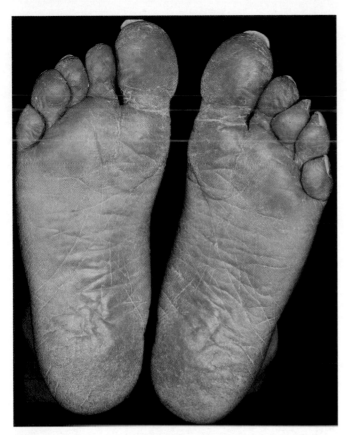

Figure 13-11 Tinea pedis. The entire plantar surface of both feet is thickened, tan colored, and covered with a fine, white scale.

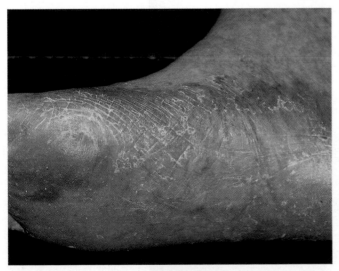

Figure 13-12 Tinea pedis. This patient has chronic inflammation of the soles that periodically flares on the dorsum and ankle.

Two feet—one hand syndrome

The two feet—one hand syndrome involves dermatophyte infection of both feet, with tinea of the right or left palm. Nail infection of the hands and feet may also be present. Most cases occur in men. The same organism infects the feet, hand, and nails. *T. rubrum* is the causative organism in most cases. The development of tinea pedis/onychomycosis generally precedes the development of tinea of the hand. Tinea manuum usually develops in the hand used to excoriate the feet or pick toenails. Patients whose occupation involves a high intensity of use of the hands are more likely to develop the disease at an earlier age.[10]

TREATMENT. The newest class of antifungal agents produces higher cure rates and more rapid responses in dermatophyte infections than do older agents such as clotrimazole. They produce a higher cure rate and lower relapse rate than the antifungal/corticosteroid combination (Lotrisone [clotrimazole/betamethasone]).[11]

Terbinafine 1% cream (Lamisil over-the-counter) applied twice daily for 1 week results in a high cure rate in interdigital tinea pedis. In one series, terbinafine gave progressive mycologic improvement; at 5 weeks after treatment, 88% of the patients were clear of infection.[12] Effective short-course therapy with potent fungicidal drugs such as terbinafine may avoid treatment failure caused by noncompliance with fungistatic agents, such as clotrimazole, that require 4 weeks of treatment. Butenafine (Mentax cream, Lotrimin Ultra over-the-counter) applied twice daily for 1 week is also highly effective in treating interdigital tinea pedis.[13] Econazole nitrate (Spectazole) has activity against several bacterial species associated with severely macerated interdigital interspaces.[14] Recurrence is prevented by wearing wider shoes and expanding the web space with a small strand of lamb's wool (Dr. Scholls' Lamb's Wool). Powders, not necessarily medicated, absorb moisture. The powders should be applied to the feet rather than to the shoes. Wet socks should be changed.

Hyperkeratotic, moccasin-type tinea of the plantar surface responds slowly to conventional therapy. Oral terbinafine 250 mg qd[15] for 2 to 6 weeks produced sustained cure rates of 71% to 94%. Griseofulvin 250 to 500 mg bid for 6 weeks resulted in a 27% to 35% cure rate.

Acute vesicular tinea pedis responds to wet Burrow's solution compresses applied for 30 minutes several times each day. Oral antifungal drugs control the acute infection. Secondary bacterial infection is treated with oral antibiotics. A vesicular id reaction sometimes occurs at distant sites during an inflammatory foot infection. Wet dressings, group V topical steroids, and, occasionally, prednisone 20 mg bid for 8 to 10 days are required for control of id reactions.

Tinea pedis has been effectively treated with pulse doses of 150 mg fluconazole once weekly, with 200 mg itraconazole qd for 2 weeks or 200 mg bid for 1 week, and with 250 mg terbinafine qd for 2 weeks.[16]

Pitted keratolysis

Pitted keratolysis, a disease mimicking tinea pedis, is an eruption of the weight-bearing surfaces of the soles. The most common sites of onset are the pressure-bearing areas, such as the ventral aspect of the toe, the ball of the foot, and the heel. Lesions are rarely seen on the non–pressure-bearing locations. Hyperhidrosis is the most frequently observed symptom. Malodor and sliminess of the skin are also distinctive features.[17]

The disease is bacterial in origin but is often misinterpreted as a fungal infection. It is characterized by many circular or longitudinal, punched-out depressions in the skin surface (Figures 13-13 and 13-14). Most cases are asymptomatic, but painful, plaquelike lesions may occur in both adults and children.[18] The eruption is limited to the stratum corneum and causes little or no inflammation. Hyperhidrosis, moist socks, or immersion of the feet favors its development. There may be a few circular pits that remain unnoticed, or the entire weight-bearing surface may be covered with annular furrows. Several bacteria have been implicated, including *Dermatophilus congolensis* and *Micrococcus sedentarius*. These bacteria produce and excrete exoenzymes (keratinase) that are able to degrade keratin and produce pitting in the stratum corneum when the skin is hydrated and the pH rises above neutrality.[19] These organisms are not easily cultured, but the filamentous and coccoid microorganisms can be demonstrated by hematoxylin and eosin staining of a formalin-fixed section of shaved stratum corneum prepared for histopathology. The clinical presentation is so characteristic that laboratory confirmation is usually not necessary.

TREATMENT. Treatment consists of promoting dryness. Socks should be changed frequently. Rapid clearing occurs with application of 20% aluminum chloride (Drysol) twice a day. Lazer Formalyde Solution (10% formaldehyde), a potent antiperspirant, is also useful. Treatment can then be applied periodically when necessary. Antibiotics are effective even without aluminum chloride or formaldehyde. The application twice a day of alcohol-based benzoyl peroxide (Panoxyl 5) may also be useful. Treatment with acne medications such as topical erythromycin solution or clindamycin solution is also curative. Mupirocin (Bactroban) ointment or cream may also be effective.[20] Oral erythromycin is an alternative.

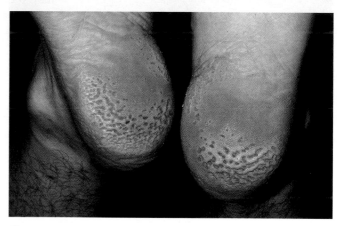

Figure 13-13 Pitted keratolysis. Deep longitudinal furrows are located primarily on weight-bearing surfaces.

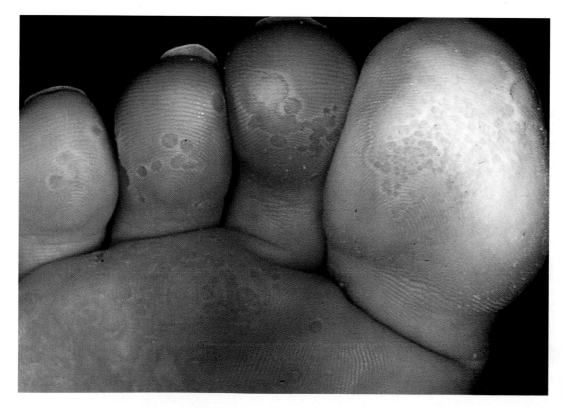

Figure 13-14 Pitted keratolysis. The skin around the deep pits is often wet and macerated.

Tinea of the groin

Tinea of the groin (*tinea cruris,* "jock itch") occurs often in the summer months after sweating or wearing wet clothing and in the winter months after wearing several layers of clothing. The predisposing factor, as with many other types of superficial infection, is the presence of a warm, moist environment. Men are affected much more frequently than are women; children rarely develop tinea of the groin. Itching becomes worse as moisture accumulates and macerates this intertriginous area.

The lesions are most often unilateral and begin in the crural fold. A half-moon–shaped plaque forms as a well-defined scaling, and sometimes a vesicular border advances out of the crural fold onto the thigh (Figure 13-15). The skin within the border turns red-brown, is less scaly, and may develop red papules. Acute inflammation may appear after a person has worn occlusive clothing for an extended period. The infection occasionally migrates to the buttock and gluteal cleft area. Involvement of the scrotum is unusual—unlike *Candida* reactions, in which it is common (Figure 13-16). Specimens for potassium hydroxide examination should be taken from the advancing scaling border.

Topical steroid creams are frequently prescribed for inflammatory skin disease of the groin, and they modify the typical clinical presentation of tinea. The eruption may be much more extensive, and the advancing, scaly border may not be present (Figure 13-35). Red papules sometimes appear at the edges and center of the lesion. This modified form (tinea incognito) may not be immediately recognized as tinea; the only clue is the history of a typical, half-moon–shaped plaque treated with cortisone cream. Scale, if present, contains numerous hyphae.

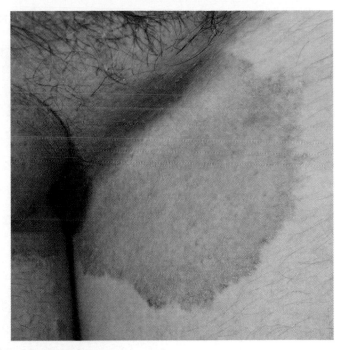

Figure 13-15 Tinea cruris. A half-moon–shaped plaque has a well-defined, scaling border.

Figure 13-16 *Candida* groin infection. Tinea cruris usually presents as a unilateral half-moon–shaped plaque that does not extend onto the scrotum. *Candida* groin infections are more extensive and often bilateral. They infect the scrotum and show the typical fringe of scale at the border and satellite pustules.

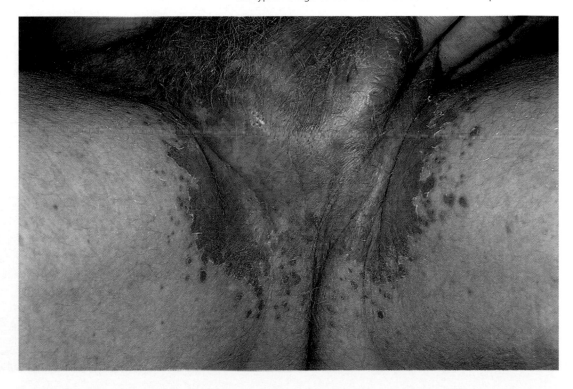

INTERTRIGO

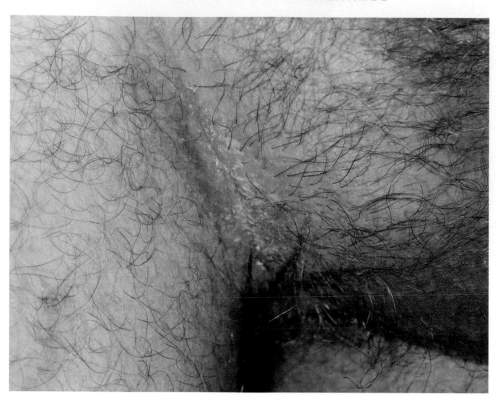

Figure 13-17 A tender, red plaque with a moist macerated surface extends to an equal extent onto the scrotum and thigh.

Figure 13-18 An advanced case with deep longitudinal fissuring in the crural fold.

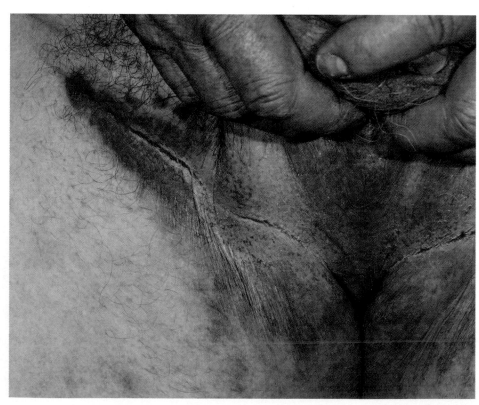

DIFFERENTIAL DIAGNOSIS

Intertrigo. A red, macerated, half-moon–shaped plaque, resembling tinea of the groin and extending to an equal extent onto the groin and down the thigh, forms after moisture accumulates in the crural fold (Figure 13-17). The sharp borders touch where the opposed skin surfaces of the skin folds of the groin and thigh meet. Obesity contributes to this inflammatory process, which may be infected with a mixed flora of bacteria, fungi, and yeast. Painful, longitudinal fissures occur in the crease of the crural fold (Figure 13-18). Groin intertrigo recurs after treatment unless weight and moisture are controlled. Psoriasis and seborrheic dermatitis of the groin may mimic intertrigo (see the section on *Candida* intertrigo).

Erythrasma. This bacterial infection (*C. minutissimum*) may be confused with tinea cruris because of the similar, half-moon–shaped plaque (Figure 13-19). Erythrasma differs in that it is noninflammatory, it is uniformly brown and scaly, and it has no advancing border. The organism produces porphyrins, which fluoresce coral-red with the Wood's light; tinea of the groin does not fluoresce. Erythrasma of the vulva may be misinterpreted as a candidal infection, especially if the Wood's light examination is negative.[21] The most common site of erythrasma is in the fourth interdigital toe space, but infection is also seen in the inframammary fold and the axillae. Gram stain of the scale shows gram-positive, rodlike organisms in long filaments. However, the scale is difficult to fix to a slide for Gram stain.

One technique is to strip the scale with clear tape and then carefully stain the taped-scale preparation. A biopsy demonstrates rods and filamentous organisms in the keratotic layer. Erythrasma responds to erythromycin (250 mg qid for 5 days) or clarithromycin[22] (single 1-gm dose) or topically to miconazole, clotrimazole, and econazole creams (but not ketoconazole). Topical acne medication such as clindamycin (Cleocin-T lotion) or erythromycin bid for 2 weeks is effective. Some topical antibiotics contain alcohol and may be irritating when applied to the groin.

TREATMENT. Tinea of the groin responds to any of the topical antifungal creams listed in the Formulary. Lesions may appear to respond quickly, but creams should be applied twice a day for at least 10 days. Moist intertriginous lesions may be contaminated with dermatophytes, other fungi, or bacteria. Antifungal creams with activity against *Candida* and dermatophytes (e.g., miconazole) are applied and covered with a cool wet Burrow's solution, water, or saline compress for 20 to 30 minutes 2 to 6 times daily until macerated, wet skin has been dried. The wet dressings are discontinued when the skin is dry, but the cream is continued for at least 14 days or until all evidence of the fungal infection has disappeared. Any residual inflammation from the intertrigo is treated with a group V through VII topical steroid twice a day for a specified length of time (e.g., 5 to 10 days). A limited amount of topical steroid cream is prescribed to discourage long-term use. Absorbent powders, not necessarily medicated (e.g., Z-Sorb), help to control moisture but should not be applied until the inflammation is gone. Resistant infections respond to any of the oral agents listed in Table 13-2.

Lotrisone solution or cream (betamethasone dipropionate/clotrimazole) may be used for initial treatment if lesions are red, inflamed, and itchy. A pure antifungal cream should be used once symptoms are controlled. Prolonged use of this steroid antifungal preparation may not cure the infection and may cause striae in this intertriginous area.

Systemic therapy is sometimes necessary. Tinea cruris is effectively treated by 50 to 100 mg fluconazole qd or 150 mg once weekly for 2 to 3 weeks, by 100 mg itraconazole qd for 2 weeks or 200 mg qd for 7 days, and by 250 mg terbinafine qd for 1 to 2 weeks.[16] Griseofulvin 500 mg qd for 4 to 6 weeks is also effective.[23]

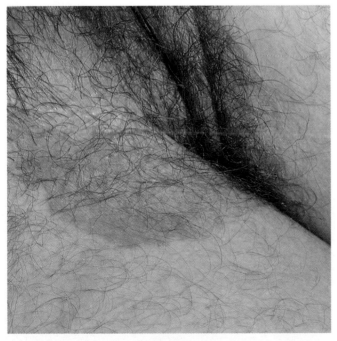

Figure 13-19 Erythrasma: a bacterial infection *(Corynebacterium minutissimum)*. The diffuse brown, scaly plaque resembles tinea cruris.

Tinea of the body and face

Tinea of the face (excluding the beard area in men), trunk, and limbs is called *tinea corporis* ("ringworm of the body"). The disease can occur at any age and is more common in warm climates. There is a broad range of manifestations, with lesions varying in size, degree of inflammation, and depth of involvement. This variability is explained by differences in host immunity and the species of fungus. An epidemic of tinea corporis caused by *Trichophyton tonsurans* was reported in student wrestlers.[24]

ROUND ANNULAR LESIONS. In classic ringworm, lesions begin as flat, scaly spots that then develop a raised border that extends out at varying rates in all directions. The advancing, scaly border may have red, raised papules or vesicles. The central area becomes brown or hypopigmented and less scaly as the active border progresses outward (Figure 13-20). However, it is not uncommon to see several red papules in the central area (Figures 13-22 and 13-24). There may be just one ring that grows to a few centimeters in diameter and then resolves or several annular lesions that enlarge to cover large areas of the body surface (Figures 13-21, 13-23, and 13-24). These larger lesions tend to be mildly itchy or asymptomatic. They may reach a certain size and remain for years with no tendency to resolve. Clear, central areas of the larger lesions are yellow-brown and usually contain several red papules. The borders are serpiginous or annular and very irregular.

Pityriasis rosea and multiple small annular lesions of ringworm may appear to be similar. However, the scaly ring of pityriasis rosea does not reach the edge of the red border as it does in tinea. Other distinguishing features of pityriasis rosea include rapid onset of lesions and localization to the trunk. Tinea from cats may appear suddenly as multiple round-to-oval plaques on the trunk and extremities.

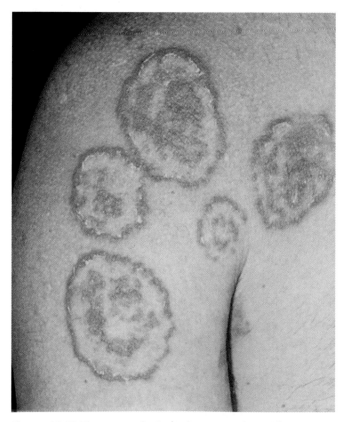

Figure 13-20 Tinea corporis. A classic presentation with an advancing red, scaly border. The reason for the designation "ringworm" is obvious.

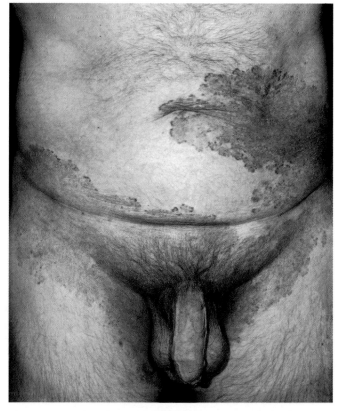

Figure 13-21 Tinea corporis. The border areas are fairly distinct and contain red papules. The central area is light brown and scaly.

TINEA OF THE FACE AND BODY

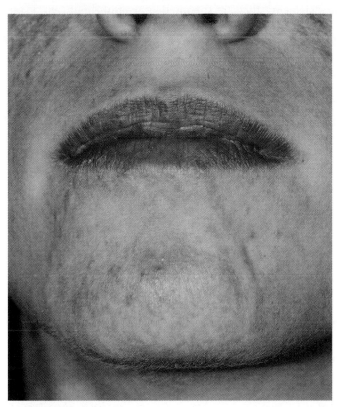

Figure 13-22 Tinea of the face. Sharply defined borders extend from the lip to the chin. The central area is hypopigmented.

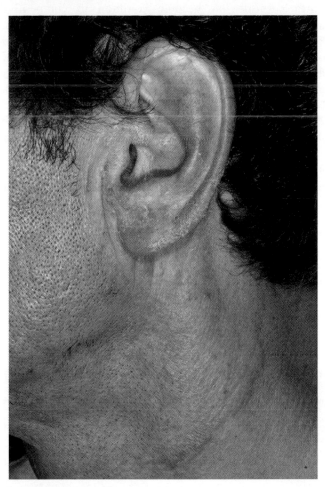

Figure 13-23 Tinea of the face. The plaque involves the entire face. A sharp border occurs on the neck.

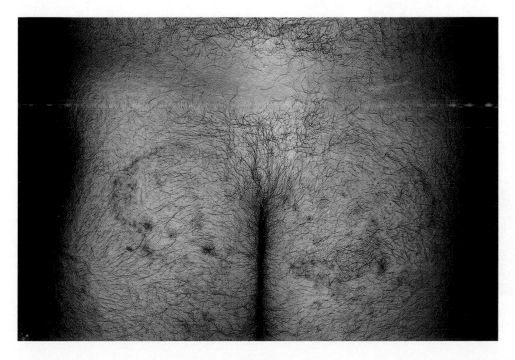

Figure 13-24 The fungal infection has extended deep into the follicles, creating a papular surface. Topical antifungal agents may not penetrate deep enough to adequately treat this process.

Tinea gladiatorum

Tinea corporis has become common in competitive wrestling. Most reported cases are caused by *T. tonsurans*. Person-to-person contact is probably the main source of transmission. The role of potential asymptomatic carriers of dermatophytes is unknown.[25,26]

DEEP INFLAMMATORY LESIONS. Zoophilic fungi such as *T. verrucosum* from cattle may produce a very inflammatory skin infection (Figures 13-25, 13-26, and 13-27).[27] The infection is more common in northern regions, where cattle are confined in close quarters during the winter. The round, intensely inflamed lesion has a uniformly elevated, red, boggy, pustular surface. The pustules are follicular and represent deep penetration of the fungus into the hair follicle (Figures 13-25 and 13-27). Secondary bacterial infection can occur. The process ends with brown hyperpigmentation and scarring (Figure 13-26). A fungal culture helps to identify the animal source of the infection.

A distinctive form of inflammatory tinea called Majocchi's granuloma[28] that is caused by *T. rubrum* and other species[29] was originally described as occurring on the lower legs of women who shave, but it is also seen at other sites on men and children. The primary lesion is a follicular papulopustule or inflammatory nodule. Intracutaneous and subcutaneous granulomatous nodules arise from these initial inflammatory tinea infections. Lesions have necrotic areas containing fungal elements; they are surrounded by epithelioid cells, giant cells, lymphocytes, and polymorphonuclear leukocytes, and they are believed to result from the rupturing of infected follicles into the dermis and subcutis: thus the term *granuloma*. There is marked variation from the usual hyphal forms. These include yeast forms, bizarre hyphae, and mucinous coatings. These variations may be a factor in allowing the dermatophytes to persist and grow in an abnormal manner.[29] Lesions are single or multiple and discrete or confluent. The area involved covers a few to 10 cm and may be red and scaly, but it is not as intensely inflamed as the *T. verrucosum* infection described earlier. The border may not be well defined. Skin biopsy with special stains for fungi is required for diagnosis if hyphae cannot be demonstrated in scale or hair.

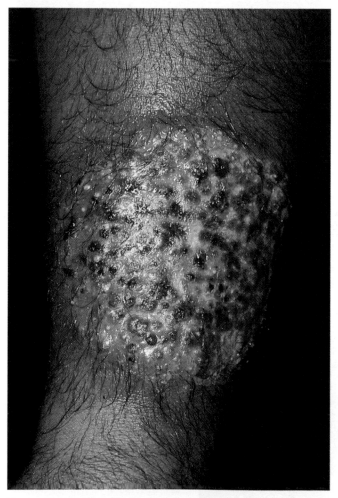

Figure 13-25 *Trichophyton verrucosum,* a zoophilic fungi from cattle that causes intense inflammation in humans.

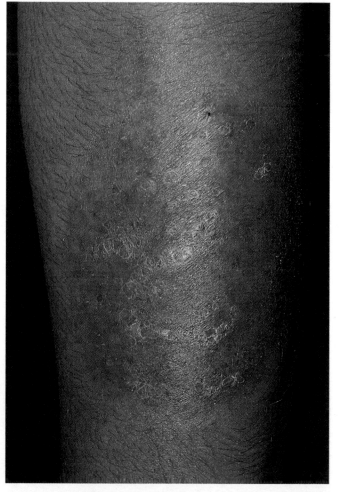

Figure 13-26 *Trichophyton verrucosum.* The deep inflammatory infection has caused brown hyperpigmentation and scarring. The hair follicles were destroyed.

TREATMENT. The superficial lesions of tinea corporis respond to the antifungal creams described in the Formulary. Lesions usually respond after 2 weeks of twice-a-day application, but treatment should be continued for at least 1 week after resolution of the infection. Extensive superficial lesions or those with red papules respond more predictably to oral therapy (see Table 13-2). Tinea corporis is treated by 50 to 100 mg fluconazole qd or 150 mg once weekly for 2 to 4 weeks, by 100 mg itraconazole qd for 2 weeks or 200 mg qd for 7 days, and by 250 mg terbinafine qd for 1 to 2 weeks.[30] The recurrence rate is high for those with extensive superficial infections. Deep inflammatory lesions require 1 to 3 or more months of oral therapy. Inflammation can be reduced with wet Burrow's solution compresses, and bacterial infection is treated with the appropriate oral antibiotics. Some authors believe that oral or topical antifungal agents do not alter the course of highly inflammatory tinea (e.g., tinea verrucosum), because the intense inflammatory response destroys the organisms. However, oral antifungals are safe, and few physicians would withhold such therapy. As with tinea capitis kerion infections, a short course of prednisone may be considered for patients who have highly inflamed kerions, such as the patient in Figure 13-25.[31]

INVASIVE DERMATOPHYTE INFECTION. Dermatophytes are typically confined within the keratinized, epithelial layer of the skin. The pathogenic potential is dependent, however, on a variety of local and systemic factors affecting the natural host resistance to dermatophytic infection. Underlying systemic conditions that cause depressed cellular immunity, such as malignant lymphomas and Cushing's disease, as well as the administration of exogenous steroids or immunosuppressive agents, can lead to atypical, generalized, or invasive dermatophyte infection. Invasive dermatophyte infection should be included in the differential diagnosis of nodular, firm, or fluctuant masses (particularly on the extremities).[32] Several dermatophyte species have caused a deep, generalized infection in which the organism invaded various visceral organs.[33]

Figure 13-27 *Trichophyton verrucosum.* "Barn itch" occurred in this farmer who rested his head against the cow while milking. Fungal infections caught from animals are often intensely inflamed.

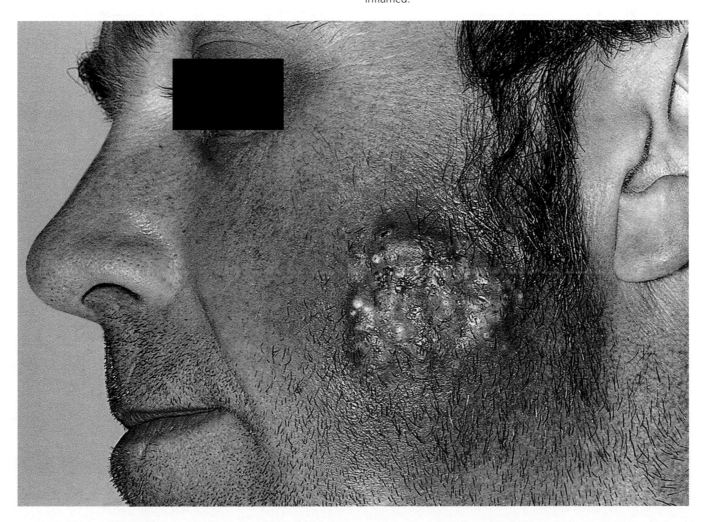

TINEA OF THE HAND

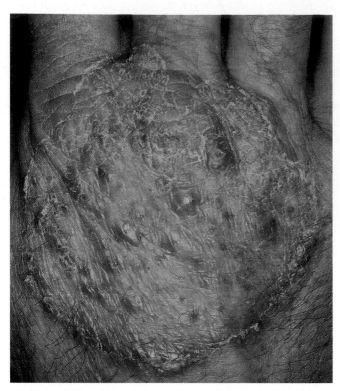

Figure 13-28 The classic "ringworm" pattern of infection with a prominent scaling border.

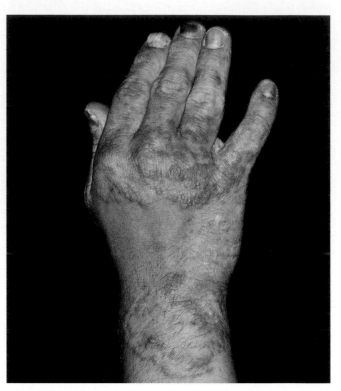

Figure 13-29 The infected areas are red with little or no scale. Note infection of the fingernails.

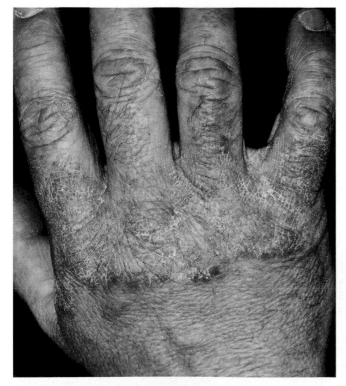

Figure 13-30 There is a well-defined red border. Scaling is present, in contrast to the case illustrated in Figure 13-29.

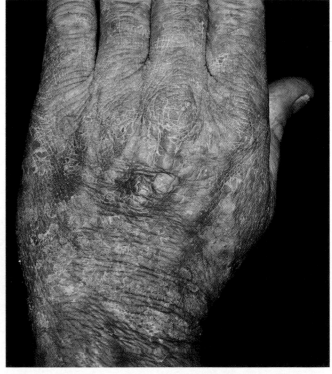

Figure 13-31 There is diffuse erythema and scaling, simulating contact dermatitis.

Tinea of the hand

Tinea of the dorsal aspect of the hand (tinea manuum) (Figures 13-28 to 13-31) has all of the features of tinea corporis; tinea of the palm (Figure 13-32) has the same appearance as the dry, diffuse, keratotic form of tinea on the soles. The dry keratotic form may be asymptomatic and the patient may be unaware of the infection, attributing the dry, thick, scaly surface to hard physical labor. Tinea of the palms is frequently seen in association with tinea pedis. The usual pattern of infection is involvement of one foot and two hands or of two feet and one hand. Fingernail infection often accompanies infection of the dorsum of the hand or palm. Treatment is the same as for tinea pedis and, as with the soles, a high recurrence rate can be expected for palm infection.

Figure 13-32 The involved palm is thickened, very dry, and scaly. The patient is often unaware of the infection and feels that these changes are secondary to dry skin or hard physical labor.

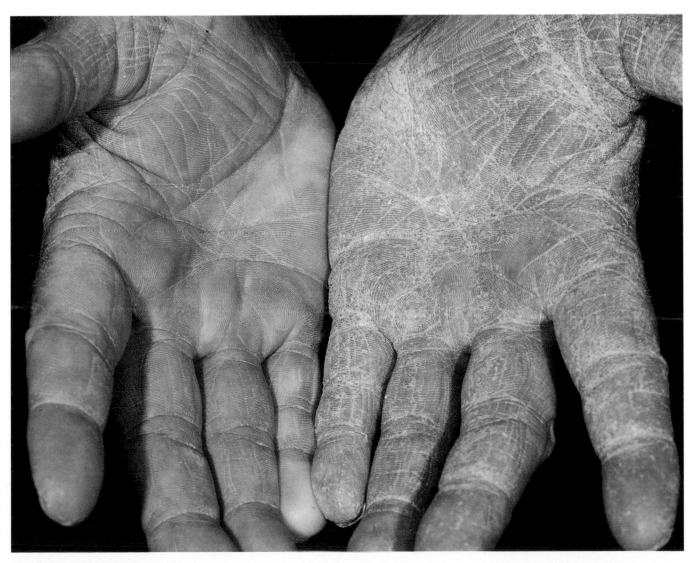

Tinea incognito

Fungal infections treated with topical steroids often lose some of their characteristic features. Topical steroids decrease inflammation and give the false impression that the rash is improving while the fungus flourishes secondary to cortisone-induced immunologic changes. Treatment is stopped, the rash returns, and memory of the good initial response prompts reuse of the steroid cream, but by this time the rash has changed. Scaling at the margins may be absent. Diffuse erythema, diffuse scale, scattered pustules (Figures 13-33, 13-34, and 13-35) or papules, and brown hyperpigmentation may all result. A well-defined border may not be present and a once-localized process may have expanded greatly. The intensity of itching is variable. Tinea incognito is most often seen on the groin (Figure 13-35), on the face, and on the dorsal aspect of the hand. Tinea infections of the hands are often misdiagnosed as eczema and treated with topical steroids. Hyphae are easily demonstrated, especially a few days after discontinuing use of the steroid cream when scaling reappears.

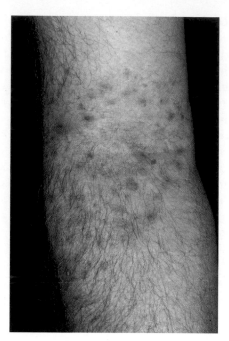

Figure 13-33 Tinea incognito. The antecubital fossa is a common area to find atopic eczema. This patient had tinea that was misdiagnosed as eczema. Potent topical steroids allowed the process to extend and penetrate deep into follicles.

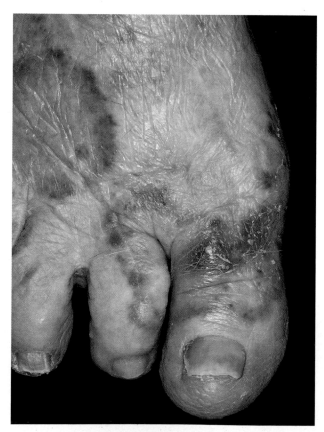

Figure 13-34 Tinea incognito. Tinea had extended out of the toe web and a diagnosis of eczema was made. Topical steroid treatment then allowed the active border to extend.

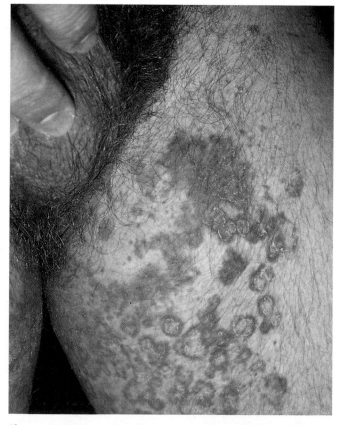

Figure 13-35 Tinea incognito. A group IV topical steroid was applied to the area of tinea cruris for 3 weeks. Characteristic features of tinea are missing.

Tinea of the scalp

Tinea of the scalp (tinea capitis) occurs most frequently in prepubertal children between 3 and 7 years of age. The infection has several different presentations.[34] The species of dermatophyte likely to cause tinea capitis varies from country to country, but anthropophilic species (found in humans) predominate in most areas. Tinea capitis is most common in areas of poverty and crowded living conditions. The infection originates from contact with a pet or an infected person. Each animal is associated with a limited number of fungal species; therefore an attempt should be made to identify the fungus by culture to help locate and treat a possible animal source.[35] Spores are shed in the air in the vicinity of the patient. Therefore direct contact is not necessary to spread infection. Unlike other fungal infections, tinea of the scalp may be contagious by direct contact or from contaminated clothing; this provides some justification for briefly isolating those with proven infection.

TRANSMISSION. Large family size, crowding, and low socioeconomic status increase the chance of infection. Infectious fungal particles that have fallen from the infected person may be viable for months. Tinea capitis can be transmitted by infected persons, fallen hairs, animals, fomites (clothing, bedding, hairbrushes, combs, hats), and furniture. Zoophilic dermatophytes are acquired from contact with pets or wild animals. Cats and dogs are the source of *M. canis*. Farmers acquire *T. verrucosum* from touching the hide of infected cattle. *Microsporum gypseum* infection comes from contaminated soil.

Asymptomatic scalp carriage of dermatophytes by classmates and adults is probably an important factor contributing to disease transmission and reinfection. The asymptomatic carriage persists for an indefinite period.

HAIR SHAFT INFECTION. Hair shaft infection is preceded by invasion of the stratum corneum of the scalp. (See diagram of hair anatomy on p. 835.) The fungus grows down through this dead protein layer into the hair follicle and gains entry into the hair in the lower intrafollicular zone, just below the point where the cuticle of the hair shaft is formed. Because of the cuticle, the fungi cannot cross over from the perifollicular stratum corneum into the hair but must go deep into the hair follicle to circumvent the cuticle.[36] This may explain why topical antifungal agents are ineffective for treating tinea capitis. The fungi then invade the keratinized, outer root sheath, enter the inner cortex, and digest the keratin contained inside the hair shaft. The growth of hyphae occurs within the hair above the zone of keratinization of the hair shaft and keeps pace with the growth of hair. Distal to this zone of active growth, arthrospores are formed within or on the surface of the hair, depending on the species of dermatophytes. Hyphae grow inside and fragment into short segments called *arthrospores*. The arthrospores remain inside the hair shaft in the endothrix pattern (Figure 13-36). In the ectothrix type, they dislodge (Figure 13-37), obscure and penetrate the surface cuticle on the hair shaft surface, and form a sheath of closely packed spheres. The arthrospores are either large (6 to 10 mm) or small (2 to 3 mm). Large spores can be seen as separate structures with the low-power microscope objective. Higher power is needed to see the small spores.

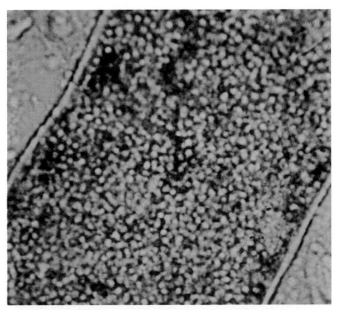

Figure 13-36 Large spore endothrix pattern of hair invasion (*Trichophyton tonsurans* "a sack of marbles").

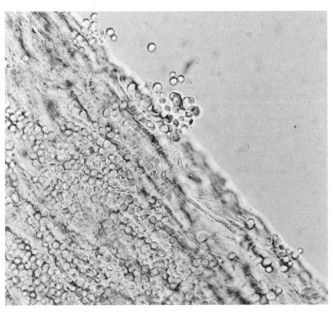

Figure 13-37 Large spore ectothrix pattern of hair invasion (*Trichophyton verrucosum*).

ENDOTHRIX PATTERN OF INVASION. Endothrix hair invasion is produced predominantly by *T. tonsurans*, *Trichophyton soudanense*, and *Trichophyton violaceum*. The fungus grows completely within the hair shaft, and the cuticle surface of the hair remains intact. The hyphae within the hair are converted to arthroconidia (spores). The spores remain in the hair shaft. In "black dot" tinea capitis caused by *T. tonsurans* and *T. violaceum*, the hair cortex is almost completely replaced by spores and swells at the infundibular level, impeding further exit of the growing hair and causing the already weakened hair to coil up inside the infundibulum, forming a black dot.[37] Endothrix infections tend to progress, become chronic, and may last into adult life.

ECTOTHRIX PATTERN OF INVASION. Ectothrix hair invasion is associated with *Microsporum audouinii*, *M. canis*, and *T. verrucosum*. Inflammatory tinea related to exposure to a kitten or puppy usually is a fluorescent small-spore ectothrix. Some of the hyphae destroy, break through the surface of the hair shaft (cuticle) and invade the keratinized inner root sheath that grows around the exterior of the hair shaft. The hyphae are subsequently converted into infectious arthrospores (arthroconidia). The arthrospores are located both on the inside of the hair shaft and on the outer surface to produce the ectothrix pattern seen under the microscope.[38] The arthroconidia that surround the hair have the appearance of a sheath.

MICROSCOPIC PATTERNS OF HAIR INVASION. There are three patterns of hair invasion: small-spored ectothrix, large-spored ectothrix, and large-spored endothrix. Infection originates inside the hair shaft in all patterns.

CLINICAL PATTERNS OF INFECTION. A systematic approach for the clinical and laboratory investigations of tinea capitis is presented in Box 13-1. The inflammatory response to infection is variable. Noninflammatory tinea of the scalp is illustrated in Figure 13-38. A severe, inflammatory reaction with a boggy, indurated, tumorlike mass that exudes pus is called a *kerion*; it represents a hypersensitivity reaction to fungus and heals with scarring and some hair loss. The hair loss is less than would be expected from the degree and depth of inflammation. Cervical or occipital lymphadenopathy occurs in all types of tinea capitis. The diagnosis of tinea capitis should be questioned if lymphadenopathy is not present. A fungal infection is rarely the cause when neither adenopathy nor alopecia is present.[39]

Box 13-1 Systematic Approach to Investigation of Tinea Capitis

Determine clinical presentation

Most forms of tinea capitis begin with one or several round patches of scale or alopecia.

Inflammatory lesions, even if untreated, tend to resolve spontaneously in a few months; the noninflammatory infections are more chronic.

Patchy alopecia plus fine dry scale plus no inflammation

    Short stubs of broken hair ("gray patch ringworm"): *M. audouinii*

    Hairs broken off at surface ("black dot ringworm"): *T. tonsurans* (most common), *T. violaceum*

    Patchy alopecia plus swelling plus purulent discharge: *M. canis*, *T. mentagrophytes* (granular), *T. verrucosum*

Kerion is a severe inflammatory reaction with boggy induration: any fungus, but especially *M. canis*, *T. mentagrophytes* (granular), *T. verrucosum*

Wood's light examination

Blue-green fluorescence of hair—only *M. canis* and *M. audouinii* have this feature. Scale and skin do not fluoresce.

Potassium hydroxide wet mount of plucked hairs

The pattern of hair invasion is characteristic for each species of fungus. Hairs that can be removed with little resistance are best for evaluation.

Large-spored endothrix pattern-chains of large spores (densely packed) within the hair, "like a sack full of marbles." *T. tonsurans*, *T. violaceum*

Large-spored ectothrix pattern: chains of large spores inside and on the surface of the hair shaft and visible with the low-power objective: *T. verrucosum*, *T. mentagrophytes*

Small-spored ectothrix pattern: small spores randomly arranged in masses inside and on the surface of the hair shaft, not visible with the low-power objective. Looks like a stick dipped in maple syrup and rolled in sand: *M. canis*, *M. audouinii*

Identification of source after species is verified by culture

Anthropophilic (parasitic on humans): infection from other humans: *M. audouinii*, *T. tonsurans*, *T. violaceum*

Zoophili (parasitic on animals)—infection from animals or other infected humans: *M. canis*—dog, cat, monkey; *T. mentagrophytes* (granular)—dog, rabbit, guinea pig, monkey; *T. verrucosum*—cattle

Trichophyton tonsurans

Since the 1950s, *T. tonsurans* (large-spored endothrix) has been responsible for more than 90% of the scalp ringworm in the United States, but *M. canis* (small-spored ectothrix) is still a major cause in some parts of the United States. The occurrence rate is equal in boys and girls, and most cases are seen in the crowded inner cities in blacks or Hispanics. Cases of tinea capitis before the 1950s was caused by *M. audouinii*, which spontaneously clears in adolescence and fluoresces green with the Wood's light. *T. tonsurans* does not fluoresce and infects people of all ages.

It can remain viable for long periods on inanimate objects such as combs, brushes, blankets, and telephones.[40] *T. tonsurans* lesions may occur outside of the scalp in patients, their families, and their close friends. These lesions serve as a reservoir for reinfection; therefore all siblings or close contacts within the family should be examined. The peak incidence of infection occurs at ages 3 through 9 years. This fungal infection does not tend to resolve spontaneously at puberty, resulting in a large population of infected carriers.

FOUR PATTERNS OF INFECTION. *T. tonsurans* has four different clinical infection patterns. There may be multiple cases within a family, and each person may have a different infection pattern. The clinical presentation may be related to specific host T-lymphocyte response. This dermatophytosis is most frequently incurred from contact with an infected child, either directly or via a variety of fomites. Current studies indicate that an asymptomatic adult carrier state exists and may provide a source for continued reinfection in children.[41,42]

Noninflammatory black dot pattern. In the black dot pattern, there are well-demarcated areas of hair loss, with hairs broken off at the follicular orifice, giving the characteristic appearance of black dots if the patient's hair is black. Red hairs will produce a "red dot" pattern. This is the most distinctive pattern. Large areas of alopecia are present without inflammation (Figures 13-38 and 13-39). There is a mild-to-moderate amount of scalp scale. Occipital adenopathy may be present. Lack of inflammation may be explained by the fact that cell-mediated immunity to *Trichophyton* antigen skin tests is negative in these patients. The infected hairs of *T. tonsurans* have arthrospores inside the hair shaft; the arthrospores weaken the hair and cause it to break off at or below the scalp surface, resulting in a black dot appearance of the scalp surface (see Figure 13-36). Broken hairs are typically less than 2 mm long. Hairs long enough to be pulled are generally not infected.

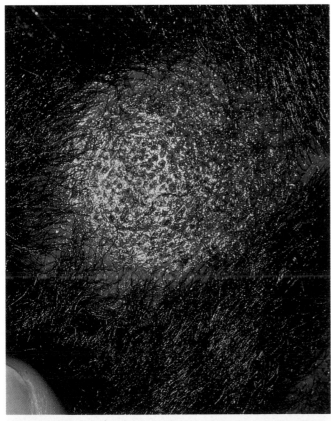

Figure 13-38 *Trichophyton tonsurans.* Black dot ringworm. There are areas of alopecia with scale but no inflammation. Arthrospores inside the shafts of infected hairs weaken the hair and cause it to break off at or below the scalp surface, resulting in the "black dot" appearance of the surface. *(From Solomon LM et al: Current Concepts 2(3):224, 1985; reproduced by permission of Blackwell Scientific Publications.)*

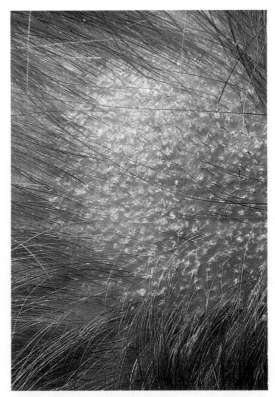

Figure 13-39 *Trichophyton tonsurans.* Noninflammatory "black dot" scaling pattern. Infection of the hair causes the shaft to fracture, leaving infected hair stubs. The color of the hair determines the color of the dots. Black hair presents with black dots. Light hair presents with white dots.

Inflammatory tinea capitis (kerion). Most patients with this infection pattern have a positive skin test to *Trichophyton* antigen, suggesting that the patient's immune response may be responsible for intense inflammation. Approximately 35% of patients infected with *T. tonsurans* have this pattern. There are one or multiple inflamed, boggy, tender areas of alopecia with pustules on and/or in surrounding skin (Figures 13-40 through 13-43). Fever, occipital adenopathy, leukocytosis, and a diffuse, morbilliform rash may occur. Potassium hydroxide wet mounts and fungal cultures are often negative because of destruction of fungal structures by inflammation, and treatment may have to be initiated based on clinical appearance.[43] Scarring alopecia may occur (Figure 13-44).

Seborrheic dermatitis type. This type is common and the most difficult to diagnosis because it resembles dandruff. There is diffuse or patchy, fine, white, adherent scale on the scalp. Close examination shows tiny, perifollicular pustules and/or hair stubs that have broken off at the level of the scalp: the black dot pattern. Less commonly, there is patchy or diffuse hair loss.[44] Adenopathy is often present. Culture is often necessary to make the diagnosis because only 29% of affected patients have a positive potassium hydroxide examination.[45]

PUSTULAR TYPE. There are discrete pustules or scabbed areas without scaling or significant hair loss. Pustules suggest bacterial infection, and patients with pustules may receive several courses of antibiotics before the correct diagnosis is made. The pustules may be sparse or numerous. As with kerions, the cultures and potassium hydroxide wet mounts may be negative.

DIFFERENTIAL DIAGNOSIS. Seborrheic dermatitis and psoriasis may be confused with tinea of the scalp. Tinea amiantacea, a form of seborrheic dermatitis that occurs in children, is frequently misdiagnosed as tinea. Tinea amiantacea is a localized 2- to 8-cm patch of large, brown, polygonal-shaped scales that adheres to the scalp and mats the hair. The matted scale grows out, attached to the hair (see Figure 8-30). There is little or no inflammation.

ID REACTION TO THERAPY. A dermatophytid (id) reaction may accompany oral antifungal therapy. The id reaction is not a widespread fungal infection but may be a cell-mediated immune response to the dermatophyte after therapy has been started. The id eruption is typically pruritic, papular or vesicular, and sometimes follicular. It usually begins on the face and spreads to the trunk. The palms and soles may be involved. A drug eruption is usually macular, papular, or urticarial and begins on the trunk. Topical steroids may be required to control symptoms. It is usually not necessary to stop the oral antifungal drug.

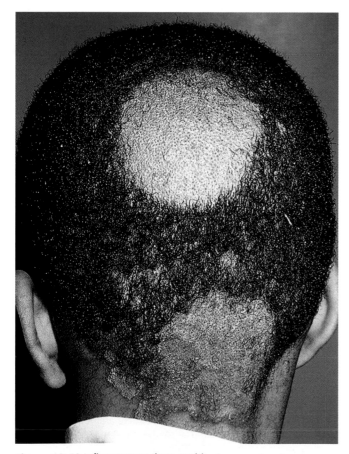

Figure 13-40 Inflammatory tinea capitis. A very extensive infection with extension onto the neck.

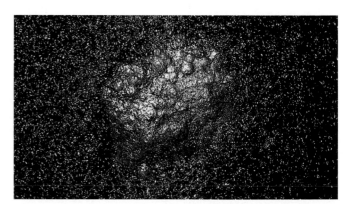

Figure 13-41 Deep, boggy, papular and pustular red lesions are called kerions. Cervical lymphadenopathy may develop.

TINEA CAPITIS

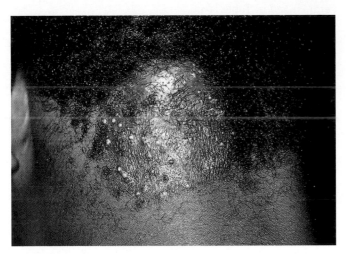

Figure 13-42 A severely inflammatory, boggy, indurated, tumor-like mass (kerion).

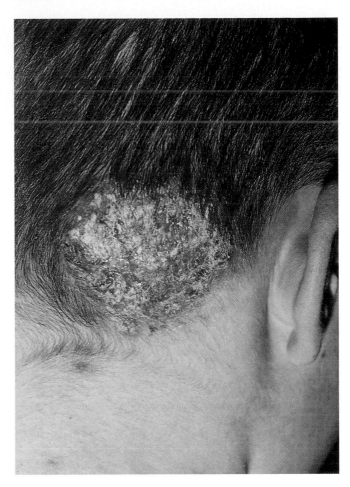

Figure 13-43 This severely inflamed deep lesion has accumulated serum and crust on the surface. Cervical lymphadenopathy was present.

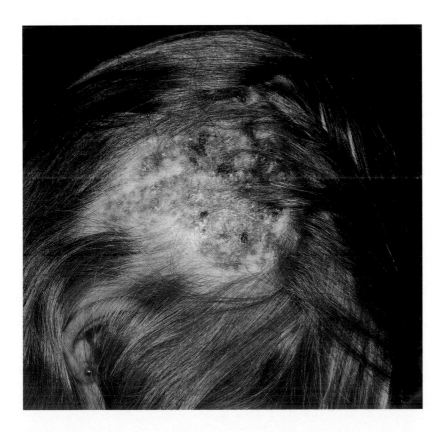

Figure 13-44 A huge kerion healed after 2 months of treatment with griseofulvin. The scalp is scarred, and hair follicles have been destroyed.

LABORATORY TECHNIQUES. The laboratory diagnosis of scalp tinea is made by first examining scale and hair on a microscope slide in a potassium hydroxide wet mount and then culturing hair and scalp scale. Wood's light examination is of little value today because most infections in the United States are caused by *T. tonsurans,* which does not fluorescence.

Potassium hydroxide wet mounts. The short hairs are traditionally collected with forceps—a tedious, time-consuming method. A better method is to firmly rub a tap water–moistened gauze[46] or a toothbrush over the involved area. Tightly woven gauze is the most effective (Topper dressing sponge). Each hair is lifted off the gauze with a needle or forceps and placed on a slide for potassium hydroxide preparation. Potassium hydroxide 10% to 20% solution is added, the slide is gently heated, and the slide is microscopically examined for fungal hyphae and spores. Early or inflammatory lesions may only contain very few hyphae. Overheating of the slide may burst the hair and make it difficult to differentiate the endothrix pattern from the ectothrix pattern.

Culture techniques. The brush-culture method involves gently rubbing a previously sterilized toothbrush in a circular motion over areas where scale is present or over the margins of patches of alopecia.[47] The brush fibers are then pressed into the culture media and the brush is discarded. A cotton swab produces similar results.[48] Cultures turn positive faster when using these collection techniques (see Figure 13-45). Sabouraud's dextrose agar or Mycosel (Mycobiotic) agar containing cycloheximide and chloramphenicol to suppress the growth of common saprophytic and bacterial contaminants are the two most commonly used culture media. DTM is similar to Mycosel (Mycobiotic) agar but contains a color indicator that changes from yellow to red in the presence of dermatophyte fungi. Accurate identification of the species of fungus is difficult with DTM.

Incubate cultures at 25°C to 30°C. Cultures usually show signs of growth in 7 to 10 days. The laboratory may incubate cultures for 30 days before reporting them negative.

Wood's light examination. Examination with Wood's ultraviolet light will show a yellow-green fluorescence with the ectothrix organisms *M. audouinii* and *M. canis. T tonsurans,* an endothrix-producing organism, does not fluorescence.

TREATMENT. The treatment of tinea capitis in children is summarized in Table 13-1.

Griseofulvin is the current drug of choice in children. It has a long track record of safety, is approved by the Food and Drug Administration for the treatment of tinea capitis in children, has the least known drug interactions, and is well tolerated.[49] Dosages of 20 to 25 mg/kg/day are prescribed for 6 to 8 weeks. Longer courses are often necessary. Newer antifungal drugs are under investigation, and their role in treating tinea capitis in children is still being defined. These drugs are concentrated in hair, skin, and nails, where they form a long-lasting reservoir. Safety, efficacy,[50] and cost data favor terbinafine for the treatment of *T. tonsurans* infections.[51] Recurrences with terbinafine are less frequent than with griseofulvin.[52]

Current data suggest that *M. canis* infections might respond better to itraconazole. Ketoconazole is not prescribed for children who may be at greater risk of liver toxicity.

A few authors have suggested suppressing the inflammation of a kerion with topical,[53] oral, or intralesional steroids. A randomized study showed that the combination of oral prednisolone with griseofulvin does not result in additional objective or subjective improvement compared with griseofulvin alone in cases with kerion.[54]

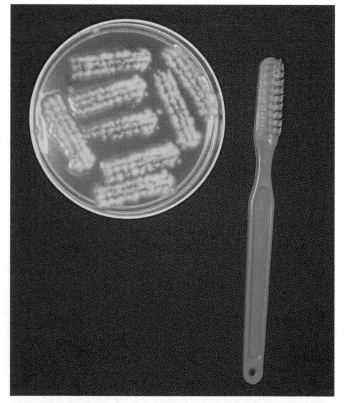

Figure 13-45 *Trichophyton tonsurans.* Culture technique for sampling dry scale in the scalp. *(From Solomon LM et al: Current Concepts 2(3):224, 1985; reproduced by permission of Blackwell Scientific Publications.)*

TREATMENT OF CARRIERS. Shampoos containing 1% to 2.5% selenium sulfide, 1% to 2% zinc pyrithione, povidone-iodine, or ketoconazole 2%[55] inhibited the growth of fungi. Povidone-iodine 4% shampoo has been shown to be effective in reducing *T. violaceum* carriage. They may be useful as adjunctive therapy to control spore loads in infected children and asymptomatic carriers.[56] These agents are lathered, massaged in well, and left on the scalp for 5 minutes. They are used 2 to 3 times each week during the course of treatment or longer.

Griseofulvin. Griseofulvin is the drug of choice for treating dermatophyte infections in infants and children. The drug is safe and well tolerated. Headaches and gastrointestinal symptoms (nausea, vomiting, heartburn) are the most common side effects, but these tend to disappear as therapy continues. It is absorbed more efficiently with a fatty meal; children can be given the medicine with ice cream or whole milk.

Patients are reexamined in 6 or 8 weeks. If the potassium hydroxide wet mount or culture is still positive or if there is little clinical improvement, treatment should be continued. Patients with tinea capitis should be treated 2 weeks beyond the time that cultures and potassium hydroxide preparations become negative. This generally requires at least 6 to 12 weeks of treatment.

Terbinafine. This drug is well absorbed after oral dosage and is well tolerated. Gastrointestinal symptoms are the most common side effects, and they subside with continuing therapy.

Fluconazole. Fluconazole is well absorbed, and its bioavailability is not influenced by food intake. There is little hepatic metabolism of fluconazole. The most common side effects are nausea and vomiting, but liver function test abnormalities are also found. Fluconazole is approved by the Food and Drug Administration for use in children older than 6 months. It is available in a pleasant-tasting liquid formula (10 and 40 mg/ml).

Itraconazole. Clinical trials have shown varying response rates. Bioavailability is improved when it is taken with a fatty meal. Itraconazole is a relatively safe drug. The frequency of side effects depends on duration of therapy. Nausea and vomiting occur with greatest frequency; abnormalities in liver functions occur in more than 1% of patients.

PREVENTION OF RECURRENCE. *T. tonsurans* spores may remain viable on furniture, combs, and brushes. Scrupulous cleaning of all possibly contaminated objects helps to prevent reinfection. All family members should be examined carefully for tinea capitis and tinea corporis.

Table 13-1 Tinea Capitis—Oral Drugs Used to Treat Children

Drug	Dosage	Duration
Griseofulvin (250-, 333-, and 500-mg tablets or suspension)	15 to 25 mg/kg/day (microsize) May increase to 25 mg/kg Or 15 mg/kg (ultramicrosize)	6 to 8+ wk
Terbinafine (250-mg tablet)	<20 kg: 62.5 mg qd 20 to 40 kg: 125 mg qd >40 kg: 250 mg qd	2 to 4 wk
Itraconazole (100-mg tablet or oral suspension) Note: The oral solution is better absorbed.	5 mg/kg/day 3 mg/kg/day (oral suspension) Capsule: simplified dosing 10 to 20 kg: 100 mg qod 21 to 30 kg: 100 qd 31 to 40 kg: 100 mg and 200 mg on alternate days 41 to 50 kg: 200 mg qd >50 kg: 200 to 300 mg qd	4- to 6-wk course or pulse dosing with 1-wk treatment intervals for 2 to 3 consecutive months
Fluconazole (50-, 100-, and 200-mg tablets or oral suspension)	5 mg/kg/day 6 mg/kg/day 8 mg/kg once weekly	4 to 6 wk 20 days 4 to 16 wk

Adapted from Elewski BE: J Am Acad Dermatol 2000:42: 1-20 and Gupta AK, et al: Pediatr Dermatol 1999:16: 171.

Tinea of the beard

Fungal infection of the beard area (tinea barbae) should be considered when inflammation occurs in this area. Bacterial folliculitis and inflammation secondary to ingrown hairs (pseudofolliculitis) are common. However, it is not unusual to see patients who have finally been diagnosed as having tinea after failing to respond to several courses of antibiotics. A positive culture for staphylococcus does not rule out tinea, in which purulent lesions may be infected secondarily with bacteria. Like tinea capitis, the hairs are almost always infected and easily removed. The hairs in bacterial folliculitis resist removal.

SUPERFICIAL INFECTION. This pattern resembles the annular lesions of tinea corporis. The hair is usually infected.

DEEP FOLLICULAR INFECTION. This pattern clinically resembles bacterial folliculitis except that it is slower to evolve and is usually restricted to one area of the beard. Bacterial folliculitis spreads rapidly over wide areas after shaving. Tinea begins insidiously with a small group of follicular pustules. The process becomes confluent in time with the development of a boggy, erythematous, tumorlike abscess covered with dense, superficial crust similar to that of fungal kerions seen in tinea capitis (Figures 13-46, 13-47, and 13-48). Hairs may be painlessly removed at almost any stage of the infec-

tion and examined for hyphae. Zoophilic *Trichophyton mentagrophytes* and *T. verrucosum* are the most common pathogens. *T. verrucosum* infection is acquired from the hide of dairy cattle and causes a severe pustular eruption on the face and neck. Many patients are dairy farmers (see Figure 13-27). Pustular tinea barbae in farmers may be mistaken for a *S. aureus* infection. Species identification by culture helps to identify the possible animal reservoir of infection.

TREATMENT. Treatment is the same as that for tinea capitis. Oral agents (Tables 13-2 and 13-3) are usually required because creams do not penetrate to the depths of the hair follicle.

Treatment of fungal infections

TOPICAL PREPARATIONS. A variety of preparations are commercially available. Studies have shown that undecylenic acid (e.g., Desenex) may be almost as effective for treating dermatophyte infections as are the newer agents.[57] Most of the medicines are available as creams or lotions; some are available as powders or aerosols. They are effective for all dermatophyte infections except for deep, inflammatory lesions of the body and scalp. They have no effect on tinea of the nail. Creams or lotions should be applied twice a day until the infection is clear. (See the Formulary for a list of the available topical agents.)

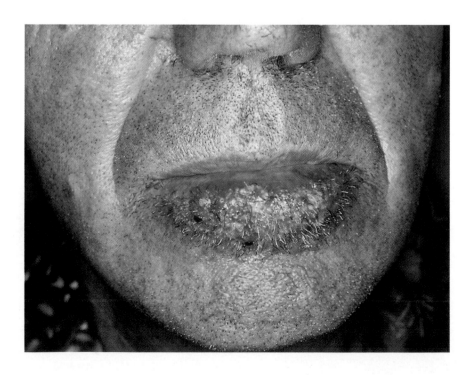

Figure 13-46 Tinea of the beard. A deep boggy infection of the follicles. The patient had been treated with several different oral antibiotics before the diagnosis of tinea was finally made. Oral antifungal agents are required to treat this deep infection.

TINEA BARBAE

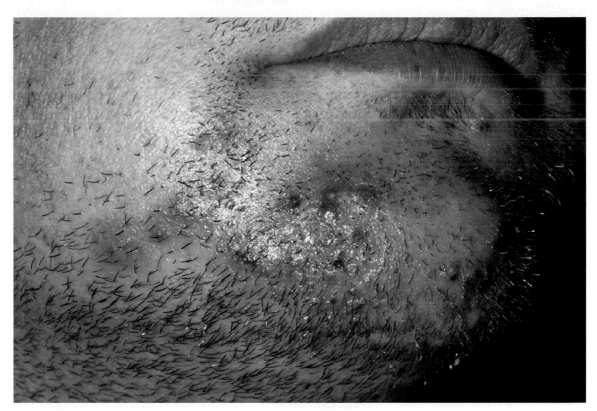

Figure 13-47 Inflamed areas are indurated and eroded on the surface. Hairs may be painlessly removed. Removal of beard hair in bacterial infections is usually painful.

Figure 13-48 This transplant patient had a subtle red scaling eruption that covered the chin and cheeks. A diagnosis of eczema was made and topical steroid treatment caused further disease extension. A KOH exam showed hyphae.

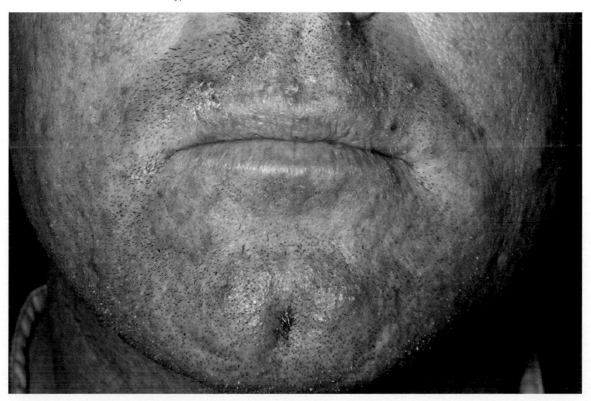

Systemic agents (see Tables 13-2 and 13-3)

GRISEOFULVIN. Griseofulvin is active only against dermatophytes; yeast infections, including those caused by *Candida* organisms and *Pityrosporum* organisms (tinea versicolor), and deep fungi do not respond. The drug has been available for more than 40 years and has been proved to be safe. Griseofulvin has a fungistatic effect; therefore it works best on actively growing dermatophytes, in which it may inhibit fungal cell wall synthesis. Griseofulvin probably diffuses into the stratum corneum from the extracellular fluid and sweat. Increased sweating may increase the concentration in the stratum corneum, thereby enhancing the drug's effect. Griseofulvin produces a sustained blood level so that a once- or twice-a-day schedule is adequate. Absorption varies from person to person; individual patients attain consistently high or low levels of the drug. Taking the drug with fatty foods may enhance absorption.

Two types of preparations are available: microsize and ultramicrosize. The newer, ultramicrosize forms are better absorbed and require approximately 50% to 70% of the dosage of the microsize form. Many brands are available in both forms. In microsize forms, the drug is supplied as 125-, 250-, and 500-mg tablets; in ultramicrosize forms, it is supplied as 125-, 250-, and 330-mg tablets. A liquid formulation is available. The recommended dosage and duration of therapy are listed in Table 13-2; the dosage should be adequate. Reported treatment failures are probably the result of using too small a dosage rather than of resistant organisms.

Adverse reactions. Griseofulvin is a safe drug. Headaches and gastrointestinal symptoms are the most common side effects. The dosage can be temporarily lowered to see if the symptoms clear, but sometimes the drug must be discontinued. Hepatotoxicity, leukopenia, and photosensitivity rarely occur[58]; therefore routine blood studies are not necessary[59] unless treatment is to last for many months or the dosage is exceptionally high. If a headache occurs, it usually does so during the first few days of treatment and may disappear as treatment is continued. A trial at a lower dosage level is warranted for those with headaches lasting longer than 48 hours. Patients with persistent headaches after a lower dosage trial need alternative treatment. Bone marrow suppression, once attributed to griseofulvin, probably never occurs, and routine complete blood cell counts are not necessary. Gastrointestinal upset, urticaria, photosensitivity, and morbilliform skin eruptions have been reported. Griseofulvin activates hepatic enzymes that cause degradation of warfarin and other drugs. Appropriate steps should be taken if combined treatment is used.

ALLYLAMINES. Allylamines, like the azoles, inhibit ergosterol synthesis, but they do so at an earlier point. The result, as with the azoles, is membrane disruption and cell death.

TERBINAFINE. Terbinafine (see Table 13-3) belongs to the allylamine class of antifungal agents. It inhibits squalene epoxidase, a membrane-bound enzyme that is not part of the cytochrome P-450 superfamily and is fungicidal to dermatophytes. Terbinafine is well absorbed, and highly lipophilic and keratophilic, and is distributed throughout adipose tissue, dermis, epidermis, and nails. The drug persists in plasma, dermis-epidermis, hair, and nails for weeks. Persistence of the drug in plasma is of concern when side effects are experienced. Terbinafine is delivered to the stratum corneum via the sebum and, to a lesser extent, through incorporation into the basal keratinocytes and diffusion through the dermis-epidermis. Terbinafine is not found in eccrine sweat. It remains in skin at concentrations above the mean inhibitory concentration (MIC) for most dermatophytes for 2 to 3 weeks after discontinuation of long-term oral therapy. After 6 and 12 weeks of oral therapy, terbinafine has been detected in the nail plate for 30 and 36 weeks, respectively, at a concentration well above the MIC for most dermatophytes. Terbinafine is metabolized in the liver. Dose adjustments may be needed for patients with liver dysfunction. In patients with renal disease, the elimination half-life can become prolonged. The dose of terbinafine should be halved when the serum creatinine exceeds 300 µmol/L, or when the creatinine clearance is less than or equal to 50 ml/min (0.83 ml/sec).

Indications. Oral terbinafine is effective for onychomycosis and other dermatomycoses (see Table 13-2).

TRIAZOLES. Triazoles are similar to imidazoles in chemical structure and mechanism of action.

Itraconazole (sporanox). Itraconazole, like the other antifungal azoles, inhibits fungal cytochrome P-450–dependent enzymes, blocking the synthesis of ergosterol, the principal sterol in the fungal cell membrane. The characteristics of itraconazole are shown in Table 13-3. Itraconazole is lipophilic and has a high affinity for keratinizing tissues. It adheres to the lipophilic cytoplasm of keratinocytes in the nail plate, allowing progressive build-up and persistence in the nail plate. The drug reaches high levels in the nails that persist for at least 6 months after discontinuation of 3 months of therapy and during pulsed cycles. The concentration in the stratum corneum remains detectable for 4 weeks after therapy. Itraconazole levels in sebum are 5 times higher than those in plasma and remain high for as long as 1 week after therapy. This suggests that secretion in sebum may account for the high concentrations found in skin. Itraconazole has an affinity for mammalian cytochrome P-450 enzymes, as well as for fungal P-450–dependent enzyme, and thus has the potential for clinically important interactions (e.g., astemizole, rifampin, oral contraceptives, H2 receptor antagonists, warfarin, cyclosporine). Absorption of itraconazole is significantly increased by the presence of food; it should be taken with a full meal.

Fluconazole (diflucan). Fluconazole is much more specific and effective at inhibiting cytochrome P-450 than are the imidazole agents. The characteristics of fluconazole are shown in Table 13-3. Fluconazole is highly water soluble and is transported to the skin through sweat and concentrated by evaporation. It achieves high concentrations in the epidermis and nails and persists for long periods of time.

Ketoconazole (nizoral). The use of ketoconazole for the treatment of dermatophyte infections has greatly diminished with the introduction of itraconazole, fluconazole, and terbinafine. These newer drugs are more effective and less likely to cause hepatic toxicity.

Table 13-2 Oral Antifungal Drug Dosages

	Griseofulvin (ultramicrosize)	Ketoconazole (Nizoral)	Fluconazole (Diflucan)	Itraconazole (Sporanox)	Terbinafine (Lamisil)
Tinea corporis and cruris	Adult: 500 mg qd 2 to 4 wk Child: 5 to 7 mg/kg/day 2 to 6 wk	200 to 400 mg/day 2 wk	150 mg once a week for 2 to 4 wk	100 mg qd 1 to 2 wk 200 mg qd 1 wk	250 mg qd 1 to 2 wk
Tinea capitis	15 to 25 mg/kg/day (microsize) Or 15 mg/kg (ultramicrosize) 6 to 8 wk	NR	5 mg/kg/day 4 to 6 wk 6 mg/kg/day 20 days 8 mg/kg once weekly 4 to 16 wk	5 mg/kg/day 4 to 6 wk 5 mg/kg/day for 1 week plus 1 to 3 pulses 3 weeks apart 3 mg/kg/day (oral suspension) for 1 week plus 1 to 3 pulses 3 weeks apart Capsule–simplified dosing: 10 to 20 kg: 100 mg qod 21 to 30 kg: 100 qd 31 to 40 kg: 100 mg and 200 mg on alternate days 41 to 50 kg: 200 mg qd >50 kg: 200 to 300 mg qd	20 to 40 kg: 125 mg qd 2 to 4 wk >40 kg: 250 mg qd 2 to 4 wk
Onychomycosis	NR	NR	150 mg once a week for 9 mo	200 mg qd Fingernails: 6 wk Toenails: 12 wk Pulse dosing: 200 mg bid 1 wk on, 3 wk off Toenails: 3 to 4 mo Fingernails: 2 to 3 mo	250 mg qd Fingernails: 6 wk Toenails: 12 wk
Tinea pedis	Adult: 500 mg qd 6 to 12 wk Child: 5 to 7 mg/kg/day 6 to 12 wk	NR	50 mg once a week for 3 to 4 wk	Moccasin tinea pedis 200 mg bid 1 week	Moccasin tinea pedis 250 mg qd 2 wk 200 mg qd 3 wk
Tinea versicolor	Not effective	400 mg single dose 200 mg qd 5 days Prophylaxis with 400 mg once monthly for recurrent disease	300 or 400 mg single dose; repeat in 2 wk if needed	200 mg qd 7 days Prophylaxis: 200 mg bid 1 day per month for 6 mo for recurrent disease	Oral not effective Topical is effective
Vaginal candidiasis	Not effective	200 to 400 mg qd 5 to q 4 days	150 mg single dose 100 mg 5 to 7 days	200 mg 3 to 5 days	Not effective

NR, Not recommended.

Table 13-3 Oral Antifungal Drugs

	Griseofulvin (ultramicrosize)	Ketoconazole (Nizoral)
Dosage forms	125-, 250-, and 333-mg ultramicronized tablets 125 mg/5 ml	200-mg tablet
Gastrointestinal absorption	Fatty foods enhance absorption	Acid environment enhances absorption. Take with breakfast with an acidic fruit juice. Absorption reduced by antiacids, histamine-2 blockers (cimetidine, ranitidine, famotidine, nizatidine), acid pump inhibitors (omeprazole, lansoprazole), and didanosine
Persistent in plasma	2 wk	2 days
Persistent in skin and nails	1 to 2 wk	Unknown
Laboratory monitoring*	Rx 6 wk CBC, LFT	Baseline CBC, LFT; repeat each month
Abnormal LFT elevations		
Adverse drug reactions mechanism	Potent inducer of microsomal cytochrome P-450 enzymes	Metabolized by and inhibits liver cytochrome P-450 enzyme
Adverse events		
Adverse drug interactions	Decreases levels of warfarin, estrogen, birth control pills Effect of alcohol is potentiated Barbiturates depress activity of griseofulvin	Raises serum levels of astemizole, cisapride, quinidine Quinidine: tinnitus, cardiac arrhythmias Anticoagulants: bleeding Sulfonylureas: hypoglycemia Cyclosporine, tacrolimus: renal toxicity Calcium channel blockers: edema—Midazolam, triazolam: increased sedation Phenytoin: dizziness, ataxia Induce synthesis of cortisol producing symptoms of hypoadrenalism (fatigue, malaise) Reduce synthesis of testosterone: impotence, gynecomastia
Adverse drug reactions	Nausea, vomiting, diarrhea, headache, dizziness, insomnia, cutaneous eruptions, photosensitivity (rare)	Gastrointestinal disturbances, disulfiram-like effect when alcohol is ingested, hepatitis (1:10,000)—stop drug if nausea, vomiting, fatigue, malaise, dark urine, pale stools, jaundice, or cutaneous eruptions occur

CBC, Complete blood cell count; LFT, liver function tests.

*Patient education regarding the symptoms of early hepatitis and advice to stop the drug at first sign of symptoms (nausea, malaise, fatigue) is essential to prevent progression to severe liver injury.

Fluconazole (Diflucan)	Itraconazole (Sporanox)	Terbinafine (Lamisil)
50-, 100-, and 200-mg tablets 150-mg tablet (for vaginal infections)	100 mg capsule	250 mg
	Acid environment enhances absorption. Take with breakfast with an acidic fruit juice. Absorption reduced by antiacids, histamine-2 blockers (cimetidine, ranitidine,famotidine, nizatidine, and acid pump inhibitors (omeprazole, lansoprazole), and didanosine	
	1 wk	4 to 6 wk
3 months	6 to 9 months lipophilic	4 to 6 wk lipophilic
For continuous therapy. Baseline CBC, LFT; repeat each 4 to 6 wk	For continuous therapy. Baseline CBC, LFT; repeat each 4 to 6 wk	Baseline CBC, LFT; repeat each 4 to 6 wk
Low incidence	2.0% pulse dosing 4.0% continuous dosing	3.3% to 7%
Metabolized by and inhibits liver cytochrome P-450 enzyme	Metabolized by liver and inhibits cytochrome P-450 enzymes	Metabolized by liver cytochrome P-450 enzymes. The Cytochrome P-450 enzyme CYP2D6 is inhibited by terbinafine.
	8.3%	10.5%
Possibly the same type of drug interactions as ketoconazole but less likely when the drug is given on an intermittent basis Cautions: Astemizole (Hismanal) Cisapride (Propulsid) Warfarin (Coumadin) Cyclosporine (Neoral) Phenytoin (Dilantin) Sulfonylureas	Drugs that induce cytochrome P-450 enzymes will increase the catabolism of and reduce the plasma concentration of itraconazole (phenytoin, rifampin, rifabutin, isoniazid, carbamazepine) May be involved in the same drug interactions as ketoconazole Cautions Atorvastatin (Lipitor) Digoxin Quinidine Warfarin (Coumadin) Cyclosporine (Neoral) Calcium channel blockers Contraindications Astemizole (Hismanal) Triazolam (Halcion) Cisapride (Propulsid) Lovastatin (Mevacor) Simvastatin (Zocor) Midazolam (Versed)	CYP2D6 is involved in the metabolism of tricyclic antidepressants and other psychotropic drugs Increases clearance and thus lowers levels of cyclosporine Decreases clearance of caffeine Terbinafine blood levels are increased by cimetidine, and decreased by rifampin and rifabutin Monitor theophylline levels
Gastrointestinal disturbances Hepatitis much less likely than with ketoconazole	Headache, gastrointestinal disturbances, cutaneous eruptions Hepatitis much less likely than with ketoconazole Peripheral edema especially if taken with calcium channel blockers	Gastrointestinal disturbances, alteration in taste (2.8%), cutaneous eruptions, neutropenia, agranulocytosis

Candidiasis (Moniliasis)

The yeastlike fungus *C. albicans* and a few other *Candida* species are capable of producing skin, mucous membrane, and internal infections. The organism lives with the normal flora of the mouth, vaginal tract, and gut, and it reproduces through the budding of oval yeast forms. Pregnancy, oral contraception, antibiotic therapy, diabetes, skin maceration, topical steroid therapy, certain endocrinopathies, and factors related to depression of cell-mediated immunity may allow the yeast to become pathogenic and produce budding spores and elongated cells (pseudohyphae) or true hyphae with septate walls. The pseudohyphae and hyphae are indistinguishable from dermatophytes in potassium hydroxide preparations (Figure 13-49). Culture results must be interpreted carefully because the yeast is part of the normal flora in many areas.

The yeast infects only the outer layers of the epithelium of mucous membrane and skin (the stratum corneum). The primary lesion is a pustule, the contents of which dissect horizontally under the stratum corneum and peel it away. Clinically, this process results in a red, denuded, glistening surface with a long, cigarette paper–like, scaling, advancing border. The infected mucous membranes of the mouth and vaginal tract accumulate scale and inflammatory cells that develop into characteristic white or white-yellow, curdy material.

Yeast grows best in a warm, moist environment; therefore infection is usually confined to the mucous membranes and intertriginous areas. The advancing infected border usually stops when it reaches dry skin.

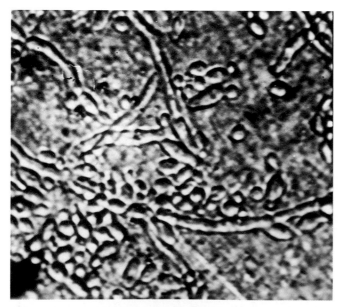

Figure 13-49 *Candida albicans.* A potassium hydroxide wet mount of skin scrapings showing both elongated pseudohyphae and budding spores.

Candidiasis of normally moist areas

Candidiasis affects normally moist areas such as the vagina, the mouth, and the uncircumcised penis. In the vagina, it causes vulvovaginitis; in the mouth, it causes thrush; and in the uncircumcised penis, it causes balanitis.

Vulvovaginitis

Vulvovaginitis has infectious (see Table 13-4) and noninfectious causes. Infectious vaginitis is the most common cause of a vaginal discharge. Common infectious causes include several species of yeasts, *Trichomonas vaginalis,* and *Gardnerella vaginalis* and its associated proliferation of anaerobic bacteria. Other causes include infectious cervicitis, a physiologic discharge, and allergic or irritant contact vaginitis. Atrophic vaginitis is the most common noninfectious cause of vaginitis in the postmenopausal woman. *Neisseria gonorrhoeae,* group A β-hemolytic *Streptococcus (Streptococcus pyogenes),* other bacteria, pinworms, and foreign bodies in the vagina are also possible causes of vaginitis in prepubertal girls.

LABORATORY STUDIES. Laboratory confirmation is provided by saline or potassium hydroxide wet mount examination, the amine whiff test, determination of the vaginal pH, and the culture. Effective therapy can then be prescribed for all forms of infectious vaginitis.

Monilial vulvovaginitis

Vaginal candidiasis is the most common cause of vaginal discharge. Greater than 50% of women older than 25 years develop vulvovaginal candidiasis at some time; fewer than 5% of these women experience recurrences. Infection is usually due to *C. albicans.* The incidence of infections due to yeasts other than *C. albicans* has increased in the last few years. Of these non-*albicans* species, *C. tropicalis* and *C. glabrata* are the most important. Currently used drug therapies (e.g., imidazoles) do not adequately eradicate non-*albicans* species. A possible explanation for the recent increased selection of these species may be the shortened antifungal therapies (1- to 3-day regimens) that suppress *C. albicans* but create an imbalance of flora that facilitates an overgrowth of non-*albicans* species.[60]

Candida is present in the normal flora of the vaginal tract and rectum in 10% of women. Candidal vaginitis develops in approximately one fourth of women in their child-bearing years. Heat and moisture are increased under large folds of fat and occlusive undergarments. Symptoms may worsen a few days before menstruation. One study showed that 30% of women treated with antibiotics developed candidal vaginitis.[61]

CLINICAL PRESENTATION. Vaginal candidiasis usually begins with vaginal itching and/or a white, thin-to-creamy discharge. Symptoms may resolve spontaneously after several days, or they may progress. The vaginal mucous membranes and external genitalia become red, swollen, and sometimes eroded and painful. They are covered with a thick, white,

Table 13-4 Vaginal Infections

	Monilial (Candida)	Bacteria vaginosis (G. vaginalis and anaerobic bacteria)	Trichomoniasis
Vaginal discharge	White, clumpy	Gray, homogeneous	Profuse greenish, sometimes frothy
Symptoms	Itching	Malodorous discharge	Malodorous discharge, itching, dyspareunia, dysuria
Saline or potassium hydroxide wet mount	Budding yeast, pseudophae 30% will be negative	Clue cells (epithelial cells) with adherent bacteria	Motile trichomonads, white blood cells (do not use potassium hydroxide)
pH	<4.5	>4.7	4.5
Amine whiff test (add 10% potassium hydroxide to discharge)		+ (fishy odor due to release of amines)	+ (strong odor because of a proliferation of anaerobic organisms)
Culture	Standard transport media	Standard transport media	Diamond's media
Treatment	Imidazole creams: Miconazole (Monistat-7) Clotrimazole (Gyne-Lotrimin) Many other products Oral agents: Fluconazole (Diflucan) Itraconazole (Sporanox) Treat sexual partners if the partners are symptomatic	Metronidazole (Flagyl) 500 mg bid 1 wk Metrogel cream Clindamycin (Cleocin) Oral or cream 2% Amoxicillin-clavulanic acid (Augmentin) Treat sexual partners if recurrent	Metronidazole (Flagyl) 500 mg bid 1 wk 250 mg tid 1 wk 2 gm single dose Combined oral and intravaginal metronidazole for resistant cases Treat sexual partner to prevent reinfection

Adapted from Vulvovaginitis. In Conn's Current Therapy. Saunders , 2000, pp 1053.

Note: The laboratory personnel can perform all of these tests if provided with sufficient material. Discharge specimens should be taken to the laboratory immediately if trichomoniasis is suspected; motility of the organism may not be visible after 15 to 30 minutes.

---

crumbly discharge, which becomes more copious during pregnancy. The infection may spread onto the thighs and anus, producing a tender, red skin surface with discrete pustules, called *satellite lesions,* that appear outside the edges of the advancing border. The diagnosis is confirmed by a potassium hydroxide preparation of the discharge.

MANAGEMENT. First-line therapy consists of antifungal creams (Table 13-5). The two alternative agents boric acid gelatin capsules and gentian violet aqueous solution are effective, especially for treating species of *Candida* other than *C. albicans.*

Oral antifungal agents include ketoconazole (Nizoral), fluconazole (Diflucan), and itraconazole (Sporanox) (see Table 13-2).

Topical antifungal agents. There are a large variety of topical medications in many forms, including tablets, creams, and tampons (see Table 13-5 and the Formulary). Clotrimazole and miconazole are the most widely used. The cure rate with polyenes (nystatin) is 70% to 80%; the cure rate with azole derivatives is 85% to 90%. Topical antimycotic therapy is free of systemic side effects. The initial application may cause local burning, especially if inflammation is severe. The burning is a local irritant reaction rather than an allergy. Treatment schedules are listed in Table 13-14 and the

Formulary. The course should be repeated if symptoms have not subsided. Cream is useful if the external areas are also infected; the cream runs out and coats the vulva. Cream may also be applied directly from the tube. There is sufficient cream supplied for both external and internal application. Nystatin (Mycostatin) has been used for years. One tablet is placed with the applicator high in the vaginal tract twice a day for 2 weeks. The duration of treatment is extended if

Table 13-5 Topical Agents Used in the Initial Therapy of Fungal Vulvovaginitis

Generic name	Trade name
Miconazole	Monistat-7
Clotrimazole	Gyne-Lotrimin, Mycelex-7
Butoconazole	Femstat
Terconazole	Terazol-3
Tioconazole	Vagistat-1
Nystatin	Mycostatin
Alternatives Gentian violet (1% aqueous solution) Boric acid (gelatin capsules)	

signs or symptoms persist. Although nystatin must be used longer than the azoles, it is still an effective and safe medicine.

Oral antifungal agents. Oral preparations include fluconazole, itraconazole, and ketoconazole. Fluconazole (Diflucan) is the preferred oral drug for candida vaginitis. A single 150-mg oral tablet was shown to be as effective as other oral and intravaginal regimens, with minimal adverse effects.[62]

ACUTE VAGINAL CANDIDIASIS. The imidazoles and triazoles are the first choice of treatment for vulvovaginal candidiasis. There is a lack of clear superiority of one azole agent or dosing regimen. Most patients are treated with a short course of intravaginal therapy (1 to 3 days) for acute, uncomplicated candidal vaginitis. The physician's judgment and the patient's preference determine the specific antifungal agent and route of administration; cost, distribution of inflammation, and medicine vehicle characteristics are factors in the decision. Many patients prefer oral treatment. Oral and vaginal medications are almost equally effective in treating acute disease. Fluconazole administered as a single 150-mg oral dose proved to be as safe and effective as 7 days of intravaginal clotrimazole therapy for *C. vaginitis.*[63]

PATIENT PREFERENCE. Half of patients prefer oral medication; only 5% prefer intravaginal therapy, and the others have no clear preference. Before treating vaginal candidiasis, the physician should ask the patient about her preference.

PARTNER TREATMENT. Vaginal candidiasis is usually not a sexually transmitted disease and routine treatment of male partners is not necessary. One study showed that treatment of male partners with a brief course of ketoconazole was not of value in reducing the incidence of relapse in women with recurrent vaginal candidiasis.[64] Partner treatment is indicated for men with balanoposthitis or for chronic recurrent cases.

SIDE EFFECTS. Side effects of treatment for vaginal candidiasis are rare.

PREGNANCY. Oral therapy should not be given to pregnant patients or to patients who are not using reliable contraceptive measures. Topical therapy during pregnancy may require longer therapy (6 to 14 days). Women who do not use reliable contraception should use oral treatment only during the first 10 days of the menstrual cycle.

Candida strains can be cultured from the vagina in 10% to 20% of pregnant women. The incidence of vaginal candidiasis in pregnancy is twice as high as in the nonpregnant state. The incidence is higher late in pregnancy. In 80% to 90% of the cases, candidiasis is caused by *C. albicans.* Treatment of vaginal candidiasis in pregnancy is indicated not only to make the woman symptom free but also to protect the fetus from a life-threatening *Candida* sepsis. Itraconazole cannot be used for oral treatment of vaginal candidiasis in pregnant women because of possible teratogenic effects.

Recurrent (resistant) disease

Vulvovaginal candidiasis is considered recurrent when at least four episodes occur in 1 year or at least three episodes unrelated to antibiotic therapy occur within 1 year. Patients with chronic and recurrent candidal vaginitis rarely have recognizable precipitating or causal factors.[65] Appearance of non-*albicans* species is possible but unusual. Relapse is due to persistent yeast in the vagina rather than to frequent vaginal reinfection. Causes include treatment-resistant *Candida* species other than *C. albicans,* frequent antibiotic therapy, contraceptive use, compromise of the immune system, increasing frequency of sexual intercourse, and hyperglycemia. Women with recurrent candidal vaginitis are more likely to use solutions for vulvoperineal cleansing or vaginal douching. Frequent yeast infections could be an early sign of HIV infection.

LABORATORY TESTS. Potassium hydroxide preparations of vaginal secretions are not sufficiently sensitive to exclude fungal infection in recurrent disease. If microscopic examination is negative but clinical suspicion is high, fungal cultures should be obtained.

TREATING RESISTANT CASES. Some women have repeated or ongoing infection even after several courses of antiyeast therapy. The pathogenesis is poorly understood and the majority of patients have no recognizable predisposing factors.

There is no definitive cure for recurrent disease, but long-term maintenance regimens with oral or topical medication are effective.

Weekly applications of terconazole 0.8% cream were effective in preventing recurrent episodes of candidal vaginitis and were well tolerated.[66]

Patients with recurrent disease should be advised to lose excess weight and to wear loose-fitting, cotton undergarments. Daily ingestion of 8 ounces of yogurt containing *L. acidophilus* decreased both candidal colonization and infection in one study.[67] The efficacy of yeast-elimination diets is unknown.

Attempts to reduce the number of attacks by treating sexual partners and suppressing a gastrointestinal tract focus with Mycostatin have failed. Many patients experience recurrences once prophylaxis is discontinued; therefore long-term therapy may be necessary. Patients are more likely to comply when antifungal therapy is administered orally.[68]

Candida should be documented by culture for any patient who has recurrent or persistent disease and a negative potassium hydroxide (potassium hydroxide) slide.

Long-term maintenance therapy schedules are listed in Table 13-6.

Resistant organisms. Vaginal candidiasis due to *C. glabrata* may not respond to any of the azole drugs. Vaginal nystatin or local application of 1% gentian violet may eradicate this species. Recurrent infections after treatment may be with more common *Candida* species.[69]

Table 13-6 Treatment Options for Acute and Recurrent Vulvovaginal Candidiasis

Agent	Dosing regimen
Treatment of acute episode	
Clotrimazole (Gyne-Lotrimin)	100-mg tablets administered intravaginally for 7 days
Terconazole 0.8% cream (Terazol 3)	One full applicator (5 gm) administered intravaginally for 3 days
Fluconazole (Diflucan)	150 mg administered orally (one dose) 100 mg administered orally for 5 to 7 days
Ketoconazole (Nizoral)	200 mg administered orally once daily for 14 days 400 mg administered orally once daily for 14 days
Itraconazole	200 mg administered orally for 3 to 5 days
Boric acid	600-mg vaginal suppository administered twice daily for 14 days (must be compounded)
Prophylaxis (maintenance)	
Clotrimazole (Gyne-Lotrimin)	Two 100-mg tablets administered intravaginally twice weekly for 6 months
Terconazole 0.8% cream (Terazol 3)	One full applicator (5 gm) administered vaginally once a week
Fluconazole (Diflucan)	150 mg administered orally once a month 100 to 200 mg weekly
Itraconazole (Sporanox)	50 to 100 mg administered daily 200 mg bid administered orally once a month
Ketoconazole (Nizoral)	Two 200-mg tablets administered orally for 5 days after the menses for six months One half of a 200-mg tablet administered orally once daily for 6 months
Boric acid	600-mg vaginal suppository administered once daily during menstruation (5-day menses)

Adapted from Ringdahl EN: Am Fam Physician 2000;61: 3306.

Oral candidiasis

C. albicans may be transmitted to the infant's oral cavity during passage through the birth canal. It is part of the normal mouth flora in many adults.

Non−*albicans Candida* species are causing an increasing number of infections. Most of these occur in immunocompromised individuals, especially in those infected with HIV. Oral candidosis is common in advanced cancer. The two most common species in a study of patients with advanced cancer were *C. albicans* and *C. glabrata,* with fewer numbers of *C. tropicalis, C. parapsilosis, C. guilliermondi,* and *C. inconspicua.* Non−*albicans Candida* yeasts are common in the mouths of patients with advanced stage cancer, and these may have reduced sensitivity to fluconazole. *Candida dubliniensis* is a recently identified yeast, mostly isolated in HIV-positive individuals with oral candidiasis.

HIV INFECTION. Oropharyngeal candidiasis may be the first manifestation of HIV infection, and more than 90% of patients with AIDS develop the disease. A concern in these patients is clinical relapse after treatment, which appears to be dependent on degree of immunosuppression and is more common with clotrimazole and ketoconazole than with fluconazole or itraconazole.

Infants. Oral candidiasis in children is called thrush. Healthy, newborn infants, especially if premature, are susceptible. In older infants, thrush usually occurs in the presence of predisposing factors such as antibiotic treatment or debilitation. In the healthy newborn, thrush is a self-limited infection, but it should be treated to avoid interference with feeding. The infection appears as a white, creamy exudate or white, flaky, adherent plaques. The underlying mucosa is red and sore. The mother should be examined for vaginal candidiasis.

Adults. In the adult, oral candidiasis occurs for several reasons; clinically, it is found in a variety of acute and chronic forms. Extensive oral infection may occur in diabetics, patients with depressed cell-mediated immunity, the elderly, and patients with cancer, especially leukemia. Prolonged corticosteroid, immunosuppressive or broad-spectrum antibiotic therapy, and inhalant steroids may also cause infection.

The acute process in adults is similar to the infection in infants. The tongue is almost always involved (Figure 13-50). Infection may spread into the trachea or esophagus and cause very painful erosions, appearing as dysphagia, or it may spread onto the skin at the angles of the mouth (perlèche). A specimen may be taken by gently scraping with a tongue blade. Pseudohyphae are easily demonstrated. In other cases, the oral cavity may be red, swollen, and sore, with little or no exudate (Figure 13-51). In this instance, pseudohyphae are often difficult to find and treatment may have to be started without laboratory verification.

Chronic infection appears as localized, firmly adherent plaques with an irregular, velvety surface on the buccal mucosa. They may occur from the mechanical trauma of cheek biting, poor hygiene of dental prostheses, pipe smoking, or irritation from dentures. A biopsy is indicated to rule out leukoplakia and lichen planus if organisms cannot be demonstrated.

Localized erythema and erosions with minimal white exudate may be caused by candidal infection beneath dentures and is commonly called *denture sore mouth*. The border is usually sharply defined. Hyperplasia with thickening of the mucosa occurs if the process is long lasting. The gums and hard palate are most frequently involved. Organisms may be difficult to find.

TREATMENT. Azoles, both topical (clotrimazole) and systemic (fluconazole, itraconazole), have largely replaced older topical antifungals (gentian violet, nystatin).

Fluconazole. Fluconazole (200 mg/day for adults) is the first-line management option for the treatment and prophylaxis of localized and systemic *C. albicans* infections. It is effective, well tolerated, and suitable for use in most patients with *C. albicans* infections, including children, the elderly, and those with impaired immunity. Prophylactic administration of fluconazole can help to prevent fungal infections in patients receiving cytotoxic cancer therapy. The increasing use of fluconazole for the long-term prophylaxis and treatment of recurrent oral candidosis in AIDS patients has led to the emergence of *C. albicans* infections that are not responsive to conventional doses. Second-line therapy with a wider spectrum antifungal, such as itraconazole, should be sought if treatment with fluconazole is not sucessful. *Candida* spp. other than *C. albicans* may develop resistance to fluconazole in a patient who is repeatedly exposed to the drug.

Itraconazole. Itraconazole solution is as effective as fluconazole but is less well tolerated as first-line therapy.[70] Itraconazole oral solution is a useful therapy in the treatment of HIV-infected patients with fluconazole-refractory oropharyngeal candidiasis. HIV-infected patients with oropharyngeal candidiasis for whom fluconazole therapy (200 mg/day) failed were treated with 100 mg of itraconazole oral solution administered twice daily (200 mg/day) for 14 days. Patients who demonstrated an incomplete response to treatment were treated for an additional 14 days (28 days total).[71]

Clotrimazole (Mycelex) troche. Children and adults are effectively treated by slowly dissolving a clotrimazole (Mycelex) troche in the mouth 5 times a day for 14 days.

Ketoconazole (Nizoral). Ketoconazole (Nizoral 200-mg oral tablet) given once a day is a second-line drug for treatment of oropharyngeal candidiasis.

Nystatin (Mycostatin) oral suspension. For infants, the dosage is 2 ml of nystatin (Mycostatin) oral suspension qid, 1 ml in each side of the mouth. For adults, the dosage is 4 to 6 ml, with one half of the dose in each side of the mouth retained as long as possible before swallowing. Treatment is continued for 48 hours after symptoms have disappeared; a 10-day course is typical. The oral suspension is useful for infants but less effective for adults, probably because the liquid may not come in contact with the entire surface of the oral cavity.

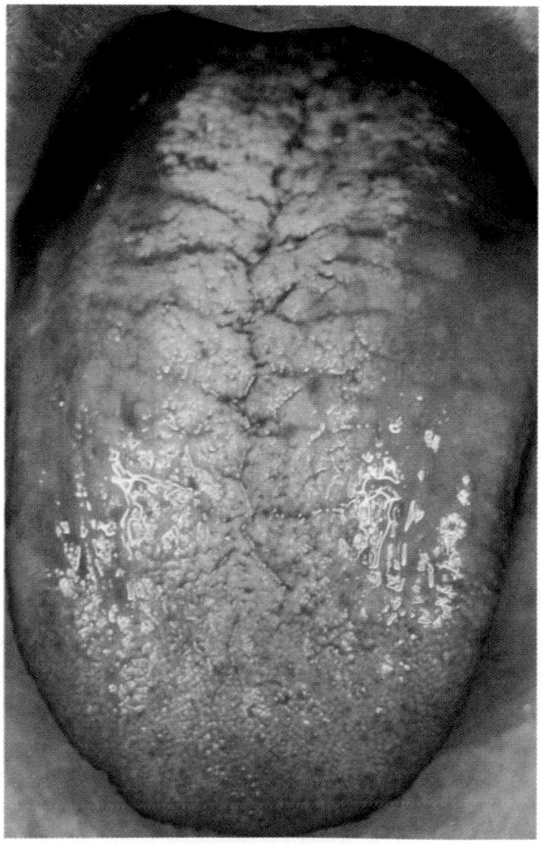

Figure 13-50 Oral candidiasis. A chronic infection with white debris covering the surface of the tongue.

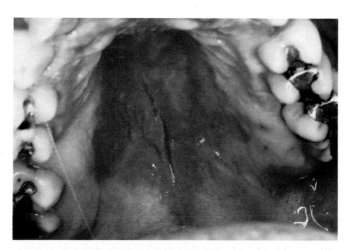

Figure 13-51 Oral candidiasis. The hard palate is red and swollen.

Candida balanitis

The uncircumcised penis provides the warm, moist environment ideally suited for yeast infection, but the circumcised male is also at risk. *Candida balanitis* sometimes occurs after intercourse with an infected female and is more common in those who had vaginal intercourse than in those who had anal intercourse within 3 months.[72] Tender, pinpoint, red papules and pustules appear on the glans and shaft of the penis. The pustules rupture quickly under the foreskin and may not be noticed (Figure 13-52). Typically, 1- to 2-mm, white, doughnut-shaped, possibly confluent rings are seen after the pustules break. In some cases pustules never evolve, and the multiple red papules may be transient, resolving without treatment. The presence of pustules is highly suggestive of candidiasis. White exudate similar to that seen in *Candida* vaginal infections may be present (Figure 13-53). The infection may occur and persist without sexual exposure.

TREATMENT. The eruption responds quickly with twice-a-day application for 7 days of miconazole, clotrimazole, or several of the other medications listed in the Formulary. Relief is almost immediate, but treatment should be continued for 7 days. Preparations containing topical steroids give temporary relief by suppressing inflammation, but the eruption rebounds and worsens, sometimes even before the cortisone cream is discontinued. A single 150-mg dose of fluconazole was comparable in efficacy and safety to clotrimazole cream applied topically for 7 days when administered to patients with balanitis.[73]

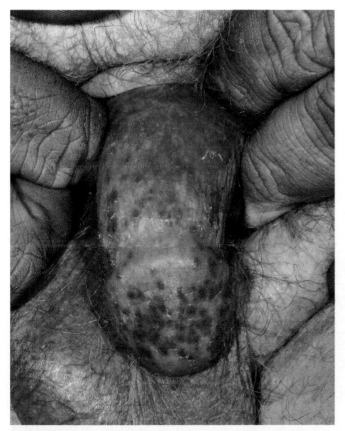

Figure 13-52 *Candida balanitis.* Multiple red, round erosions are present on the glans and shaft of the penis. There is a white exudate.

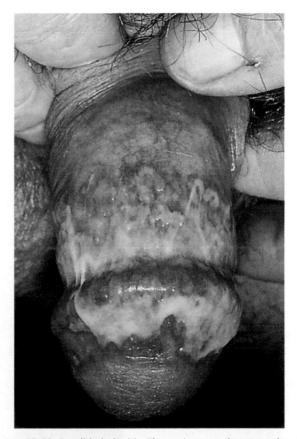

Figure 13-53 *Candida balanitis.* The moist space between the skin surfaces of the uncircumcised penis is an ideal environment for *Candida* infection. This thick white exudate is typical of a severe acute infection.

Candidiasis of large skin folds

Candidiasis of large skin folds (*Candida* intertrigo) occurs under pendulous breasts, between overhanging abdominal folds, in the groin and rectal area, and in the axillae. *Skin folds* (intertriginous areas where skin touches skin) contain heat and moisture, providing the environment suited for yeast infection. Hot, humid weather; tight or abrasive underclothing; poor hygiene; and inflammatory diseases occurring in the skin folds, such as psoriasis, make a yeast infection more likely.

There are two presentations. In the first type, pustules form but become macerated under apposing skin surfaces and develop into red papules with a fringe of moist scale at the border. Intact pustules may be found outside the apposing skin surfaces (Figures 13-54 and 13-55). The second type consists of a red, moist, glistening plaque that extends to or just beyond the limits of the apposing skin folds (Figure 13-56). The advancing border is long, sharply defined, and has an ocean wave–shaped fringe of macerated scale (see Figure 13-49). The characteristic pustule of candidiasis is not observed in intertriginous areas because it is macerated away as soon as it forms. Pinpoint pustules do appear outside the advancing border and are an important diagnostic feature when present (Figures 13-54, 13-55, and 13-57). There is a tendency for painful fissuring in the skin creases.

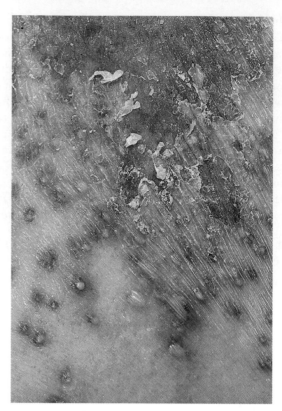

Figure 13-54 Candidiasis under the breast. There are several moist, red papules and pustules with a fringe of white scale.

Figure 13-55 *Candida* intertrigo. An acute infection. The fringe of scale is present on the opposing borders. There are numerous satellite pustules beyond the intertriginous area.

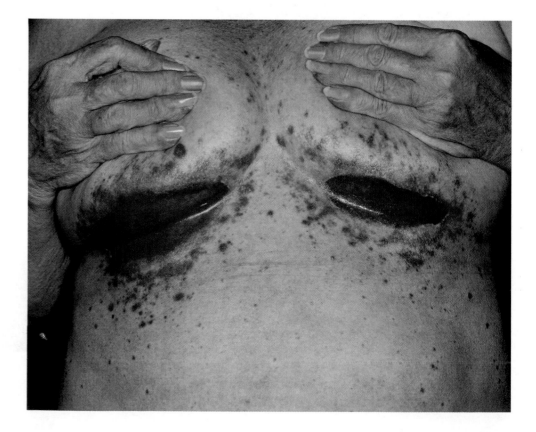

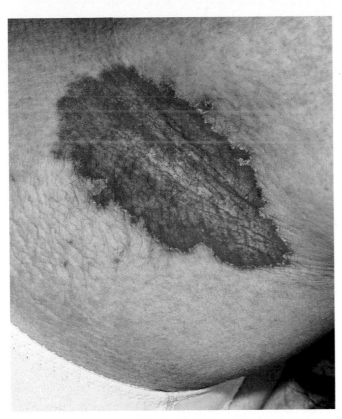

Figure 13-56 Candidiasis of the axillae. A prominent fringe of scale is present at the border.

TREATMENT. Eradication of the yeast infection must be accompanied by maintained dryness of the area. A cool, wet Burrow's solution, water, or saline compress is applied for 20 to 30 minutes several times each day to promote dryness. Antifungal cream is applied in a thin layer twice a day until the rash clears. Some of these medicines are also available in lotion form, but the liquid base may cause stinging when applied to intertriginous areas. Miconazole nitrate (Monistat-Derm lotion) is the least irritating. Application of compresses should be continued until the skin remains dry. Heat from a gooseneck lamp held several inches away from the involved site is sometimes useful to enhance drying. An absorbent powder, not necessarily medicated, such as Z-Sorb, may be applied after the inflammation is gone. The powder absorbs a small amount of moisture and acts as a dry lubricant, allowing skin surfaces to slide freely, thus preventing moisture accumulation in a potentially stagnant area.

Figure 13-57 *Candida* intertrigo. The overhanging abdominal fold and groin area are infected in this obese patient.

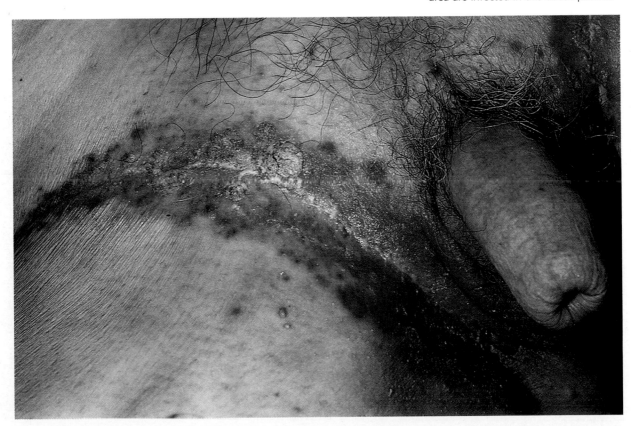

Diaper candidiasis

An artificial intertriginous area is created under a wet diaper, predisposing the area to a yeast infection with the characteristic red base and satellite pustules as described earlier (Figure 13-58). Diaper dermatitis is often treated with steroid combination creams and lotions that contain antibiotics. Although these medications may contain the antiyeast agent clotrimazole, its concentration may not be sufficient to control the yeast infection. The cortisone component may alter the clinical presentation and prolong the disease. A nodular, granulomatous form of candidiasis in the diaper area, appearing as dull, red, irregularly shaped nodules, sometimes on a red base, has been described and may represent an unusual reaction to *Candida* organisms or to a *Candida* organism infection modified by steroids (Figure 13-59). Although dermatophyte infections are unusual in the diaper area, they do occur.[74] Every effort should be made to identify the organism and treat the infection appropriately.

TREATMENT. Dryness should be maintained by changing the diaper frequently or leaving it off for short periods. Antifungal creams should be applied twice a day until the eruption is clear, in approximately 10 days. Some erythema from irritation may be present after 10 days; this can be treated by alternately applying 1% hydrocortisone cream followed in a few hours by creams active against yeasts (see the Formulary). Apply each agent twice a day. Baby powders may help prevent recurrence by absorbing moisture. Mupirocin ointment 2% (Bactroban) applied 3 or 4 times daily is effective for severe *Candida* and bacterial diaper dermatitis.[75]

DIFFERENTIAL DIAGNOSIS. Any recalcitrant diaper dermatitis must be further investigated to uncover underlying disease. Inflammation in the diaper area can be caused by psoriasis, seborrheic dermatitis, Langerhans cell histiocytosis (Letterer-Siwe disease), acrodermatitis enteropathica (zinc deficiency), biotin deficiency, Kawasaki disease, and HIV infection.

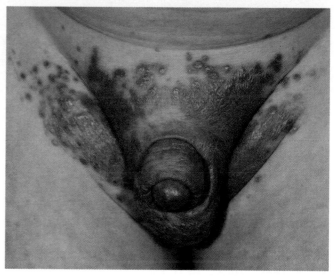

Figure 13-58 Diaper candidiasis, an advanced case. The skin folds are deeply erythematous. The urethral meatus is infected and numerous satellite pustules are on the lower abdominal area.

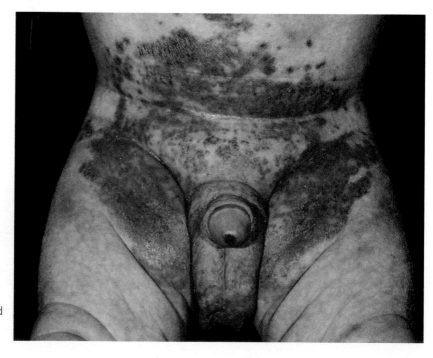

Figure 13-59 Nodular candidiasis of the diaper area. Red nodules are present on a red base and beyond the diffusely inflamed area. The patient had been treated with a cream containing corticosteroids and antifungal agents.

Candidiasis of small skin folds
Finger and toe webs

Web spaces are like small intertriginous areas. Cooks, bartenders, dishwashers, dentists, and others who work in a moist environment are at risk. White, tender, macerated skin erodes, revealing a pink, moist base (Figures 13-60, 13-61, and 13-62). Candidiasis of the toe webs occurs most commonly in the narrow interspace between the fourth and fifth toes, where it may coexist with dermatophytes and gram-negative bacteria. Clinically and in potassium hydroxide preparations, infection by *Candida* and dermatophytes may appear to be identical. Macerated, white scale becomes thick and adherent. Diffuse candidiasis of the webs and feet is unusual. Both areas are treated with any of the antifungal creams or lotions listed in the Formulary. Strands of lamb's wool (Dr. Scholl's Lamb's Wool) can be placed between the toe webs to separate and promote dryness.

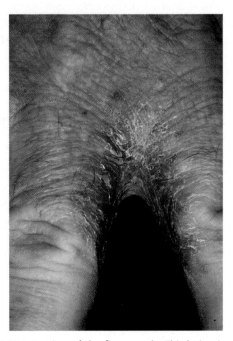

Figure 13-60 Intertrigo of the finger web. This lesion is not wet and macerated like that in Figure 13-61. This eczematous process occurred in a bartender whose hands were constantly wet.

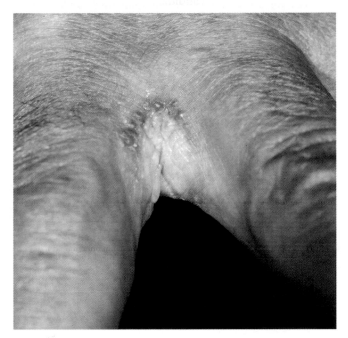

Figure 13-61 Candidiasis of the finger web. The acute phase with maceration of the web. Pustules are present at the border.

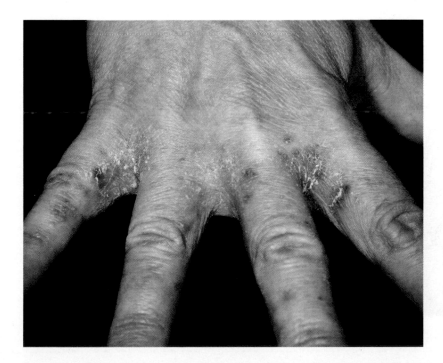

Figure 13-62 Candidiasis of the finger webs. All webs are infected except the wide space between the thumb and index finger.

Angles of the mouth

Angular cheilitis or perlèche, an inflammation at the angles of the mouth, can occur at any age. Patients may have the misconception that they have a vitamin B deficiency; yeast and bacteria may be involved in the process. Lip licking, biting the corners of the mouth, or thumb sucking causes perlèche in the young. Continued irritation may lead to eczematous inflammation. The presence of saliva at the angles of the mouth is the most important factor. Excess saliva occurs as a result of mouth breathing secondary to nasal congestion and of malocclusion resulting from poorly fitting dentures and compulsive lip licking. Aggressive use of dental floss may cause mechanical trauma to mouth angles.[76] A moist, intertriginous space forms in skin folds at the angles of the mouth as a result of advancing age, congenital excessive-angle skin folds, sagging that occurs with weight loss, or abnormal vertical shortening of the lower one third of the face from loss of teeth and resultant resorption of the alveolar bone. Capillary action draws fluid from the mouth into the fold, creating maceration, chapping, fissures, erythema, exudation, and secondary infection with *Candida* organisms and/or staphylococci.

The infection starts as a sore fissure in the depth of the skin fold (Figure 13-63). Erythema, scale, and crust form at the sides of the fold (Figure 13-64). Patients lick and moisten the area in an attempt to prevent further cracking. This attempt at relief only aggravates the problem and may lead to eczematous inflammation, staphylococcal infection, or hypertrophy of the skin fold.

Consider contact dermatitis, diabetes mellitus, and HIV infection in chronic treatment—resistant cases.

TREATMENT. Treatment consists of applying antifungal creams (see the Formulary), followed in a few hours by a group V steroid cream with a nongreasy base (e.g., triamcinolone acetonide [Aristocort A] 0.1%) until the area is dry and free of inflammation. As an alternative, Lotrisone lotion may be applied twice a day until symptoms resolve. Patients should discontinue topical steroids when inflammation has resolved. Thereafter, a thick, protective lip balm (e.g., Chap Stick) is applied frequently. Zyplast collagen injected at the mouth angles can decrease the depth of the grooves[77] and fill the depression that often occurs below the lateral lower lip, thereby correcting the anatomic defect causing the problem. Culture resistant cases for bacteria and yeast. Mupirocin ointment or cream 2% (Bactroban) applied 3 or 4 times daily may be effective for both yeast and bacteria.[75]

Chronic mucocutaneous candidiasis

Chronic mucocutaneous candidiasis (CMC) is a rare syndrome that is characterized by recurrent and persistent *Candida* infection of the skin, nails, and mucous membranes without disseminated candidiasis. It is usually recognized in infancy or childhood, and there are frequently underlying genetic, endocrine, or immunologic features. The diagnosis is often made initially by failure of a child with oral candidiasis to respond to topical anti-*Candida* treatment. Autosomal dominant or recessive predisposition and endocrinopathy (e.g., hypoparathyroidism or hypoadrenalism) and hypothyroidism are all associated conditions. Patients may have a variety of immune defects mainly involving defects in T-lymphocyte function. There are three categories based on the age of the patient at onset[78] and many subtypes.

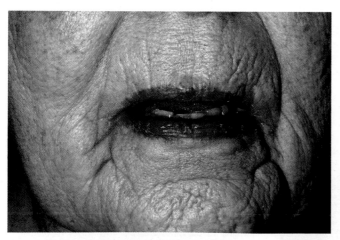

Figure 13-63 Angular cheilitis (perlèche). Skin folds at the angles of the mouth are red and eroded.

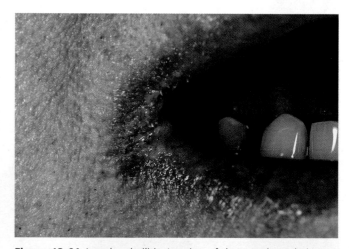

Figure 13-64 Angular cheilitis. Interigo of the mouth angle is a combination of eczema, *Candida,* and bacteria infection.

Tinea Versicolor

Tinea versicolor is a common fungal infection of the skin caused by the dimorphic lipophilic yeast *Pityrosporum orbiculare* (round form) and *Pityrosporum ovale* (oval form). Some authors believe these are different forms of the same organism. (Both were previously called *Malassezia furfur*.) The organism is part of the normal skin flora and appears in highest numbers in areas with increased sebaceous activity. It resides within the stratum corneum and hair follicles, where it thrives on free fatty acids and triglycerides. Certain predisposing endogenous factors (adrenalectomy, Cushing's disease, pregnancy, malnutrition, burns, corticosteroid therapy, immunosuppression, depressed cellular immunity, oral contraceptives) or exogenous factors (excess heat, humidity) cause the yeast to convert from budding yeast form to its mycelial form, leading to the appearance of tinea versicolor. Whether the disease is contagious is unknown. The disease may occur at any age, but it is much more common during the years of higher sebaceous activity (i.e., adolescence and young adulthood). Some individuals, especially those with oily skin, may be more susceptible.

CLINICAL PRESENTATION. The individual lesions and their distribution are highly characteristic. Lesions begin as multiple small, circular macules of various colors (white, pink, or brown) that enlarge radially (Figures 13-65 to 13-68). Tinea versicolor infections produce a spectrum of clinical presentations and colors that include (1) red to fawn-colored macules, patches, or follicular papules that are predominantly caused by a hyperemic inflammatory response; (2) hypopigmented lesions; and (3) tan to dark brown macules and patches. Melanocyte damage appears to be the basis for hypopigmentation. Dicarboxylic acids produced by the *Pityrosporum* may have a cytotoxic effect of melanocytes and inhibit the dopa-tyrosinase reaction. There is a reduction in number, size, and aggregation of melanosomes in melanocytes and in surrounding keratinocytes. The lesions may be hyperpigmented in blacks. The color is uniform in each individual. The lesions may be inconspicuous in fair-complexed individuals during the winter. White hypopigmentation becomes more obvious as unaffected skin tans. The upper trunk is most commonly affected, but it is not unusual for lesions to spread to the upper arms, neck, and abdomen. Involvement of the face, back of the hands, and legs can occur. Facial lesions are more common in children; the forehead is the site of facial involvement usually affected. The eruption may itch if it is inflammatory, but it is usually asymptomatic. The disease may vary in activity for years, but it diminishes or disappears with advancing age. The differential diagnosis includes vitiligo, pityriasis alba, seborrheic dermatitis, secondary syphilis, and pityriasis rosea.

Figure 13-65 Tinea versicolor. Numerous circular, scaly lesions. The eruption is light brown or fawn colored in fair-complected, untanned skin.

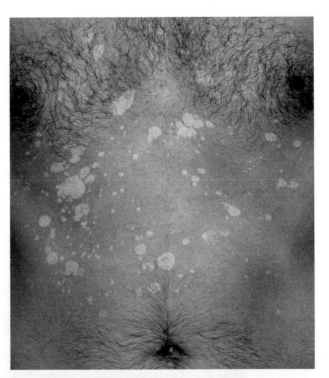

Figure 13-66 The classic presentation of tinea versicolor with white, oval, or circular patches on tan skin.

TINEA VERSICOLOR

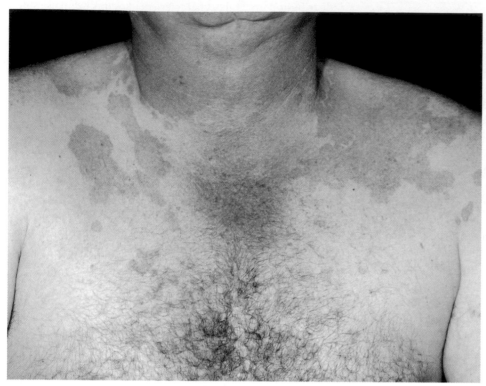

Figure 13-67 Broad confluent scaly patches in a fair-skinned individual.

Figure 13-68 Scaling macules coalesce to form broad areas of irregularly shaped areas that can be either lighter or darker than the surrounding skin.

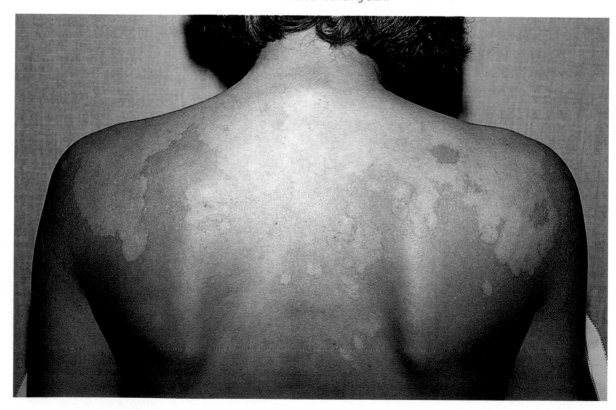

DIAGNOSIS. A powdery scale that may not be obvious on inspection can easily be demonstrated by scraping lightly with a #15 surgical blade (Figure 13-69). Potassium hydroxide examination of the scale shows numerous hyphae that tend to break into short, rod-shaped fragments intermixed with round spores in grapelike clusters, giving the so-called spaghetti-and-meatballs pattern (Figure 13-70). Wood's light examination shows irregular, pale, yellow-to-white fluorescence that fades with improvement. Some lesions do not fluoresce. Culture is possible but rarely necessary.

TREATMENT. Griseofulvin is not active against tinea versicolor. A variety of medicines eliminate the fungus, but relief is usually temporary and recurrences are common (40% to 60%). Patients must understand that the hypopigmented areas will not disappear immediately after treatment. Sunlight accelerates repigmentation. The inability to produce powdery scale by scraping with a #15 surgical blade indicates the fungus has been eradicated. Fungal elements may be retained in frequently worn garments that are in contact with the skin;

discarding or boiling such clothing might decrease the chance of recurrence. Patients without obvious involvement who have a history of multiple recurrences might consider repeating a treatment program just before the summer months to avoid uneven tanning.

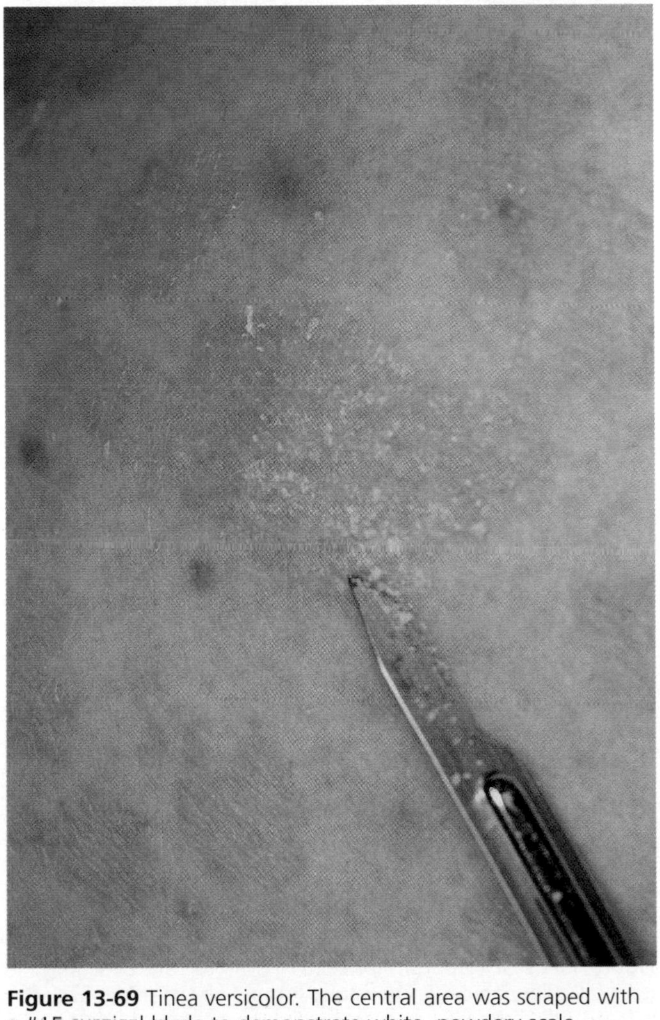

TOPICAL TREATMENT. Topical treatment is indicated for limited disease. Recurrence rates are high.

Ketoconazole shampoo. Ketoconazole 2% shampoo, used as a single application or daily for 3 days, is highly effective and is the treatment of first choice. Apply the shampoo to the entire skin surface from the lower posterior scalp area down to the thighs. The shampoo is left in place for 5 minutes and then rinsed thoroughly.[79] Wash the scalp with the shampoo at the same time.

Selenium sulfide suspension 2.5%. When applied for 10 minutes every day for 7 consecutive days, the suspension (available as Selsun or in generic forms) resulted in an 87% cure rate at a 2-week follow-up evaluation.[80] Blood and urine levels determined during this study showed that no significant absorption of selenium took place.[80] The suspension is applied to the entire skin surface from the lower posterior scalp area down to the thighs. Another commonly recommended schedule is to apply the lotion and wash it off in 24 hours. This is repeated once each week for a total of 4 weeks. There are many suggested variations of this treatment schedule. Wash the scalp with the lotion at the same time.

Terbinafine solution (lasmisil soluntion 1% spray bottle). Application of the spray to the effected areas twice a day for 1 week is effective. Lamisil spray is available as an over-the-counter product.

Figure 13-69 Tinea versicolor. The central area was scraped with a #15 surgical blade to demonstrate white, powdery scale.

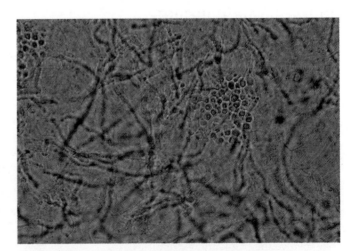

Figure 13-70 Tinea versicolor. A potassium hydroxide wet mount. A low-power view showing numerous short, broad hyphae and clusters of budding cells, which have been described as having the appearance of "spaghetti and meatballs."

Antifungal antibiotics. Miconazole, ketoconazole, clotrimazole, econazole, or ciclopirox olamine is applied to the entire affected area 1 or 2 times a day for 2 to 4 weeks. The creams are odorless and nongreasy but expensive.

ORAL TREATMENT (SEE TABLE 13-2). Oral treatment may be used in patients with extensive disease and those who do not respond to conventional treatment or have frequent recurrences.

Itraconazole. Itraconazole 200 mg qd for 7 days provided an 89% mycologic cure rate at the end of 4 weeks.[81] A double-blind, placebo-controlled study was conducted to evaluate prophylactic treatment. All patients received itraconazole 200 mg qd for 7 days. Prophylactic treatment with itraconazole 200 mg bid 1 day per month for 6 consecutive months was administered to one group; the other group received placebo. At the prophylactic treatment end point (6 months), mycologic cure was 88% in the itraconazole group and 57% in the placebo group.[82]

Fluconazole. Fluconazole, 300 or 400 mg given as a single dose and repeated if needed after 2 weeks, was very effective.[83]

Ketoconazole. A single dose of 400 mg of ketoconazole is effective. Prophylaxis with 400 mg once monthly resulted in no recurrence during follow-up of 4 to 15 months. Efficacy can be enhanced by refraining from antacids and taking the drug at breakfast with fruit juice. The patient should not bathe for at least 12 hours after treatment; this allows the medication to accumulate in the skin.

Terbinafine and griseofulvin. Terbinafine or griseofulvin taken orally is not effective.

PREVENTING RECURRENCES. Once-weekly application of ketoconazole 2% shampoo (Nizoral), applied as a lotion to the neck, trunk, and proximal extremities 5 to 10 minutes before showering, may help prevent recurrences.

Pityrosporum folliculitis

Pityrosporum folliculitis is an infection of the hair follicle caused by the yeast *P. orbiculare,* the same organism that causes tinea versicolor. The typical patient is a young woman with asymptomatic or slightly itchy follicular papules and pustules localized to the upper back and chest, upper arms, and neck.[84] Occlusion and greasy skin may be important predisposing factors. It is frequently diagnosed as acne (Figure 13-71). Diabetes mellitus and administration of broad-spectrum antibiotics or corticosteroids are predisposing factors. Follicular occlusion may be a primary event, with yeast overgrowth as a secondary occurrence.[85] Hodgkin's disease may predispose to pityrosporum folliculitis.[86] These patients complain of severe generalized pruritis; the eruption may involve the trunk and extremities.

Pityrosporum is very common in the tropics, where it presents as a polymorphous eruption with the following characteristics.[87] The primary lesion is a keratinous plug that underlies four clinical types of lesion: follicular papules (dome-shaped papules with a central depression), pustules, nodules, and cysts. The lesions evolve from follicular plugs colonized by *Pityrosporum.* The face is often affected—this is the most common site in female patients and the second most common in male patients. The lesions are localized to the mandible, chin, and sides of the face. This is in contrast to the usually more central facial location of acne vulgaris. Lesions also are found on the nape of the neck, abdomen, buttocks, and thighs. Both young men and young women are equally affected. Their active sebaceous glands presumably provide the lipid-rich environment required by the yeast.

A potassium hydroxide examination reveals abundant round, budding yeast cells, and sometimes hyphae. Treatment is the same as for tinea versicolor. Combined ketoconazole shampoo and systemic ketoconazole (200 mg qd for 4 weeks) produced clearance of the lesions in 100% of patients, whereas systemic therapy resulted in only a 75% clearance rate. Topical econazole and miconazole failed in 90%.[88] Salicylic acid wash (Sal Ac) is keratolytic and effective.[89]

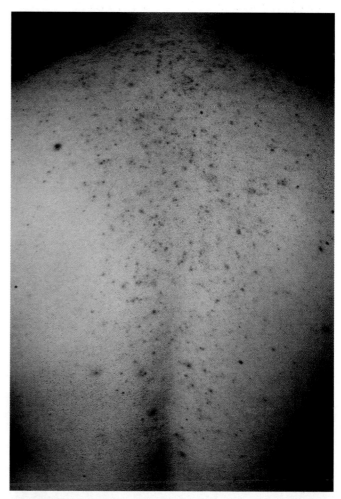

Figure 13-71 Pityrosporum folliculitis. Asymptomatic or slightly itchy follicular papules and pustules located on the upper back. It is frequently diagnosed as acne.

References

1. Sorensen GW, Jones HE: Immediate and delayed hypersensitivity in chronic dermatophytosis, Arch Dermatol 1976;112: 40.

2. Burke WA, Jones BE: A simple stain for rapid office diagnosis of fungus infection of the skin, Arch Dermatol 1984;120:1519.

3. Brodell RT, Helms SF, Snelson ME: Office dermatologic testing: the potassium hydroxide preparation, Am Fam Physician 1991;43: 2061.

4. Head ES, Henry JC, MacDonald EM: The cotton swab technic for the culture of dermatophyte infections: its efficacy and merit, J Am Acad Dermatol 1984;11: 797.

5. Kearse HJ, Miller OF: Tinea pedis in prepubertal children: does it occur? J Am Acad Dermatol 1988;19: 619.

6. McBride A, Cohen BA: Tinea pedis in children, Am J Dis Child 1992;146: 844.

7. Svejgaard E, Christophersen J, Jelsdorf HM: Tinea pedis and erythrasma in Danish recruits: clinical signs, prevalence, incidence, and correlation to atopy, J Am Acad Dermatol 1986;14: 993.

8. Kates SG, et al: Microbial ecology of interdigital infections of toe web spaces, J Am Acad Dermatol 1990;22: 578.

9. Dahl MV: Suppression of immunity and inflammation by-products produced by dermatophytes, J Am Acad Dermatol 1993;28: S19.

10. Daniel Cr, et al: Two feet-one hand syndrome: a retrospective multicenter survey, Int J Dermatol 1997;36: 658.

11. Smith EB, et al: Double-blind comparison of naftifine cream and clotrimazole/betamethasone dipropionate cream in the treatment of tinea pedis, J Am Acad Dermatol 1992;26: 125.

12. Berman R, et al: Efficacy of a 1-week, twice-daily regimen of terbinafine 1% cream in the treatment of interdigital tinea pedis: results of placebo-controlled, double-blind, multicenter trials, J Am Acad Dermatol 1992;26: 956.

13. Savin R, et al: One-week therapy with twice-daily butenafine 1% cream versus vehicle in the treatment of tinea pedis: a multicenter, double-blind trial, J Am Acad Dermatol 1997;36(2 Pt 1): S15.

14. Kates SG, et al: The antibacterial efficacy of econazole nitrate in interdigital toe web infections, J Am Acad Dermatol 1990;22: 583.

15. White JE, Perkins PJ, Evans EJ: Successful 2-week treatment with terbinafine (Lamisil) for moccasin tinea pedis and tinea manuum, Br J Dermatol 1991;125: 260.

16. Lesher JJ: Oral therapy of common superficial fungal infections of the skin, J Am Acad Dermatol 1999;40(6 pt 2): S31.

17. Takama H, et al: Pitted keratolysis: clinical manifestations in 53 cases, Br J Dermatol 1997;137(2): 282.

18. Shah AS, Kamino H, Prose NS: Painful, plaque-like, pitted keratolysis occurring in childhood, Pediatr Dermatol 1992;9: 251.

19. Hanel H, et al: Quantification of keratinolytic activity from Dermatophilus congolensis, Med Microbiol Immunol 1991;180: 45.

20. Vazquez-Lopez F, Perez-Oliva N: Mupirocine ointment for symptomatic pitted keratolysis (letter), Infection 1996;24: 55.

21. Mattox TF, et al: Nonfluorescent erythrasma of the vulva, Obstet Gynecol 1993;81: 862.

22. Wharton J, Wilson P, Kincannon J: Erythrasma treated with single-dose clarithromycin, Arch Dermatol 1998;134: 671.

23. Faergemann J, et al: A multicentre (double-blind) comparative study to assess the safety and efficacy of fluconazole and griseofulvin in the treatment of tinea corporis and tinea cruris, Br J Dermatol 1997;136: 575.

24. Stiller MJ, et al: Tinea corporis gladiatorum: an epidemic of Trichophyton tonsurans in student wrestlers, J Am Acad Dermatol 1992;27: 632.

25. el Fari M, et al: An epidemic of tinea corporis caused by Trichophyton tonsurans among children (wrestlers) in Germany, Mycoses 2000;43: 191.

26. Adams B: Tinea corporis gladiatorum: a cross-sectional study, J Am Acad Dermatol 2000;43: 1039.

27. Powell FC, Muller SA: Kerion of the glabrous skin, J Am Acad Dermatol 1982;7: 490.

28. Janniger CK: Majocchi's granuloma, Cutis 1992;50: 267.

29. Smith KJ, et al: Majocchi's granuloma, J Cutan Pathol 1991;18: 28.

30. Lesher JJ: Oral therapy of common superficial fungal infections of the skin, J Am Acad Dermatol 1999;40(6 pt 2): S31.

31. Weksberg F, Fisher BF: Unusual tinea corporis caused by Trichophyton verrucosum, Int J Dermatol 1986;25: 653.

32. Barson WJ: Granuloma and pseudogranuloma of the skin due to microsporum canis, Arch Dermatol 1985;121: 895.

33. Hironaga M, et al: Trichophyton mentagrophytes granulomas: unique systemic dissemination to lymph nodes, testes, vertebrae, and brain, Arch Dermatol 1983;119: 482.

34. Albert AA: Tinea capitis, Arch Dermatol 1988;124: 1554.

35. Jacobs PH: Dermatophytes that infect animals and humans, Cutis 1988;42: 330.

36. Shelley WB, Shelley ED, Burneister V: The infected hairs of tinea capitis due to Microsporum canis: demonstration of uniqueness of the hair cuticle by scanning electron microscopy, J Am Acad Dermatol 1987;16: 354.

37. Lee JY, Hsu ML: Pathogenesis of hair infection and black dots in tinea capitis caused by Trichophyton violaceum: a histopathological study, J Cutan Pathol 1992;19: 54.

38. Okuda C, et al: Fungus invasion of human hair tissue in tinea capitis caused by Microsporum canis: light and electron microscopic study, Arch Dermatol Res 1989;281: 238.

39. Hubbard T: The predictive value of symptoms in diagnosing childhood tinea capitis, Arch Pediatr Adolesc Med 1999;153: 1150.

40. Hebert AA, Head ES, MacDonald EM: Tinea capitis caused by Trichophyton tonsurans, Pediatr Dermatol 1985;2: 219.

41. Babel DE, Baughman SA: Evaluation of the adult carrier state in juvenile tinea capitis caused by Trichophyton tonsurans, J Am Acad Dermatol 1989;21: 1209.

42. Babel DE, Rogers AL, Beneke ES: Dermatophytosis of the scalp: incidence, immune response, and epidemiology, Mycopathologia 1990;109: 69.

43. Frieden IL: Diagnosis and management of tinea capitis, Pediatr Ann 1987;16: 39.

44. Rippon JW: Tinea capitis: current concepts. Special symposia. Identification of dermatophytes in the clinical office, Pediatr Dermatol 1985;2: 224.

45. Gan VN, Petruska M, Ginsburg CM: Epidemiology and treatment of tinea capitis: ketoconazole vs. griseofulvin, Pediatr Infect Dis J 1987;6: 46.

46. Borchers SW: Moistened gauze technic to aid in diagnosis of tinea capitis, J Am Acad Dermatol 1985;13: 672.

47. Hubbard TW, de Triquet JM: Brush-culture method for diagnosing tinea capitis, Pediatrics 1992;90: 416.

48. Friedlander S, et al: Use of the cotton swab method in diagnosing tinea capitis, Pediatrics 1999;104(2 pt 1): 276.

49. Bennett M, et al: Oral griseofulvin remains the treatment of choice for tinea capitis in children, Pediatr Dermatol 2000;17: 304.

50. Caceres-Rios H, et al: Comparison of terbinafine and griseofulvin in the treatment of tinea capitis, J Am Acad Dermatol 2000;42 (1 pt 1): 80.

51. Krafchik B, Pelletier J: An open study of tinea capitis in 50 children treated with a 2-week course of oral terbinafine, J Am Acad Dermatol 1999;41: 60.

52. Caceres-Rios H, Rueda M, Ballona R, et al: Comparison of terbinafine and griseofulvin in the treatment of tinea capitis, J Am Acad Dermatol 2000;42(1 pt 1): 80.

53. Stephens CJ, Hay RJ, Black MM: Fungal kerion-total scalp involvement due to Microsporum canis infection, Clin Exp Dermatol 1989;14: 442.

54. Hussain I, et al: A randomized, comparative trial of treatment of kerion celsi with griseofulvin plus oral prednisolone vs. griseofulvin alone, Med Mycol 1999;37: 97.

55. Greer D: Successful treatment of tinea capitis with 2% ketoconazole shampoo, Int J Dermatol 2000;39: 302.

56. Pomeranz A, et al: Asymptomatic dermatophyte carriers in the households of children with tinea capitis, Arch Pediatr Adolesc Med 1999;153: 483.

57. Landau JW: Commentary: undecylenic acid and fungus infections, Arch Dermatol 1983;119: 351.

58. Blank H: Commentary: treatment of dermatomycoses with griseofulvin, Arch Dermatol 1982;118: 835.

59. Sherertz EF: Are laboratory studies necessary for griseofulvin therapy? J Am Acad Dermatol 1990;22: 1103.

60. Horowitz BJ, Giaquinta D, Ito S: Evolving pathogens in vulvovaginal candidiasis: implications for patient care, J Clin Pharmacol 1992;32: 248.

61. Bluestein D, Rutledge C, Lunsden L: Predicting the occurrence of antibiotic-induced candidal vaginitis (AICV), Fam Pract Res J 1991;11: 319.

62. Patel HS, Peters M 2nd, Smith CL: Is there a role for fluconazole in the treatment of vulvovaginal candidiasis? Ann Pharmacother 1992;26: 350.

63. Sobel J, et al: Single oral dose fluconazole compared with conventional clotrimazole topical therapy of Candida vaginitis. Fluconazole Vaginitis Study Group. Am J Obstet Gynecol 1995;172(4 pt 1): 1263.

64. Fong IW: The value of treating the sexual partners of women with recurrent vaginal candidiasis with ketoconazole, Genitourin Med 1992; 68:174.

65. Sobel JD: Pathogenesis and treatment of recurrent vulvovaginal candidiasis, Clin Infect Dis 1992;14: S148.

66. Kunzelmann V, et al: [Prerequisites for effective therapy of chronic recurrent vaginal candidiasis], Mycoses 1996;39 Suppl 1: 65.

67. Hilton E, et al: Ingestion of yogurt containing Lactobacillus acidophilus as prophylaxis for candidal vaginitis, Ann Intern Med 1992;116: 353.

68. Sobel J, et al: Single oral dose fluconazole compared with conventional clotrimazole topical therapy of Candida vaginitis. Fluconazole Vaginitis Study Group, Am J Obstet Gynecol 1995;172(4 pt 1): 1263.

69. White DJ, Johnson EM, Warnock DW: Management of persistent vulvo vaginal candidosis due to azole-resistant Candida glabrata, Genitourin Med 1993;69: 112.

70. Quan M: Vaginitis: meeting the clinical challenge, Clin Cornerstone 2000;3: 36.

71. Martin M: The use of fluconazole and itraconazole in the treatment of Candida albicans infections: a review, J Antimicrob Chemother 1999;44: 429.

72. Stary A, et al: Comparison of the efficacy and safety of oral fluconazole and topical clotrimazole in patients with candida balanitis, Genitourin Med 1996;72: 98.

73. Abdennader S, et al: [Balanitis and infectious agents. A prospective study of 100 cases], Ann Dermatol Venereol 1995;122: 580.

74. Jacobs AH, O'Connell BM: Tinea in tiny tots, Am J Dis Child 1986;140: 1034-1038.

75. de Wet P, et al: Perianal candidosis—a comparative study with mupirocin and nystatin, Int J Dermatol 1999;38: 618.

76. Kahana M, Yahalom R, Schewach-Miller M: Recurrent angular cheilitis caused by dental flossing, J Am Acad Dermatol 1986;15: 113.

77. Chernosky ME: Collagen implant in management of perlèche (angular cheilosis), J Am Acad Dermatol 1985;12: 493.

78. Kirpatrick CH, Windhorst DB: Mucocutaneous candidiasis and thymoma, Am J Med 1979;66: 939.

79. Lange D, et al: Ketoconazole 2% shampoo in the treatment of tinea versicolor: a multicenter, randomized, double-blind, placebo-controlled trial, J Am Acad Dermatol 1998;39: 944.

80. Sanchez JL, Torres VM: Selenium sulfide in tinea versicolor: blood and urine levels, J Am Acad Dermatol 1984;11: 238.

81. Hickman J: A double-blind, randomized, placebo-controlled evaluation of short-term treatment with oral itraconazole in patients with tinea versicolor, J Am Acad Dermatol 1996;34(5 pt 1): 785.

82. Faergemann J, et al: Efficacy of itraconazole in the prophylactic treatment of pityriasis (tinea) versicolor, Arch Dermatol 2002; 138: 69.

83. Amer M: Fluconazole in the treatment of tinea versicolor. Egyptian Fluconazole Study Group, Int J Dermatol 1997;36: 940.

84. Back O, Faergemann J, Hornqvist R: Pityrosporum folliculitis: a common disease of the young and middle-aged, J Am Acad Dermatol 1985;12: 56.

85. Hill MK, et al: Skin surface electron microscopy in Pityrosporum folliculitis: the role of follicular occlusion in disease and the response to oral ketoconazole, Arch Dermatol 1990;126: 1071.

86. Helm KF, Lookingbill DP: Pityrosporum folliculitis and severe pruritus in two patients with Hodgkin's disease (letter), Arch Dermatol 1993;129: 380.

87. Jacinto-Jamora S, Tamesis J, Katigbak ML: Pityrosporum folliculitis in the Philippines: diagnosis, prevalence, and management, J Am Acad Dermatol 1991;24: 693.

88. Abdel-Razek M, et al: Pityrosporum (Malassezia) folliculitis in Saudi Arabia—diagnosis and therapeutic trials, Clin Exp Dermatol 1995;20: 406.

89. Hartmann AA: The influence of various factors on the human resident skin flora, Semin Dermatol 1990;9: 305.

❏ **Exanthems**
   Measles
   Hand, foot, and mouth disease
   Scarlet fever
   Rubella
   Erythema infectiosum
   Roseola infantum
   Enteroviruses: echovirus and coxsackievirus
      exanthems
   Kawasaki syndrome
   Superantigen toxin-mediated illnesses
   Toxic shock syndrome
   Cutaneous drug reactions

❏ **Drug eruptions: clinical patterns and most**
   frequently causal drugs
   Exanthems (maculopapular)
   Urticaria
   Pruritus

❏ **Drug eruptions**
   Acute generalized exanthematous pustulosis
   Acneiform (pustular) eruptions
   Eczema
   Blistering drug eruptions
   Erythema multiforme and toxic epidermal
      necrolysis
   Exfoliative erythroderma
   Fixed drug eruptions
   Lichenoid (lichen planus–like drug
      eruptions)
   Lupus erythematosus–like drug eruptions
   Photosensitivity
   Pigmentation
   Vasculitis
   Lymphomatoid drug eruptions
   Chemotherapy-induced acral erythema
   Skin eruptions associated with specific drugs

The word *exanthem* means a skin eruption that bursts forth or blooms. Exanthematous diseases are characterized by widespread, symmetric, erythematous, discrete, or confluent macules and papules that initially do not form scale. Exanthematous disease is one of the few diseases for which the term *maculopapular* is an appropriate descriptive term. Other lesions, such as pustules, vesicles, and petechiae, may form, but most of the exanthematous diseases begin with red macules or papules. Widespread red eruptions such as guttate psoriasis or pityriasis rosea may have a similar beginning and are often symmetric, but these conditions have typical patterns of scale and are therefore referred to as *papulosquamous eruptions*. Diseases that begin with exanthems may be caused by bacteria, viruses, or drugs. Most have a number of characteristic features such as a common primary lesion, distribution,[1] duration, and systemic symptoms. Some are accompanied by oral lesions that are referred to as *enanthems*. Pediatric exanthems are summarized in Table 14-1.

Exanthems were previously consecutively numbered according to their historical appearance and description: first disease, measles; second disease, scarlet fever; third disease, rubella; fourth disease, "Dukes' disease" (probably coxsackievirus or echovirus); fifth disease, erythema infectiosum; and sixth disease, roseola infantum.

Table 14-1 Exanthems

Disease	Age group	Prodrome incubation	Morphology
Measles (rubeola)	0 to 20 yr	Rhinitis, cough, fever, conjunctivitis, Koplick's spots 8 to 12 days	Erythematous macules and papules later becomes confluent; turns coppery-colored
German measles (rubella)	5 to 25 yr	Mild URI symptoms 14 to 23 days	Generalized maculopapular becomes pinpoint
Roseola (exanthem subitum HHV-6)	0 to 3 yr	High fever for 3 to 5 days Diarrhea, cough 5 to 15 days	Pale pink almond-shaped macules and papules
Erythema infectiosum (fifth disease parvovirus B-19)	4 yr (1 to 17 yr) Nonimmune adults	Nonspecific fever and malaise 13 to 18 days	Macular erythema on face (1 to 4 days), erythematous macular eruption for first week followed by lacy erythema
Unilateral laterothoracic exanthem	12 to 63 mo	URI symptoms	Discrete mild pruritic 1-mm (erythematous papules and morbilliform, eczematous plaques) Spontaneous resolution after 5 wk
Papular-purpuric gloves and socks syndrome (parvovirus B-19)	Children, mean age 24 mo	Fever	Finely papular, purpuric, petechial edema and erythema; resolves spontaneously within 1 to 2 wk
Chickenpox (varicella)	1 to 14 yr	Fever, malaise, headache, anorexia, abdominal pain for 48 hours	Erythematous macules that evolve into vesicles containing serous fluid Different stages of lesions present simultaneously
Kawasaki (mucocutaneous syndrome lymph node syndrome)	Usually <5 yr	High fever Irritability	Erythematous maculopapular, Desquamation of the tips of the fingers (morbilliform or vesiculobullous form) and toes
Gianotti-Crosti syndrome (papular acrodermatitis of childhood)	Peak 1 to 6 yr; can occur in adults	URI Generalized adenopathy	Lichenoid, flesh-colored to red papules May form plaques
Meningococcemia (Neisseria meningitidis)	<2 yr	Hepatosplenomegaly Fever, malaise, URI symptoms	Petechiae, purpura, bullous lesions seen
Rocky Mountain spotted fever (Rickettsia rickettsii)	Any age	Fever, malaise, headache	Pale red or rose colored macules Evolves to petechiae and purpura
Henoch-Schonlein (purpura)	6 mo to young	Arthralgia or abdominal pain	Symmetric palpable purpura
Erythema multiforme	10 to 30 yr	Infection with HSV or mycoplasma may precede; drug exposure	Erythematous macules with darker center "target lesion"
Scarlet fever	1 to 10 yr	2 to 4 days	Pinpoint papules Desquamation of the tips of the fingers and toes

Adapted from Gable EK, et al: Prim Care June 2000; 27:353.

Twenty-five percent of all children may be group A streptococcal carriers.

Distribution of rash	Associated findings	Laboratory findings
Begins in hairline on neck and face Moves down and covers entire body Becomes confluent as it fades and leaves a brownish hue with fine desquamation	Koplik's spots, exudative conjunctivitis, photophobia, and severe cough; pneumonia, swelling of the hands and feet Otitis media, encephalitis 1:1000, subacute sclerosing panencephalitis (late)	WBC count and ESR are low Measles immunoglobulin M (IgM) titer
Begins on face Migrates to trunk	Tender retroauricular, posterior cervical, and occipital adenopathy Slight fever Transient polyarthralgia and polyarthritis in adolescents and adults, especially females	Nasal culture for virus Antibody titer
Trunk, neck, and proximal extremities	Rash appears as fever resolves Irritability, febrile seizures possible	Leukocytosis at onset of fever, but leukopenia as the temperature increases
Face ("slapped cheek") followed by extremities; lacy rash over extensor surfaces Rash can recur	Spontaneous abortion (from severe fetal anemia and hydrops fetalis) Aplastic crises in sickle cell disease Women may develop arthralgia or arthritis	IgM antibodies CBC Evaluate the immune status of exposed pregnant women (IgG)
Predominantly unilateral Begins close to axilla and spreads to become bilateral Retains a unilateral predominance on trunk or flexures and may become bilateral	Fever, upper respiratory tract infection, vomiting, diarrhea	Relative lymphocytosis 37%
Sharply demarcated gloves and socks distribution Groin, buttock, antecubital, and popliteal fossae Nose may be involved	Fever, lymphadenopathy, oral lesions Clears in 1 to 2 weeks	Leukopenia
Begins on face scalp or trunk Spreads peripherally	Pruritus present Lesions seen on mucous membranes	Culture of vesicle Acute and convalescent serum samples for IgG
Most prominent on the trunk and extremities Perineal accentuation typical of KS but fades abruptly without residual of measles Desquamation around perineum and fingertips after first week	Conjunctivitis; strawberry tongue, fissured lips, adenopathy; coronary artery aneurysms Swelling of the hands and feet No hypotension or renal involvement	WBC count and ESR are high Thrombocytosis during the second to third week Sterile pyuria in the first week
Face, buttocks, extremities	Fever, malaise, diarrhea	Skin biopsy Some cases, surface antigenemia Elevation of serum transaminase and alkaline phosphatase without hyperbilirubinemia
Trunk, extremities, palms, and soles	Temperature >40° C Shock DIC	Culture blood and CSF Antigen detection in CSF
Begins on wrists, ankles; spreads centrally; seen on palms and soles	Hepatosplenamegaly, hyponatremia, myalgias, CNS involvement	Any of the rickettsial group-specific serologic tests
Buttocks, extensor extremities	Gastrointestinal, musculoskeletal, renal involvement	Skin biopsy H&E Immunofluorescences
Extensor surfaces of extremities, palms, and soles can be involved	May progress to involve mucous membranes, Stevens-Johnson syndrome	Skin biopsy
Generalized; spares palms and soles	Exudative pharyngitis	Group A streptococcal positive throat culture Elevated WBC count and ESR

Continued

Table 14-1 Exanthems—cont'd

Disease	Age group	Prodrome incubation	Morphology
Toxic shock syndrome	Children with burns and tracheitis	Sudden onset	Macular erythroderma, desquamation of the tips of the fingers and toes
Drug exanthem	Any age	7 to 10 days after the drug is first taken	Maculopapular, urticarial, pruritus
Hand, foot, and mouth disease (coxsackievirus A16 and others)	Children	4 to 6 days, 50% fever, malaise	Vesiculopustules
Staphylococcal scalded skin syndrome	<5 yr	Malaise, fever, irritability	Tender, generalized macular erythema becomes vesicular and bullous

Adapted from Gable EK, et al: Prim Care June 2000; 27:353.
Twenty-five percent of all children may be group A streptococcal carriers.

Exanthems

Measles

Measles (rubeola or morbilli) is a highly contagious viral disease transmitted by contact with droplets from infected individuals who cough. These droplets may remain suspended in the air in nonventilated physicians' waiting rooms and infect patients even after the infected patient has left.[2] Most cases have a benign course, but encephalitis occurs in 1:2000 individuals; survivors frequently have permanent brain damage and mental retardation. Death, predominantly from respiratory and neurologic causes, occurs in 1:3000 reported measles cases. The risk of death is known to be greater for infants and adults than for children and adolescents. Measles occurring during pregnancy may affect the fetus. Most commonly, this involves premature labor, moderately increased rates of spontaneous abortion, and low birth weight infants. Measles infection in the first trimester of pregnancy may be associated with an increased rate of congenital malformation.[3] In the prevaccine era, most measles cases affected preschool and young school-age children. In 1980, more than 60% of cases in which the age was known occurred among persons 10 years or older.

INCIDENCE. The World Health Organization (WHO) has estimated that 777,000 children died as a result of measles during 2000. During 1990 to 2000, implementation of national vaccination and surveillance programs reduced measles incidence in the Americas by 99%. Haiti and Venezuela are the last countries in the Americas where measles is endemic. Measles can be imported to measles-free countries from countries where measles is endemic; therefore, all countries in the Americas must maintain the highest possible population immunity (i.e., >95% among infants and children). Measles is the leading cause of vaccine-preventable death in Africa.

VACCINE. Lifelong immunity is established with a single injection of live measles virus vaccine given at approximately 15 months of age. From 1963 to 1967, both live and inactivated measles vaccines were in use; since 1968 only the live vaccine has been used. Susceptible persons include those who were vaccinated between 1963 and 1967 with inactivated vaccine, patients given live measles virus vaccine before their first birthdays, and those patients who have never had measles. Prior recipients of killed measles vaccine may develop atypical measles syndrome when exposed to natural measles and should be revaccinated with live measles virus.

Typical measles

The incubation period of measles (rubeola) (Figure 14-1) averages 10 to 12 days from exposure to prodrome and 14 days from exposure to rash (range, 7 to 18 days). The disease is spread by respiratory droplets and can be communicated from slightly before the beginning of the prodromal period to 4 days after appearance of the rash; communicability is minimal after the second day of the rash. Prodromal symptoms of severe, brassy cough; coryza; conjunctivitis; photophobia; and fever appear 3 to 4 days before the exanthem and increase daily in severity. The nose and eyes run continuously: the classic sign of measles. Koplik's spots (blue-white spots with a red halo) appear on the buccal mucous membrane opposite the premolar teeth 24 to 48 hours before the exanthem and remain for 2 to 4 days.

ERUPTIVE PHASE. The rash begins on the fourth or fifth day on the face and behind the ears, but in 24 to 36 hours, it spreads to the trunk and extremities (Figure 14-2). It reaches maximum intensity simultaneously in all areas in approximately 3 days and fades after 5 to 10 days. The rash consists of slightly elevated maculopapules that vary in size from 0.1 to 1.0 cm and vary in color from dark red to a purplish hue. They are frequently confluent on both the face and body, a feature

Distribution of rash	Associated findings	Laboratory findings
Diffuse	Hypotension, renal involvement, a focus of infection	Elevations of the serum creatinine phosphokinase level
Generalized, symmetric, often spares the face Palms and soles may be involved	Periorbital edema, fever	ESR is low
Hands, feet, buttock Erosions on mouth	Submandibular and/or cervical lymphadenopathy Dysphagia 90%	Biopsy
Face, neck, axilla, and groin	Staphylococcal infection of nasopharynx or conjunctiva	Elevated WBC count and ESR

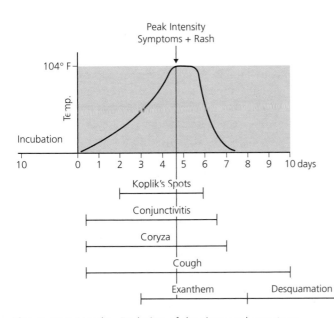

Figure 14-1 Measles. Evolution of the signs and symptoms.

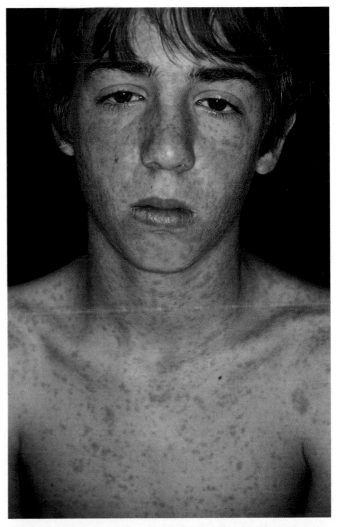

Figure 14-2 Measles. Early eruptive stage with involvement of the face and trunk. Eruption has become confluent on the face.

that is such a distinct characteristic of measles that eruptions of similar appearance in other diseases are termed *morbilliform*. The early rash blanches on pressure; the fading rash is yellowish-brown with a fine scale, and it does not blanch. Supportive treatment is the only necessity unless complications, such as bacterial infection or encephalitis, appear.

The disease can be severe and is most frequently complicated by diarrhea, middle ear infection, or bronchopneumonia. Encephalitis occurs in approximately 1 of every 1000 reported cases; survivors of this complication often have permanent brain damage and mental retardation. Death occurs in 1 to 2 of every 1000 reported measles cases in the United States. The risk for death from measles or its complications is greater for infants, young children, and adults than for older children and adolescents. The most common causes of death are pneumonia and acute encephalitis. In developing countries, measles is often more severe, and the case-fatality rate can be as high as 25%.

Management of measles

Vitamin A deficiency impairs epithelial integrity and systemic immunity and increases the incidence and severity of infections during childhood. Vitamin A supplementation is effective in reducing total mortality and complications from measles infections; it is likely to be more effective in populations with nutritional deficiencies.[4]

VITAMIN A TREATMENT. Vitamin A, retinol-binding protein (RBP), and albumin are significantly reduced early in the exanthem. Treatment with vitamin A reduces morbidity and mortality in measles,[4] and all children with severe measles should be given vitamin A supplements regardless of whether they are thought to have a nutritional deficiency.[5,6] Vitamin A–treated children recover more rapidly from pneumonia and diarrhea, have less croup, and spend fewer days in the hospital.[7] Treated patients have an increase in the total number of lymphocytes and measles IgG antibody.[9] The risk of death or a major complication during a hospital stay is half that of untreated patients.

The appropriate dose regimens for safe administration of vitamin A in complicated measles are for age under 6 months, 50,000 IU; for age between 6 months and 2 years, 100,000 IU; and for age over 2 years, 200,000 IU, administered via mouth on admission. A repeated dose can be administered on the next day.

VACCINATION

Immunity. Persons are considered immune if they have documentation of adequate immunization with live measles vaccine on or after the first birthday, physician-diagnosed measles, or laboratory evidence of measles immunity. Most persons born before 1957 are likely to have been naturally infected and generally need not be considered susceptible. Routine serologic screening to determine measles immunity is not recommended.

Individuals exposed to disease. Live vaccine, if given within 72 hours of measles exposure, may provide protection and is preferable to the use of human immunoglobulin in persons at least 12 months of age if there is no contraindication.

USE OF HUMAN IMMUNOGLOBULIN. Human immunoglobulin can be given to prevent or modify measles in a susceptible person within 6 days after exposure. The recommended dose of IG is 0.25 ml/kg (0.11 ml/lb) of body weight (maximum dose, 15 ml).

REVACCINATION RISKS. There is no enhanced risk from administering live measles vaccine to persons who are already immune to measles.

Pregnancy. Live measles vaccine should not be given to women known to be pregnant or who are considering becoming pregnant within 3 months after vaccination. This precaution is based on the theoretical risk of fetal infection.

Hand, foot, and mouth disease

Hand, foot, and mouth disease (HFMD), which has no relation to hoof-and-mouth disease in cattle, is a contagious enteroviral infection occurring primarily in children and characterized by a vesicular palmoplantar eruption and erosive stomatitis. It is most often caused by coxsackievirus A16 and enterovirus 71. Enteroviruses are believed to be spread via the fecal-oral and perhaps respiratory routes. This disease may occur as an isolated phenomenon, or it may occur in epidemic form. It is more common among children.

CLINICAL PRESENTATION. The incubation period is 4 to 6 days. There may be mild symptoms of low-grade fever, sore throat, and malaise for 1 or 2 days. Twenty percent of patients develop submandibular and/or cervical lymphadenopathy.

ERUPTIVE PHASE. Oral lesions, present in 90% of cases, are generally the initial sign. Aphthaelike erosions varying from a few to 10 or more appear anywhere in the oral cavity and are most frequently small and asymptomatic (Figure 14-3). The cutaneous lesions, which occur in approximately two thirds of patients, appear less than 24 hours after the enanthem. They begin as 3- to 7-mm, red macules that rapidly become pale, white, oval vesicles with a red areola (Figure 14-4). There may be a few inconspicuous lesions, or there may be dozens. The vesicles occur on the palms, soles (Figure 14-5), dorsal aspects of the fingers and toes, and occasionally on the face, buttocks, and legs. They heal in approximately 7 days, usually without crusting or scarring.

Nail matrix arrest was reported in a small group of children after HFMD.

Beau's lines (transverse ridging) and/or onychomadesis (nail shedding) followed HFMD by 3 to 8 weeks.[9]

HAND, FOOT, AND MOUTH DISEASE

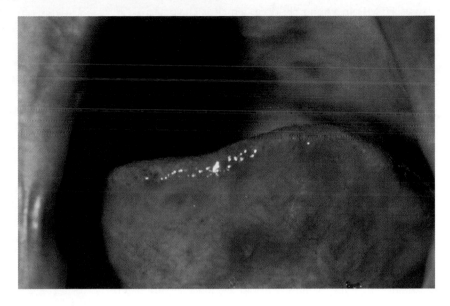

Figure 14-3 Aphthae-like erosions may appear anywhere in the oral cavity.

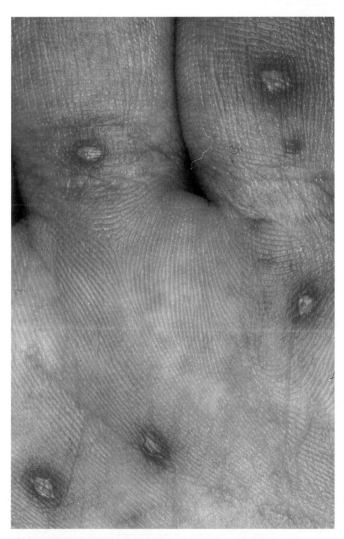

Figure 14-4 Cloudy vesicles with a red halo are highly characteristic of this disease.

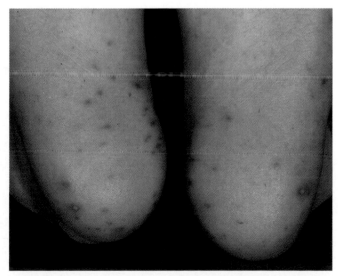

Figure 14-5 A cluster on the soles of a young boy. The pale, white, oval vesicles with a red areola are a distinguishing feature of this disease.

FATAL CASES IN AN EPIDEMIC. Enterovirus 71 infection causes HFMD in young children, which is characterized by several days of fever (100%) and vomiting, oral ulcers (66%), and vesicles on the backs of the hands and feet (62%). The illness rapidly progresses to include seizures (28%), flaccid limb weakness (17%), or cardiopulmonary symptoms (chest radiographs showing pulmonary edema and echocardiograms showing left ventricular dysfunction), resulting in cardiopulmonary arrest soon after hospitalization (median time, 9 hours).[10]

The initial illness resolves but is sometimes followed by aseptic meningitis, encephalomyelitis, or even acute flaccid paralysis similar to paralytic poliomyelitis. In 1998 an epidemic of enterovirus 71 infection caused HFMD and herpangina in thousands of people in Taiwan, some of whom died. The chief neurologic complication was rhombencephalics, which had a fatality rate of 14%. The most common initial symptoms were myoclonic jerks, and magnetic resonance imaging usually showed evidence of brainstem involvement.[11]

Most of those who died were young, and the majority died of pulmonary edema and pulmonary hemorrhage.[12] Hyperglycemia is the most important prognostic factor.[13]

DIFFERENTIAL DIAGNOSIS. When cutaneous lesions are absent, the disease may be confused with aphthous stomatitis. The oral erosions of HFMD are usually smaller and more uniform. The vesicles of herpes appear in clusters, and those of varicella endure longer and always crust. Both varicella and herpes have multinucleated, giant cells in smears taken from the moist skin exposed when a vesicle is removed (Tzanck smear). Giant cells are not present in lesions of HFMD.

TREATMENT. Symptomatic relief and reassurance are all that are required.

Scarlet fever

Scarlet fever (scarlatina) is an endemic, contagious disease produced by a streptococcal, erythrogenic toxin. The circulating toxin is responsible for the rash and systemic symptoms. The infection may originate in the pharynx or skin and is most common in children (ages 1 to 10 years) who lack immunity to the toxin. Scarlet fever was a feared disease in the nineteenth and early twentieth centuries, when it was more virulent, but presently scarlet fever is usually benign. Virulent strains may appear in the future. New waves of scarlet fever are associated with an increase in frequency of *Streptococcus pyogenes* clones carrying variant gene alleles encoding streptococcal pyrogenic exotoxin A (scarlet fever toxin).[14] Previous exposure to the toxin is required for expression of disease. Streptococcal pyrogenic exotoxin A causes disease by enhancing delayed-type hypersensitivity to streptococcal products.

INCUBATION PERIOD. The incubation period of scarlet fever (Figure 14-6) is 2 to 4 days.

PRODROMAL AND ERUPTIVE PHASE. The sudden onset of fever and pharyngitis is followed shortly by nausea, vomiting, headache, and abdominal pain. The entire oral cavity may be red, and the tongue is covered with a yellowish-white coat through which red papillae protrude. Diffuse lymphadenopathy may appear just before the onset of the eruption. The systemic symptoms continue until the fever subsides. The rash begins about the neck and face and spreads in 48 hours to the trunk and extremities; the palms and soles are spared (Figure 14-7). The face is flushed except for circumoral pallor, whereas all other involved areas exhibit a vivid scarlet hue with innumerable pinpoint papules that give a sandpaper quality to the skin (Figure 14-8). The rash is more limited and less dramatic in milder cases. Linear petechiae (Pastia's sign) are characteristic; they are found in skin folds, particularly the antecubital fossa and inguinal area. The tongue sheds the white coat to reveal a red, raw, glazed surface with engorged papillae (Figure 14-9).

Figure 14-6 Scarlet fever. Evolution of signs and symptoms.

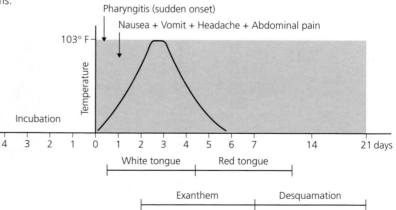

SCARLET FEVER

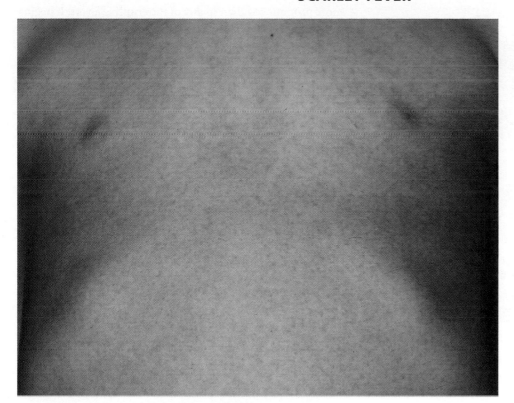

Figure 14-7 Early eruptive stage on the trunk showing numerous pinpoint red papules.

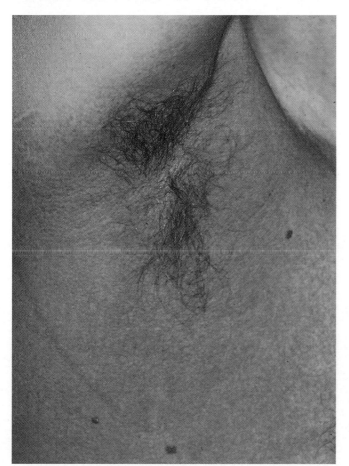

Figure 14-8 Fully evolved eruption. Numerous papules giving a sandpaper-like texture to the skin.

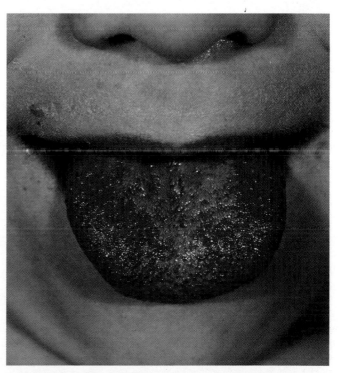

Figure 14-9 Portions of the white coat remain in the center, but the remainder of the tongue is red with engorged papillae ("strawberry tongue").

SCARLET FEVER

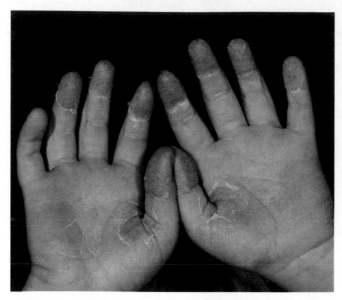

Figure 14-10 Desquamation of the hands.

The fever and rash subside and desquamation appears, more pronounced than in any of the eruptive fevers. It begins on the face, where it is sparse and superficial; progresses to the trunk, often with a circular, punched-out appearance; and finally spreads to the hands (Figure 14-10) and feet (Figure 14-11), where the epidermis is the thickest. Clinically, the hands and feet appear normal during the initial stages of the disease. Large sheaths of epidermis may be shed from the palms and soles in a glovelike cast, exposing new and often tender epidermis beneath. A transverse groove may be produced in all of the nails (Beau's lines) (Figure 14-12). The pattern of desquamation of the palms and soles and grooving of the nails is such a distinct characteristic of scarlet fever that it is helpful in making a retrospective diagnosis in cases where the eruption is minimal. A rising antistreptolysin-*O* titer constitutes additional supporting evidence for a recent infection. Desquamation is generally complete in 4 weeks, but it may last for 8 weeks. Recurrence rates of scarlet fever as high as 18% have been reported.

TREATMENT. Treat with penicillin, cephalosporins, erythromycin, ofloxacin, rifampin, or the newer macrolides.

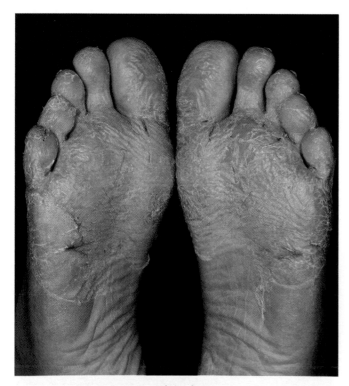

Figure 14-11 Desquamation of the feet.

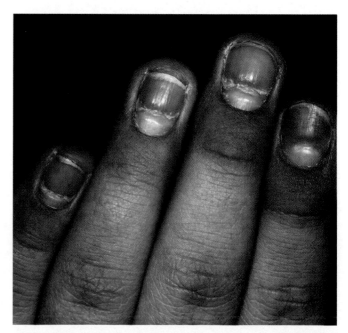

Figure 14-12 Beau's lines: transverse grooves on all nails several weeks after skin signs of scarlet fever have cleared.

Rubella

Rubella (German measles, 3-day measles) is a benign, contagious exanthematous viral infection characterized by nonspecific signs and symptoms including transient erythematous and sometimes pruritic rash, postauricular or suboccipital lymphadenopathy, arthralgia, and low-grade fever. Clinically similar exanthematous illnesses are caused by parvovirus, adenoviruses, and enteroviruses. Moreover, 25% to 50% of rubella infections are subclinical. The most important consequences of rubella are the miscarriages, stillbirths, fetal anomalies, and therapeutic abortions that result when rubella infection occurs during early pregnancy, especially during the first trimester.

CONGENITAL RUBELLA SYNDROME. Pregnant women who have rubella early in the first trimester may transmit the disease to the fetus, which may consequently develop a number of congenital defects (congenital rubella syndrome).

The anomalies most commonly associated with congenital rubella syndrome are auditory (e.g., sensorineural deafness), ophthalmic (e.g., cataracts, micro-ophthalmia, glaucoma, chorioretinitis), cardiac (e.g., patent ductus arteriosus, peripheral pulmonary artery stenosis, atrial or ventricular septal defects), and neurologic (e.g., microcephaly, meningoencephalitis, mental retardation). Infants frequently exhibit both intrauterine and postnatal growth retardation.

The number of women susceptible to rubella is substantial.[15] The incidence of the congenital rubella syndrome is increasing. Presently, most women who plan a pregnancy have the rubella titer measured. Many women have had a subclinical infection and already have an adequate titer. Women with no evidence of previous infection should be immunized and warned that pregnancy must be avoided for 2 months, during which time attenuated virus may be present in the tissues. Women of unknown immune status who conceive and are subsequently exposed to rubella or develop an exanthem that in any way resembles rubella should have a titer measured immediately and again 7 to 14 days later. If infection is likely and therapeutic abortion is unacceptable, then passive immunization with immune serum globulin (0.25 mg/lb) should be given. The value of this prophylactic treatment is unknown.

REINFECTION WITH RUBELLA. Reinfection with rubella during pregnancy is rare. It may occur in previously immunized or infected women whose hemagglutinin titers are lower than 1/64. The disease is asymptomatic in some of these women. In general, reinfection does not result in fetal injury,[16] but cases have been described in which infants of mothers infected during pregnancy were born with varying degrees of congenital rubella syndrome.[17,18] In questionable cases, cordocentesis or amniocentesis is performed[19] for culture and antibody titers before a decision is made regarding interruption of pregnancy.[20] The measurement of IgG avidity (avidity-ELISA) can differentiate between acute or recent primary rubella (low IgG avidity) from preexisting rubella immunity (high IgG avidity), including rubella reinfections.[21]

INCUBATION PERIOD. The incubation period of rubella (Figure 14-13) is 18 days, with a range of 14 to 21 days.

PRODROMAL PHASE. Mild symptoms of malaise, headache, and moderate temperature elevation may precede the eruption by a few hours or a day. Children are usually asymptomatic. Lymphadenopathy, characteristically postauricular, suboccipital, and cervical, may appear 4 to 7 days before the rash and be maximal at the onset of the exanthem. In 2% of cases, petechiae on the soft palate occur late in the prodromal phase or early in the eruptive phase.

ERUPTIVE PHASE. The eruption begins on the neck or face and spreads in hours to the trunk and extremities. The lesions are pinpoint to 1 cm, round or oval, pinkish or rosy red macules or maculopapules. The color is less vivid than that of scarlet fever and lacks the blue or violaceous tinge seen in measles. The lesions are usually discrete but may be grouped or coalesced on the face or trunk. The rash fades in 24 to 48 hours in the same order in which it appeared and may be followed by a fine desquamation.

Among adults infected with rubella, transient polyarthralgia or polyarthritis occur frequently. These manifestations are particularly common among women.

Arthritis, affecting primarily the phalangeal joints of women, may occur in the prodromal period and may last for 2 to 3 weeks after the rash has disappeared. No treatment is required.

Central nervous system complications (e.g., encephalitis) occur at a ratio of 1:6000 cases and are more likely to affect adults. Thrombocytopenia occurs at a ratio of 1:3000 cases and is more likely to affect children.

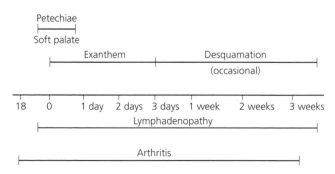

Figure 14-13 Rubella. Evolution of signs and symptoms.

Erythema infectiosum (parvovirus B19 infection)

PARVOVIRUS B19 INFECTION. Parvovirus B19 is associated with many disease manifestations that vary with the immunologic and hematologic status of the patient. The main target of B19 infection is the red cell receptor globoside (blood group P antigen) of erythroid progenitor cells of the bone marrow. People who do not have the virus receptor (erythrocyte P antigen) are naturally resistant to infection with this virus.[22]

Infection causes erythema infectiosum in immunocompetent patients. It is the primary cause of transient aplastic crisis in patients with underlying hemolytic disorders. Persistent infection in immunosuppressed patients may present as red cell aplasia and chronic anemia. In utero infection may result in hydrops fetalis or congenital anemia. There is no evidence of reinfection in immunocompetent individuals.

Seroprevalence is 2% to 10% in children younger than 5 years, 40% to 60% in adults older than 20 years, and 85% or more in those older than 70 years. The average annual seroconversion rate of women of childbearing age is 1.5%.

The virus may be transmitted via the respiratory route and via the transfusion of infected blood and blood products. Nosocomial transmission has been well documented. Individuals are not viremic or infectious at the rash or arthropathy stage of disease.

ERYTHEMA INFECTIOSUM. Erythema infectiosum (fifth disease) is caused by the B19 parvovirus. It is relatively common and mildly contagious and appears sporadically or in epidemics. Peak attack rates occur in children between 5 and 14 years of age. Asymptomatic infection is common.[23]

INCUBATION PERIOD. The incubation period of erythema infectiosum (Figure 14-14) is 13 to 18 days.[24] Viremia occurs after the incubation period and reticulocyte numbers fall, resulting in a temporary drop in hemoglobin concentration of 1 g/dl in a normal person.

There is a nonspecific prodromal illness, followed by a three-stage erythematous disease.

PRODROMAL SYMPTOMS. Symptoms are usually mild or absent. Pruritus, low-grade fever, malaise, and sore throat precede the eruption in approximately 10% of cases. Lymphadenopathy is absent. Older individuals may complain of joint pain.

ERUPTIVE PHASE. There are three distinct, overlapping stages.

Facial erythema ("slapped cheek"). Red papules on the cheeks rapidly coalesce in hours, forming red, slightly edematous, warm, fiery red, erysipelas-like plaques that are symmetric on both cheeks and spare the nasolabial fold and the circumoral region (Figure 14-15). The "slapped cheek" appearance fades in 4 days. The classic slapped cheek is much more common in children than in adults.

Net pattern erythema. This unique characteristic eruption—erythema in a fishnetlike pattern—begins on the extremities approximately 2 days after the onset of facial erythema and extends to the trunk and buttocks, fading in 6 to 14 days (Figure 14-16). At times, the exanthem begins with erythema and does not become characteristic until irregular clearing takes place. This second-stage rash may vary from very faint erythema to a florid exanthem. Livedo reticularis has a similar netlike pattern, but it does not fade quickly.

Recurrent phase. The eruption may fade and then reappear in previously affected sites on the face and body during the next 2 to 3 weeks. Temperature changes, emotional upsets, and sunlight may stimulate recurrences. The rash fades without scaling or pigmentation. There may be a slight lymphocytosis or eosinophilia.

Figure 14-14 Erythema infectiosum. Evolution of signs and symptoms.

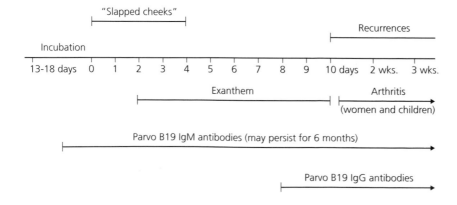

PAPULAR-PURPURIC "GLOVES AND SOCKS" SYNDROME.
This febrile dermatosis is characterized by fever, pruritic edema, followed by pain and petechial involvement of hands and feet with sharp demarcation at the wrists and ankles, and an enanthem of petechiae and oral erosions. The histopathologic findings are nonspecific and consist of an interface dermatitis with a superficial perivascular inflammatory infiltrate mostly composed of lymphocytes, with numerous extravasated erythrocytes. Acute infection by parvovirus B19 is demonstrated in several cases.[25] Medications may be another factor in the pathogenesis.[26]

POLYARTHROPATHY SYNDROME AND PRURITUS

Adults. Women exposed to the parvovirus during outbreaks may develop itching and arthralgia or arthritis. Men are not affected. The itching varies from mild to intense and is localized or generalized. In most cases a nonspecific macular eruption occurs without the appearance of the typical netlike pattern before the arthritis.

Women develop moderately severe, symmetric polyarthritis that may evolve to a form that is often indistinguishable from rheumatoid arthritis.[27] Most have involvement of the knees and other joints, as well as migratory arthritis.[28,29]

B19 patients present with the sudden onset of symmetric peripheral polyarthropathy of moderate severity. B19 infection mimics rheumatoid arthritis in the acute stage, and the rheumatoid factor test can be positive.

The joints can be painful, with accompanying swelling and stiffness. Symptoms continue for 1 to 3 weeks. In some women, arthropathy or arthritis may persist or recur for months or years.

There are striking similarities between B19 infection and systemic lupus erythematosus: both may present with malar rash, fever, arthropathy, myalgia, cytopenia, hypocomplementemia, and anti-DNA and antinuclear antibodies (ANA).[30]

The differential diagnosis includes acute rheumatoid arthritis, seronegative arthritis, Lyme disease, and lupus.[31] Parvovirus infection should be considered when an adult woman has acute polyarthropathy associated with pruritus, especially if she has been exposed to children with erythema infectiosum.

The demonstration of anti−parvovirus-B19 immunoglobulins (IgM) and anti−parvovirus-B19 IgG is a most important diagnostic finding. Measurement of IgM must be done within the first months, as it disappears later on. Immunosuppressive agents used to treat rheumatoid arthritis may prolong persistence of virus and disease in parvovirus-B19−induced arthritis/arthropathy.

B19 infection is not associated with joint destruction seen in rheumatoid arthritis.[32] Prolonged symptoms do not correlate with serologic studies, such as the duration of B19 immunoglobulin M (IgM) response, or persistent viremia.

Adult flulike symptoms and arthropathies begin coincident with IgG antibody production in 18 to 24 days after exposure and are probably immune-complex mediated.

Children. Both male and female children may develop joint symptoms. Most cases have acute arthritis of brief duration; a few have arthralgias. Two patterns are seen: olyarticular, affecting more than five joints; and pauciarticular, affecting four or fewer joints. Large joints are affected more often than small joints. The knee is the most common joint affected (82%). Laboratory findings are normal. The duration of joint symptoms is usually less than 4 months, but some have persistent arthritis for 2 to 13 months, which fulfills the criteria for the diagnosis of juvenile rheumatoid arthritis.[33]

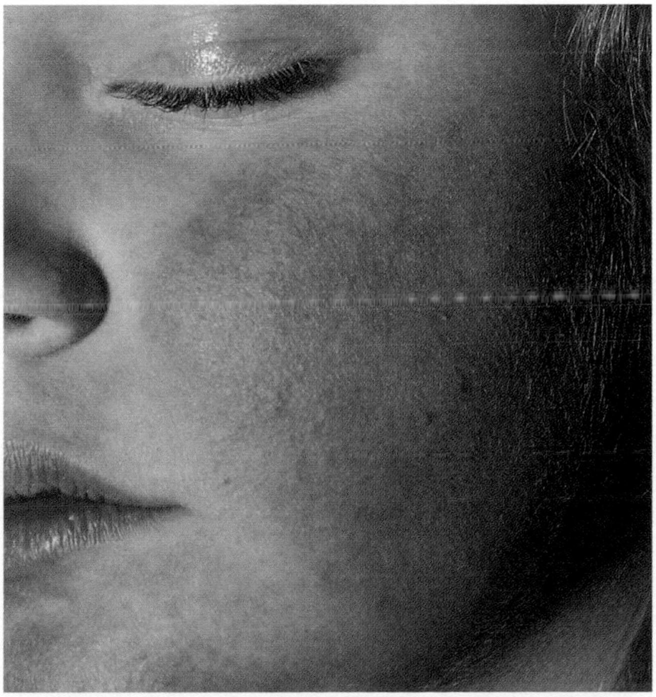

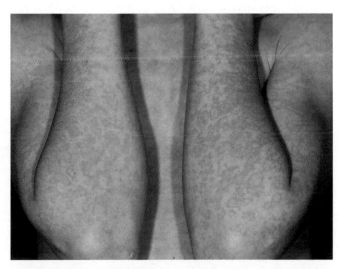

Figure 14-15 Erythema infectiosum. Facial erythema "slapped cheek." The red plaque covers the cheek and spares the nasolabial fold and the circumoral region.

Figure 14-16 Erythema infectiosum. Netlike pattern of erythema.

INFECTION IN THE PREGNANT WOMAN (INTRAUTERINE INFECTION AND SPONTANEOUS ABORTION). In pregnant women, infection can, but usually does not, lead to fetal infection (Box 14-1). Fetal infection sometimes causes severe anemia, congestive heart failure, generalized edema (fetal hydrops), and death. Many fetuses dying because of this infection are not noticeably hydropic.[34]

Parvovirus B19 probably causes 10% to 15% of all cases of nonimmune hydrops. If the fetus survives fetal hydrops caused by B19, there usually are no long-term sequelae.

The fetus has a high rate of red-cell production; its immature immune system may not be able to mount an adequate immune response. Parvovirus has been implicated as a cause of spontaneous abortion (from severe fetal anemia and hydrops fetalis).[35,36]

Maternal infection in the first half of pregnancy is associated with 10% excess fetal loss and hydrops fetalis in 3% of cases (of which up to 60% resolve spontaneously or with appropriate management). B19-associated congenital abnormalities have not been reported among several hundred liveborn infants of B19-infected mothers. The overall risk of serious adverse outcome from occupational exposure to parvovirus B19 infection during pregnancy is low (excess early fetal loss in 2 to 6:1000 pregnancies and fetal death from hydrops in 2 to 5:10,000 pregnancies). It is not recommended that susceptible pregnant women be excluded routinely from working with children during epidemics.[37]

The polymerase chain reaction is a sensitive and rapid method for the diagnosis of intrauterine infection.[38]

ANEMIA. The virus has the propensity to infect and lyse erythroid precursor cells and interrupt normal red-cell production. In a person with normal hematopoiesis, B19 infection produces a self-limited red-cell aplasia that is clinically inapparent. In patients who have increased rates of red-cell destruction or loss and who depend on compensatory increases in red cell production to maintain stable red-cell indices, B19 infection may lead to transient aplastic crisis. Patients at risk for transient aplastic crisis include those with hemoglobinopathies (sickle cell disease, thalassemia, hereditary spherocytosis, and pyruvate kinase deficiency) and those with anemias associated with acute or chronic blood loss. B19 infection accounts for most, if not all, aplastic crises in sickle cell disease, but at least 20% of infections do not result in aplasia.[39,40] Up to 30% of hospital staff members may be infected when exposed to infected sickle cell patients.[41] In immunodeficient persons and those with AIDS,[42] B19 may persist, causing chronic red-cell aplasia, which results in chronic anemia. Some of these patients may be cured with immune globulin therapy.[43]

LABORATORY. IgM antibodies are the most sensitive indicator of acute B19 infection in immunologically normal persons. IgM antibody to B19 appears about 10 to 14 days after infection and is detectable for as long as 3 months after exposure. IgG antibody also appears about 2 weeks after infection; the IgG response persists for life and levels rise with reexposure.

MANAGEMENT. Parents need only to be assured that this unusual eruption will fade and does not require treatment. Most health departments do not recommend exclusion from school for children with fifth disease. Many infections are inapparent, and exposure may occur in the community, as well as in school.

Evaluate the immune status of exposed pregnant women. The risks are nil if the women is IgG positive. If she is not immune (although the risk of the fetus's being affected is very low), fetal surveillance by repeated ultrasonographic examination and immune status reevaluation is recommended.

Because the major immune response appears to be humoral, patients with chronic infection have been treated with immune globulin. These patients often respond with a marked reduction in the level of B19 viremia and with reticulocytosis, followed within a few weeks by resolution of the anemia. Patients with persistent infection should be monitored for evidence of relapse by observation of the reticulocyte counts and by assays for B19 viremia when indicated.

Box 14-1 Facts and Recommendations for Pregnant Women Exposed to B19 Parvovirus

Risk of maternal infection during an epidemic: 30% to 65%
Infected women may be asymptomatic

Nurses and school teachers: high rate of infection if exposed
People with fifth disease are contagious before they develop the rash; therefore exposure at the onset of an outbreak cannot be avoided
Pregnant personnel should remain at home until 2 to 3 weeks after the last identified case

Laboratory tests
IgM tests for symptomatic exposed women
Fetal ultrasonography for confirmed or suspected cases
Polymerase chain reaction testing (if available) of amniotic fluid and fetal serum—a sensitive and rapid method for diagnosis of intrauterine infection
Monitor alpha-fetoprotein* in exposed and infected women
Ultrasonography when alpha-fetoprotein levels are increased
Abnormal ultrasound: fetal blood sampling as a guide for possible fetal transfusion
Teratogenic effects not demonstrated
Therapeutic abortion not indicated

Adapted from Levy M, Stanley ER: Can Med Assoc J 1990; 143:849.
*Maternal serum alpha-fetoprotein is a marker for fetal aplastic crisis during intrauterine human parvovirus infection.

Roseola infantum (human herpes virus 6 and 7 infection)

Roseola infantum (exanthem subitum, "sudden rash," sixth disease, rose rash of infants, 3-day fever) is caused primarily by human herpes virus 6 (HHV-6), which is epidemiologically and biologically similar to cytomegalovirus.[44] As with other herpes viruses, HHV-6 shows persistent and intermittent or chronic shedding in the normal population, making the unusually early infection of children (seroconversion in the first year of life in up to 80% of all children) understandable. The virus remains latent in monocytes and macrophages and probably in the salivary glands. Virus may infect infants through the saliva mainly from mother to child. A severe, infectious mononucleosis–like syndrome in adults may be caused by a primary infection with HHV-6.[45] HHV-6 has also been implicated in idiopathic pneumonitis in immunocompromised hosts.[46]

Most cases are asymptomatic or present with fever of unknown origin and occur without a rash.[47,48] The disease is sporadic, and the majority of cases occur between the ages of 6 months and 4 years. Primary HHV-7 infection occurs later in childhood (at approximately 3 years of age) and also causes exanthema subitum, although less often than HHV-6. HHV-6 antibody is present in 90% to 100% of the population over age 2. The development of high fever, as is seen in roseola, is worrisome, but the onset of the characteristic rash is reassuring.

One study showed that HHV-6 was responsible for 10% of hospital visits for acute illness in infants younger than 25 months of age and 33% of the febrile seizures occuring in children younger than 2 years

In infants and young children HHV-6 is a major cause of visits to the emergency department, febrile seizures, and hospitalizations.[48]

INCUBATION PERIOD. The incubation period of roseola infantum (Figure 14-17) is 12 days, with a range of 5 to 15 days.

PRODROMAL SYMPTOMS. There is a sudden onset of high fever of 103° to 106° F with few or minor symptoms. Most children appear inappropriately well for the degree of temperature elevation, but they may experience slight anorexia or one or two episodes of vomiting, running nose, cough, and hepatomegaly. Seizures (but more frequently general cerebral irritability) may occur before the eruptive phase. Most recover without sequelae.[49] Cases of encephalitis/encephalopathy with abnormal electroencephalograms and cerebral computed tomograms have been reported; epilepsy developed in one case and another died.[50] HHV-6 DNA has been detected in the cerebrospinal fluid (CSF); this suggests that HHV-6 may invade the brain during the acute phase.[50] HHV-6 infection should be suspected in infants with febrile convulsions, even those without the exanthem.[51] Mild-to-moderate lymphadenopathy, usually in the occipital regions, begins at the onset of the febrile period and persists until after the eruption has subsided.

Figure 14-17 Roseola infantum. Evolution of signs and symptoms.

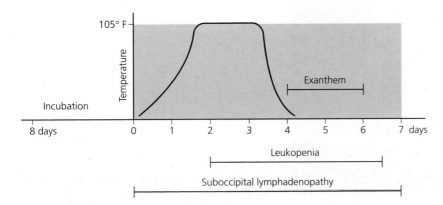

ERUPTIVE PHASE. The rash begins as the fever subsides. The term *exanthem subitum* indicates the sudden "surprise" of the blossoming rash after the fall of the fever. Numerous pale pink, almond-shaped macules appear on the trunk and neck, become confluent, and then fade in a few hours to 2 days without scaling or pigmentation (Figures 14-18 and 14-19). The exanthem may resemble rubella or measles, but the pattern of development, distribution, and associated symptoms of these other exanthematous diseases are different.

LABORATORY EVALUATION. Leukocytosis develops at the onset of fever, but leukopenia with a granulocytopenia and relative lymphocytosis appears as the temperature increases and persists until the eruption fades.[52] Seroconversion during the convalescent phase can be detected with immunofluorescence or enzyme immunoassays.

TREATMENT. Control temperature with aspirin and provide reassurance. HHV-6 is inhibited by several antiviral drugs in the laboratory, including ganciclovir and foscarnet. Treatment may be considered for patients with serious HHV-6—associated disease confirmed with virologic tests.[53]

ROSEOLA INFANTUM

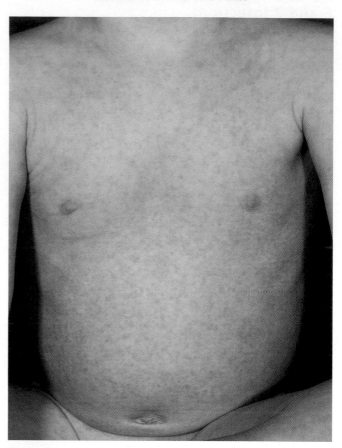

Figure 14-18 Numerous pale pink, almond-shaped macules.

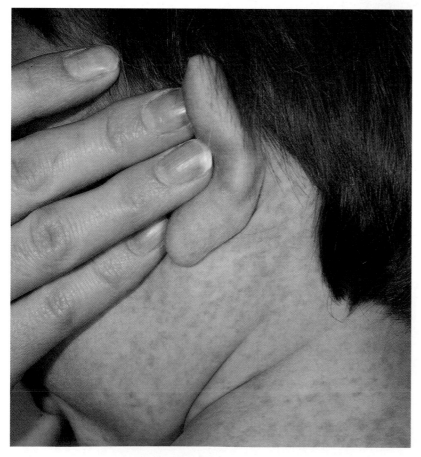

Figure 14-19 Pale pink macules may appear first on the neck.

Enteroviruses: echovirus and coxsackievirus exanthems

The previously described diseases characteristically display a predictable set of signs and symptoms. Roseola and erythema infectiosum are relatively common. Many physicians never see cases of measles, German measles, or scarlet fever. The most common exanthematous eruptions are caused by the enteroviruses, echovirus, and coxsackievirus. A large number of these viruses may begin with a skin eruption. Some of these eruptions are characteristic of the virus type, but in most cases one must be satisfied with the diagnosis of "viral rash." In many cases, drug eruptions cannot be distinguished from the nonspecific exanthems of these enteroviruses.

SYSTEMIC SYMPTOMS. Many are possible, such as fever, nausea, vomiting, and diarrhea, along with typical viral symptoms of photophobia, lymphadenopathy, sore throat, and possibly encephalitis.

EXANTHEM. The rash may appear at any time during the course of the illness, and it is usually generalized. Lesions are erythematous maculopapules with areas of confluence, but they may be urticarial, vesicular, or sometimes petechial (Figure 14-20). The palms and soles may be involved. The eruptions are more common in children than in adults. In most cases, the rash fades without pigmentation or scaling.

TREATMENT. Treatment consists of relieving symptoms.

Figure 14-20 Viral exanthem. Symmetric erythematous maculopapular eruption.

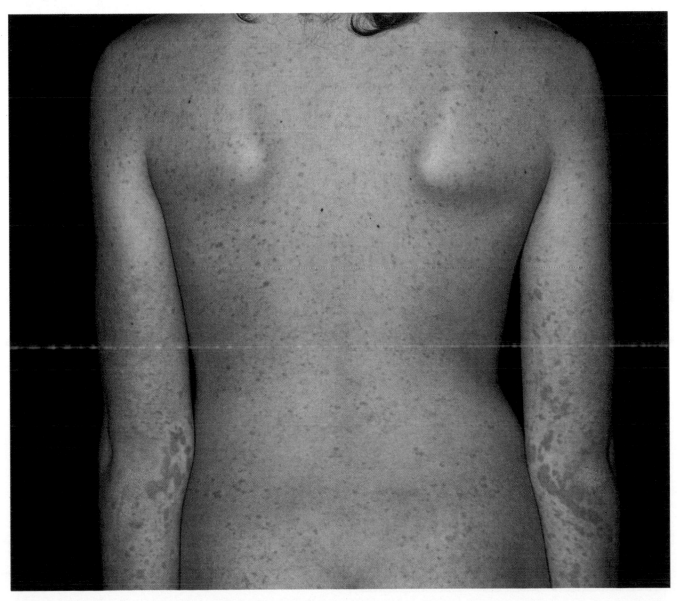

Kawasaki syndrome

Kawasaki syndrome (KS), or mucocutaneous lymph node syndrome, was first described in Japan in 1967 but now is reported in both endemic and epidemic forms worldwide.[58,59] Patients' ages range from 7 weeks to 12 years (mean, 2.6 years); rare adult cases are reported. Kawasaki syndrome is an acute multisystem vasculitis of unknown etiology that is associated with marked activation of T cells and monocyte/macrophages. An infectious agent is strongly suggested by its occurrence primarily in young children (who apparently lack immunity) and by the existence of outbreaks. The agent may trigger genetically influenced immune responses. Recurrences are rare. The major causes of short- and long-term morbidity are the cardiovascular manifestations. The histopathologic features of vasculitis involving arterioles, capillaries, and venules appear in the earliest phase of the disease.

THREE CLINICAL PHASES

Acute. The acute febrile phase lasts seven to 14 days and ends with the resolution of fever. There is conjunctival injection, mouth and lip changes, swelling and erythema of the hands and feet, rash, and cervical lymphadenopathy.

Subacute. The subacute phase covers the period from the end of the fever to about day 25. There are desquamation of the fingers and toes, arthritis and arthralgia, and thrombocytosis.

Convalescent. The convalescent phase begins when clinical signs disappear and continues until the erythrocyte sedimentation rate (ESR) becomes normal, usually 6 to 8 weeks after the onset of illness.

CLINICAL MANIFESTATIONS. There is no single clinical finding or laboratory test that is diagnostic, but the diagnosis should be considered in children with rash and fever of unknown origin.[60,61] The Centers for Disease Control and Prevention (CDC) definition is shown in Table 14-2. The evolution of signs and symptoms is shown in Figure 14-21. Children have high fever for 1 to 2 weeks, rash, and edema of the extremities that is painful and interferes with walking, and they are extremely irritable.

MAJOR DIAGNOSTIC FEATURES

Fever. The fever, without chills or sweats, is a constant feature (range, 5 to 30 days; mean, 8.5 days) in untreated patients. It begins abruptly and spikes from 101° to 104° F (usually 39° C) and does not respond to antibiotics or antipyretics. KS should be in the differential diagnosis of prolonged fever in infants; occasionally, prolonged fever is the only manifestation of KS. In patients treated with aspirin at 80 to 100 mg/kg/day and a single 2-g/kg dose of intravenous gamma-globulin (IVGG), fever usually resolves in 1 or 2 days.

Conjunctival injection. Self-limited, bilateral congestion of the bulbar and sometimes the palpebral conjunctivae is an almost constant feature. Typically, the inflammation spares the area of the conjunctiva around the limbus. Uveitis occurs in 70% of cases. There is no discharge or ulceration, as seen in Stevens-Johnson syndrome.

Oral mucous membrane changes. The lips and oral pharynx become red 1 to 3 days after the onset of the fever. The lips become dry, fissured, cracked, and crusted (Figure 14-22). Secondary infection of the lips can occur. Hypertrophic tongue papillae result in the "strawberry tongue" typically seen in scarlet fever. There is no sore throat, but small ulcerations may form. Cough occurs in 25% of patients.

Extremity changes. Within 3 days of the onset of fever, the palms and soles become red, and the hands and feet become edematous (Figure 14-23, A). The edema is nonpitting. The tenderness can be severe enough to limit walking and use of the hands. The edema lasts for approximately 1 week. Peeling of the hands and feet occurs 10 to 14 days after the onset of fever (Figure 14-23, B). The peeling is similar to that seen in scarlet fever. Generalized desquamation of the skin is uncommon. The skin peels off in sheets, beginning about the nails and fingertips and progressing down to the palms and soles. The skin of children with diaper area inflammation peels at the margins of the rash and on the labia and scrotum. One to 2 months after the onset of KS, transverse grooves across the nails may develop (Beau's lines).

Table 14-2 Kawasaki Syndrome Centers for Disease Control and Prevention Diagnostic Criteria	
Symptom	Occurrence (%)
Fever lasting >5 days plus at least four of the following:	100
1. Bilateral conjunctival injection	92
2. Mucous membrane changes (≥1)	100
Red or fissured lips	84
Red pharynx	72
"Strawberry" tongue	32
3. Lower extremity changes (≥1)	
Erythema of palms or soles	72
Edema of hands or feet	48
Desquamation (generalized or periungual)	56
4. Rash—erythematous exanthema	100
5. Cervical lymphadenopathy (≥1 node >1.5 cm)	72

Data from Velez-Torres R, Callen JP: Int J Dermatol 1987; 26:96.

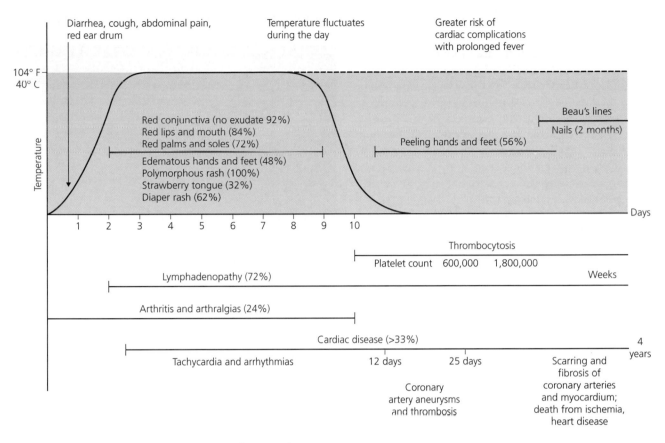

Diarrhea, cough, abdominal pain, red ear drum

Temperature fluctuates during the day

Greater risk of cardiac complications with prolonged fever

104° F
40° C

Temperature

Red conjunctiva (no exudate 92%)
Red lips and mouth (84%)
Red palms and soles (72%)
Edematous hands and feet (48%)
Polymorphous rash (100%)
Strawberry tongue (32%)
Diaper rash (62%)

Beau's lines
Nails (2 months)
Peeling hands and feet (56%)

Days

1 2 3 4 5 6 7 8 9 10

Thrombocytosis
Platelet count   600,000   1,800,000

Lymphadenopathy (72%)

Weeks

Arthritis and arthralgias (24%)

Cardiac disease (>33%)

4 years

Tachycardia and arrhythmias

12 days   25 days

Coronary artery aneurysms and thrombosis

Scarring and fibrosis of coronary arteries and myocardium; death from ischemia, heart disease

Figure 14-21 Kawasaki syndrome. Evolution of signs and symptoms.

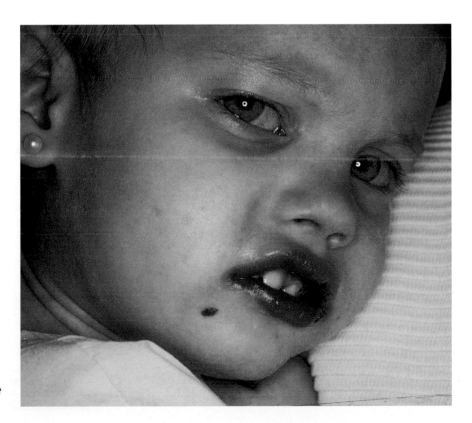

Figure 14-22 Kawasaki syndrome. Nonpurulent conjunctival injection and "cherry red" lips with fissuring and crusting are early signs of the disease. *(Courtesy Anne W. Lucky, M.D.)*

Rash. A rash appears soon after the onset of fever. Several symptoms have been described. The most common forms are urticarial and a diffuse, deep red, maculopapular eruption (Figure 14-24, A). Less often the rash resembles erythema multiforme, scarlet fever, or the erythema marginatum seen in rheumatic fever. Dermatitis in the diaper area is common. The perineal rash usually occurs in the first week of the onset of symptoms. Red macules and papules become confluent (Figure 14-24, B). Desquamation occurs within 5 to 7 days. Perineal desquamation occurs 2 to 6 days before desquamation of the fingertips and toes (Figure 14-24, C). Vesiculopustules may develop over the elbows and knees.

Cervical lymphadenopathy. Firm, nontender, nonsuppurative lymphadenopathy is often limited to a single node and occurs in only 50% to 75% of patients. Children with acute cervical adenitis unresponsive to antibiotic therapy may have KS.

OTHER CLINICAL FEATURES

Abdominal symptoms. Acute distention of the gallbladder (hydrops) is common and presents with a right upper quadrant mass, jaundice, and pain or guarding in the first or second week of the illness; ultrasound is useful. It resolves in a few days without surgery.

Urethritis. Inflammation of the mucosa of the urethra causes sterile pyuria and is seen in more than 75% of patients.

Arthritis and arthralgias. A polyarticular arthritis or arthralgia of the feet and hands often develops in the first 10 days. This process may evolve to a pauciarticular arthritis that involves the larger joints such as the knees and hips. Early-onset arthritis is associated with synovial fluid WBC counts of 100,000 to 300,000/μL with a PMN predominance; late-onset arthritis has a lower synovial WBC count of approximately 50,000/μL with 50% mononuclear cells.

Aseptic meningitis. Approximately 25% have irritability or severe lethargy and stiff neck. Lumbar puncture reveals 25 to 100 WBCs/μL, predominantly lymphocytes, and normal glucose and normal to mildly elevated protein levels.

KAWASAKI SYNDROME—HAND LESIONS

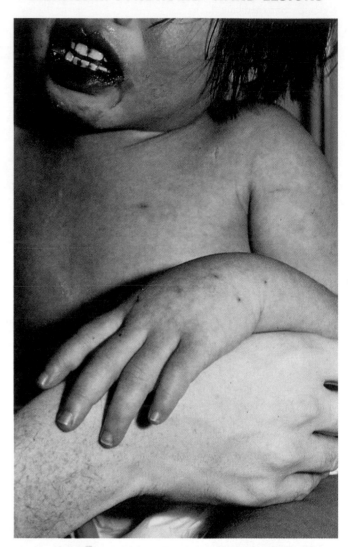

A

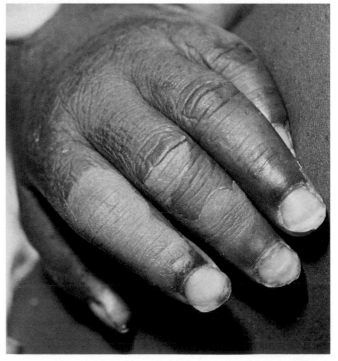

B

Figure 14-23 A, The hands become red and swollen. **B,** The hands peel approximately 2 weeks after the onset of fever. *(Courtesy Nancy B. Esterly, M.D.)*

CARDIAC AND OTHER ORGAN VESSEL INVOLVEMENT.
Kawasaki syndrome is the major cause of acquired heart disease in children in the United States. Cardiovascular manifestations are the leading cause of morbidity and mortality. Coronary artery abnormalities develop in 25% of untreated children. Aneurysms occur 1 to 3 weeks after the onset of fever. Risk factors for coronary aneurysms are fever for more than 10 days; recurrence of fever following an afebrile period of more than 48 hours; arrhythmias other than first-degree heart block; male gender; age of less than 1 year; cardiomegaly; and low platelet count, hematocrit, and serum albumin at presentation. Coronary aneurysms resolve within 5 to 18 months in approximately 50% of patients. The remaining patients may show decreased size of aneurysms and coronary obstruction or stenosis.

Arterial changes are seen at various other sites and organs as part of systemic arteritis. Aneurysms may be found in the axillary, common iliac, celiac, and mesenteric arteries. Arterial involvement of organs such as the kidney is well documented.

KAWASAKI SYNDROME—EXANTHEM

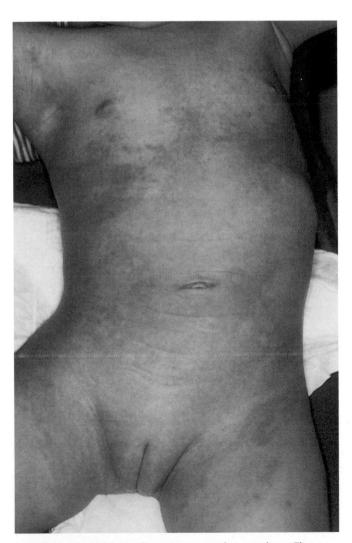

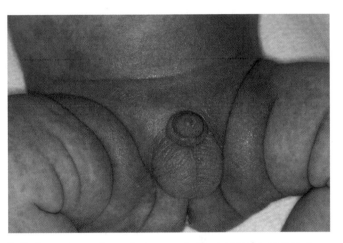

B, Red macules and papules appear in the perineal area 3 to 4 days after the onset of the illness. The rash becomes confluent and desquamates within 5 to 7 days. Desquamation of the fingertips and toes occurs 2 to 6 days later.

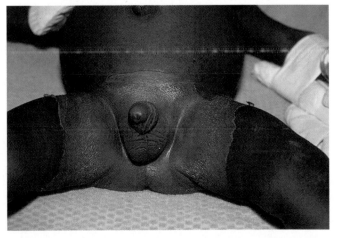

A, Diffuse, blanching, erythematous, macular exanthem. The eruption is frequently concentrated in the perineal area.

C, The skin of children with diaper-area inflammation peels at the margin of the rash. *(Courtesy Anne W. Lucky, M.D.)*

Figure 14-24

LABORATORY EVALUATION. The acute phase is characterized by marked inflammation and immune activation. Leukocytosis (20,000 to 30,000) with a shift to the left (80%), thrombocytosis, anemia, and T-cell and monocyte-macrophage activation occur. Acute-phase reactants, such as ESR (90%), C-reactive protein, and serum alpha$_1$-antitrypsin, are elevated with the onset of fever and persist for up to 10 weeks after onset of illness. Other findings include mild transaminase elevations, abnormal urinalysis consisting of sterile pyuria (68%), and CSF pleocytosis (25%). Thrombocytosis is a distinctive sign of this disease. The platelet count begins to rise on the tenth day of the illness, peaks at 600,000 to 1.6 million, and returns to normal by the thirtieth day of the illness. Echocardiography is obtained as soon as the diagnosis is suspected.

TREATMENT

Acute stage. Treatment of patients with KS in the first 10 days of illness with intravenously administered gamma-globulin (IVGG) and aspirin reduces the prevalence of coronary abnormalities from 20%-25% to 2%-4%.[62,63] A large, single dose of IVGG is more effective than daily doses. Treat with a 2 g/kg dose of IVGG given over 10 to 12 hours and aspirin 80 to 100 mg/kg/day given every 6 hours. A serum salicylate level of approximately 20-25 mg/dl is desirable. Aspirin is reduced to antithrombotic doses of 3 to 5 mg/kg/day as a single daily dose when fever has resolved at approximately day 14 of the illness. Aspirin can be discontinued after six to eight weeks if echocardiograms show no evidence of coronary artery abnormalities. If coronary artery abnormalities are detected, low-dose aspirin therapy should be continued indefinitely. IVGG improves myocardial function, reduces the prevalence of coronary disease, and leads to rapid defervescence and more rapid normalization of acute phase reactants. Aspirin is used for its antiinflammatory and antithrombotic effects and to reduce fever. Patients who present with desquamation and a history consistent with KS who are afebrile are not treated with IVGG because IVGG is unlikely to prevent coronary disease after the acute inflammatory response has subsided. Patients with fever 48 hours after IVGG infusion may benefit from additional IVGG. Live parenteral virus vaccines (i.e., measles, mumps, rubella, and varicella) should be delayed 6 to 11 months after IVGG. The use of corticosteroid therapy is controversial.

After acute stage. Repeat the echocardiogram, CBC, and ESR at 2 to 3 weeks and again at 6 to 8 weeks. Discontinue aspirin if the ESR and echocardiogram are normal at 6 to 8 weeks. Patients with coronary dilatation or aneurysm formation receive aspirin indefinitely.

Superantigen toxin-mediated illnesses

Streptococcus and *Staphylococcus* can produce circulating toxins that cause clinical disease. Many of these toxins function as superantigens.

Pyrogenic toxin superantigens comprise a large family of exotoxins made by *Staphylococcus* aureus and group A streptococci. These toxins include toxic shock syndrome toxin-1, the staphylococcal enterotoxins, and the streptococcal pyrogenic exotoxins (synonyms: scarlet fever toxins and erythrogenic toxins), all of which have the ability to cause toxic shock syndromes and related illnesses (Box 14-2).

SUPERANTIGENS. Normally antigens are processed inside antigen-presenting cells. A protein fragment of the antigen is then expressed on the cell surface in the groove of the major histocompatibility type II complex (MHCII). The antigen-MHCII complex then interacts with a receptor on a T cell, which results in cytokine production.[64]

Superantigens are proteins with a special chemical structure that are manufactured by bacteria and viruses that are not processed by antigen presenting cells. They bind directly to the MHCII complex outside of the groove and cause a nonspecific stimulation of T cells.

Conventional antigens activate 0.01% or more of the body's T cells. A superantigen–T cell interaction activates 5% to 30% of the entire T-cell population. This leads to massive cytokine production, especially that of tumor necrosis factor-α (TNF-α), interleukin-1 (IL-1), and interleukin-6 (IL-6). Fever, emesis, hypotension, shock, tissue injury, and cutaneous signs including strawberry tongue, acral erythema with desquamation, and erythematous eruption with perineal accentuation are the result of massive cytokine production.

The best-characterized superantigens are staphylococcal enterotoxins A through E, toxic shock syndrome toxin 1, and exfoliating toxin; these are all toxins released from *S. aureus*. Other bacterial proteins known to have superantigen properties are streptococcal pyrogenic exotoxins A through C and streptococcal M protein.

Box 14-2 Toxin-Mediated Streptococcal and Staphylococcal Diseases

Necrotizing fasciitis
Recalcitrant erythematous desquamating disorder
Scarlet fever
Staphylococcal scalded-skin syndrome
Streptococcal toxic shock syndrome (STSS)
Toxic shock syndrome
Atopic dermatitis*
Guttate psoriasis*
Kawasaki syndrome*
*Possibly toxin mediated.

Toxic shock syndrome

Toxic shock syndrome (TSS), originally described in 1978, is a rare, potentially fatal, multisystem illness associated with *S. aureus* infection and production of superantigen toxins. Early cases were associated with tampon use. Most cases now occur in the postoperative setting,[65] but TSS has been described in association with influenza, sinusitis, tracheitis, postpartum state,[66] intravenous drug use, HIV infection, cellulitis, burn wounds, and allergic contact dermatitis.[67]

Infected burn wounds in hospitalized children and bacterial tracheitis are relatively high-risk settings for pediatric TSS.

SUPERANTIGEN PRODUCTION. Five enterotoxins are elaborated by staphylococci (SE A to E) plus TSS toxin-1 (TSST-1). Many cases of TSS are mediated by TSST-1 and enterotoxin B and C production, which is associated with massive release of cytokines (TNF-α and IL-1). These cytokines produce fever, rash, hypotension, tissue injury, and shock. Absence of antibody to TSST-1 is a major risk factor for acquisition of TSS.

Erythrogenic toxins (pyrogenic exotoxins) A, B, and C produced by group A β-hemolytic streptococci (*S. pyogenes*) may cause a disease with all the defining criteria for TSS. Streptococci toxic shock syndrome (STSS) differs from that due to *S. aureus* in two ways. A focus of infection in soft tissue and skin[68] is usually present in STSS, and many patients have bacteremia.[69]

CLINICAL MANIFESTATIONS. The criteria for diagnosis of both forms of TSS are listed in Boxes 14-3 and 14-4. The evolution of signs and symptoms is illustrated in Figure 14-25. The CDC definition of TSS requires a temperature greater than 38.9° C, hypotension with a systolic blood pressure less than 90 mm Hg, or postural dizziness, rash, desquamation, evidence of multiple organ system involvement, and exclusion of other reasonable pathogens. Recurrences occur in as many as 30% to 40% of cases.

DERMATOLOGIC MANIFESTATIONS. The dermatologic manifestations are listed in Box 14-5. The disease has several features in common with KS and scarlet fever. A diffuse scarlatiniform erythroderma, bulbar conjunctiva hyperemia, and palmar edema are highly characteristic early signs. Desquamation of the tips of the fingers and toes occurs 1 to 2 weeks after the onset in exactly the same manner as is seen in scarlet fever and KS.

LABORATORY. Important laboratory abnormalities are listed in Box 14-6.

DIFFERENTIAL DIAGNOSIS. TSS can mimic many diseases.[70] The differential diagnosis of TSS is drug eruptions, KS, scarlet fever, staphylococcal scalded skin syndrome, toxic epidermal necrolysis, and viral exanthems.

Figure 14-25 Toxic shock syndrome. Evolution of signs and symptoms.

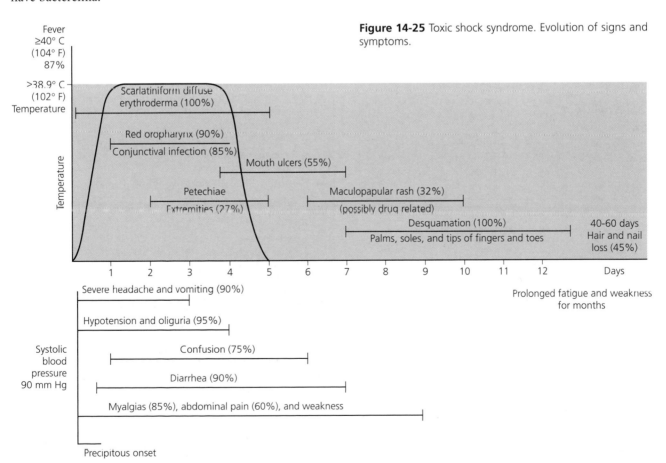

Box 14-3 Toxic Shock Syndrome Centers for Disease Control and Prevention Clinical Case Definition 1997

An illness with the following clinical manifestations
1. Fever: temperature ≥102.0° F (≥38.9° C)
2. Rash: diffuse macular erythroderma
3. Desquamation: 1 to 2 weeks after onset of illness, particularly on the palms and soles
4. Hypotension: systolic blood pressure ≤90 mm HG for adults or less than fifth percentile by age for children aged <16 years; orthostatic drop in diastolic blood pressure ≥15 mmHg from lying to sitting, orthostatic syncope, or orthostatic dizziness

Multisystem involvement (three or more of the following):
- Gastrointestinal: vomiting or diarrhea at onset of illness
- Muscular: severe myalgia or creatine phosphokinase level at least twice the upper limit of normal
- Mucous membrane: vaginal, oropharyngeal, or conjunctival hyperemia
- Renal: blood urea nitrogen or creatinine at least twice the upper limit of normal for laboratory or urinary sediment with pyuria (>5 leukocytes per high-power field) in the absence of urinary tract infection
- Hepatic: total bilirubin, alanine aminotransferase enzyme, or asparate aminotransferase enzyme levels at least twice the upper limit of normal for laboratory
- Hematologic: platelets <100,000/mm³
- Central nervous system: disorientation or alterations in consciousness without focal neurologic signs when fever and hypotension are absent

Laboratory criteria

Negative results on the following tests, if obtained:
- Blood, throat, or cerebrospinal fluid cultures (blood culture may be positive for *Staphylococcus aureus*)
- Rise in titer to Rocky Mountain spotted fever, leptospirosis, or measles

Case classification

Probable: a case that meets the laboratory criteria and in which four of the five clinical findings described above are present

Confirmed: a case that meets the laboratory criteria and in which all five of the clinical findings described above are present, including desquamation, unless the patient dies before desquamation occurs

Box 14-4 Streptococcal Toxic Shock Syndrome: Centers for Disease Control and Prevention Clinical Case Definition 1996

Clinical description

Streptococcal toxic shock syndrome (STSS) is a severe illness associated with invasive or noninvasive group A streptococcal *(Streptococcus pyogenes)* infection. STSS may occur with infection at any site but most often occurs in association with infection of a cutaneous lesion. Signs of toxicity and a rapidly progressive clinical course are characteristic, and the case-fatality rate may exceed 50%.

Clinical case definition

An illness with the following clinical manifestations occurring within the first 48 hours of hospitalization or, for a nosocomial case, within the first 48 hours of illness:
- Hypotension defined by a systolic blood pressure less than or equal to 90 mm Hg for adults or less than the fifth percentile by age for children aged less than 16 years.
- Multiorgan involvement characterized by two or more of the following:
1. Renal impairment: creatinine greater than or equal to 2 mg/dL (greater than or equal to 177 µmol/L) for adults or greater than or equal to twice the upper limit of normal for age. In patients with preexisting renal disease, a greater than twofold elevation over the baseline level.
2. Coagulopathy: platelets less than or equal to 100,000/mm³ (less than or equal to 100 × 10⁶/L) or disseminated intravascular coagulation, defined by prolonged clotting times, low fibrinogen level, and the presence of fibrin degradation products.
3. Liver involvement: alanine aminotransferase, aspartate aminotransferase, or total bilirubin levels greater than or equal to twice the upper limit of normal for the patient's age. In patients with preexisting liver disease, a greater than twofold increase over the baseline level.
4. Acute respiratory distress syndrome: defined by acute onset of diffuse pulmonary infiltrates and hypoxemia in the absence of cardiac failure or by evidence of diffuse capillary leak manifested by acute onset of generalized edema, or pleural or peritoneal effusions with hypoalbuminemia.
5. A generalized erythematous macular rash that may desquamate.
6. Soft-tissue necrosis, including necrotizing fasciitis or myositis, or gangrene.

Laboratory criteria for diagnosis

Isolation of group A *Streptococcus*.

Case classification

Probable: a case that meets the clinical case definition in the absence of another identified etiology for the illness and with isolation of group A *Streptococcus* from a nonsterile site.

Confirmed: a case that meets the clinical case definition and with isolation of group A *Streptococcus* from a normally sterile site (e.g., blood or cerebrospinal fluid or, less commonly, joint, pleural, or pericardial fluid).

Box 14-5 Dermatologic Manifestations of Toxic Shock Syndrome

Erythroderma (100%)
Diffuse scarlatiniform involving chest, abdomen or back, and extremities

Desquamation (100%)
Palms, soles, tips of fingers and toes without scarring

Edema of the hands and feet (50%)
Nonpitting edema not associated with synovitis

Petechiae (27%)
Primarily on the extremities

Conjunctival injection (85%)
Bilateral, nonpurulent palpebral and bulbar conjunctivitis

Oropharyngeal hyperemia (90%)
Beefy red without exudate or membrane formation, strawberry tongue; some have multiple, punctate, nonpurulent buccal ulcerations

Vaginal hyperemia (100%)
Frequently tender external genitalia

Loss of hair and nails (45%)
Telogen effluvium occurs 2½ months after onset

Data from Chesney PJ, et al: JAMA 1981; 246:741.

Box 14-6 Toxic Shock Syndrome: Important Laboratory Abnormalities

Present in >85% of patients in the first 2 days of hospitalization
Coagulase-positive staphylococci cultured from specific sites, not from blood

Immature and mature polys >90% of WBC

Total lymphocyte count <650/mm³

Total serum protein level <5.6 gm/dl

Serum albumin level <3.1 mg/dl

Serum calcium level <7.8 mg/dl

Serum creatinine clearance <1.0 mg/dl

Serum bilirubin value >1.5 mg/dl

Serum cholesterol level <120 mg/dl

Prothrombin time >12 sec

Present in >70% of patients in the first 2 days of hospitalization
Platelet count <150,000/mm³

Pyuria of >5 WBC per high-power field

Proteinuria >2+

BUN >20 mg/dl

SGOT >41 U/L

From Chesney PJ, et al: JAMA 1981; 246:741.

DIAGNOSIS. The diagnosis is made when the clinical criteria mentioned in Box 14-3 are met. The important laboratory findings are listed in Box 14-6. A biopsy may be helpful in the early stages to establish the diagnosis. Assays for toxin and antibody can be performed.

TREATMENT. Treatment of TSS includes hydration, vasopressors, removal of tampons, and incision and drainage of abscesses. Treat intravenously, (10 to 14 days) with an antistaphylococcal penicillin or first-generation cephalosporin (oxacillin, nafcillin, cloxacillin, cefazolin). Penicillin-allergic patients are treated with vancomycin or erythromycin. It is possible that sublethal concentrations of silver sulfadiazine cream leads to increased toxin production by *S. aureus*; therefore mupirocin ointment or povidone-iodine solution are used if topical treatment is required. Treatment of STSS includes immediate debridement and both intravenous penicillin and clindamycin for 10 to 14 days. Penicillin allergic patients are treated with erythromycin or ceftriaxone. Human immunoglobulins (IGIV 2 gm/kg daily for 2 days) decreases mortality.[71] Antibodies that are capable of neutralizing toxins are present in commercially available IVIG preparations. These antibodies can facilitate patient improvement through toxin neutralization. There are many anecdotal examples of the effectiveness of IVIG as a part of staphylococcal TSS therapy. IVIG may be useful in managing TSS patients whose disease is due to methicillin-resistant *S. aureus* infections.[72] Most methicillin-resistant *S. aureus* infections in the United States produce staphylococcal enterotoxins B or C in very high concentrations. These preparations allow for neutralization of toxin until appropriate antibiotic therapy can be determined. Patients at nearly all stages of illness appear to respond positively to IVIG-neutralization of pyrogenic toxin superantigens.

Cutaneous drug reactions

INCIDENCE. Rashes are among the most common adverse reactions to drugs. They occur in many forms and mimic many dermatoses. They occur in 2% to 3% of hospitalized patients[73-75] (Table 14-3); in those patients there is no correlation between the development of an adverse reaction and the patients's age, diagnosis, or survival. The last Boston Collaborative Drug Surveillance Project estimated that approximately 30% of hospitalized patients experience adverse events attributable to drugs and that from 3% to 28% of all hospital admissions are related to adverse drug eruptions.[73]

Any dermatologic condition that appears within 2 weeks of starting a medication should include "drug-induced" in the differential.

Online and Other Resources: Pdr.net and MEDLINE provide current information on drug interactions. *The Drug Eruption Reference Manual* by Jerome Litt is available in paperback and online (www.drugeruptiondata.com). Drug interaction information is found at www.drug-interactions.com.

The mechanisms of adverse drug reactions are listed in Box 14-7. The proposed immunologic mechanisms of adverse drug reactions are listed in Table 14-4.

When drug-specific IgE antibodies bind to corresponding mast cell or basophil surface receptors, vasoactive mediators are released within minutes, causing an immediate-type reaction, clinically noted as pruritus, erythema, urticaria, angioedema, or anaphylaxis.

The drugs that commonly trigger this IgE mechanism are the beta-lactam antibiotics (especially the penicillins and first-generation cephalosporins) or autologous sera. These reactions are not dose dependent and require that the patient be sensitized before the "allergic" episode. On discontinuance or dissipation of the triggering agent, the cutaneous reaction usually resolves spontaneously within 48 hours.

MECHANISM. Two groups of mechanisms are involved in the pathogenesis of drug reactions: immunologic, with all four types of hypersensitivity reactions described; and nonimmunologic, accounting for at least 75% of all drug reactions.

Toxic epidermal necrolysis and other severe cutaneous adverse drug reactions may be linked to an inherited defect in the detoxification of drug metabolites. In a few predisposed patients a drug metabolite may bind to proteins in the epidermis and trigger an immune response leading to immunoallergic cutaneous adverse drug reactions. The drugs most often responsible for the eruptions are antimicrobial agents and antipyretic/antiinflammatory analgesics.[74]

Table 14-3 Rates of Allergic Skin Reactions to Specific Drugs (Urticaria, Generalized Maculopapular Eruption, Generalized Pruritus)

Drug or Substance	Reactions (%)
Platelet	45
Amoxicillin	5
Trimethoprim-sulfamethoxazole	3
Ampicillin	3
Ipodate	3
Blood	2
Penicillin	2
Cephalosporins	2
Erythromycin	2
Dihydralazine hydrochloride	2
Cyanocobalamin	2
Quinidine	1
Hyoscine butylbromide	1
Cimetidine	1
Phenylbutazone	1
Data from Bigby M, et al: JAMA 1986; 256:3358.	

Box 14-7 Mechanisms of Adverse Drug Reactions

Overdose
Accumulation
Pharmacologic side effects
Drug-drug interactions
Idiosyncrasy
Microbial imbalance
Exacerbation of existing latent or overt disease
Jarisch-Herxheimer reaction
Hypersensitivity
Autoimmune-like reaction
Teratogenic effect
Interaction of the drug and sunlight or other light sources
Other unknown mechanisms
Adapted from Beltrani VS: Immunol Allergy Clin North Am 1998; 18. The proposed immunologic mechanisms of adverse drug reactions are listed in Table 14-4.

Table 14-4 Proposed Immunologic Mechanisms of Adverse Drug Reactions of the Skin

T-cell mediated	Immune complexes	Toxic (not immunologic)	Mast cell degranulation, immunologic, nonimmunologic, others
Erythroderma	Fixed drug eruptions	Acneiform	Urticaria
Fixed drug eruptions	Erythema nodosum		
Photoallergic	Erythema multiforme		
Erythema nodosum	Pigmented purpura		
Toxic epidermal necrolysis	Vasculitis		
Pigmented purpura	Serum sickness		
Lichenoid	Maculopapular		
Eczema			
Vesicular/bullous			
Maculopapular			

Adapted from Beltrani VS: Immunol Allergy Clin North Am 1998; 18.

CLINICAL CHARACTERISTICS. The most common types of reactions are maculopapular (exanthematous eruptions), urticarial, and fixed drug eruptions.[75] Toxic epidermal necrolysis, erythema multiforme, and fixed drug eruptions share similar pathologic features and are caused by many of the same drugs. Photoallergic drug reactions require the interaction of drugs, UV irradiation, and the immune system. Eruptions seen in serum sickness include exanthem, urticaria, vasculitis, urticarial vasculitis, and erythema multiforme.[76]

The typical patient seen by the dermatologist is a hospitalized patient who is on several medications. A fever occurs and hours later a diffuse maculopapular rash, hives, and/or generalized pruritus develop; the attending physician stops all medications and consults the dermatologist. Although maculopapular and urticarial eruptions are the most common examples of a drug eruption, several other patterns occur.

Knowledge of these patterns and the drugs that commonly cause them helps to solve what is often a difficult problem when patients take many drugs simultaneously (Box 14-8).

CLINICAL DIAGNOSIS. Examine the patient and determine the primary lesion and distribution. Then ask when did it start? Does it itch? Drugs can cause skin symptoms without a rash (itching, burning, pain). Maculopapular and urticarial eruptions are the most frequent patterns. Maculopapular eruptions occur suddenly, often with fever, 7 to 10 days after the drug is first taken. They are generalized, symmetric, and often pruritic. Drug eruptions are always suspected when hives are present. One must be familiar with the many other patterns of skin eruptions and the types of eruptions caused by specific drugs in order to diagnose drug-related disease (see Box 14-8). Knowledge of the frequency with which certain drugs cause allergic drug reactions also helps to identify offending agents. The clinical characteristics of each type of reaction are described here.

Box 14-8 Cutaneous Patterns of Drug Eruptions

Acneiform	Photosensitivity
Alopecia	Pigmentation
Eczema	Pityriasis rosea–like
Erythema multiforme	Purpura
Erythema nodosum	Seborrheic dermatitis–like
Exanthems (maculo-papular, morbilliform)	Toxic epidermal necrolysis
Exfoliative erythroderma	Urticarial vasculitis
Fixed eruption	Vesiculobullous (pemphigus-like)
Lichenoid (lichen planus–like)	Lupus erythematosus–like

Box 14-9 Diagnostic Tests to Consider in the Evaluation of a Possible Drug Eruption

- Skin biopsy to categorize an eruption (i.e., urticaria, perivascular dermatitis, leukocytoclastic vasculitis) or to differentiate it from psoriasis, lichen planus, or cutaneous T-cell lymphoma.
- Drug levels for overdose or in a comatose or noncommunicative patient.
- Patch test for allergic contact dermatitis.
- Prick, radioallergosorbent test (RAST), or intradermal testing are indicated only for IgE-induced, immediate-type (urticarial) reactions (e.g., penicillin, insulin, papain, protamine, streptokinase, heterologous antisera, tetanus toxoid, cephalosporins). These require expertise for antigen selection.
- Serum tryptase levels are associated with acute anaphylaxis with or without itching, flushing, or urticaria, especially in severe reactions with cardiovascular involvement. For less severe acute reactions, negative serum tryptase does not rule out drug-induced anaphylaxis.
- Immunoassays for drug-specific antibody isotypes other than IgE high titers of drug-specific IgG antibodies have been associated with drug-induced immune complex syndromes (e.g., serum sickness).

DIAGNOSTIC TESTS. Box 14-9 lists tests to consider.

Serum tryptase. Serum tryptase is a biochemical marker of the release of mast-cell granules that occurs during an allergic reaction.

Mast cells release histamine and tryptase. Tryptase is secreted exclusively by mast cells. It is not detectable in the serum of healthy or allergic individuals. Tryptase levels greatly increase after an anaphylactic reaction caused by drugs, insect venom, and food. Serum tryptase levels have been associated with acute anaphylaxis with or without itching, flushing, or urticaria, especially in severe reactions with cardiovascular involvement. For less severe acute reactions, negative serum tryptase does not rule out drug-induced anaphylaxis.

Tryptase may be used to verify an anaphylactic event due to allergen or drug exposure. Patients with allergic urticaria and those with idiosyncratic responses to acetylsalicylic acid (ASA) exhibited a small increase in serum tryptase. Increased levels of tryptase can be detected up to three to six hours after the anaphylactic reaction. Tryptase is stable and may even be determined on post mortem serum (up to 24 hours) if anaphylaxis is suspected as the cause of death. Serial measurements may be needed to confirm mast-cell participation in milder reactions. Levels return to normal within 12 to 14 hours after release.

MANAGEMENT. The management of patients suspected of having a drug eruption is listed in the Box 14-10.

Box 14-10 Management of Patients with a Suspected Dermatologic Drug Reaction

- Make a flow sheet documenting time of onset of eruption, drugs, dosages, duration, and interruptions in the use of drugs.
- Determine the frequency of adverse reactions to the drug in the general population.
- Is the drug likely to be responsible for the cutaneous reaction, or is the eruption an unrelated dermatologic disease?
- Determine time of onset. Most cutaneous drug reactions occur 1 to 2 weeks after starting the drug.
- Consider ordering drug levels. Some cutaneous reactions may be dependent on dose or cumulative toxicity.
- Discontinue suspected offending drugs. Most adverse dermatologic reactions to drugs will improve when the drug is stopped.
- Rechallenge is the most accurate way to identify the offending drug. The decision to rechallenge a patient is made on an individual basis. Rechallenge in patients who have had urticarial-, bullous-, or erythema multiforme–like eruptions can be very dangerous. A reaction that fails to recur on rechallenge with a drug is unlikely to be caused by that agent.
- Symptomatic relief is provided with antihistamines and group V topical steroids.

Drug Eruptions: Clinical Patterns and Most Frequently Causal Drugs

Exanthems (maculopapular)

Maculopapular eruptions, the most frequent of all cutaneous drug reactions, are often indistinguishable from viral exanthems. They are the classic ampicillin and amoxicillin drug rashes, but practically any drug can trigger a maculopapular eruption (see Box 14-11). Red macules and papules become confluent in a symmetric, generalized distribution that often spares the face (Figures 14-26, 14-27, and 14-28). Itching is common. Mucous membranes, palms, and soles may be involved. Fever may be present from the onset. These eruptions are identical in appearance to a viral exanthem and routine laboratory tests usually fail to differentiate the two diseases. Onset is 7 to 10 days after starting the drug but may not occur until after the drug is stopped. The rash lasts for 1 to 2 weeks and fades in some cases even if the drug is continued. Lesions clear rapidly following withdrawal of the implicated agent and may progress to a generalized exfoliative dermatitis if use of the drug is not discontinued. The pathogenesis is unknown.

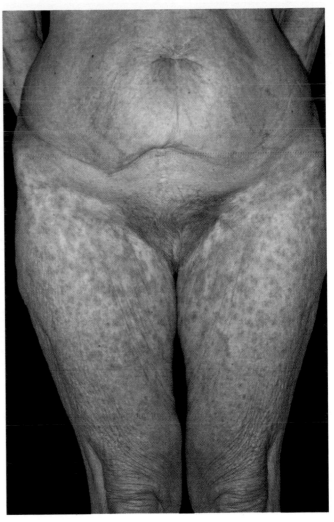

Figure 14-27 Maculopapular exanthems are the most common drug eruption pattern. They occur 7 to 10 days after starting the drug. Exanthems are often widespread and symmetric and spare the face, palms, and soles.

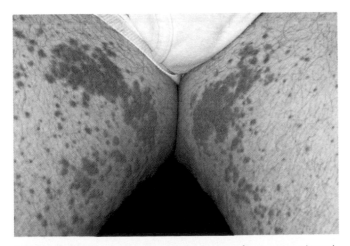

Figure 14-26 Maculopapular exanthems are often symmetric and present with confluent erythematous macules and papules.

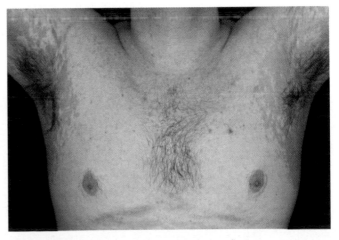

Figure 14-28 Symmetric distribution of a confluent maculopapular drug eruption.

Box 14-11 Drug Reactions and the Drugs that Cause Them

Maculopapular (exanthematous) eruptions
Ampicillin
Barbiturates
Diflunisal (Dolobid)
Gentamicin
Gold salts
Isoniazid
Meclofenamate (Meclomen)
Phenothiazines
Phenylbutazone
Phenytoin
(5% of children—dose dependent)
Quinidine
Sulfonamides
Thiazides
Thiouracil
Trimethoprim-sulfamethoxazole
(in patients with AIDS)

Anaphylactic reactions
Aspirin   Sera (animal derived)
Penicillin   Tolmetin (Tolectin)
Radiographic dye

Serum sickness
Aspirin   Sulfonamides
Penicillin   Thiouracils
Streptomycin

Acneiform (pustular) eruptions
Bromides   Iodides
Hormones   Isoniazid
ACTH   Lithium
Androgens   Phenobarbital (aggravates acne)
Corticosteroids   Phenytoin
Oral contraceptives

Alopecia
Allopurinol   Indomethacin
Anticoagulants   Levodopa
Antithyroid drugs   Oral contraceptives
Chemotherapeutic agents   Propranolol
Alkylating agents   Quinacrine
Antimetabolites   Retinoids
Cytotoxic agents   Thallium
Colchicine   Vitamin A
Hypocholesteremic drugs

Erythema nodosum
Iodides
Oral contraceptives
Sulfonamides

Exfoliative erythroderma
Allopurinol   Hydantoins
Arsenicals   Isoniazid
Barbiturates   Lithium
Captopril   Mercurial diuretics
Cefoxitin   Paraaminosalicylic acid
Chloroquine   Phenylbutazone
Cimetidine   Sulfonamides
Gold salts   Sulfonylureas

Fixed drug eruptions
Aspirin   Phenylbutazone
Barbiturates   Sulfonamides
Methaqualone   Tetracyclines
Phenazones   Trimethoprim-sulfamethoxazole
Phenolphthalein   Many others reported

Lichen planus-like eruptions
Antimalarials   Methyldopa
Arsenicals   Penicillamine
Beta-blockers   Quinidine
Captopril   Sulfonylureas
Furosemide   Thiazides
Gold salts

Erythema multiforme-like eruptions
Allopurinol   Penicillin
Barbiturates   Phenolphthalein
Carbamazepine   Phenothiazines
Hydantoins   Rifampin
Minoxidil   Sulfonamides
Nitrofurantoin   Sulfonylureas
Nonsteroidal   Sulindac agents
  anti-inflammatory

Lupus-like eruptions

Common	Probable
Hydralazine	Acebutolol
Procainamide	Carbamazepine
Uncommon	Ethosuximide
Chlorpromazine	Lithium carbonate
Hydrochlorothiazide	Penicillamine
Isoniazid	Phenytoin
Methyldopa	Propylthiouracil
Quinidine	Sulfasalazine

Photosensitivity
Amiodarone
Carbamazepine
Chlorpropamide

Box 14-11 Drug Reactions and the Drugs that Cause Them—cont'd

Photosensitivity—cont'd

Furosemide

Griseofulvin

Lomefloxacin

Methotrexate (sunburn reactivation)

Nalidixic acid

Naproxen

Phenothiazines

Piroxicam (Feldene)

Psoralens

Quinine

Sulfonamides

Tetracyclines

Demeclocycline

Doxycycline
   (less frequently with tetracycline and minocycline)

Thiazides

Tolbutamide

Skin pigmentation

ACTH (brown as in Addison's disease)

Amiodarone (slate-gray)

Anticancer drugs

Bleomycin (30%—brown, patchy, linear)

Busulphan (diffuse as in Addison's disease)

Cyclophosphamide (nails)

Doxorubicin (nails)

Antimalarials (blue-gray or yellow)

Arsenic (diffuse, brown, macular)

Chlorpromazine (slate-gray in sun-exposed areas)

Clofazimine (red)

Heavy metals (silver, gold, bismuth, mercury)

Methsergide maleate (red)

Minocycline (patchy or diffuse blue-black)

Oral contraceptives (chloasma-brown)

Psoralens

Rifampin—very high dose (red man syndrome)

Pityriasis rosea-like eruptions

Arsenicals

Barbiturates

Bismuth compounds

Captopril

Clonidine

Gold compounds

Methoxypromazine

Metronidazole

Pyribenzamine

Toxic epidermal necrolysis

Large areas of skin become bright red, then slough at the dermoepidermal border. This is a life-threatening reaction (see Chapter 18).

Allopurinol

Phenylbutazone

Phenytoin

Sulfonamides

Sulindac

Small vessel cutaneous vasculitis

Allopurinol

Diphenylhydantoin

Hydralazine

Penicillin

Piroxicam (Feldene) (Henoch-Schönlein purpura)

Propylthiouracil

Quinidine

Sulfonamides

Thiazides

Vesicles and blisters

Barbiturates (pressure areas—comatose patients)

Bromides

Captopril (pemphigus–like)

Cephalosporins (pemphigus–like)

Clonidine (cicatricial pemphigoid–like)

Furosemide (phototoxic)

Iodides

Nalidixic acid (phototoxic)

Naproxen (like porphyria cutanea tarda)

Penicillamine (pemphigus foliaceus–like)

Phenazones

Piroxicam (Feldene)

Sulfonamides

Ocular pemphigoid

Demecarium bromide

Echothiophate iodide

Epinephrine

Idoxuridine

Pilocarpine

Timolol

Chemotherapy-induced acral erythema

Cyclophosphamide

Cytosine arabinoside

Doxorubicin

Fluorouracil

Hydroxyurea

Mercaptopurine

Methotrexate

Mitotane

AMPICILLIN RASHES. Two types of skin reactions occur: an urticarial reaction mediated by skin-sensitizing antibody and a much more common exanthematous maculopapular reaction for which no allergic basis can be established. Ampicillin and other penicillins should not be given to patients who have had previous urticarial reactions while taking ampicillin. Ampicillin may safely be given to patients who have previously had a maculopapular ampicillin rash. The exanthematous reaction occurs in 50% to 80% of patients with infectious mononucleosis who take ampicillin. One study reported a high rate of drug exanthems in patients taking ampicillin in combination with allopurinol, but another study found no increased rate.[77]

CLINICAL PRESENTATION. The rash begins 5 to 10 days (range, 1 day to 4 weeks) after beginning the drug and may occur after the drug is terminated.

Latent periods of 2 to 3 weeks are seen with allopurinol, nitrofurantoin, and phenytoin. Eruptions may subside with continued use of the drug and may not recur on repeat exposure.

The rash starts on the trunk as a mildly pruritic, red, maculopapular, sometimes confluent eruption and spreads in hours in a symmetric fashion to the face and extremities (Figure 14-29). The palms, soles, and mucous membranes are spared. Lesions appear confluent in intertriginous areas (axilla, groin, and inframammary skin). Pruritus occurs frequently, and the intensity varies. A transient mild-to-moderate fever is common. Previously sensitized patients develop fever within hours of drug administration. Transient lymphadenopathy can accompany severe cases. Sometimes the eruption progresses to generalized erythroderma or exfoliative dermatitis. The rash begins to fade in 3 days and is gone in 6 days, even if the drug is continued.

DIFFERENTIAL DIAGNOSIS. Viral eruptions look and feel like drug-induced maculopapular eruptions. Drug maculopapular eruptions can be scarlitiniform, rubelliform (lentil-sized macules and faint papules), or morbilliform (look like measles). Drug eruptions usually develop within 1 week of starting treatment and last 1 to 2 weeks. Features that support a viral exanthem are hemorrhage and the absence of tissue eosinophilia.

Drug-induced morbilliform eruptions are common with ampicillin, amoxicillin, allopurinol, and TMP-SMX (in AIDS patients).

DIAGNOSIS. The histology is nonspecific. Skin biopsy may rule out other diseases. Rechallenge for diagnostic purposes is not a routine practice.

MANAGEMENT. Stop the offending drug and provide symptomatic relief. Group V topical corticosteroid creams and cool compresses are soothing and control itching. Treat severe itching or an extensive eruption with prednisone (0.5 to 1.0 mg/kg/day) for 7 to 10 days. Antihistamines provide sedation but are usually not effective at controlling itching because histamine does not cause maculopapular lesions. Stop treatment of any drug causing a generalized, symmetric maculopapular rash, and do not retreat with the same drug. Skin-test patients who require ampicillin if the nature of a previous reaction is unknown and there is no adequate substitute drug.

Urticaria

Urticaria is frequently caused by drugs, and most drugs can induce hives. Aspirin, penicillin, and blood products are the most frequent causes of urticarial drug eruptions, but almost any drug can cause hives. Hives are itchy, red, edematous plaques that are usually generalized and symmetric. There is no scaling or vesiculation. Wheals vary in size from small papules to huge plaques. The hives typically fade in less than 24 hours only to recur in another area. *Angioedema* refers to urticarial swelling of deep dermal and subcutaneous tissues and mucous membranes; the reaction may be life threatening. There are three mechanisms of drug-induced urticaria: anaphylactic and accelerated reactions (immunologic histamine release), nonimmunologic histamine release, and serum sickness.

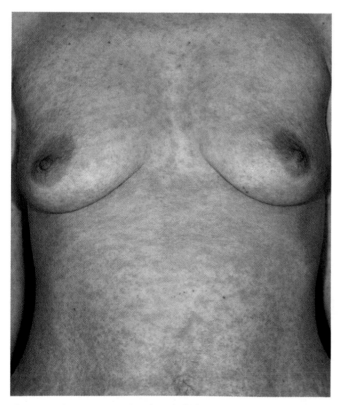

Figure 14-29 Drug eruption (ampicillin). Asymmetric, confluent maculopapular eruption.

ANAPHYLACTIC AND ACCELERATED REACTIONS. These IgE-dependent reactions occur within minutes (immediate reactions) to hours (accelerated reactions) of drug administration. Penicillin and its derivatives are the most common causes.

IgE-induced mast cell degranulation (anaphylaxis) occurs within minutes of exposure. From 1% to 5% of patients treated with beta-lactam antibiotics (penicillin, semisynthetic penicillins such as amoxicillin, cephalosporins, carbapenems) develop hives.

Most patients who give a history of allergy to penicillin do not have evidence of allergy when skin tested. Patients with a history of a reaction with past penicillin treatment who require penicillin treatment should be skin tested within days of a planned therapeutic course of penicillin. RAST testing is not reliable to rule out allergy. Patients with a positive skin test have a 50% chance of developing an immediate reaction if given penicillin. From 97% to 99% of patients with a negative test will tolerate penicillin. Many patients with documented allergy to penicillin lose it with time; about 25% may maintain the allergy indefinitely.

Both cephalosporins and penicillins have a beta-lactam ring. Clinically significant cross-reactivity occurs in less than 5% or less of patients with positive skin tests to penicillin who are subsequently given cephalosporins. Most cross-reactions involve first- and second-generation cephalosporins. Patients allergic to cephalosporins may have antibodies directed to side chain structures rather than to the beta-lactam ring; therefore patients who develop an urticarial reaction to cephalosporin rarely react to penicillin. Cephalosporin skin testing is not a standard practice.

SERUM SICKNESS. Circulating immune complexes cause serum sickness. Urticaria occurs 4 to 21 days after drug ingestion. The drug is ingested, antibody is formed over the next few days, and drug and antibody combine to form circulating immune complexes. Fever, hematuria, lymphadenopathy, and arthralgias follow (see Chapter 6).

NONIMMUNOLOGIC HISTAMINE RELEASERS. Reaction can occur in minutes. The drug may exert a direct action on the mast cell or on other pathways.

NON–IgE-INDUCED (ASPIRIN AND NSAIDS) URTICARIA. Nonimmunologic anaphylactoid reactions usually have a latency of 30 minutes to 24 hours. Angioedema or urticaria may occur. Urticaria frequently appears on the face and spreads caudad. Reactions may be dose dependent; small doses may be tolerated.

Aspirin- and NSAID-induced urticaria occurs in 25% to 50% of patients with chronic idiopathic urticaria. Fifty percent of patients with ASA- or NSAID-induced urticaria are atopic.[78] The mechanism of these reactions is thought to be cyclooxygenase inhibition, which results in the augmented production of leukotrienes. Therefore antihistamines are less effective for ASA-induced urticaria or angioedema. Preservatives (benzoic acid) and dyes (tartrazine) produce the same effect. ASA desensitization is not recommended.

Patients with ASA or NSAID hypersensitivity may use acetaminophen, disalicylic acid (e.g., salsalate, Disalcid) or choline magnesium trisalicylate (Trilisate).

RADIOCONTRAST MEDIA REACTIONS. Reaction rates to radiocontrast media (RCM) range from 4% to 12%. The histamine release is slower than that produced by IgE activation and begins 10 minutes after exposure and peaks at 45 minutes. Most reactions occur from the hyperosmolar agents. Patients who have had a past reaction to RCM have a 20% to 30% chance of a repeat reaction with subsequent exposure. Non–IgE-induced urticaria with histamine release from both basophils and mast cells occurs in 3%, itching in 3%, and flushing in 1% of patients receiving the hyperosmolar agents. Patients at risk of RCM reactions may be given doxepin (an H_1/H_2 antagonist) 10 to 25 mg 1 to 2 hours before administration of RCM to prevent an anaphylactoid reaction.

OPIATES. Opiates induce mast cells of the skin (not mucosal surfaces) to degranulate by a direct effect on the cell and release histamines. Pretreatment with antihistamines prevents pruritus, urticaria, and flushing that occurs with morphine infusion.

Other nonimmunologic histamine releasers include polymyxin B, lobster, and strawberries.

Pruritus

Most drug eruptions itch but itching can be the only manifestation of a drug reaction (e.g., gold, sulfonamides). Histamine in the skin almost always results in an urticarial reaction or, at lower concentrations, flushing. Histamine is the predominant mediator of IgE-induced reactions (with greater potential for life-threatening anaphylaxis), and these are more responsive to antihistamine (an H1 and, at times, concomitant administration of an H2 antagonist may be rewarding) therapy. Histamine is not the only mediator of itch released during inflammatory reactions. Kinins, leukotrienes, prostaglandins, and serotonin are also mediators of itching and itching induced by these mediators would not respond to antihistamines. Oral contraceptives can produce itching similar to pruritus gravidarum. Opiates can directly cause mast cell degranulation. Itching induced by opiates responds to the narcotic antagonist naloxone, rather than antihistamines.

Drug Eruptions

Acute generalized exanthematous pustulosis

Acute generalized exanthematous pustulosis (AGEP) is characterized by acute onset often following drug intake with fever and numerous nonfollicular sterile pustules on an erythematous background predominantly in the folds and/or on the face and elevated blood neutrophils (Figure 14-30). Most cases of AGEP are drug induced. The most frequently implicated agents are calcium channel blockers, NSAIDs, anticonvulsants, and antimicrobials, particularly those with beta-lactam and macrolide properties. Acute infections with enteroviruses are also a reported cause. Pustules resolve spontaneously in less than 15 days. Withdraw the drug and consider treatment with systemic steroids. Distinction from generalized pustular psoriasis is important. AGEP has a more acute course with fever, relationship to drug therapy, and rapid spontaneous resolution following drug withdrawal. The biopsy shows subcorneal pustules that resemble those of pustular psoriasis.[79,80]

Acneiform (pustular) eruptions

These pustular eruptions mimic acne but comedones are absent. Treatment with oral corticosteroids and abuse of anabolic steroids are possible causes (Box 14-10).

Eczema

A patient who develops contact dermatitis with a topical agent develops either a focal flare at sites of previous inflammation or a generalized cutaneous eruption if exposed orally or by inhalation to the same or chemically related medication (the so-called external-internal sensitization) (Table 14-5). The symptoms develop within 2 to 24 hours after ingestion of the drug. Continued use of the medication can intensify the reaction and lead to generalization of the eruption. Antibiotics and oral hypoglycemic agents are most commonly implicated. The term "baboon syndrome" describes a distinctive form of systemic contact dermatitis with symmetric erythema in flexural areas including the elbows, axilla, eyelids, and sides of the neck accompanied by bright red anogenital lesions.[81]

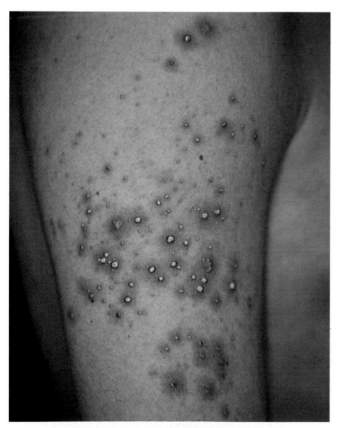

Figure 14-30 Acute generalized exanthemous pustulosis is characterized by the acute onset of fever and generalized erythema with numerous, small, discrete, sterile, nonfollicular pustules. Pustules may appear in a few days of starting the drug. Pustules resolve in less than 15 days followed by desquamation.

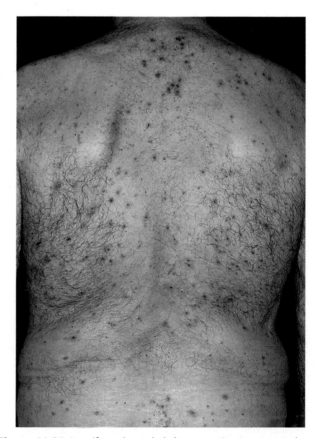

Figure 14-31 Acneiform (pustular) drug eruptions occur on the upper body. In contrast to acne vulgaris, comedones are absent.

Blistering drug eruptions

Blisters may develop alone, as part of other eruptions (e.g., erythema multiforme, toxic epidermal necrolysis, and fixed drug eruptions), or with exanthemic drug eruptions (Box 14-10). Drug-induced linear IgA dermatosis presents as a papulovesicular eruption, but mucosal and conjunctival lesions are absent. Drugs may cause a blistering eruption that mimics superficial pemphigus (pemphigus foliaceous). A morbilliform or urticarial eruption precedes the blisters. Direct and indirect immunofluorescence findings resemble non–drug-induced pemphigus. Bullous pemphigoid, an autoimmune blistering dermatosis usually seen in the elderly, presents with tense blisters on an urticarial base. Circulating antibodies are present in most cases. Direct immunofluorescent testing shows linear IgG and C3 along the dermoepidermal junction. Pseudoporphyria resembles porphyria cutanea tarda at a clinical, light microscopic, and direct immunofluorescent level, but porphyrin tests are normal. NSAIDs are the most common cause.

Erythema multiforme and toxic epidermal necrolysis

Reactions occur on the skin and mucous membranes; they include multiple, symmetric, persistent macules, papules, vesicles, and bullae. The iris or target lesion is the classic presentation for erythema multiforme, which presents with central duskiness in an expanding erythematous macule or papule. Severe forms are often caused by medications. Less severe forms are caused by mycoplasmal pneumonia, herpes simplex infections, and medication. Loss of a major portion of the cutaneous surface (toxic epidermal necrolysis) is severe and fatal in up to 30% of cases. The cause of death is loss of large areas of skin, resulting in fluid loss and sepsis. The drugs most often involved are long-acting sulfonamides, NSAIDs, and anticonvulsants. Toxic metabolites (i.e., circulating immune complexes) in predisposed individuals may be the cause of a cell-mediated cytotoxic reaction. Readministration of the responsible drug produces a recurrence. See Box 14-10 and Chapter 18.

Exfoliative erythroderma

Patients may develop erythema involving the entire skin surface from drug therapy (see Box 14-10 and Figure 14-32). Erythroderma may also occur in pityriasis rubra pilaris, psoriasis, and cutaneous T-cell lymphoma. Generalized erythema and scaling may occur if an offending agent is not withdrawn. The reaction is potentially life threatening.

Table 14-5 Eczematous Eruptions (External-Internal Sensitization*)	
Topical medication	**Oral medication**
Aminophylline suppositories	Ethylenediamine antihistamines
Benadryl cream	Benadryl, Dramamine
Caladryl lotion	Benadryl, Dramamine
Formaldehyde	Methenamine
Neomycin sulfate	Streptomycin, kanamycin, gentamicin
Thiuram and disulfiram (rubber and insecticide compounds)	Antabuse
Benzocaine, glyceryl PABA sunscreens (paraamino compounds)	Azo dyes in foods and drugs, acetohexamide, tolbutamide, chlorpropamide, chlorothiazide, paraaminosalicylic acid

Adapted from Fisher AA: Contact Dermatitis, ed 3, Philadelphia, 1986, Lea & Febiger.

*Patients allergic to certain topical medications develop focal or generalized eruptions when exposed to a chemically related oral medication.

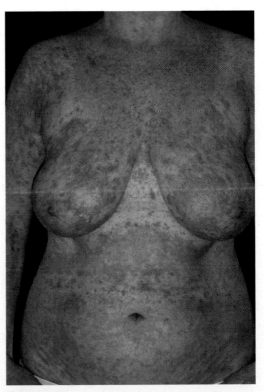

Figure 14-32 Exfoliative erythroderma. Erythroderma (red skin) may be caused by drugs, malignancy, psoriasis, and other conditions.

Fixed drug eruptions

Fixed drug eruptions are a unique form of drug allergy that produce red plaques or blisters that recur at the same cutaneous site each time the drug is ingested[82] (see Box 14-10). The clinical pattern and distribution of lesions may be influenced by the drug in question, and the study of the pattern may provide useful information in selecting the most likely causative drug. Tetracycline[83] and co-trimoxazole commonly cause lesions limited to the glans penis.[84] Cases of familial occurrence suggest that a genetic predisposition might be an important causal factor.[85,86]

CLINICAL MANIFESTATIONS. Single or multiple, round, sharply demarcated, dusky red plaques appear soon after drug exposure and reappear in exactly the same site each time the drug is taken (Figure 14-33). The lesions are generally preceded or accompanied by itching and burning, the intensity of which is usually proportionate to the severity of the inflammatory changes. Pruritus and burning may be the only manifestations of reactivation in an old patch. The area often blisters and then erodes; desquamation or crusting (after bullous lesions) follows, and brown pigmentation (Figure 14-34) forms with healing. Nonpigmenting reactions have been documented. Pseudoephedrine classically causes a nonpigmenting fixed drug eruption.[87] Lesions can occur on any part of the skin or mucous membrane,[88] but the glans penis (Figure 14-35) is the most common site. Regional lymphadenopathy is absent.

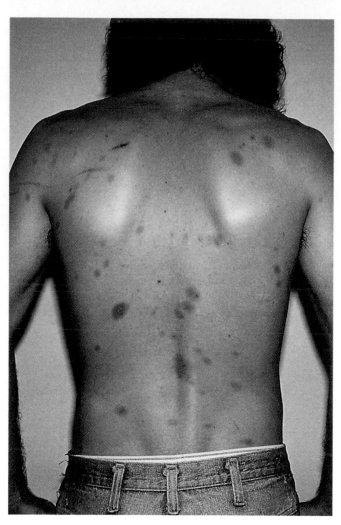

Figure 14-34 Fixed drug eruption. Multiple round, sharply demarcated plaques appeared shortly after methaqualone (Quaalude) was taken. The plaques healed with brown hyperpigmentation. *(Courtesy David W. Knox, M.D.)*

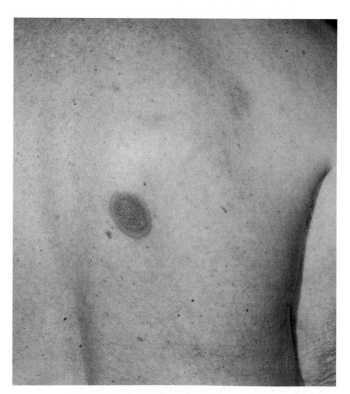

Figure 14-33 Fixed drug eruption. A single sharply demarcated, round plaque appeared shortly after trimethoprim was taken.

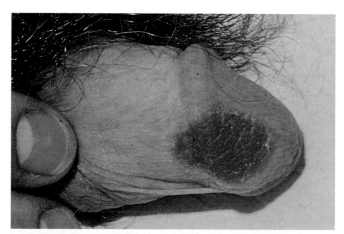

Figure 14-35 Fixed drug eruption. The glans penis is the most common site.

REACTIVATION AND REFRACTORY PHASE. The length of time from the reexposure to a drug and the onset of symptoms is 30 minutes to 8 hours (mean, 2.1 hours).[89] Following each exacerbation, some patients demonstrate a refractory period (weeks to several months),[90] during which the offending drug does not activate the lesions.

CROSS-SENSITIVITY. Ingestion of a drug with a similar chemical structure may precipitate exacerbations. This phenomenon has been reported with tetracycline derivatives and sulfonamides. There is greater cross-reactivity between tetracycline and doxycycline, both of which have one methylamino group at the fourth carbon position, than between those two antibiotics and minocycline, which has two methylamino groups at the fourth and seventh carbon positions.[91] Drugs of different chemical structures also can precipitate exacerbations. Three different, pharmacologically unrelated anticonvulsants evoked an eruption at the same site.[92]

DIAGNOSIS. A careful history is important because patients often do not relate their complaints to the use of a drug that they may be taking such as a laxative (phenolphthalein)[93] or headache remedy. Provoking the lesion with the suspected drug confirms the diagnosis, prevents recurrences, and allays the anxiety of the patient regarding venereal origin of the disease. The challenge dose should be smaller than the normal therapeutic dose,[94] but it can be cautiously increased up to the normal therapeutic dose until the reaction is elicited. In some cases 2 to 3 times the original dose may be required to elicit a repeat reaction. Some authors do not recommend these tests because of the possible risk of generalized bullous eruptions. Topical and intradermal[95] provocation tests have been used as an alternative to systemic provocation tests. Patch tests are performed on the patient's normal and prelesional skin with the drug in a petrolatum base. In one study, a positive reaction occurred only at the previous lesional site.[96]

A biopsy shows hydropic degeneration of the epidermal basal cells and pigmentary incontinence.

Lichenoid (lichen planus–like drug eruptions)

Clinically and histologically these mimic generalized lichen planus. There are multiple flat-topped, itchy violaceous papules; oral lesions may be present. The mean age of patients with lichen planus is approximately 50 years; the mean age for lichenoid drug eruptions is approximately 60 years. The latent period between the beginning of administration of a drug and the eruption is between 3 weeks and 3 years.[97] The lesions are chronic and persist for weeks or months after the offending drug is stopped. Lesions heal with brown pigmentation. Gold and antimalarials are most often associated with drug-induced lichen planus (see Box 14-10).

Lupus erythematosus–like drug eruptions

The reaction has been reported with a number of drugs,[98] but most frequently with procainamide and hydralazine (see Box 14-10). The reaction is dose related. A variety of skin signs can occur, including erythema with a "butterfly" rash, urticaria, livedo reticularis, and vasculitis, but they all are infrequently seen in drug-induced lupus.

Clinical presentation includes arthritis, arthralgias, and elevated ESR. Fever, renal involvement, and CNS disease are rare. The ratio of females to males is 4:1. The ANAs, antihistone, and anti–single-stranded DNA antibodies are markers for lupus-like drug eruptions. The predominant nuclear antibodies are directed against histone proteins. In one study ANAs occurred in 83% of patients receiving procainamide for cardiac arrhythmias; they had no symptoms of a connective tissue disease. Significant elevation of antibody binding to single-stranded DNA and double-stranded DNA was seen; 65.4% had antibodies to total histones.[99] Serum complement levels remained normal. Dermoepidermal junction immunofluorescence, as measured by the "lupus-band test" was positive in 6% of patients with procainamide-induced lupus, compared with positive test results in 54% of patients with idiopathic systemic lupus erythematosus (SLE).[100] A genetic predisposition exists. Both drugs are inactivated by acetylation; most patients have the slow acetylation phenotype. The combination of HLA-DRW-4, female sex, slow acetylator status, and a minimum dosage of 200 mg/day of hydralazine inevitably leads to the syndrome.[101] Susceptible patients may be identified by determination of acetylator type and DR status. Stopping the drug results in rapid clinical improvement and gradual (months) disappearance of autoantibodies. Drug-induced subacute cutaneous lupus erythematosus has been described in patients taking calcium channel blockers. They develop typical photoinduced annular papulosquamous eruptions and antibodies to Ro, La, and centromere antigens and positive ANAs.[102]

Photosensitivity

Photosensitivity eruptions represent 8% of all adverse cutaneous drug reactions. Both systemic and topical medications can induce photosensitivity. There are two main types: phototoxicity and photoallergy.

Phototoxic reactions are related to drug concentration and can occur in anyone. The drug absorbs radiation and enters an excited state, producing species including reactive oxygen radicals that react with other cellular constituents. The rash occurs within a few hours following the first exposure to a drug and resembles an exaggerated sunburn with blistering, desquamation, and hyperpigmentation. The eruption is confined to sun-exposed areas. The reaction can occur on first administration and subsides when the drug is stopped.

Photoallergic reactions are less common and are not concentration related. They occur in only a small fraction of people exposed and may spread to involve areas that have not been exposed to the sun, possibly from an autosensitization phenomenon. They are a form of delayed hypersensitivity reaction and appear within 24 to 48 hours of antigenic challenge. They occur in sun-exposed areas, sparing the submental and retroauricular areas and upper eyelids. On rare occasions, the reaction can persist for years, even without further drug exposure.

Onycholysis (separation of the nail plate from the nail bed) may occur from drug photosensitivity and has occurred with tetracyclines, psoralens, and fluoroquinolones.

Pigmentation

Pigmentation can result from drugs that increase production of melanin, causing pigment incontinence by damaging epidermal keratinocytes or melanocytes in the basal layer or by deposition (see Box 14-10).

Vasculitis

Small vessel necrotizing vasculitis (palpable purpura) may be precipitated by drugs (see Box 14-10). Lesions are most often concentrated on the lower legs but may be generalized and involve the kidneys, joints, and brain. Any drug can evoke vasculitis in a predisposed patient.

Lymphomatoid drug eruptions

Any patient who develops an atypical lymphoid infiltrate should have a drug-based etiology excluded before the diagnosis of cutaneous lymphoma is made.[103] Lesions that resemble mycosis fungoides have been reported with phenytoin (Dilantin), phenothiazines, barbiturates, beta-blockers, angiotensin-converting enzyme inhibitors, calcium channel blockers, H1 and H2 antagonists, benzodiazepines, and antidepressants.

Chemotherapy-induced acral erythema

Chemotherapy-induced acral erythema occurs most commonly with cytosine arabinoside, fluorouracil, doxorubicin, and, less often, other drugs (see Box 14-10).[104] It appears to be dose dependent, and a direct toxic effect of the drug is likely. Tingling on the palms and soles is followed in a few days by painful, symmetric, well-defined swelling and erythema. Cytosine arabinoside has a predilection to progress to blisters; doxorubicin and fluorouracil are much less likely to cause blisters.[105] Treatment is supportive, with elevation and cold compresses. Systemic steroids have been used with variable success. Cooling the hands and feet during treatment to decrease blood flow may attenuate the reaction. Modification of the dosage schedule may also help.

Skin eruptions associated with specific drugs

CUTANEOUS COMPLICATIONS OF CHEMOTHERAPEUTIC AGENTS. Cancer chemotherapeutic agents adversely affect rapidly dividing cells. Stomatitis, alopecia, onychodystrophy, chemical cellulitis, phlebitis, and hyperpigmentation occur with several agents. Self-limited palmar-plantar erythema, occasionally with bulla formation, has been reported (see earlier).

ANTICONVULSANT HYPERSENSITIVITY SYNDROME. This syndrome has a variable spectrum of clinical and laboratory findings: fever, rash, lymphadenopathy, and hepatitis (hepatomegaly and increase in serum aminotransferase), with leukocytosis and eosinophilia. The three most commonly used anticonvulsants—phenytoin, phenobarbital, and carbamazepine—can each produce the reaction. Cutaneous reactions to phenytoin occur in up to 19% of patients. These vary from morbilliform eruptions to erythroderma, erythema multiforme, and toxic epidermal necrolysis. A small percentage of patients develop a hypersensitivity syndrome that presents with a macular or papular rash or erythroderma and, rarely, pustules.[106] The outcome depends on the severity of the hepatic injury and the presence of other complications. The reaction is serious and may result in death.

References

1. Sison-Fonacier L, Bystryn J-C: Regional variations in antigenic properties of skin: a possible cause for disease-specific distribution of skin lesions, J Exp Med 1986; 164:2125.

2. Remington PL, et al: Airborne transmission of measles in a physician's office, JAMA 1985; 253:1574.

3. Jespersen CS, Littauer J, Sagild U: Measles as a cause of fetal defects, Acta Paediatr Scand 1977; 66:367.

4. Villamor E, Fawzi W: Vitamin A supplementation: implications for morbidity and mortality in children, J Infect Dis 2000; 182 Suppl 1:S122.

5. Fawzi WW, et al: Vitamin A supplementation and child mortality: a meta-analysis, JAMA 1993; 269:898.

6. Hussey GD, Klein M: A randomized, controlled trial of vitamin A in children with severe measles, N Engl J Med 1990; 323:160.

7. Caballero B, Rice A: Low serum retinol is associated with increased severity of measles in New York City children, Nutr Rev 1992; 50:291.

8. Coutsoudis A, et al: Vitamin A supplementation enhances specific IgG antibody levels and total lymphocyte numbers while improving morbidity in measles, Pediatr Infect Dis J 1992; 11:203.

9. Clementz G, Mancini A: Nail matrix arrest following hand-foot-mouth disease: a report of five children, Pediatr Dermatol 2000; 17:7.

10. Chan L, et al, for the Outbreak Study Group: Deaths of children during an outbreak of hand, foot, and mouth disease in Sarawak, Malaysia: clinical and pathological characteristics of the disease, Clin Infect Dis 2000; 31:678.

11. Huang C, et al: Neurologic complications in children with enterovirus 71 infection, N Engl J Med 1999; 341:936.

12. Ho M, et al: An epidemic of enterovirus 71 infection in Taiwan. Taiwan Enterovirus Epidemic Working Group, N Engl J Med 1999; 341:929.

13. Chang L, et al: Clinical features and risk factors of pulmonary oedema after enterovirus-71-related hand, foot, and mouth disease, Lancet 1999; 354:1682.

14. Knoll H, et al: Scarlet fever and types of erythrogenic toxins produced by the infecting streptococcal strains, Int J Med Microbiol 1991; 276:94.

15. Lee SH, et al: Resurgence of congenital rubella syndrome in the 1990s: report on missed opportunities and failed prevention policies among women of childbearing age, JAMA 1992; 267:2616.

16. Zolti M, et al: Rubella-specific IgM in reinfection and risk to the fetus, Gynecol Obstet Invest 1990; 30:184.

17. Best JM, et al: Fetal infection after maternal reinfection with rubella: criteria for defining reinfection, Br Med J 1989; 299:773.

18. Miron D, On A: Congenital rubella syndrome after maternal immunization, Harefuah 1992; 122:291.

19. Skvorc-Ranko R, et al: Intrauterine diagnosis of cytomegalovirus and rubella infections by amniocentesis, Can Med Assoc J 1991; 145:649.

20. Hedman K, Rousseau SA: Measurement of avidity of specific IgG for verification of recent primary rubella, J Med Virol 1989; 27:288.

21. Enders G, Knotek F: Rubella IgG total antibody avidity and IgG subclass-specific antibody avidity assay and their role in the differentiation between primary rubella and rubella reinfection, Infection 1989; 17:218.

22. Brown KE, et al: Resistance to parvovirus B19 infection due to lack of virus receptor (erythrocyte P. antigen), N Engl J Med 1994; 330:1192.

23. Brown K, Young N: Parvovirus B19 in human disease, Annu Rev Med 1997; 48:59.

24. Joseph PR: Incubation period of fifth disease, Lancet 1986; 2:1390.

25. Grilli R, et al: Papular-purpuric "gloves and socks" syndrome: olymerase chain reaction demonstration of parvovirus B19 DNA in cutaneous lesions and sera, J Am Acad Dermatol 1999; 41(5 Pt 1):793.

26. van RM, et al: [Drug-induced papular-purpuric gloves and socks syndrome], Hautarzt 1999; 50:280.

27. Naides SJ: Parvovirus B19, Rheum Dis Clin North Am 1993; 19:457.

28. White DG, et al: Human parvovirus arthropathy, Lancet 1985; 1:419.

29. Naides SJ, et al: Rheumatologic manifestations of human parvovirus B19 infection in adults, Arthritis Rheum 1990, 33.1297.

30. Nesher G, Osborn T, Moore T: Parvovirus infection mimicking systemic lupus erythematosus, Semin Arthritis Rheum 1995; 24:297.

31. Mayo DR, Vance DW Jr: Parvovirus B19 as the cause of a syndrome resembling Lyme arthritis in adults, N Engl J Med 1991; 324:419.

32. Speyer I, Breedveld F, Dijkmans B: Human parvovirus B19 infection is not followed by inflammatory joint disease during long term follow-up: a retrospective study of 54 patients, Clin Exp Rheumatol 1998; 16:576.

33. Nocton JJ, et al: Human parvovirus B19-associated arthritis in children, J Pediatr 1993; 122:186.

34. Wright C, Hinchliffe S, Taylor C: Fetal pathology in intrauterine death due to parvovirus B19 infection, Br J Obstet Gynaecol 1996; 103:133.

35. Kovacs BW, et al: Prenatal diagnosis of human parvovirus B19 in nonimmune hydrops fetalis by polymerase chain reaction, Am J Obstet Gynecol 1992; 167:461.

36. Sheikh AU, et al: Long-term outcome in fetal hydrops from parvovirus B19 infection, Am J Obstet Gynecol 1992; 167:337.

37. Gilbert G: Parvovirus B19 infection and its significance in pregnancy, Commun Dis Intell 2000; 24 Suppl:69.

38. Torok TJ, et al: Prenatal diagnosis of intrauterine infection with parvovirus B19 by the polymerase chain reaction technique, Clin Infect Dis 1992; 14:149.

39. Serjeant GR, et al: Human parvovirus infection in homozygous sickle cell disease, Lancet 1993; 341:1237.

40. Rao SP, et al: Transient aplastic crisis in patients with sickle cell disease: B19 parvovirus studies during a 7-year period, Am J Dis Child 1992; 146:1328.

41. Bell LM, et al: Human parvovirus B19 infection among hospital staff members after contact with infected patients, N Engl J Med 1989; 321:485.

42. Naides SJ, et al: Parvovirus B19 infection in human immunodeficiency virus type 1-infected persons failing or intolerant to zidovudine therapy, J Infect Dis 1993; 168:101.

43. Kurtzman G, et al: Pure red-cell aplasia of 10 years' duration due to persistent parvovirus B19 infection and its cure with immunoglobulin therapy, N Engl J Med 1989; 321:519.

44. Okada K, et al: Exanthema subitum and human herpesvirus 6 infection: clinical observations in fifty-seven cases, Pediatr Infect Dis J 1993; 12:204.

45. Akashi K, et al: Brief report: severe infectious mononucleosis-like syndrome and primary human herpesvirus 6 infection in an adult, N Engl J Med 1993; 329:168.

46. Cone RW, et al: Human herpesvirus 6 in lung tissue from patients with pneumonitis after bone marrow transplantation, N Engl J Med 1993; 329:156.

47. Pruksananonda P, et al: Primary human herpesvirus 6 infection in young children, N Engl J Med 1992; 326:1445.

48. Breese C, et al: Human herpes virus-6 infection in children, N Engl J Med 1994; 331:432.

49. Hayashi M, et al: Long-term neurological outcome in children with convulsions during exanthema subitum, No To Hattatsu 1993; 25:53.

50. Suga S, et al: Clinical and virological analyses of 21 infants with exanthem subitum (roseola infantum) and central nervous system complications, Ann Neurol 1993; 33:597.

51. Segondy M, et al: Herpesvirus 6 infection in young children, N Engl J Med 1992; 327:1099.

52. Wiersbitzky S, et al: The blood picture in exanthema subitum (Zahorsky): critical 3-day fever-exanthema in young children, Kinderarztl Prax 1991; 59:258.

53. Leach C: Human herpesvirus-6 and -7 infections in children: agents of roseola and other syndromes, Curr Opin Pediatr 2000; 12:269.

54. Deleted in proofs.

55. Deleted in proofs.

56. Deleted in proofs.

57. Deleted in proofs.

58. Burns J, et al: Kawasaki disease: a brief history, Pediatrics 2000; 106:E27.

59. Burns J: Kawasaki disease, Adv Pediatr 2001; 48:157.

60. Nasr I, Tometzki A, Schofield O: Kawasaki disease: an update, Clin Exp Dermatol 2001; 26:6.

61. Rowley A, Shulman S: Kawasaki syndrome, Pediatr Clin North Am 1999; 46:313.

62. Leung D, Meissner H: The many faces of Kawasaki syndrome, Hosp Pract (Off Ed) 2000; 35:77.

63. Taubert K, Shulman S: Kawasaki disease, Am Fam Physician 1999; 59:3093-3102, 3107.

64. McCormick J, Yarwood J, Schlievert P: Toxic shock syndrome and bacterial superantigens: an update, Annu Rev Microbiol 2001; 55:77.

65. Odom S, et al: Postoperative staphylococcal toxic shock syndrome due to pre-existing staphylococcal infection: case report and review of the literature, Am Surg 2001; 67:745.

66. Davis D, Gash-Kim T, Heffernan E: Toxic shock syndrome: case report of a postpartum female and a literature review, J Emerg Med 1998; 16:607.

67. Issa N, Thompson R: Staphylococcal toxic shock syndrome: suspicion and prevention are keys to control, Postgrad Med 2001; 110:55.

68. Torres-Martinez C, et al: Streptococcus associated toxic shock, Arch Dis Child 1992; 67:126.

69. Hauser A: Another toxic shock syndrome: streptococcal infection is even more dangerous than the staphylococcal form, Postgrad Med 1998; 104:31.

70. Herzer C: Toxic shock syndrome: broadening the differential diagnosis, J Am Board Fam Pract 2001; 14:131.

71. Stevens D: Rationale for the use of intravenous gamma globulin in the treatment of streptococcal toxic shock syndrome, Clin Infect Dis 1998; 26:639.

72. Schlievert P: Use of intravenous immunoglobulin in the treatment of staphylococcal and streptococcal toxic shock syndromes and related illnesses, J Allergy Clin Immunol 2001; 108(4 Suppl):S107.

73. Bigby M, et al: Drug-induced cutaneous reactions: a report from the Boston collaborative drug surveillance program on 15,438 consecutive inpatients, 1975 to 1982, JAMA 1986; 256:3358.

74. Roujeau JC, Stern RS: Severe adverse cutaneous reactions to drugs, N Engl J Med 1994; 331:1272.

75. Alanko K, Stubb S, Kauppinen K: Cutaneous drug reactions-clinical types and causative agents: a five-year survey of inpatients (1981-1985), Acta Derm Venereol (Stockh) 1989; 69:223.

76. Bigby M, et al: Allergic cutaneous reactions to drugs, Prim Care 1989; 16:713.

77. Hoigne R, et al: Occurrence of exanthems in relation to aminopenicillin preparations and allopurinol, N Engl J Med 1987; 316:1217.

78. Grzelewska-Rzymowska I, Szmidt M, Rozniecki J: Aspirin-induced urticaria—a clinical study, J Investig Allergol Clin Immunol 1992; 2:39.

79. Britschgi M, et al: T-cell involvement in drug-induced acute generalized exanthematous pustulosis, J Clin Invest 2001; 107:1433.

80. Sidoroff A, et al: Acute generalized exanthematous pustulosis (AGEP): a clinical reaction pattern [record supplied by publisher], J Cutan Pathol 2001; 28:113.

81. Wakelin S, et al: Amoxycillin-induced flexural exanthem, Clin Exp Dermatol 1999; 24:71.

82. Sehgal VH, Gangwani OP: Genital fixed drug eruptions, Genitourin Med 1986; 62:56.

83. Thankappan TP, Zachariah J: Drug-specific clinical pattern in fixed drug eruptions, Int J Dermatol 1991; 30:867.

84. Gaffoor PM, George WM: Fixed drug eruptions occurring on the male genitals, Cutis 1990; 45:242.

85. Hatzis J, et al: Fixed drug eruption in a mother and her son, Cutis 1992; 50:50.

86. Pellicano R, et al: Familial occurrence of fixed drug eruptions, Acta Derm Venereol 1992; 72:292.

87. Hindioglu U, Sahin S: Nonpigmenting solitary fixed drug eruption caused by pseudoephedrine hydrochloride, J Am Acad Dermatol 1998; 38:499.

88. Jain VK, et al: Fixed drug eruption of the oral mucous membrane, Ann Dent 1991; 50:9.

89. Korkij W, Soltani K: Fixed drug eruption: a brief review, Arch Dermatol 1984; 120:520.

90. Sehgal VN, Gangwani OP: Fixed drug eruption: current concepts, Int J Dermatol 1987; 26:67.

91. Tham S, Kwok Y, Chan H: Cross-reactivity in fixed drug eruptions to tetracyclines, Arch Dermatol 1996; 132:1134.

92. Chan H, Tan K: Fixed drug eruption to three anticonvulsant drugs: an unusual case of polysensitivity, J Am Acad Dermatol 1997; 36(2 Pt 1):259.

93. Zanolli MD, et al: Phenolphthalein-induced fixed drug eruption: a cutaneous complication of laxative use in a child, Pediatrics 1993; 91:1199.

94. Kanwar AJ, et al: Ninety-eight fixed drug eruptions with provocation tests, Dermatologica 1988; 177:274.

95. Osawa J, et al: Evaluation of skin test reactions in patients with non-immediate type drug eruptions, J Dermatol 1990; 17:235.

96. Lee AY, Lee YS: Provocation tests in a chlormezanone-induced fixed drug eruption, Drug Intell Clin Pharm 1991; 25:604.

97. Halevy S, Shai A: Lichenoid drug eruptions, J Am Acad Dermatol 1993; 29:249.

98. Hess EV: Drug-related lupus, Curr Opin Rheumatol 1991; 3:809.

99. Mongey AB, et al: Serologic evaluation of patients receiving procainamide, Arthritis Rheum 1992; 35:219.

100. Batchelor JR, et al: Hydralazine-induced systemic lupus erythematosus: influence of HLA-DB and sex on susceptibility, Lancet 1980; 1:1107.

101. Kauppinen K, Stubb S: Drug eruptions: causative agents and clinical types-series of inpatients during a 10-year period, Acta Derm Venereol (Stockh) 1984; 64:320.

102. Crowson A, Magro C: Subacute cutaneous lupus erythematosus arising in the setting of calcium channel blocker therapy, Hum Pathol 1997; 28:67.

103. Crowson A, Magro C: Recent advances in the pathology of cutaneous drug eruptions, Dermatol Clin 1999; 17:537.

104. Baack BR, Burgdorf WHC: Chemotherapy-induced acral erythema, J Am Acad Dermatol 1991; 24:457.

105. Waltzer JF, Flowers FP: Bullous variant of chemotherapy-induced acral erythema, Arch Dermatol 1993; 129:43.

106. Kleier RS, et al: Generalized pustulation as a manifestation of the anticonvulsant hypersensitivity syndrome, Arch Dermatol 1991; 127:1361.

❑ **Scabies**
Anatomic features, life cycle, and immunology
Scabies in long-term care facilities

❑ **Pediculosis**
Biology and life cycle

❑ **Caterpillar dermatitis**

❑ **Spiders**
Black widow spider
Brown recluse spider

❑ **Ticks**
Lyme disease and erythema migrans
Rocky Mountain spotted and spotless fever
Tick bite paralysis
Removing ticks

❑ **Cat-scratch and related diseases**
Neurologic complications
Bacillary angiomatosis

❑ **Animal and human bites**

❑ **Stinging insects**
Toxic reactions
Allergic reactions
Indications for venom skin testing and
    immunotherapy

❑ **Biting insects**
Papular urticaria
Fleas
Myiasis
Mosquitoes

❑ **Creeping eruption**

❑ **Ants**
Fire ants

❑ **Dermatitis associated with swimming**
Swimmer's itch (fresh water)
Nematocyst stings
Florida, Caribbean, Bahamas
Echinoderms (sea urchins and starfish)

Scabies

Human scabies is a highly contagious disease caused by the mite *Sarcoptes scabiei* var. *hominis.* The mite is an obligate parasite to humans. Scabies is not primarily a sexually transmitted disease; 30-year cycles of scabies do not exist. Scabies spreads in households and neighborhoods in which there is a high frequency of intimate personal contact or sharing of inanimate objects, and fomite transmission is a major factor in household and nosocomial passage of scabies.[1] Dogs and cats may be infested by almost identical organisms; these sometimes may be a source for human infestation.[2] In the past, scabies was attributed to poor hygiene. Most contemporary cases, however, appear in individuals with adequate hygiene who are in close contact with numbers of individuals, such as schoolchildren. Blacks rarely acquire scabies; the reason is unknown.

SARCOPTES SCABIEI

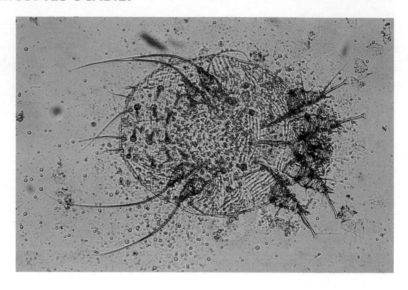

Figure 15-1 *Sarcoptes scabiei* in a potassium hydroxide wet mount *(×* 40).

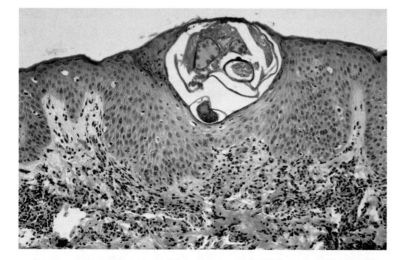

A, Cross-section of a mite in the stratum corneum.

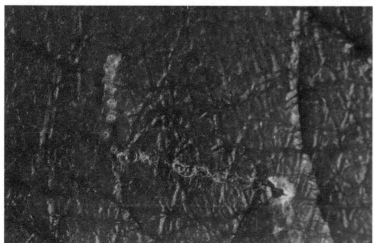

B, Burrow. The mite excavates a burrow in the stratum corneum (the dead, horny layer of the epidermis).

Figure 15-2

Anatomic features, life cycle, and immunology

Anatomic features

The adult mite is $\frac{1}{3}$-mm long and has a flattened, oval body with wrinklelike, transverse corrugations and eight legs (Figure 15-1). The front two pairs of legs bear claw-shaped suckers and the two rear pairs end in long, trailing bristles. The digestive tract fills a major portion of the body and is readily observed when the mite is seen in cross-section of histologic specimens (Figure 15-2, A).

INFESTATION AND LIFE CYCLE. Infestation begins when a fertilized female mite arrives on the skin surface. Within an hour, the female excavates a burrow in the stratum corneum (dead, horny layer) (Figure 15-2, B). During the mite's 30-day life cycle, the burrow extends from several millimeters to a few centimeters in length. The burrow does not enter the underlying epidermis except in the case of hyperkeratotic Norwegian scabies, a condition in which scaly, thick skin develops in retarded, immunosuppressed, or elderly patients in the presence of thousands of mites. Eggs laid at the rate of two or three a day (Figure 15-3) and fecal pellets (scybala) are deposited in the burrow behind the advancing female. Scybala are dark, oval masses that are seen easily with the eggs when burrow scrapings are examined under a microscope. Scybala may act as an irritant and may be responsible for some of the itching. The larvae hatch, leaving the egg casings in the burrow, and reach maturity in 14 to 17 days. The adult mites copulate and repeat the cycle. Therefore, 3 to 5 weeks after infestation, there are only a few mites present. This life cycle explains why patients experience few if any symptoms during the first month after contact with an infested individual. After a number of mites (usually less than 20) have reached maturity and have spread by migration or the patient's scratching, the initial, minor, localized itch evolves into intense, generalized pruritus.

IMMUNOLOGY. A hypersensitivity reaction rather than a foreign-body response may be responsible for the lesions, which may delay recognition of symptoms of scabies. Elevated IgE titers develop in some patients infested with scabies, along with eosinophilia, and an immediate-type hypersensitivity reaction to an extract prepared from female mites.[3] IgE levels fall within a year after infestation. Eosinophilia returns to normal shortly after treatment. The fact that symptoms develop much more rapidly when reinfestation occurs supports the claim that the symptoms and lesions of scabies are the result of a hypersensitivity reaction.

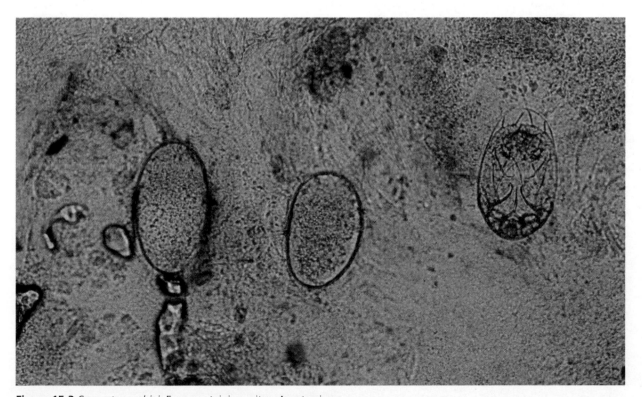

Figure 15-3 *Sarcoptes scabiei.* Eggs containing mites. A potassium hydroxide wet mount (× 40).

Clinical manifestations

Transmission of scabies occurs during direct skin contact with an infected person.

A mite can possibly survive for days in normal home surroundings after leaving human skin.[4] Mites survive up to 7 days in mineral oil microscopic slide mounts.

The disease begins insidiously. Symptoms are minor at first and are attributed to a bite or dry skin. Scratching destroys burrows and removes mites, providing initial relief. The patient remains comfortable during the day but itches at night. Nocturnal pruritus is highly characteristic of scabies. Scratching spreads mites to other areas and after 6 to 8 weeks the once localized area of minor irritation has become a widespread, intensely pruritic eruption.

The most characteristic features of the lesions are pleomorphism and a tendency to remain discrete and small. Primary lesions are soon destroyed by scratching.

Primary lesions

Mites are found in burrows and at the edge of vesicles but rarely in papules.

BURROW. The linear, curved, or S-shaped burrows are approximately as wide as #2 suture material and are 2 to 15 mm long (Figure 15-2, B). They are pink-white and slightly elevated. A vesicle or the mite, which may look like a black dot at one end of the burrow, often may be seen. Scratching destroys burrows; therefore they do not appear in some patients. Burrows are most likely to be found in the finger webs, wrists, sides of the hands and feet, penis, buttocks, scrotum, and the palms and soles of infants.

VESICLES AND PAPULES. Vesicles are isolated, pinpoint, and filled with serous rather than purulent fluid. The fact that they remain discrete is a key point in differentiating scabies from other vesicular diseases such as poison ivy. The finger webs are the most likely areas to find intact vesicles (Figure 15-4). Infants may have vesicles or pustules on the palms and soles. Small, discrete papules may represent a hypersensitivity reaction and rarely contain mites.

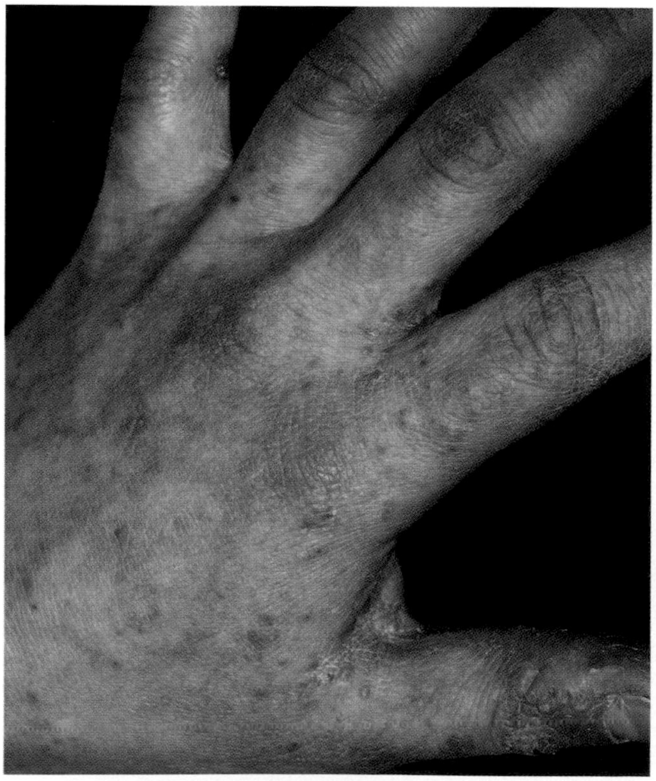

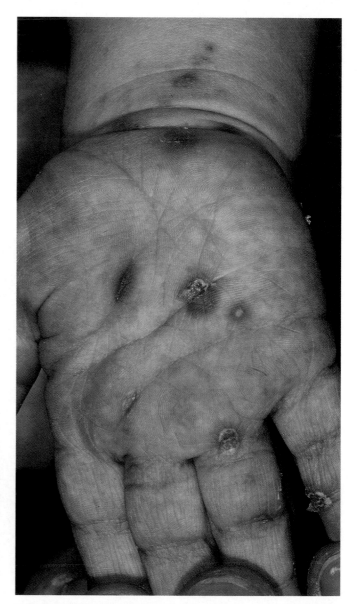

Figure 15-4 Scabies. Tiny vesicles and papules in the finger webs and on the back of the hand.

Figure 15-5 Scabies. Pustules on the palms of an infant. Note the papular lesions on the wrist.

SCABIES—GENITAL

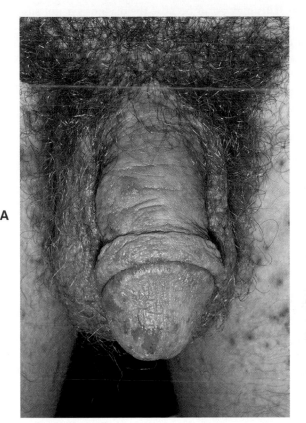

A

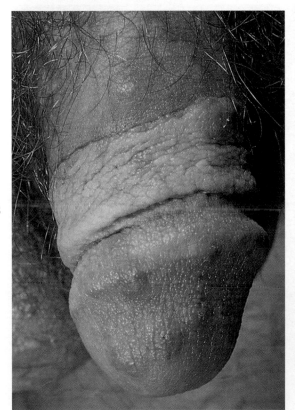

B

Secondary lesions

Secondary lesions result from infection or are caused by scratching. They often dominate the clinical picture. Pinpoint erosions are the most common secondary lesions. Pustules are a sign of secondary infection (Figure 15-5). Scaling, erythema, and all stages of eczematous inflammation occur as a response to excoriation or to irritation caused by overzealous attempts at self-medication. Nodules occur in covered areas such as the buttocks, groin, scrotum, penis, and axillae. The 2- to 10-mm indolent, red papules and nodules sometimes have slightly eroded surfaces, especially on the glans penis (Figure 15-6). Nodules may persist for weeks or months after the mites have been eradicated. They may result from persisting antigens of mite parts.[5]

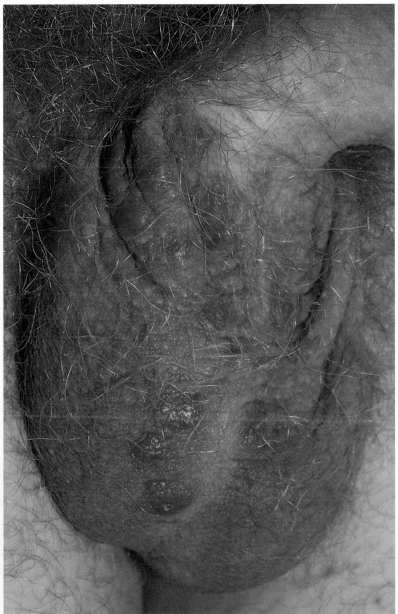

C

Figure 15-6 A, The genital and groin are acutely inflamed with a widespread infestation. **B,** Eroded papules on the glans is a highly characteristic sign of scabies. **C,** An established infestation of the penis and scrotum. Large papules may remain after appropriate therapy and sometimes require treatment with intralesional steroids.

Distribution

Lesions of scabies are typically found in the finger webs, wrists, extensor surfaces of the elbows and knees, sides of the hands and feet, axillary areas, buttocks, waist area, and ankle area (Figures 15-7 and 15-8). In men, the penis and scrotum are usually involved; in women, the breast, including the areola and nipple, may be infested. Lesions, often vesicular or pustular, may be most numerous on the palms and soles of infants. The scalp and face, rarely involved in adults, occasionally are infested in infants.

The number and type of lesions and the extent of involvement vary greatly among patients. Some patients have a few itchy vesicles in the finger webs early in the course of their disease. Many patients in these early stages attempt self-treatment and are encouraged by the relief obtained from over-the-counter, antipruritic lotions. Topical steroids offer greater relief but mask the progressive disease by suppressing inflammation. Delay of proper treatment allows the eruption to extend into all of the characteristic areas, as well as onto the trunk, arms, legs, and occasionally the face. Extensive involvement is often accompanied by erythema, scaling, and infection. Infants and children have diffuse scabies more often than do adults. Symptoms vary from periods of nocturnal pruritus to constant, frantic itching. Untreated scabies can last for months or years.

Infants

Infants, more frequently than adults, have widespread involvement. This may occur because the diagnosis is not suspected and proper treatment is delayed while medication is given for other suspected causes of itching, such as dry skin, eczema, and infection. Infants occasionally are infested on the face and scalp, something rarely seen in adults. Vesicles are common on the palms and soles; this is a highly characteristic sign of scabies in infants (Figure 15-9). Secondary eczematization and impetiginization are common, but burrows are difficult to find. Nodules may be seen in the axillae and diaper area.

The elderly

Elderly patients may have few cutaneous lesions but itch severely. The decreased immunity associated with advanced age may allow the mites to multiply and survive in great numbers. These patients have few cutaneous lesions other than excoriations, dry skin, and scaling, but they experience intense itching. Eventually papules and nodules appear and may become numerous. Entire nursing home populations may be infested (see treatment section). A skin scraping from any scaling area may show numerous mites at all stages of development.

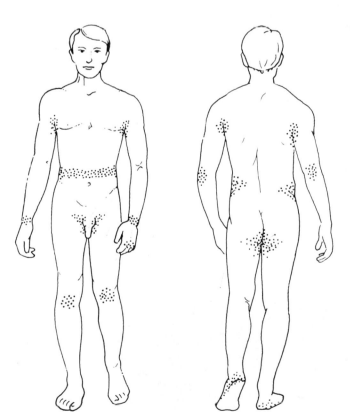

Figure 15-7 Scabies. Distribution of lesions.

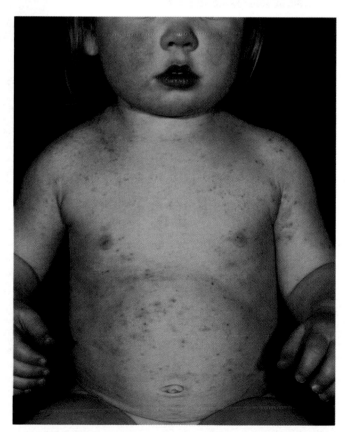

Figure 15-8 Diffuse scabies on an infant. The face is clear. The lesions are most numerous around the axillae, chest, and abdomen.

Crusted (Norwegian) scabies

The term *Norwegian scabies* was first used in 1848 to describe an overwhelming scabies infestation of patients with Hansen's disease. In patients with crusted scabies, lesions tend to involve hands and feet with asymptomatic crusting rather than the typical inflammatory papules and vesicles. There is thick, subungual, keratotic material and nail dystrophy. Digits and sites of trauma may show wartlike formations. Gray scales and thick crusts may be present over the trunk and extremities. Desquamation of the facial skin may occur. The hair may shed profusely. Crusted scabies occurs in people with neurologic or mental disorders (especially Down's syndrome), senile dementia, nutritional disorders, infectious diseases, leukemia, and immunosuppression (such as patients with acquired immunodeficiency syndrome). Itching may be absent or severe. A lack of immunity and indifference to pruritus have been suggested as reasons for the development of this distinct clinical picture. A mineral oil or potassium hydroxide examination of crusts shows numerous mites at all stages of development.

Diagnosis

The diagnosis is suspected when burrows are found or when a patient has typical symptoms with characteristic lesions and distribution (Box 15-1).

A definite diagnosis is made when any of the following products are obtained from burrows or vesicles and identified microscopically: mites, eggs, egg casings (hatched eggs), or feces (scybala).

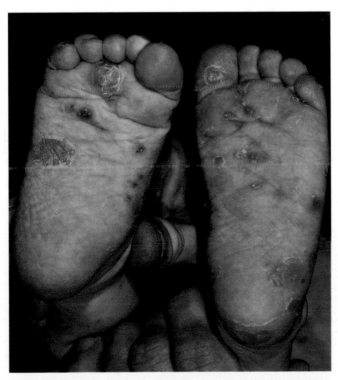

Figure 15-9 Scabies. Infestation of the palms and soles is common in infants. The vesicular lesions have all ruptured.

Burrow identification

Initially, the areas most apt to contain burrows are observed. To enhance burrows for better viewing, the surface should be touched with a drop of mineral or immersion oil or a blue or black fountain or felt-tip pen (the ink method dyes the burrow; surface ink may be removed with an alcohol swab). The burrow absorbs the ink and is highlighted as a dark line (Figure 15-10). The accentuated lesions are smoothly scraped away with a curved #15 scalpel blade and transferred to a glass microscope slide for examination.

Papules and vesicles

Nonexcoriated papules and vesicles may be sampled but do not usually contain the eggs and egg casings found in an established burrow.

Sampling techniques and slide mount preparation

Various techniques are available for obtaining diagnostic material. In most cases the suspected lesion can be sampled easily if it is shaved or scraped with a no. 15 surgical blade and the material is transferred to a microscope slide for direct examination.

MINERAL OIL MOUNTS. A drop of mineral oil may be placed over the suspected lesion before removal. Skin scrapings adhere, feces are preserved, and the mite remains alive and motile in clear oil. Squamous cells do not separate when heated in a clear oil mount, and mites under a clump of squamous cells may be missed.

POTASSIUM HYDROXIDE WET MOUNTS. The scrapings are transferred directly to a glass side, a drop of potassium hydroxide is added, and a cover slip is applied. If diagnostic material is not found, the preparation is gently heated and the cover slip is pressed to separate squamous cells. Feces remain intact for short periods but may be dissolved quickly when the mount is heated. Skin biopsy is rarely necessary to make the diagnosis.

Box 15-1 Signs and Symptoms of Scabies
Nodules on the penis and scrotum
Rash present for 4 to 8 weeks has suddenly become worse
Pustules on the palms and soles of infants
Nocturnal itching
Generalized, severe itching
Pinpoint erosions and crusts on the buttocks
Vesicles in the finger webs
Diffuse eruption sparing the face
Patient becomes better, then worse, after treatment with topical steroids
Rash is present in several members of the same family
Patient (especially an infant) develops more extensive rash despite treatment with antibiotics and topical medications

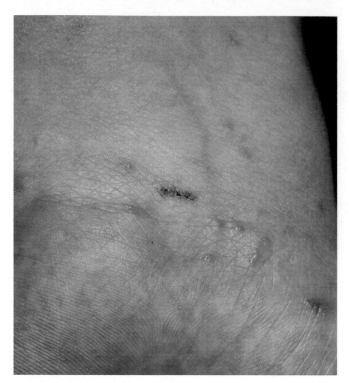

Figure 15-10 Felt-tipped ink pen has penetrated and highlighted a burrow. The ink is retained after the surface is wiped clean with an alcohol swab.

Treatment and management
Permethrin

Permethrin (Elimite cream, Acticin cream) is a synthetic pyrethrin that demonstrates extremely low mammalian toxicity. It is the drug of choice for the treatment of scabies in children and adults of all ages. Several studies show that it is more effective than lindane. A diminished sensitivity to permethrin has been documented. One application is said to be effective but a second treatment 1 week after the first application is now standard practice. The over-the-counter permethrin preparation (Nix) is lower in strength (1%) and ineffective against scabies. Unlike lindane, permethrin undergoes insignificant absorption (2%), after which it is rapidly degraded.

Lindane

Lindane is the generic name for the chemical gamma benzene hexachloride, a compound chemically similar to an agricultural pesticide also referred to as lindane. It is a central nervous system stimulant that produces seizures and death in the scabies mite. Kwell is one brand name for lindane. Generic lindane is available. Lindane is available as a cream, shampoo, and lotion. Lotion dispensed from bulk containers may not be agitated; therefore the concentration of lindane may be inadequate. Reports of lindane resistance have appeared. A second treatment 1 week after the first application is standard practice. A follow-up examination at 2 to 4 weeks is recommended. Approximately 10% of lindane is absorbed through intact skin. Lindane accumulates in fat and binds to

brain tissue. Pruritus may persist for weeks. Additional, unprescribed applications, without documented evidence of persistent infestation, may be dangerous. Lindane should be avoided in children younger than 2 years of age, pregnant or nursing women, and patients with human immunodeficiency virus or acquired immunodeficiency syndrome. Children with severe, underlying, cutaneous disease may be at greater risk for toxicity. This is also true for premature, emaciated, or malnourished children and those with a history of seizure disorders.[6]

APPLICATION TECHNIQUE FOR PERMETHRIN AND LINDANE. The cream or lotion is applied to all skin surfaces below the neck and the face in children. Patients with relapsing scabies and the elderly should be treated from head (including the scalp) to toe. One ounce is usually adequate for adults. Reapply medicine to the hands if hands are washed. The nails should be cut short and medication applied under them vigorously with a toothbrush. A hot, soapy bath is not necessary before application. Moisture increases the permeability of the epidermis and increases the chance for systemic absorption. If a patient has bathed before lindane administration, the skin must be allowed to completely dry to prevent excessive absorption. Adults should wash 12 hours after application, and infants should be washed 8 to 12 hours after application. One application of either medicine is considered adequate. Many clinicians prefer two applications 1 week apart. Patients should be told that it is normal to continue to itch for days or weeks after treatment and that further application of medication is usually not necessary and worsens itching by causing irritation. Bland lubricants may be applied to relieve itching.

Ivermectin

Ivermectin is an antiparasitic agent used for the treatment and prevention of onchocerciasis ("river blindness") and other filarial diseases. Ivermectin (6-mg tablet) is a promising alternative for the treatment of scabies. There is uncertainty whether optimal therapy is 200 to 250 ug/kg given on day 1 and day 8 or whether it is a one-dose treatment of 400 ug/kg.[7] Either regimen may eradicate the scabietic nymphs. Many clinicians routinely prescribe the two-dose regimen. The average adult dose is 12 mg as a single dose or 12 mg on day 1 and 12 mg on day 8. Resolution of pruritus occurs within 48 hours of treatment. Patients with thick, crusted lesions do better with a combination of ivermectin and topical treatment such as permethrin cream. Ivermectin may prove useful for the treatment of patients in nursing homes.

Sulfur

Sulfur has been used to treat scabies for more than 150 years. The pharmacist mixes 6% (5% to 10% range) precipitated sulfur in petrolatum or a cold cream base. The compound is applied to the entire body below the neck once each day for 3 days. The patient is instructed to bathe 24 hours after each application. Sulfur applied in this manner is highly effective, but these preparations are messy, have an unpleasant odor, stain, and cause dryness.[8] Sulfur in petrolatum was thought to be safer than lindane for treating infants, but the safety of topical sulfur has never been established.[9]

Crotamiton (Eurax lotion)

A study of children with scabies showed an 89% cure rate after 4 weeks with permethrin 5% cream (Elimite) and a 60% cure rate with crotamiton cream.[10] The toxicity of crotamiton is unknown. Reported cure rates for once-a-day application for 5 days range from 50% to 100%. Crotamiton may have antipruritic properties, but this has been questioned.

Eradication program for nursing homes

Scabies is a problem in nursing homes.[11,12] The severity is greater than that in an ambulatory population. The face and scalp can be involved, and multiple treatments may be necessary. The first problem is proper diagnosis. The elderly have an atypical presentation with few lesions other than excoriations, dry skin, and scaling, but they experience intense itching. Lesions are located on the back and buttocks rather than the web spaces, axilla, and groin. A plan for eradication of scabies in nursing homes is outlined Box 15-2.

Management of complications

ECZEMATOUS INFLAMMATION AND PYODERMA. Patients with signs of infection should be started on systemic antibiotics that treat *Staphylococcus aureus* and *Streptococcus pyogenes*. A group V topical steroid may be applied three times a day to all red, scaling lesions for 1 or 2 days before the application of lindane.

POSTSCABIETIC PRURITUS. Pruritus may persist for weeks after treatment and may be attributed to a hypersensitivity response to remaining dead mites and mite products.

Itching usually decreases substantially 24 hours after treatment and then gradually decreases during the following week or two. Patients with persistent itching may be treated with oral antihistamines, and, if inflammation is present, they may be treated with topical steroids. Intractable itching responds to a short course of systemic corticosteroids.

Box 15-2 Management of Scabies Epidemic in an Extended-Care Facility

1. Educate patients, staff, family, and frequent visitors about scabies and the need for cooperation in treatment.
2. Apply scabicide to all patients, staff, contact staff, and frequent visitors, symptomatic or not. Treat symptomatic family members of staff and visitors.
3. Launder all bedding and clothes worn in the last 48 hours in hot water (or dry clean).
4. Clean beds and floors with routine cleaning agents just before scabicide is removed.
5. Reexamine for treatment failures in 1 week and 4 weeks.

NODULAR SCABIES. Persistent nodular lesions, most commonly found on the scrotum, are treated with intralesional steroids (e.g., triamcinolone acetonide [Kenalog] 10 mg/mL).

ENVIRONMENTAL MANAGEMENT. Intimate contacts and all family members in the same household should be treated. The spread of scabies via inanimate objects occurs. Live mites have been recovered from dust samples, chairs, and bed linens in the homes of patients with scabies up to 96 hours after being isolated from the host. Clothing that has touched infected skin should be washed. Wash all clothing, towels, and bed linen (in a normal washing machine cycle) that have touched the skin. It is not necessary to rewash clean clothing that has not yet been worn. Bed linens, floors, and chairs should be vacuumed and cleaned. It is especially important to thoroughly clean the rooms of patients who are confined in single rooms in long-term care facilities.

Scabies in long-term care facilities

Scabies in a nursing home can be highly disruptive. The staff, families, and patients become anxious about issues of treatment, origin of infestation, hygiene, and communicability. Everyone has a sense of urgency. Diagnosis is often a problem.

Diagnosis

It is important to confirm the diagnosis microscopically before committing large financial resources to treatment. The diagnosis of scabies should be considered in any nursing home resident with an unexplained generalized rash. The clinical presentation may vary in older, immunocompromised, or cognitively impaired persons. Erythematous, papulosquamous lesions are predominantly truncal. Pruritus is often absent.

Treatment

Residents with cognitive impairment and restricted mobility may be treatment resistant. All infested individuals should be treated within the same 24- to 48-hour period to reduce the risk of reinfestation. Permethrin is the drug of choice in the nursing home population. Many patients will require repeat therapy 1 week following the initial application. Follow-up evaluation 2 weeks after treatment is necessary to detect new lesions and the presence of live mites. Residents with dementia and severe functional impairment who fail to respond to Permethrin cream (5%) may benefit from treatment with oral Ivermectin.[13] Treatment with two 12-mg doses of ivermectin given 2 weeks apart and procedures for environmental disinfection led to almost complete control of a nursing home outbreak.[14] Cure rates may increase if both permethrin and ivermectin are used simultaneity in the same patient.[15] Additional applications of permethrin and mechanical clearing of hyperkeratotic subungual areas may be necessary. Clean infested patient rooms at the same time patients are treated.

Pediculosis

Infestation with lice is called pediculosis. Lice are transmitted by close personal contact and contact with objects such as combs, hats, clothing, and bed linen. Infestation is usually symptomless and is not associated with serious disease. Lice cannot jump or fly. Pets are not vectors. Diagnosis is made by seeing the lice or their eggs. Treatment with lindane, permethrin, pyrethrins and malathion is used, but resistance to all medications has been documented in various countries.

Biology and life cycle

Lice are obligate human parasites that cannot survive off their host for more than 10 days (adults) to 3 weeks (fertile eggs). Actual survival rates may be shorter than this. Lice are called ectoparasites because they live on, rather than in, the body. They are classified as insects because they have six legs. Three kinds of lice infest humans: *Pediculus humanus* var. *capitis* (head louse), *Pediculus humanus* var. *corporis* (body louse), and *Pthirus pubis* (pubic or crab louse). All three have similar anatomic characteristics. Each is a small (less than 2 mm), flat, wingless insect with three pairs of legs located on the anterior part of the body directly behind the head. The legs terminate in sharp claws that are adapted for feeding and permit the louse to grasp and hold firmly on to hair or clothing. The body louse is the largest and is similar in shape to the head louse (Figure 15-11). The crab louse is the smallest, with a short, oval body and prominent claws resembling sea crabs (Figure 15-12).

Lice feed approximately five times each day by piercing the skin with their claws, injecting irritating saliva, and sucking blood. They do not become engorged like ticks, but, after feeding, they become rust colored from the ingestion of blood; their color is an identifying characteristic. Lice feces can be seen on the skin as small, rust-colored flecks. Saliva and, possibly, fecal material can induce a hypersensitivity reaction and inflammation. Lice are active and can travel quickly, which explains why they can be transmitted so easily. The life cycle from egg to egg is approximately 1 month.

Nits

The female lays approximately six eggs, or nits, each day for up to 1 month, then dies. The louse incubates, hatches in 8 to 10 days, and reaches maturity in approximately 18 days. Nits are 0.8 mm long and are firmly cemented to the bases of hair shafts close to the skin to acquire adequate heat for incubation (Figure 15-13). Nits are very difficult to remove from the hair shaft.

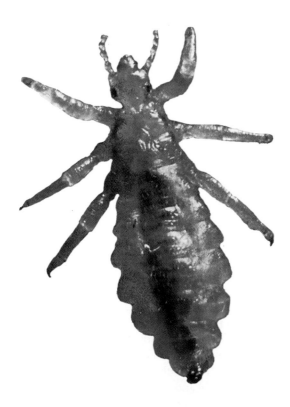

Figure 15-11 Body louse. The largest of three lice infesting humans. *(Courtesy Ken Gray, Oregon State University Extension Services.)*

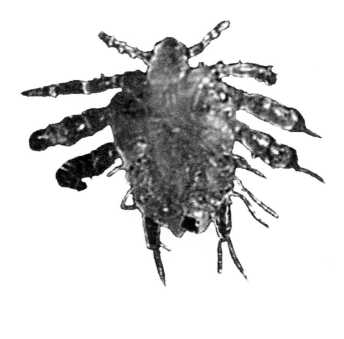

Figure 15-12 Crab louse has a short body and large claws used to grasp hair. *(Courtesy Ken Gray, Oregon State University Extension Services.)*

Clinical manifestations
Pediculosis capitis

The head louse effectively infests only the human head and is distinct from body and pubic lice. Lice infestation of the scalp is most common in children. More girls than boys are afflicted and American blacks rarely have head lice. Head lice can be found anywhere on the scalp, but are most commonly seen on the back of the head and neck and behind the ears (Figure 15-14). The average patient carries less than 20 adult lice. Less than 5% of patients will have more than 100 lice in the scalp. Scratching causes inflammation and secondary bacterial infection, with pustules, crusting, and cervical adenopathy. Sensitization to the lice toxin, feces, or body parts takes 3 to 8 months and is a cause of pruritus. Posterior cervical adenopathy without obvious disease is characteristic of lice. The eyelashes may be involved, causing redness and swelling. Examination of the posterior scalp shows few adult organisms but many nits. Nits are cemented to the hair, whereas dandruff scale is easily moved along the hair shaft. Head lice can survive away from the human host for about 3 days, and nits can survive for up to 10 days. The primary source of transmission is direct contact with an infested person but fomite transmission (hats, brushes, combs, earphones, bedding, furniture) is common. Head lice do not carry or transmit any human disease.

Pediculosis corporis

Infestation by body lice is uncommon. Typhus, relapsing fever, and trench fever are spread by body lice during wartime and in underdeveloped countries. Pediculosis corporis is a disease of the unclean. Body lice live and lay their nits in the seams of clothing and return to the skin surface only to feed. They run and hide when disturbed and are rarely seen. Body lice induce pruritus that leads to scratching and secondary infection.

EYELASH INFESTATION. Infestation of the eyelashes is seen almost exclusively in children. The lice are acquired from other children or from an infested adult with pubic lice. Eyelash infestation may induce blepharitis with lid pruritus, scaling, crusting, and/or purulent discharge. Eyelash infestation may be a sign of childhood sexual abuse.

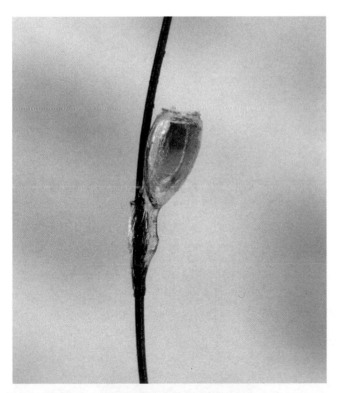

Figure 15-13 Louse egg (nit) is cemented to a hair shaft.

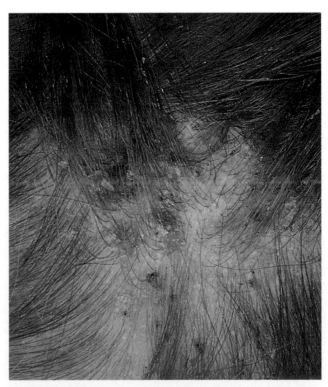

Figure 15-14 *Pediculosis capitis.* A heavy infestation with secondary pyoderma.

Pediculosis pubis

Pubic lice are the most contagious sexually transmitted problem known. Up to 30% of patients infested with pubic lice have at least one other sexually transmitted disease. The chance of acquiring pubic lice from one sexual exposure with an infested partner is more than 90%, whereas the chance of acquiring syphilis or gonorrhea from one sexual exposure with an infected partner is approximately 30%. Blacks are affected with the same frequency as whites. The pubic hair is the most common site of infestation, but lice frequently spread to the hair around the anus. On hairy persons, lice may spread to the upper thighs, abdominal area, axillae (Figure 15-15), chest, and beard. Infested adults may spread pubic lice to the eyelashes of children.

The majority of patients complain of pruritus. Many patients are aware that something is crawling on the groin, but are not familiar with the disease and have never seen lice. Approximately 50% of patients have little inflammation, but those who delay seeking help may develop widespread inflammation and infection of the groin with regional adenopathy. Occasionally, gray-blue macules (maculae ceruleae)[16] (Figure 15-16) varying in size from 1 to 2 cm are seen in the groin and at sites distant from the infestation. Their cause is not known, but they may represent altered blood pigment.

Diagnosis

Lice are suspected when a patient complains of itching in a localized area without an apparent rash. Scalp and pubic lice will be apparent to those who carefully examine individual hairs; they are not apparent with only a cursory examination. Finding nits does not indicate active infestation. Nits may persist for months after successful treatment. Live eggs reside within a quarter inch of the scalp.

Combing

Combing the hair with a fine-toothed "nit," or detection, comb is effective for detecting and removing live lice. The comb is inserted near the crown until it touches the scalp, and then drawn firmly down. The teeth of the comb should be 0.2 to 0.3 mm apart to trap lice. The entire head of hair should be combed at least twice; the comb should be examined for lice after each stroke. It usually takes 1 minute to find the first louse.

Lice and nits can be seen easily under a microscope. Live nits fluoresce and can be detected easily by Wood's light examination, a technique that is especially useful for rapid examination of a large group of children. Nits that contain an unborn louse fluoresce white. Nits that are empty fluoresce gray.

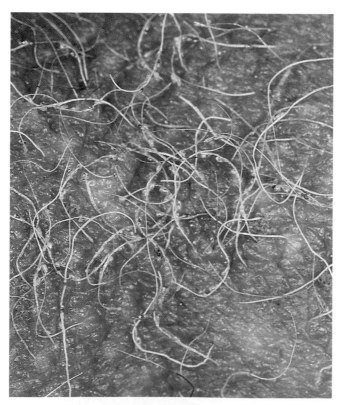

Figure 15-15 *Pediculosis pubis.* A heavy infestation with numerous nits and lice on the scrotum.

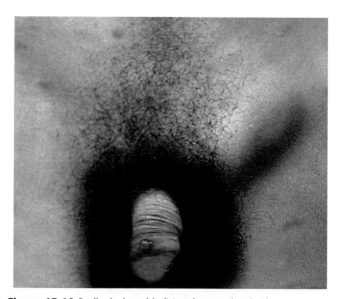

Figure 15-16 *Pediculosis pubis (Maculae ceruleae).* Blue-gray macules can be seen with lice infestation.

Treatment
Head, body, and pubic lice

Resistance to all topical medications has been documented. Some head lice in the United States have become resistant to 1% lindane, Nix, and pyrethrins. Ovide was the only pediculicide in the United States that had not become less effective.[17] Insecticides kill both lice and eggs. A fine-toothed comb should be used a day or two after the final application of insecticide to confirm that the treatment has been successful. The presence of live (moving) lice of all sizes suggests resistance to treatment, whereas finding only one adult-sized louse suggests reinfestation. Regular weekly detection combing is recommended for several weeks after cure. Household members and those in close contact with the patient should be screened and treated as necessary. Environmental cleaning is probably unwarranted, although combs and brushes should be washed in hot water.

PERMETHRIN. Permethrin is the most effective over-the-counter treatment.[18] It paralyzes the nerves that allow the lice to breathe. Lice can close down their respiratory airways for 30 minutes when immersed in water. Therefore all insecticides are put on dry hair. The cream rinse (Nix) is applied to the scalp after the hair is shampooed and dried. The medication is rinsed out with water after 10 minutes. Permethrin is not 100% ovicidal, and higher cure rates may be obtained by a second application 1 week after the first treatment. Developing eggs have no central nervous system during the first 4 days of life. Insecticides that act on the metabolism of neural tissue must have residual activity to be ovicidal. Permethrin has a clinical efficacy of 95%. Lindane and pyrethrin have cure rates less than 90%. Permethrin, unlike pyrethrin and all other topical insecticides, remains active for 2 weeks and is detectable on the hair for 14 days. Cream rinses and conditioning shampoos coat the hairs and protect the lice from the insecticide. Do not use these products for 2 weeks after permethrin treatment. Patients who fail to respond may respond to the prescription strength cream (5% permethrin; Elimite). The medication is left on overnight under a shower cap.

PYRETHRIN. Pyrethrin (RID, A-200, R & C) is available as a liquid, gel, and shampoo. The shampoos are applied, lathered, and washed off in 5 minutes. Lotions are used for treating body and pubic hair infestation. They are applied over the entire affected area and washed off in 10 minutes. Treatment should be repeated in 7 to 10 days. It does not kill all nits and has no residual activity. It is used a second time 1 week after the initial application.

MALATHION (OVIDE). Malathion is rapidly pediculicidal and ovicidal and is useful for lice resistant to pyrethrins and permethrin. It binds to hair and has residual activity. One treatment is usually sufficient. The lotion is applied to dry hair until the hair and scalp are wet. It need not be applied to the ends of long hair below the level of the shirt collar. It is left on for 8 to 12 hours and then washed out. Nits are removed with a comb. The treatment is repeated in 7 to 9 days if lice are still present. The alcoholic preparation Ovide is flammable until dry. Malathion is available by prescription in the United States but is over the counter in the United Kingdom.

It is not recommended for infants and neonates.

LINDANE. Lindane 1% shampoo is indicated for patients who have failed to respond to the above medications or who are intolerant to other lice therapies. Resistance of the louse to lindane is reported.

IVERMECTIN. Ivermectin causes paralysis and death of lice. The drug has selective activity against parasites, without systemic effects in mammals. A single, oral dose of ivermectin (Stromectol) 200 mug/kg repeated in 10 days is effective. The drug is available as a 6-mg pill. A single dose of 12 mg (two 6-mg pills) is generally used for an average-sized adult.[19] The efficacy is 73% after a single dose. Results were more favorable when ivermectin was used in combination with the LiceMeister comb (www.licemeister.org).[20]

TRIMETHOPRIM/SULFA (BACTRIM, SEPTRA). A rare patient with severe hair matting and dense infestation may not respond to conventional treatment. The two remaining options are shaving the head or treatment with trimethoprim/sulfa (TMP/SMX). One study of 20 females with pediculosis capitis showed that one tablet of Bactrim or Septra (80 mg of trimethoprim plus 400 mg of sulfamethoxazole) twice daily for 3 days resulted in a cure. Within 12 to 48 hours after treatment, the lice migrated to the bed linen and died.[21] Trimethoprim/sulfa probably works by killing essential bacteria in the louse's gut. Co-trimoxazole has no effect on nits; therefore a second course must be given 7 to 10 days later.

A combination of 1% permethrin creme rinse (two weekly applications) and TMP/SMX (10-day course) was effective in one study for treating children from 2 to 13 years old. Dual therapy can be reserved for cases of multiple treatment failures or suspected cases of lice-related resistance to therapy.[22]

Nit removal

All preparations kill lice, but some nits may survive. Even dead nits remain attached to the hair until removed. Nits are difficult to remove. Over-the-counter "nit looseners" or "nit removers" are probably not very effective. Applying hair conditioner and then gripping the hair with the index finger and thumb and sliding the nits off is effective.

A special comb, the licemeister (www.licemeister.org), has $1\frac{1}{2}$-inch long metal teeth that go through more hair with each pass collecting both lice and nits. It is available online and at pharmacies. As many nits as possible should be removed to prevent reinfestation. A close haircut may be considered for patients with hundreds of nits.

WET COMBING. Mechanical removal of lice with a wet comb is an alternative to insecticides. The combing procedure is the same as for diagnosis but is done on wet hair with added lubricant (hair conditioner or olive oil) and continued until no lice are found (15 to 30 minutes per session or longer for long, thick hair). Combing is repeated once every three to four days for several weeks and should continue for 2 weeks after any session in which an adult louse is found. This approach cured 38% of cases in a trial in which treatment was carried out by parents, but it was only half as effective as malathion lotion.[23]

"No nit" policies

Exclusion from school for head lice is a common practice. Three fourths of children with nits alone are not infested, and no-nit policies are therefore excessive. Exclusion from school based on the presence of lice or nits is not recommended by the American Public Health Association. A child can return to school immediately after completion of the first application of a normally effective insecticide or the first wet combing session, regardless of the presence of nits. It would be useful to provide a letter of explanation to the school nurse.[23]

POMADES. Petrolatum, mayonnaise, and pomades immobilize lice and kill them in about 10 minutes. Copious amounts must be used to ensure inundation of the adult lice in the scalp hair. These non-insecticidal therapies do not kill the eggs (nits), which take 8 to 10 days to hatch. These therapies must be repeated weekly for 4 weeks unless one is able to remove all the nits by combing.

FOMITE CONTROL. Fomite control is important to prevent reinfestations. Clean bed linens, pillows, towels, clothing, and hats. Rugs, furniture, mattresses, and car seats should be thoroughly vacuumed.

Eye infestation

Several methods are used for treating eye infestation. The most practical and effective method is to place petrolatum (Vaseline) on the fingertips, close the eyes, and rub the petro-latum slowly into the lids and brows three times each day for 5 days. A simple alternative is to close the eyes and apply baby shampoo to the lashes and brows with a cotton swab three times each day for 5 days. Some patients are so mortified by the presence of lice close to their eyes that they demand immediate removal. To do so, the reclining patient closes the eyes and the lice are plucked from the eyelashes with forceps. Older children tolerate this simple procedure. Fluorescein drops (10% to 20%) applied to the lids and lashes produce an immediate toxic effect on the lice.[24] Oral ivermectin should be considered for resistant cases.[19]

Caterpillar Dermatitis

Caterpillars are the larvae of butterflies or moths. Many species of caterpillars possess short hairs (setae) that can irritate the skin (Figure 15-17). Outbreaks of caterpillar dermatitis are seasonal; they occur shortly after the young caterpillars have appeared. Contact with the setae occurs by direct exposure to the caterpillar or windblown setae. Whether the pruritic cutaneous reaction that follows contact is secondary to mechanical irritation, the injection of vasoactive substances, or a hypersensitivity reaction remains unclear.[25]

The brown tail moth and the gypsy moth are found in the northeastern states. Gypsy moth caterpillars hang from trees on long threads. Suspension in the air allows setae to float away on the wind and land on skin or clothing hung out to dry. The puss caterpillar, also known as the wooly slug, is found in the southeastern states. It is approximately 1 inch long and its back and sides are completely covered with fine bristles.[26] The Io moth caterpillar is found east of the Rocky Mountains. It is 2 to 3 inches long and pale green with reddish stripes. Each body segment is armed with tufts of spines. The saddleback caterpillar is found east of Texas and south of Massachusetts. It is approximately 1 inch long, green, and fleshy. The characteristic marking is a brown or purple saddle-shape on the midback. Stout spines are located at each end and along the sides; these spines are hollow and contain a toxin.

Clinical manifestations

Erythema, papules, and vesicles may appear shortly after contact. Irritation may result from mechanical stimulation or from release of irritating substances on the hairs (Figure 15-18). The sting of the puss caterpillar produces an immediate, severe, shooting, burning pain in practically all cases. Some patients experience delayed symptoms such as itching and may develop papules and vesicles similar to insect bites 12 hours after exposure. Closed patch testing with gypsy moth caterpillar hairs has revealed that a delayed hypersensitivity response develops in these patients, similar to that in poison ivy contact dermatitis.[27]

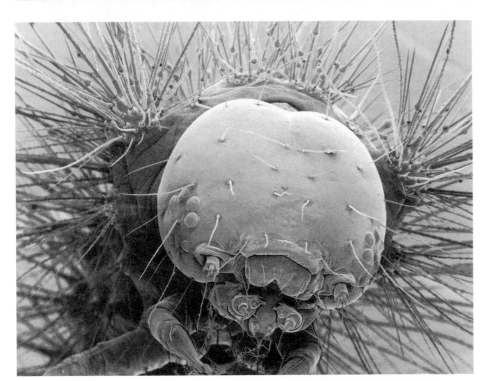

Figure 15-17 Gypsy moth caterpillar. The caterpillar is covered with numerous hairlike structures. *(Courtesy Kathleen Shields, Ph D., United States Department of Agriculture, Hamden, Conn.)*

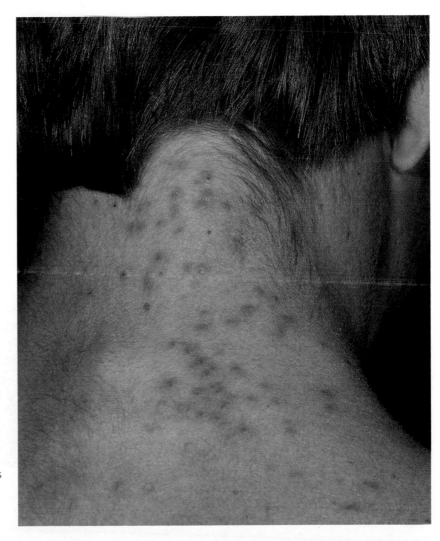

Figure 15-18 Gypsy moth dermatitis. A group of papules and vesicles occurred shortly after a gypsy moth caterpillar was dropped on the neck of this young boy.

Distribution

Linear lesions are noted where caterpillars crawl on the skin. Eruptions secondary to windblown hairs that become embedded in clothing are localized around the collar region, the inside surfaces of the arms and legs, the abdominal flank, and the feet. A unique, gridlike track may be left on the skin after contact with the puss caterpillar. In addition to cutaneous signs, some patients develop rhinitis, conjunctivitis, and wheezing. No deaths from caterpillar contact have been reported in the United States.

Diagnosis

The diagnosis is suspected when a rash of the above description is seen in the early spring. The diagnosis can be confirmed by demonstrating caterpillar hairs on the skin surface. The technique is as follows. The sticky side of a strip of clear tape is applied to the affected area of skin. The tape is then turned sticky side down onto a microscope slide and observed under low power. Short, straight, threadlike hairs are diagnostic of caterpillar dermatitis.[28]

Treatment

Most cases resolve spontaneously within a few days to 2 weeks. For puss caterpillar stings, the immediate, gentle application of adhesive or clear tape helps to remove remaining spines. Calamine lotion may be helpful, and antihistamines sometimes bring relief if used immediately. Group V topical steroids are useful for persistent or pruritic lesions. Puss caterpillar stings often produce severe pain, which may require potent analgesics. Clothing should not be hung out to dry when thread-suspended caterpillars such as the gypsy moth caterpillar appear in the spring.

Spiders

Spiders are carnivorous arthropods that have fangs and venom, which they use to catch and immobilize or kill their prey. Most spiders are small and their fangs are too short to penetrate human skin. Spiders are not aggressive and bite only in self-defense. Spider bites may not be felt at the instant they occur. Localized pain, swelling, itching, erythema, blisters, and necrosis may occur. Most spider venoms are composed of the harmless, enzyme-spreading factor hyaluronidase and a toxin that is distributed by the spreading factor. Most toxins simply cause pain, swelling, and inflammation; however, brown recluse spider toxin causes necrosis, and black widow spider toxin causes neuromuscular abnormalities. Spider bites are common, but of the 50 species of spiders in the United States that have been known to bite humans, only the black widow and the brown recluse spider are capable of producing severe reactions.[29] The diagnosis of a spider bite cannot be made with certainty unless the act is witnessed or the spider is recovered.

Most spider bites cause pain at the instant they occur. A hivelike swelling appears at the bite site and expands radially, usually for just a few centimeters; however, the swelling can sometimes reach gigantic proportions. Occasionally, two puncta or fang marks can be found on the skin surface. The warmth and deep erythema of a bite may resemble bacterial cellulitis, but the hivelike swelling and small, satellite hives are not characteristic of bacterial infection. A biopsy, although usually not necessary for diagnosis, may show mouth parts and intense inflammation. The lesion resolves spontaneously, but itching and swelling can be controlled with cool compresses and antihistamines.

Black widow spider

The black widow spider, *Latrodectus mactans* ("shoe-button spider") is so named because the female attacks and then consumes her mate shortly after copulation. The black widow is found in every state except Alaska and is especially numerous in the rural South.

Black widow spiders have a shiny, fat abdomen that looks like a big black grape or shoe button, with the longest legs extending out in front. There is a red hourglass marking on the underside of the abdomen. This marking may appear as triangles, spots, or an irregular blotch. Adult females have a total length of 4 cm (Figure 15-19) and are the only spiders capable of envenomation. The venom contains a neurotoxin, alpha-latrotoxin. It binds to specific receptors at the neuromuscular motor end plate of both sympathetic and parasympathetic nerves, resulting in increased synaptic concentrations of catecholamines. This results in clinically migratory muscle cramps and spasm, with nausea, vomiting, hypertension, weakness, malaise, and tremors, usually lasting from days to a week. Normally shy, black widow spiders are found in woodpiles, barns, and garages, but they migrate indoors, into closets and cupboards, during cold weather. They usually do not bite when away from the web because they are clumsy and need the web for support. The web has an unmistakable crinkling, crackling sound when it is disrupted.

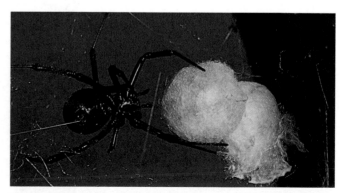

Figure 15-19 Female black widow spider with a red hourglass marking on the underside of her abdomen. Note the haphazard, randomly arranged threads of the web. *(Courtesy Ken Gray, Oregon State University Extension Services.)*

Clinical manifestations

The bite may produce an immediate, sharp pain or may be painless. The subsequent reaction is minimal, with slight swelling and the appearance of a set of small, red fang marks. The symptoms that follow are caused by lymphatic absorption and vascular dissemination of the neurotoxin and are collectively known as latrodectism. The most common presenting complaints are generalized abdominal, back, and leg pain. Fifteen minutes to 2 hours after the bite, a dull muscle cramping or severe pain with numbness gradually spreads from the inoculation site to involve the entire torso but is usually more severe in the abdomen and legs. Any or all of the skeletal muscles may be involved. Severe abdominal pain and spasm simulating a surgical abdomen are the most prominent and distressing features of latrodectism (Figure 15-20). The abdominal muscles assume a boardlike rigidity, but tenderness and distension usually do not occur. There is a generalized increase in the deep tendon reflexes. Other symptoms include dizziness, headache, sweating, nausea, and vomiting. The symptoms increase in severity for several hours (up to 24 hours), slowly subsiding and gradually decreasing in severity in 2 or 3 days.[30-32] Residual symptoms such as weakness, tingling, nervousness, and transient muscle spasm may persist for weeks or months after recovery from the acute stage. Recovery from one serious attack usually offers complete systemic immunity to subsequent bites. Convulsions, paralysis, shock, and death occur in approximately 5% of cases, usually in the young or the debilitated elderly.[33]

Treatment

IMMEDIATE FIRST AID. If the patient is seen within a few minutes of being bitten, ice may be applied to the bite site to help restrict the spread of venom. Pain relief is achieved with either black widow spider–specific antivenin alone or a combination of intravenous opioids and muscle relaxants.

ANTIVENIN. The use of antivenin significantly shortens the duration of symptoms in severe envenomations. Latrodectus mactans or black widow spider antivenin (Merck & Co., Inc.) is effective regardless of which species of *Latrodectus* causes the bite. The dose consists of the entire contents of one vial (2.5 mL) given intramuscularly or, in severe cases when the patient is under 12 years old or in shock, intravenously in 10 to 100 mL of saline over 15 to 50 minutes. Antivenin may be given intramuscularly for 1 or 2 days. The antivenin is prepared from horse serum and is therefore supplied with a 1-mL vial of normal horse serum for eye-sensitivity testing. The symptoms usually subside in 30 minutes to 3 hours after treatment; occasionally, a second dose is necessary. Hospitalization and treatment with antivenin are indicated for patients who are less than 16 years of age, older than 60 to 65 years of age, are pregnant, or who have hypertensive heart disease, respiratory distress, or symptoms and signs of severe latrodectism. One ampule is sufficient and relieves most of the symptoms within 1 to 2 hours. The administration of antivenin to patients with prolonged or refractory symptoms of latrodectism, even after 90 hours after a bite, may alleviate discomfort and weakness.[34]

Healthy patients between ages 16 and 60 years of age usually respond to muscle relaxants and recover spontaneously. In emergencies, the local or state poison center or the Department of Public Health may be called for information about the closest source of antivenin.

MUSCLE RELAXANTS. Although calcium gluconate was once the first-line treatment of severe envenomations, it was found in one large series to be ineffective for pain relief compared with a combination of IV opioids and benzodiazepines.[35] Calcium gluconate (10%; 10 mL given intravenously) acts as a muscle relaxant. The administration is repeated only once if pain persists or recurs after 1 to 2 hours.[36] Intravenous Valium may be used and later replaced with Valium pills. Alternatively, diazepam or 1 or 2 gm of methocarbamol (100 mg/mL of Robaxin in 10-mL vials) may be administered undiluted over 5 to 10 minutes. Oral doses may be used thereafter, and they usually sustain the relief initiated by the injection.

ANALGESICS. Aspirin or, if pain is severe, intravenous morphine may be given. Morphine should be used with caution, since the venom is a neurotoxin and may cause respiratory paralysis.

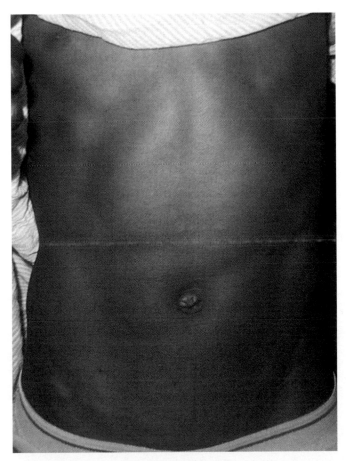

Figure 15-20 Latrodectism. Severe abdominal muscle spasms occurring hours after a black widow spider bite.

Brown recluse spider

The brown recluse spider, *Loxoscelidae reclusus* ("fiddle-back spider"), is small, approximately 1.5 cm in overall length. Its color ranges from yellowish-tan to dark brown. A characteristic, dark, violin- or fiddle-shaped marking is located on the spider's back. The broad base of the violin is near the head and the violin stem points toward the abdomen (Figure 15-21). The spider is a timid recluse, avoiding light and disturbances and living in dark areas (under woodpiles and rocks and inside human habitations, often in closets, behind picture frames, under porches, and in barns and basements). Its web is small, haphazard, and woven in cracks, crevices, or corners. It bites only when forced into contact with the skin, such as when a person puts on clothing in which the spider is residing or rummages through stored material harboring the spider. The brown recluse is usually found in the southern half of the United States, but some have been found as far north as Connecticut.[37]

Clinical manifestations

Patients infrequently present with a spider for positive identification. There is no laboratory test for diagnosis. A summary of bite severity and treatment are found in Table 15-1. Brown recluse spider bites frequently induce necrotic, slowly healing lesions. Maximum lesion severity is a predictor of time to complete healing.[38] Most bites are on an extremity. The bite produces a minor stinging or burning or an instantaneous sharp pain resembling a bee sting. Most bite reactions are mild and cause only minimal swelling and erythema[39] (Figure 15-22). Site location seems to be a factor in the severity of the local bite reaction; fatty areas such as the proximal thigh and buttocks show more cutaneous reaction. Severe bites may become necrotic within 4 hours.

The first and most characteristic cutaneous change in necrotic arachnidism, or loxoscelism, is the development and rapid expansion of a blue-gray, macular halo around the puncture site; this halo represents local hemolysis. Violaceous skin discoloration is an indication of incipient necrosis and can be used as a guide to early initiation of therapy, when it is most effective. A cyanotic pustule or vesicle/bulla may also appear at the bite site. The lesion may have an oblong, irregular configuration area at the bite site and a sudden increase in tenderness. At this stage, the superficial skin may be rapidly infarcting and the pain is severe. The necrotizing, blue macule widens and the center sinks below the normal skin surface ("sinking infarct") (Figure 15-23). The extent of the infarct is variable. Most patients experience localized reactions, but the depth of the necrotic tissue may extend to the muscle and over broad areas of skin, sometimes involving most of an extremity. The dead tissue sloughs, leaving a deep, indolent ulcer with ragged edges. Ulcers take weeks or months to heal; scarring is significant.

A severe progressive reaction that begins with moderate to severe pain at the bite site develops in a few people. Within 4 hours, the pain is unbearable and the initial erythema gives way to pallor. Within 12 to 14 hours after the bite, the victims often experience fever, chills, nausea, vomiting, weakness, joint and muscle pains, and hives or measle-like rashes. The toxin may produce severe systemic reactions such as thrombocytopenia or hemolytic anemia with generalized hemolysis, disseminated intravascular coagulation, renal failure, and sometimes death. Severe systemic reactions are rare and occur most frequently in children. Serial complete blood cell counts should be analyzed for hemolysis, thrombocytopenia, and leukocytosis. Serial urinalyses evaluates the possibility of hemoglobinuria.

A bite during pregnancy does not appear to lead to unusual risks to mother or fetus.

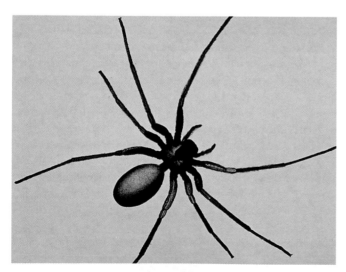

Figure 15-21 The brown recluse spider. A dark, violin-shaped marking is located on the spider's back.

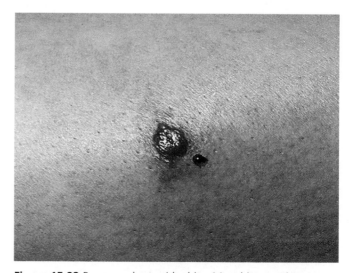

Figure 15-22 Brown recluse spider bite. Most bite reactions are mild and cause only minimal swelling and erythema.

Table 15-1 *L. reclusa* **Bite Severity and Treatment**

Severity	Clinical appearance/signs	Symptoms	Treatment
Mild	Erythema, punctum, no necrosis	Pruritus	RICE, antihistamine, aspirin, tetanus
Moderate	Erythema, mild edema, vesicle, necrosis <1 cm²	Pain, other	Add analgesic, antibiotic, consider dapsone
Severe	Erythema, edema, (hemorrhagic) bullae, ulcer, necrosis >1 cm²	Pain, other	Add dapsone, 50 mg PO QD, then 50 mg BID with G6PD
Systemic*	Rash, fever, hemolysis, thrombocytopenia, DIC	Myalgia, headache, malaise, nausea	Support; serial CBC and U/A, vigorous hydration, systemic steroids, transfusion

Adapted from Sams HH, et al: J Am Acad Dermatol 2001; 44:561.

CBC, Complete blood cell count; *DIC,* disseminated intravascular coagulation; *G6PD,* glucose-6-phosphate dehydrogenase; *RICE,* rest, ice compresses, elevation; *U/A,* urinalysis.

*Systemic symptoms are possible with bites of all cutaneous severity.

Management

Experience has shown that most bites are mild and should be treated conservatively with the following measures:

1. Bite sites are treated with RICE (Rest, Ice bags [15 min/h], Elevation).
2. An aspirin a day helps counteract platelet aggregation and thrombosis.
3. Tetanus toxoid is given if necessary.

The application of cold packs to bite sites markedly reduces inflammation, slows lesion evolution, and improves all other combinations of therapy. The application of heat to brown recluse bite sites makes lesions much worse.[40] Immediate surgery is avoided.

MODERATE TO SEVERE SKIN NECROSIS. Serious bites are usually obvious within the first 24 to 48 hours and need medical, but not surgically aggressive, treatment.

- Antibiotics (e.g., cephalosporins) should be used as infection prophylaxis in ulcerating lesions.
- Analgesics are usually required.
- Dapsone 50 mg every day and order glucose-6-phosphate dehydrogenase, then increase to 50 mg twice daily.

Secondary infection increases localized skin temperature that increases enzymatic activity and leads to further tissue damage; therefore, routine use of antibiotics is suggested.

DAPSONE. Immediate surgical excision of brown recluse bite sites induced more complications than did the use of dapsone with or without delayed excision and/or repair.[41] Dapsone 50 to 100 mg/day may be helpful in severe cutaneous reactions to prevent extensive necrosis, even if it is administered 48 hours after the bite.[42,43] Dapsone may help prevent the venom-induced perivasculitis with polymorphonuclear leukocyte infiltration that occurs with extensive cutaneous necrosis.[44] Order a glucose 6-phosphate dehydrogenase and complete blood cell count.

STEROIDS. There is little evidence that oral and intralesional steroids decrease the severity of the progressive reaction. Patients with necrosis greater than 1 cm should be tested to see if progressive hemolytic anemia, manifested by an increasing level of free serum hemoglobin or thrombocytopenia, has developed. Severe systemic loxoscelism may be treated with prednisone (1 mg/kg) given as early as possible in the development of systemic symptoms to treat hematologic abnormalities.

SURGERY. Early excision of necrotic areas was once thought to help prevent both the spread of the toxin and further necrosis. This practice is probably ineffective and should be discouraged.[45] If a proven or suspected brown recluse spider bite does not become clinically necrotic within 72 hours, a serious wound healing problem rarely develops.

Sharp debridement or excision of spider bite lesions should be vigorously discouraged. Gentle eschar removal may be performed after the wound has stabilized and inflammation has subsided (approximately 6-10 weeks).[46] Surgery is reserved for debridement of necrotic lesions.

ANTIVENIN. An antivenom has been developed. Inquire about availability.

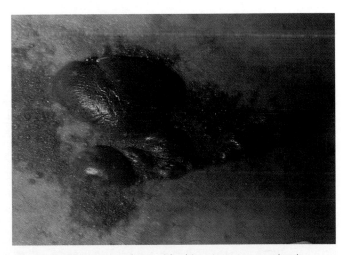

Figure 15-23 Brown recluse spider bite. A severe reaction in which infarction, bleeding, and blistering have occurred.

Ticks

Ticks are blood-sucking ectoparasites that act as vectors for rickettsial, spirochetal, bacterial, and parasitic infections. Adult ticks of some species can reach 1 cm in length; they have eight legs, and the front two are curved forward, as in crabs. The large oval or teardrop-shaped body is flat and saclike and has a leathery outer surface. There are two families of ticks: hard-bodied ticks (*Ixodidae*) and soft-bodied ticks (*Argasidae*). They are distinguished by the consistency of their bodies. Hard (ixodid) ticks are of greatest concern because they are vectors for most of the serious tickborne diseases. They can inflict local reactions such as pain, erythema, and nodules, and they are more difficult to remove than the soft (argasid) ticks. Ticks should be removed from the host as soon as possible after they are discovered to reduce the chance of infection. Proper removal of the tick, however, is just as important in reducing the chance of infection as timely removal.

Ticks perch on grass tips and bushes and wait for a warm-blooded host to pass by. They insert their recurved teeth into the skin, produce a gluelike secretion that tightens their grip, suck blood (Figure 15-24), and become engorged, sometimes tripling in size. Hard ticks may remain attached to the host for up to 10 days, whereas soft ticks release in a few hours. The bite itself is painless, but within hours an urticarial wheal appears at the puncture site and may cause itching. Ticks may go unnoticed, particularly in children, for several hours after attachment to an inconspicuous area such as the scalp.

Ticks and their associated diseases are listed in Table 15-2.

The deer tick (*Ixodes dammini*) transmits human babesiosis and Lyme disease; it is found in areas such as Massachusetts, Connecticut, New Jersey, and the islands of coastal New England. This tick is common in many areas of southern Connecticut, where it parasitizes three different host animals during its 2-year life cycle. Larval and nymphal ticks have parasitized 31 different species of mammals and 49

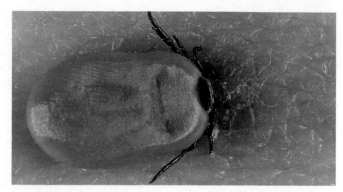

Figure 15-24 Tick. Mouth parts are deeply imbedded in the skin, and the tick is fully engorged with blood.

species of birds. White-tailed deer appear to be crucial hosts for adult ticks. All three feeding stages of the tick parasitize humans, although most infections are acquired from feeding nymphs in May through early July. Reservoir hosts for the spirochete include rodents, other mammals, and even birds. White-footed mice are particularly important reservoirs, and, in parts of southern Connecticut where Lyme disease is prevalent in humans, *Borrelia* are universally present during the summer in these mice. Prevalence of infected ticks has ranged from 10% to 35%. Isolates of *B. burgdorferi* from humans, rodents, and I. dammini are usually indistinguishable, but strains of *B. burgdorferi* with different major proteins have been identified.[47] The recent expansion of the geographic range has been attributed to the proliferation of deer in North America. The spotted fever tick (*Dermacentor variabilis*) is found in sections of the United States other than the Rocky Mountain region. Most *Dermacentor* ticks have white anterodorsal ornamentation. The Rocky Mountain wood tick (*Dermacentor andersoni*) is the vector for Rocky Mountain spotted fever in the west.

Table 15-2 Major Tickborne Diseases in the United States

Disease	Causative agent	Classification	Major vector	Region
Lyme disease	*Borrelia burgdorferi*	Bacteria (spirochete)	*Ixodes*	Northeast, Wisconsin, Minnesota, California
Relapsing fever	*Borrelia* species	Bacteria (spirochete)	*Ornithodoros*	West
Tularemia	*Francisella tularensis*	Bacteria	*Dermacentor, Amblyomma*	Arkansas, Missouri, Oklahoma
Rocky Mountain spotted fever	*Rickettsia rickettsii*	Rickettsia	*Dermacentor*	Southeast, West, South central
Ehrlichiosis	*Ehrlichia chaffeensis*	Rickettsia	*Dermacentor, Amblyomma*	South central, south Atlantic
Colorado tick fever	*Coltivirus* species	Virus	*Dermacentor*	West
Babesiosis	*Babesia* species	Protozoa	*Ixodes*	Northeast
Tick paralysis	Toxin	Neurotoxin	*Dermacentor, Amblyomma*	Northwest, South

From Spach DH et al: N Engl J Med 1993; 329:936.

Lyme disease and erythema migrans

Currently, approximately 15,000 cases of Lyme disease are reported each year. Lyme disease and erythema migrans (EM), which means "chronic migrating red rash," are caused by the spirochete *Borrelia burgdorferi* and are transmitted by the bite of certain *Ixodes* ticks of the *Iricinus* complex and possibly by other ticks. There are at least three different species of *B. burgdorferi* and this may explain why there are differences in the clinical spectrum of Lyme disease in Europe and the United States. *Ixodes* ticks have *B. burgdorferi* in their gastrointestinal systems. Lyme disease is named after Lyme, Connecticut, where the initial cluster of children with arthritis (brief but recurrent attacks of asymmetric swelling and pain in a few large joints, especially the knee, over a period of years) was reported in 1975. Like syphilis, the disease affects many systems, occurs in stages, and mimics other diseases. Cases have since been reported from all parts of the country, and people of all ages are affected. A disproportionate number of children contract Lyme disease because they spend more time in wooded areas than adults. The rapid emergence of focal epidemics is possible.[48] Antigenic differences between European and American strains of the organism may explain some of the minor differences in the clinical presentation of the disease, such as the more prominent skin involvement in European cases.

Geographic distribution

Lyme disease is now recognized on six continents and in at least 20 countries. Most cases in the United States are clustered in three regions (Figure 15-25): the Northeast coastal regions; Minnesota and Wisconsin; and parts of California, Oregon, Utah, and Nevada (see illustration below).

Eight states (Connecticut, Rhode Island, New York, New Jersey, Delaware, Pennsylvania, Maryland and Wisconsin) account for 90% of the cases reported. The geographic distribution suggests that *Borrelia* spreads when infested ticks are transported by migratory birds. *Ixodes dammini* (Figures 15-26 and 15-27) is the vector of disease in the Northeast and Midwest, and *Ixodes pacificus* in the West. The disease is reported throughout Europe. Most cases occur in the summer or early fall when people are outdoors, wearing shorts, and walking barefoot through the woods and grass. In the Northeast, they infest the white-tailed deer and white-footed mouse.

Cutaneous manifestations

There are three cutaneous lesions associated with Lyme disease: erythema migrans (formally referred to as erythema chronicum migrans), *Borrelia* lymphocytoma, and acrodermatitis chronica atrophicans. There is some evidence that several other cutaneous diseases are associated with *B. burgdorferi* infection.[49,50]

***BORRELIA* LYMPHOCYTOMA.** *Borrelia* lymphocytoma (BL) generally presents as a bluish-red nodule during the early stages of infection. It most commonly appears on the earlobe or nipple. Histologically there is a dense polyclonal lymphocytic infiltrate, which may appear after erythema migrans (EM) or as the first manifestation of Lyme borreliosis. EM and BL are early, localized cutaneous manifestations, but sometimes extracutaneous signs or symptoms of disseminated disease may appear simultaneously with either of these lesions. BL is rare; the prevalence ranges from 0.6% to 1.3% of cases of Lyme disease.[51]

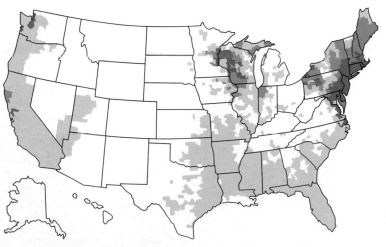

Figure 15-25 Reported cases of Lyme disease, 1993.

Areas of predicted Lyme disease transmission	High risk	Low risk
	Moderate risk	Minimal or no risk

DEER TICK

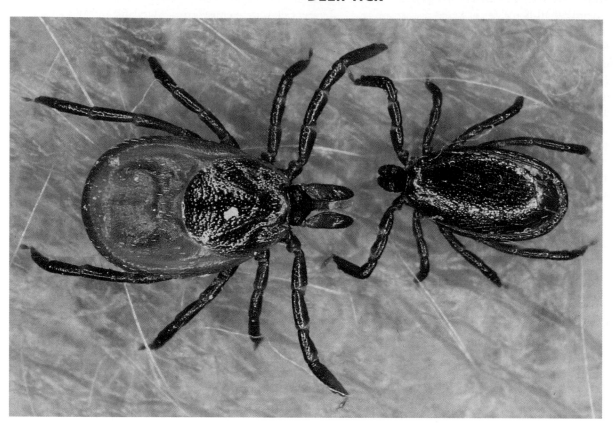

Figure 15-26 The deer tick *(Ixodes dammini)*, partly engorged (left) and unengorged (right).

Figure 15-27 The deer tick *(Ixodes dammini)*, one of the vectors for transmitting Lyme disease. This tick is very small and can easily go unnoticed when fixed to the skin in an unengorged state.

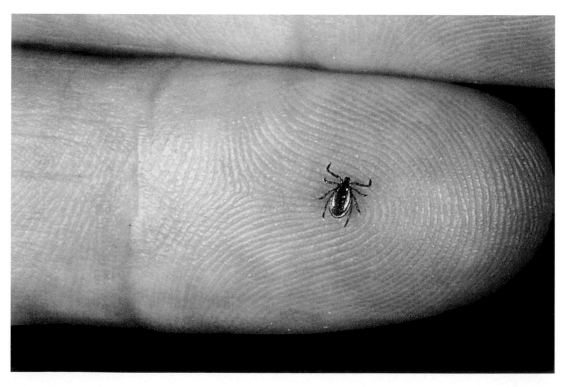

ACRODERMATITIS CHRONICA ATROPHICANS. During late infection, acrodermatitis chronica atrophicans, an erythematous, atrophic plaque unique to Lyme disease, may appear. It has been described in approximately 10% of patients with Lyme disease in Europe, but it is rarely seen in the United States. It starts with an early inflammatory phase with localized edema and bluish-red discoloration on the extensor surfaces of the hands, feet, elbows, and knees. Years to decades later there may be an atrophic phase where the skin becomes atrophic and dull red and may have a cigarette paper-like appearance.[52]

ERYTHEMA MIGRANS. The skin lesion erythema migrans (EM) is the most characteristic aspect of Lyme disease. It is described in detail below.

EARLY AND LATE DISEASE. Early Lyme borreliosis includes localized infection, entailing erythema migrans and *Borrelia* lymphocytoma without signs or symptoms of disseminated infection; regional lymphadenopathy and/or minor constitutional symptoms may be present; early disseminated infection, entailing multiple erythema migrans-like skin lesions and early manifestations of neuroborreliosis, arthritis, carditis, or other organ involvement. Late Lyme borreliosis includes chronic infection, entailing acrodermatitis chronica atrophicans; neurologic, rheumatic, or other organ manifestations that are persistent or remit for at least 12 (or 6) months.[53,54]

Three stages of infection

Lyme disease is divided into three stages that are determined by the duration of the infection from the time of the tick bite (see the diagram on p. 521).

EARLY LOCALIZED DISEASE (ERYTHEMA MIGRANS AND FLU-LIKE SYMPTOMS). Up to 90% of patients have the pathognomonic rash. It is a spontaneously healing red lesion occurring at the site of *Borrelia* inoculation. The average interval between the infectious bite and the appearance of the skin lesion is approximately 7 days (range: 3 to 30 days). The lesion begins as a small papule at the bite site. The papule forms into a slowly enlarging ring, while the central erythema gradually fades and leaves a surface that is usually normal but may be slightly blue. The ring remains flat, blanches with pressure, and does not desquamate, vesiculate, or have scale at the periphery, as ringworm does. The most common configuration of the lesion is circular, but as migration proceeds over skin folds, distortions of the configuration occur. The border of the lesion may be slightly raised.[55] Some patients complain of burning or itching. Over several days, the erythema expands rapidly away from the central bite puncture, centrifugally forming a broad, round-to-oval area of erythema measuring 5 to 10 cm (Figure 15-28). Within 1 week, it clears centrally, leaving a red, 1- to 2-cm ring that advances for days or weeks and may reach a diameter of 50 cm; 20% to 50% of cases have multiple concentric rings.[56] Tenderness is

present and itching is minimal. Even in untreated patients, lesions usually fade within 3 to 4 weeks. Within days or weeks, the spirochete may spread in the blood or lymph (stage 2). Secondary lesions or *Borrelia* lymphocytoma may occur. Multiple lesions, occurring as a result of hematogenous spread, are the cutaneous markers of disseminated spirochetal disease. A transient erythema may develop after an uninfected tick bite. It does not expand more than 1 cm in diameter and resolves in a day or two. Spider bites may also cause painful expanding red lesions.

The acute illness begins with malaise, fatigue, fever up to 105°F, the skin lesion, headache, stiff neck, myalgias, and arthralgias. Influenza will be suspected at this stage if the rash is absent. The complete blood count and erythrocyte sedimentation rate are normal. The electrocardiogram may show signs of carditis.

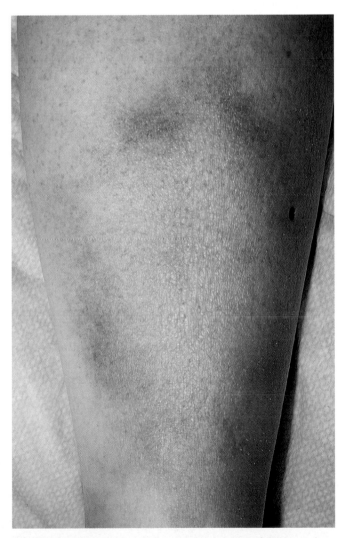

Figure 15-28 Erythema migrans. Broad oval area of erythema has slowly migrated from the central area.

EARLY DISSEMINATED DISEASE (CARDIAC AND NEUROLOGIC DISEASE). Early disseminated Lyme disease develops within 1 to 9 months of infection and can occur without EM.

Cardiac disease. Cardiac manifestations occur in 8% of untreated adults. They include fluctuating degrees of atrioventricular nodal block, mild pericarditis, and mild left ventricular dysfunction. Syncope, dizziness, shortness of breath, chest pain, or palpitations, occurs with higher degrees of block. Conduction block may resolve without antibiotics. The prognosis is excellent with treatment.

Neurologic disease. Within weeks, signs of acute neuroborreliosis develop in approximately 15% of untreated patients. These include lymphocytic meningitis with episodic headache and mild neck stiffness, subtle encephalitis with difficulty with mentation, cranial neuropathy (particularly unilateral or bilateral facial palsy), motor or sensory radiculoneuritis, mononeuritis multiplex, cerebellar ataxia, or myelitis.[57] Spinal fluid examination may reveal lymphocytic pleocytosis and elevated levels of protein with oligoclonal immunoglobulins.

Acute neurologic abnormalities typically improve or resolve within weeks or months, even in untreated patients.

LATE DISEASE (ARTHRITIS AND CHRONIC NEUROLOGIC SYNDROMES). Late Lyme disease may occur without evidence of early disease.

Joint disease. Months after the onset of illness, approximately 80% of untreated patients begin to have intermittent attacks of joint swelling and pain, primarily in large joints, especially the knee. The joints are warm but not red. After several brief attacks of arthritis, some patients may have persistent joint inflammation. In about 10% of patients, particularly those with HLA-DRB1, the arthritis persists in the knees for months or several years even after 30 days of intravenous antibiotic therapy or 60 days of oral antibiotic therapy.[58]

The joint fluid contains 10,000 to 25,000 white blood cells/mm³ (neutrophils predominate; most patients with Lyme arthritis are seropositive for anti-*B. burgdorferi* (ELISA). False-positive test results occur. Specific antibodies in the synovial fluid help confirm that the synovitis is due to B burgdorferi. Patients with Lyme arthritis usually have higher *Borrelia*-specific antibody titers than patients with any other manifestation of the illness, including late neuroborreliosis. The infection can persist for years in areas such as the joints and nervous system.

Neurologic disease. In up to 5% of untreated patients, *B. burgdorferi* may cause chronic neuroborreliosis, sometimes after long periods of latent infection. A chronic axonal polyneuropathy may develop, manifested as spinal radicular pain or distal paresthesias. Lyme encephalopathy, manifested primarily by subtle cognitive disturbances, is a possible late manifestation. There are no inflammatory changes in the cerebrospinal fluid. Computed tomography of the brain is not helpful. In patients with central nervous system involvement, the most sensitive diagnostic test is the demonstration of production of anti-*Borrelia burgdorferi* antibody in the spinal fluid.[57] Lyme encephalopathy may be treated successfully with a one-month course of intravenous ceftriaxone therapy.

Persistent infection

Some authors have documented persistent infection after treatment with currently recommended schedules. Approximately half the patients continue to experience minor symptoms, such as headache, musculoskeletal pain, and fatigue, after antibiotic treatment. Patients with severe cardiac involvement who do not respond quickly to antibiotic therapy may respond to steroids.

The Lyme disease spirochete may spread transplacentally to organs of the fetus. Women who acquire Lyme disease while pregnant should be treated promptly.[59]

Laboratory diagnosis

Diagnosis without the rash may be difficult. Routine laboratory studies are not helpful in confirming the diagnosis.

SEROLOGY. Serology is the only practical laboratory aid in diagnosis. Tests are insensitive during the first several weeks of infection, 20% to 30% of patients have positive responses, usually of the IgM isotype, during this period but by convalescence 2 to 4 weeks later, approximately 70% to 80% have seroreactivity, even after antibiotic treatment.[58] After antibiotic treatment, antibody titers fall slowly, but IgG and even IgM responses may persist for many years after treatment.

Examination of a single specimen does not discriminate between previous and ongoing infection. Because of a background false positivity even among healthy populations of nonendemic regions, serologic testing is recommended only when there is at least a one in five chance, in the physician's estimation, that the patient has active Lyme disease. New assays are becoming available, but the two-test approach, in which a positive or indeterminate result with a standardized, sensitive enzyme-linked immunosorbent assay (ELISA) test is followed by verification with a more specific Western blot assay, still provides the physician with a reasonably accurate and reliable assessment of the presence of antibodies to *B. burgdorferi*.[60]

Cultivation of *B. burgdorferi* from a skin lesion or blood is expensive and lacks sensitivity.

FALSE-POSITIVE TEST RESULTS. False-positive ELISA titer levels occur with syphilis, infectious mononucleosis, Rocky Mountain spotted fever, rheumatoid arthritis, and systemic lupus erythematosus, and in 7% of normal blood bank donors. Syphilis serologic test results for *Treponema pallidum*, such as rapid plasma reagin, venereal disease research laboratory (VDRL), or microhemagglutination assays are usually negative in Lyme disease, but the fluorescent *Treponema* antibody absorption test result may be frequently positive. Some false-positive results may be due to prior subclinical infections with *B. burgdorferi*.

LYME BORRELIOSIS

3 Stages with Remissions and Exacerbations

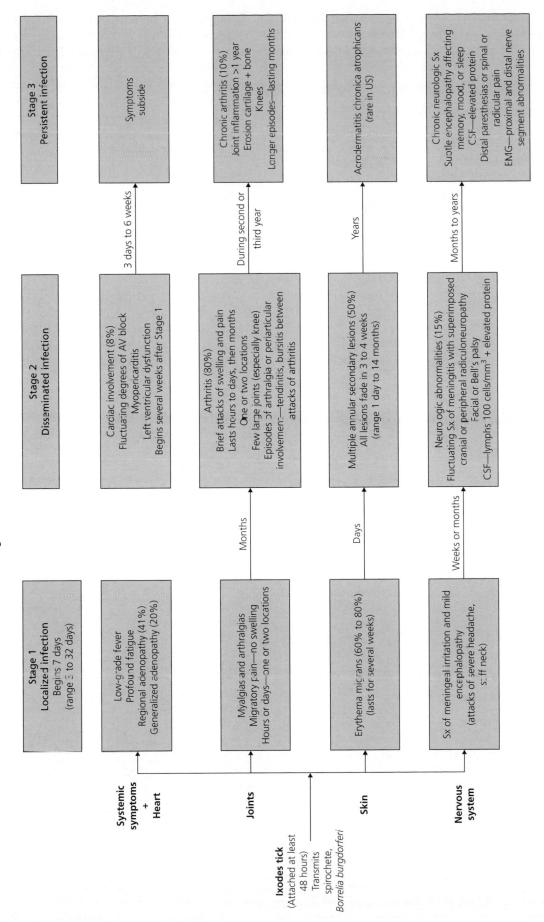

Stage 1
Localized infection
Begins 7 days
(range 3 to 32 days)

Stage 2
Disseminated infection

Stage 3
Persistent infection

Ixodes tick
(Attached at least
48 hours
Transmits
spirochete,
Borrelia burgdorferi

Systemic symptoms + Heart

Low-grade fever
Profound fatigue
Regional adenopathy (41%)
Generalized adenopathy (20%)

Cardiac involvement (8%)
Fluctuating degrees of AV block
Myopericarditis
Left ventricular dysfunction
Begins several weeks after Stage 1

— 3 days to 6 weeks →

Symptoms subside

Joints

Myalgias and arthralgias
Migratory pain—no swelling
Hours or days—one or two locations

— Months →

Arthritis (80%)
Brief attacks of swelling and pain
Lasts hours to days, then months
One or two locations
Few large joints (especially knee)
Episodes of arthralgia or periarticular
involvement—tendinitis, bursitis between
attacks of arthritis

— During second or third year →

Chronic arthritis (10%)
Joint inflammation >1 year
Erosion cartilage + bone
Knees
Longer episodes—lasting months

Skin

Erythema migrans (60% to 80%)
(lasts for several weeks)

— Days →

Multiple annular secondary lesions (50%)
All lesions fade in 3 to 4 weeks
(range 1 day to 14 months)

— Years →

Acrodermatitis chronica atrophicans
(rare in US)

Nervous system

Sx of meningeal irritation and mild
encephalopathy
(attacks of severe headache,
stiff neck)

— Weeks or months →

Neurologic abnormalities (15%)
Fluctuating Sx of meningitis with superimposed
cranial or peripheral radiculoneuropathy
Facial or Bell's palsy
CSF—lymphs 100 cells/mm³ + elevated protein

— Months to years →

Chronic neurologic Sx
Subtle encephalopathy affecting
memory, mood, or sleep
CSF—elevated protein
Distal paresthesias or spinal or
radicular pain
EMG—proximal and distal nerve
segment abnormalities

CULTURE AND BIOPSY. The culture or direct visualization of *B. burgdorferi* from patient specimens is possible but difficult. With Warthin-Starry silver stain, the *Ixodes dammini* spirochete was found, usually in the papillary dermis, in 86% of erythema migrans lesions.[61]

THE OVERDIAGNOSIS OF LYME DISEASE. In areas where anxiety about the disease is high, patients and physicians often ascribe clinical concerns to Lyme disease. Incorrect diagnosis often leads to unnecessary antibiotic treatment. Anxiety about possible late manifestations of Lyme disease has made Lyme disease a "diagnosis of exclusion" in many endemic areas. Persistence of mild to moderate symptoms after adequate therapy and misdiagnosis of fibromyalgia and fatigue may incorrectly suggest persistence of infection, leading to further antibiotic therapy. Attention to patients' anxiety and increased awareness of these musculoskeletal problems after therapy should decrease unnecessary therapy of previously treated Lyme disease.[62,63]

THE UNDERDIAGNOSIS OF LYME DISEASE. Most symptoms of *B. burgdorferi* infection are not pathognomonic. Nonspecific symptoms may persist for months even after treatment and it may take months or years for the late features of Lyme disease to resolve. Expanding erythema of EM resembles a spider bite. Radiculoneuropathy is diagnosed as a herniated cervical disc. Lymphocytic meningitis is misdiagnosed as viral meningitis. Monarthritis may be diagnosed as atypical rheumatoid arthritis or septic arthritis. Physicians in endemic areas must have a high index of suspicion for this confusing disease that can mimic so many other diseases.

Treatment

RISK OF INFECTION. The risk of Lyme disease after a deer-tick bite in areas with a high incidence of Lyme disease is 3.2%. Ticks must become at least partially engorged with blood (i.e., they must feed for many hours) before *B. burgdorferi* is transmitted. Erythema migrans developed more frequently after untreated bites from nymphal ticks than after bites from adult female ticks (8 of 142 bites [5.6%] vs. 0 of 97 bites [0%]), and particularly after bites from nymphal ticks that were at least partially engorged with blood (8 of 81 bites [9.9%]), as compared with 0 of 59 bites from unfed, or flat, nymphal ticks (0%). Among subjects bitten by

---

Table 15-3 Treatment of Lyme Disease*

Signs/symptoms	Drug	Adult dosage	Pediatric dosage[†]
Erythema migrans	Doxycycline[‡] (Vibramycin, and others)	100 mg PO bid × 21 d	>8 yr: 1-2 mg/kg bid
	OR Amoxicillin (Amoxil, and others)	500 mg PO tid × 21 d	50 mg/kg/day divided tid
	OR Cefuroxime axetil (Ceftin)	500 mg PO bid × 21 d	30 mg/kg/day divided bid
Neurologic disease Facial nerve palsy	Doxycycline[‡] OR Amoxicillin	100 mg PO bid × 21-28 d 500 mg PO tid × 21-28 d	25-50 mg/kg/day divided tid
More serious CNS disease	Ceftriaxone (Rocephin) OR Cefotaxime (Claforan) OR Penicillin G	2 gm/day IV × 14-28 d 2 gm IV q8h × 14-28 d 20-24 million units/day IV × 14-28 d	75-100 mg/kg/day IV 150-200 mg/kg/day in 3-4 doses 300,000 units/kg/day IV
Cardiac disease Mild (first degree AV block)	Doxycycline[‡] OR Amoxicillin	100 mg PO bid × 21-28 d 500 mg PO tid × 21-28 d	25-50 mg/kg/day divided tid
More serious	Ceftriaxone OR Penicillin G	2 gm/day IV × 14-21 d 18-24 million units/day IV × 14-21 d	50-75 mg/kg/day IV 300,000 units/kg/day IV
Arthritis[§]			
Oral	Doxycycline[‡] OR Amoxicillin	100 mg PO bid × 28 d 500 mg PO tid × 28 d	50 mg/kg/day divided tid
Parenteral	Ceftriaxone OR Penicillin G	2 gm/day IV × 14-28 d 18-24 million units/day IV × 14-28 d	50-75 mg/kg/day IV 300,000 units/kg/day IV

From The Medical Letter 2000; 42(1077).

*The duration of treatment is not well established. Relapse has occurred with all of these regimens; patients who relapse may need a second course of treatment. There is no evidence that either repeated or prolonged treatment benefits subjective symptoms attributed to Lyme disease.

[†]Should not exceed adult dosage

[‡]Neither doxycycline nor any other tetracycline should be used for children less than eight years old or for pregnant or lactating women.

[§]In late disease, the response to treatment may be delayed for several weeks or months.

nymphal ticks, the risk of Lyme disease was 25% if the tick had fed for 72 hours or longer and 0% if it had fed for less than 72 hours.[64]

PROPHYLACTIC DOXYCYCLINE. A single 200-mg dose of doxycycline given within 72 hours after an *I. scapularis* tick bite can prevent the development of Lyme disease (Box 15-3).[64] Anxiety about Lyme disease may be the most potent factor that drives decision making about chemoprophylaxis. Educating patients with tick bites about the excellent prognosis even if Lyme disease develops may be a better for anxiety than doxycycline.

It may be reasonable to administer doxycycline to persons bitten by ticks in areas where the incidence of Lyme disease is high and when the tick is a nymphal deer tick that is at least partially engorged with blood.[65,73]

ACTIVE DISEASE. Serologic testing has poor sensitivity in early disease. The presence of erythema migrans offers physicians the best opportunity for diagnosis. Aggressive antibiotic treatment may be initiated solely on the basis of this early clinical finding. The most recent recommendations are listed in Table 15-3.

ERYTHEMA MIGRANS. Oral antibiotic therapy shortens the duration of the rash and usually prevents development of late sequelae. Cefuroxime axetil appears to be as effective as doxycycline. Amoxicillin is also effective and is preferred for children and for pregnant or lactating women. The duration of therapy is guided by the clinical response. Relapse has occurred with all of the recommended regimens; patients who relapse may need a second course of treatment. Recommended treatment schedules are successful in preventing late sequelae in children; new episodes of erythema migrans were, however, reported in 11% of those patients 1 to 4 years after the initial episode.[66] Other studies show that major late manifestations of Lyme disease are unusual after appropriate early antibiotic therapy.[67-69]

Box 15-3 Strategies to Prevent Lyme Disease

Educate patients to check for and promptly remove attached ticks
Provide prophylactic treatment of tick bites in certain situations
  Within 72 hours after the discovery of a deer tick that is obviously engorged, or that was attached for more than 72 hours, on an adult from an area where Lyme disease is endemic; administer 200 mg doxycycline as a single dose
  Within 72 hours after the discovery of a deer tick that was attached for 36 to 72 hours, consider 200 mg doxycycline as a single dose
  When the tick was attached for less than 36 hours, it is not necessary to treat the bite
  In children, dosing and efficacy of prophylactic treatment have not been evaluated
Learn to recognize and promptly treat erythema migrans and other early manifestations of Lyme disease

Adapted from: Hayes EB, Piesman J: N Engl J Med 2003; 348: 2424

ARTHRITIS. Oral therapy with doxycycline or amoxicillin for 1 month is usually effective for treatment of Lyme arthritis. Patients who have not responded to oral treatment may respond to a second 1-month course of oral therapy or to IV therapy with penicillin G or ceftriaxone. For refractory arthritis of the knee, arthroscopic synovectomy may be helpful.

CARDIAC DISEASE. Cardiac conduction abnormalities are usually self-limited, but a temporary pacemaker may be necessary. Patients with minor cardiac involvement (first-degree atrioventricular block but PR interval less than 0.30 seconds) can usually be treated with oral doxycycline or amoxicillin. Those with more severe cardiac involvement (including first-degree atrioventricular block with PR interval greater than 0.30 seconds) should receive IV ceftriaxone or penicillin G.

NEUROLOGIC DISEASE. Patients with facial nerve palsy alone respond to oral doxycycline or amoxicillin. Patients with meningitis, other cranial or peripheral neuropathies, or encephalitis should be treated with intravenous (IV) penicillin G, ceftriaxone or cefotaxime. The same drugs may be effective for late neurologic complications, including cognitive deficits and polyneuropathies.

PERSISTENT INFECTION. Treatment with intravenous and oral antibiotics for 90 days did not improve symptoms more than placebo in patients with persistent symptoms despite previous antibiotic treatment for acute Lyme disease.[70]

JARISCH-HERXHEIMER–LIKE REACTION. Fourteen percent of patients, generally those with more severe disease, have an intensification of symptoms during the first 24 hours after the start of therapy. This Jarisch-Herxheimer–like reaction[71] (severe chills, myalgias, headache, fever, increased heart and respiratory rate lasting for hours, and increased visibility of the rash) usually occurs a few hours after treatment is begun.[72] Regardless of the antibiotic agent given, nearly half of the patients experience minor late complications—recurrent episodes of lethargy and headache or pain in joints, tendons, bursae, or muscles.

Prevention

Tick repellents are divided into those applied to the skin and those applied to clothing. The insect repellent N,N-diethyl-meta-toluamide (DEET) used on the skin repels a variety of insects, including ticks. It is especially important to detect and to remove ticks as soon as possible, since transmission of *B. burgdorferi* is unlikely if a deer tick is removed within 48 hours of attachment.[75,76]

LYME DISEASE VACCINE. The human recombinant outer-surface-protein vaccine (LYMErix-SmithKline Beecham) was licensed in 1998 for persons 15 to 70 years of age who live or work in moderate- to high-risk areas. The vaccine was withdrawn because of lack of use.

Rocky Mountain spotted and spotless fever

The name Rocky Mountain spotted fever (RMSF) was coined to describe a disease that was first observed in the Bitter Root Valley of western Montana. The disease occurs in many areas of the United States (Figure 15-29).

Four states (North Carolina, Oklahoma, Tennessee, and South Carolina) account for 48% of the reports.

Rickettsia rickettsii and ticks

Rocky Mountain spotted fever is caused by *R. rickettsii* and is transmitted by tick bites. *Rickettsiae* are released from tick salivary glands during the 6 to 10 hours they are attached to the host.

Not all tick species are effective vectors of *Rickettsia,* and even in the vector species, not all ticks are infected. Generally, only 1% to 5% of vector ticks in an area are infected. Several tick vectors may transmit RMSF organisms, but the primary ones are the American dog ticks: *Dermacentor variabilis* in the eastern United States and the Rocky Mountain wood tick, *Dermacentor andersoni,* in the West. Most cases occur in eastern states such as Tennessee and North Carolina. Adults of both tick species feed on a variety of medium-to-large mammals and on humans. Ticks are often brought into close contact with people via pet dogs or cats (dog ticks may also feed on cats).

Incidence

The age group with the highest incidence of disease are those 5 to 9 years of age. Ninety-five percent of patients report onset of illness between April 1 and September 30, the period when ticks are most active.

Pathology

Rickettsia infect the endothelium and vessel wall, not the cerebral tissue. RMSF is a rickettsial infection primarily of endothelial cells that normally have a potent anticoagulant function. As a result of endothelial cell infection and injury, the hemostatic system shows changes that vary widely from a minor reduction in the platelet count (frequently) to severe coagulopathies, such as deep venous thrombosis and disseminated intravascular coagulation (rarely). After the tick bites, organisms disseminate via the bloodstream and multiply in vascular endothelial cells, resulting in multisystem manifestations. The effects of disseminated infection of endothelial cells include increased vascular permeability, edema, hypovolemia, hypotension, prerenal azotemia, and, in life-threatening cases, pulmonary edema, shock, acute tubular necrosis, and meningoencephalitis.

Clinical manifestations

One week (range, 3 to 21 days) after the bite, there is abrupt onset of fever (94%), severe headache (88%), myalgia (85%), and vomiting (60%). The signs at onset of infection are difficult to distinguish from those of self-limited viral infections.

The rash is reported in 83% of cases and typically begins on the fourth day. It progresses through a sequence of stages and distribution that are never pathognomonic. It erupts first on the wrists and ankles. In hours it involves the palms and soles (73%), then it becomes generalized. The rash is discrete, macular, and blanches with pressure at first; it becomes petechial in 2 to 4 days (Figure 15-30). The rash is very difficult to see in African Americans, which may explain the higher fatality rate for African Americans (16%) as compared with whites (3%). In approximately 15% of cases, the rash does not

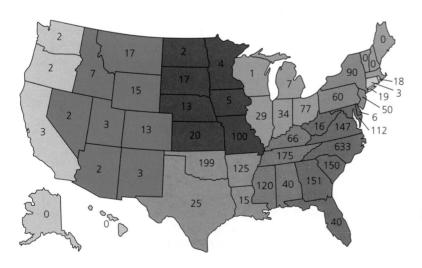

Figure 15-29 Reported cases and incidence rates of Rocky Mountain spotted fever, 1990.

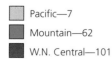 Pacific—7	W.S. Central—364	Mid. Atlantic—200
Mountain—62	E.S. Central—401	New England—40
W.N. Central—101	E.N. Central—148	S. Atlantic—1260

appear; the disease is then referred to as Rocky Mountain spotless fever.[77] Rashless disease is much more common in adults. Splenomegaly is present in one half of the cases. The fever subsides in 2 to 3 weeks, and the rash, if present, fades with residual hyperpigmentation. Although the overall mortality rate fluctuates between 3% and 7%, the mortality rate for untreated persons may exceed 30%.

Death usually results from visceral and CNS dissemination leading to irreversible shock.[78] Many of those who die have a fulminant course and are dead in 1 week. Interstitial nephritis is found at autopsy in most cases. The presence of acute renal failure is strongly associated with death.[79] Significant long-term morbidity (e.g., paraparesis; hearing loss; peripheral neuropathy; bladder and bowel incontinence; cerebellar, vestibular, and motor dysfunction; language disorders) is common in patients with severe illness caused by RMSF.[80]

In its early stages, RMSF may resemble other diseases. Only 3% to 18% of patients present with rash, fever, and a history of tick exposure on their first visit. RMSF should be suspected in patients in endemic areas who report fever, headache, and myalgias without a rash. Cough, rales, nausea, vomiting, abdominal pain, stupor, and meningismus are also RMSF symptoms. Thrombocytopenia and hyponatremia should raise the possibility of RMSF.

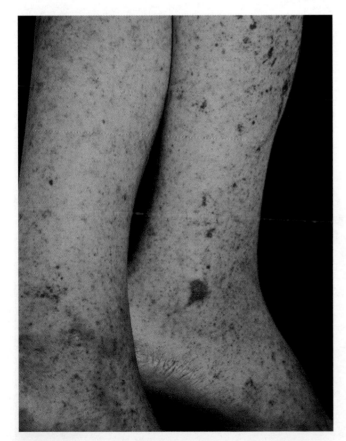

Figure 15-30 Rocky Mountain spotted fever. A generalized petechial eruption that involves the entire cutaneous surface, including the palms and soles.

Diagnosis

Delayed diagnosis and late initiation of specific antirickettsial therapy (e.g., on or after day 5 of the illness) is associated with substantially greater risk for a fatal outcome. The diagnosis must rely on clinical (fever, headache, rash, myalgia) and epidemiologic (tick exposure) criteria because laboratory confirmation cannot occur before 10 to 14 days after the onset of illness. The leukocyte count is normal or low. There is thrombocytopenia, increased serum hepatic aminotransferase level, and hyponatremia. The blood urea nitrogen (BUN) level may be increased, indicating prerenal azotemia or interstitial nephritis. Abnormalities on neuroimaging studies are not common and when present are subtle.[81]

LABORATORY. The clinical diagnosis, which is difficult, is rarely assisted by laboratory findings because antibodies are usually detected only in convalescence, and immunohistologic methods for detection of rickettsiae are unavailable in most clinics. Indirect fluorescent antibody (IFA) tests on acute and convalescent sera (a fourfold increase) are fairly accurate[82] and can be used later to confirm the diagnosis. Increase in the titre confirms the diagnosis. A single convalescent titer of 1:64 or higher (IFA) in a clinically compatible case also suggests the diagnosis. Diagnosis can also be confirmed by blood or tissue culture isolation of spotted fever group rickettsiae or by fluorescent antibody staining of biopsy or autopsy specimens, but this is not practical and is rarely performed. False-positive latex agglutination assay results occur during pregnancy. The incidence increases with the duration of pregnancy and reaches 12.1% in the third trimester.[83]

Treatment

Until reliable early diagnostic tests become available, a therapeutic trial of a tetracycline should be considered for any patient in an endemic geographic area during the summer months who has fever, myalgia, and headache. Most broad-spectrum antibiotics, including penicillins, cephalosporins, and sulfa-containing antimicrobials, are ineffective treatments for RMSF. Doxycycline is the treatment of choice except for pregnant women. Tetracycline, chloramphenicol, or a fluoroquinolone are also effective. They should be given in full dosages early in the course of the disease. Other causes of central nervous system infections such as *Neisseria meningitidis* or *Haemophilus influenzae* should be considered in the differential diagnosis, especially in the young. In these cases when diagnosis is uncertain, initial empirical therapy with chloramphenicol may be indicated.

Doxycycline is the most favorable agent for the treatment of RMSF in children younger than 9 years of age because of its documented effectiveness, broader margin of safety, reduced risk of drug-related adverse effects in young children, and convenient dosing schedule. For patients with RMSF reinfection, up to five courses of doxycycline may be administered with minimal risk of dental staining.[84]

Patients with RMSF who received antirickettsial therapy within 5 days of the onset of symptoms were significantly less likely to die than were those who received treatment after the fifth day of illness. Predictors of failure by the physician to initiate therapy the first time a patient was seen were absence of a rash and presentation within the first 3 days of illness.[85] In severe cases, fluid management is a challenge.

Tick bite paralysis

Tick bite paralysis probably results from a neurotoxin in tick saliva that is injected while the tick is feeding. The disease is most common in children, especially girls with long, thick hair. The tick, which hides on the scalp, groin, or other inconspicuous areas, must be attached for approximately 5 to 7 days before symptoms appear. It usually begins with weakness of the lower limbs, progressing in hours to falling down and incoordination, which is due to muscle weakness.[86]

Then, cranial nerve weakness with dysarthria and dysphagia leads to bulbar paralysis, respiratory failure, and death. Children may present with restlessness, irritability, and malaise. The patient complains of fatigue, irritability, and leg paresthesias, followed by loss of coordination and an ascending paralysis within 24 hours. There is no pain or fever in the early stages. Death from respiratory failure can occur if the tick is not found and removed. Recovery occurs 24 hours after the tick is detached. Tick bite paralysis is most commonly seen in the Pacific Northwest and is caused by the Rocky Mountain weed tick *Dermacentor andersoni.* In the southeastern United States, the American dog tick, *Dermacentor variabilis,* is the main cause of tick-induced paralysis.

Figure 15-31 TICKED OFF. A plastic tool used to extract ticks. The entire tick, including the mouth parts, is removed.

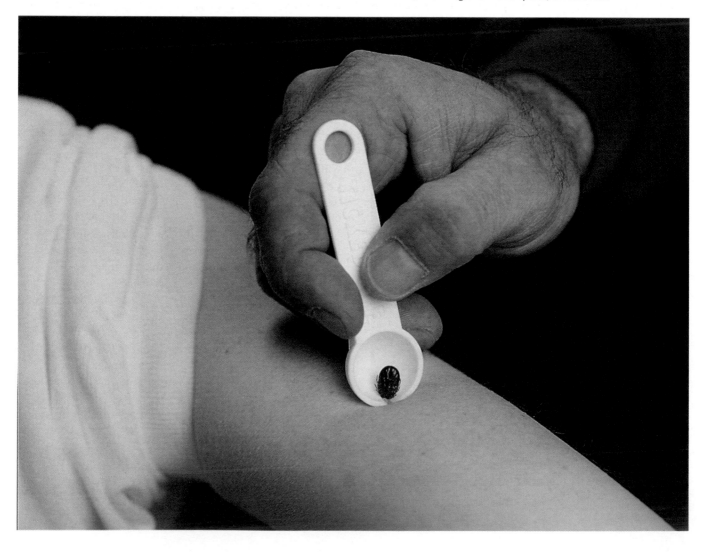

Removing ticks

A simple plastic tool called TICKED OFF removes ticks, including the mouth parts (Figure 15-31). Embedded ticks are removed completely, in one motion, while the bowl contains the tick for disposal. The tool can be used in any direction to remove ticks from the front, back, or side. TICKED OFF is held vertically. Applying slight pressure downward on the skin pushes the tick remover forward so it surrounds the tick on three sides, the small part of the "V" framing the tick. Continuous sliding motion of the notched area releases the tick. These inexpensive tools are now generally available.

Another technique for removing ticks is described in Box 15-4. Ixodid ticks are difficult to remove because they cement their mouth parts into the skin (Figure 15-32). Mechanical removal may or may not remove the cement. If no cement, or "fleshlike" material, is attached to the mouth parts after extraction, the cement is still in the skin, and attempts should be made to remove it to prevent subsequent irritation and infection. Ticks continue to salivate after extraction and must be disposed of immediately. In one study the application of petroleum jelly, fingernail polish, isopropyl alcohol, or a hot kitchen match failed to induce detachment of ticks. Hot objects may induce the ticks to salivate or regurgitate infected fluids into the wound.[87]

Ticks should not be removed by direct finger contact because of the danger of contracting a rickettsial infection. Dermacentor ticks are removed by gentle, steady, firm traction; the mouth parts usually come away attached to the tick. Ixodes dammini can rarely be removed intact by manual extraction. If detached, the mouth parts remain below the skin surface. The residual parts may be walled off and cause little harm or they may produce chronic irritation or stimulate a foreign-body reaction, resulting in a nodule known as a tick-bite granuloma. Twisting or jerking the tick during removal may break off the mouth parts. Manipulating a tick's body may cause infectious fluids to escape and enter the skin of the host or of the person removing the tick. The body of the tick should not be squeezed because additional fluid may be injected into the skin.

Box 15-4 Recommended Procedure for Tick Removal
Use blunt curved forceps, tweezers, or a thread. If fingers are used, shield them with a rubber glove or thick cloth.
Grasp the tick with forceps as close to the skin surface as possible and pull upward with steady, even pressure.
Do not twist or jerk the tick because this may cause the mouth parts and cement to be left embedded in the skin. Alternatively, take a thread (out in the woods find a loose thread in the seam of clothing), make a loop knot, pull it over the tick, and draw it tight around the smallest part of the tick at the skin surface. Pull both ends hard enough to lift up the skin. Hold this tension with thread or forceps for 3 or 4 minutes and the tick will slowly back out. Take care not to squeeze, crush, or puncture the body of the tick because its fluids (saliva, hemolymph, and gut contents) may contain infective agents.
Do not handle the tick with bare hands because infectious agents may enter via mucous membranes or breaks in the skin. This precaution is particularly directed to individuals who "detick" domestic animals using unprotected fingers. Children should not be permitted to perform this procedure. After removing the tick, thoroughly disinfect the bite site and wash hands with soap and water.

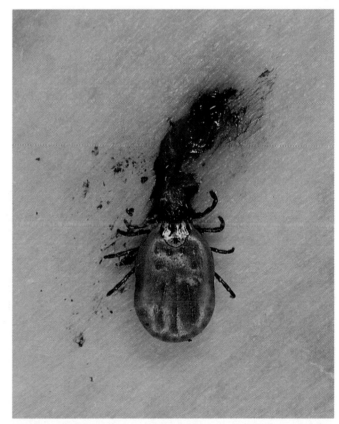

Figure 15-32 This tick was improperly extracted by grasping and pulling on the body. A large piece of tissue was torn away by the embedded mouth parts.

Cat-Scratch and Related Diseases

Cat-scratch disease is usually a benign, self-limited disease caused by *Bartonella henselae.* Cat contact is documented in 99% of cases, and in most cases the cat is immature. Cat-scratch disease is not easily acquired. Usually just one member of a family is affected, and adults rarely show symptoms, even when all family members are exposed to the same animal. The bacterium is transmitted to humans by scratches or bites; the role of fleas is possible but is not yet documented. Cats do not have to scratch to transmit the disease. In immunocompetent patients, that bacterium is responsible for cat-scratch disease, characterized by a localized lymph nodes enlargement in the vicinity of the entry site of the bacteria. In 5% to 13% of cases, the disease is more severe, including hepatitis, Parinaud's oculoglandular syndrome, neurological complications, or stellate retinitis. In immunocompromised patients, *B. henselae* is responsible for bacillary angiomatosis, bacillary peliosis hepatitis and splenitis, acute and relapsing bacteremia, or endocarditis.

Bartonella henselae

The causative agent is a pleomorphic, gram-negative bacillus, *Bartonella* (formerly Rochalimaea) *henselae* carried by cats. Cats are healthy, asymptomatic carriers and can be bacteremic for months or years. *B. henselae* can be transmitted from cat to cat by the cat flea. Approximately 10% to 16% of pet cats and 33% to 50% of stray cats carry this bacterium in their blood. This disease is more likely to occur in pet cats less than 1 year old that are infested with fleas.

Clinical manifestations

In one study, the primary inoculation site was observed in 93% of cases.[88] A red macule appears at the contact site and evolves into a nonpruritic papule (insect bites itch, but the papule of cat-scratch disease does not) 3 to 5 days after exposure to a cat; later the papule evolves into a vesicle filled with sterile fluid. The papule evolves through the vesicular and crust stage in 2 to 3 days.

Regional lymphadenopathy appears in 1 or 2 weeks. Location of lymphadenopathy depends on the site of inoculation and is seen most often in the axilla, neck, jaw, and groin. The papule may go unnoticed or be attributed to injury, and lymphadenopathy may not be appreciated. The lesion persists for 1 to 3 weeks, with a few persisting for 3 months, and ends with a scar resembling chicken pox. The enlarged nodes may persist for months with gradual resolution. In 12% of the cases, the lymph nodes undergo focal necrosis within 5 weeks. Consider the possibility of cat-scratch disease in adults with chronic lymphadenopathy who own cats.

Most patients experience mild symptoms of generalized aching, malaise, and anorexia. The temperature is usually normal, but in approximately one third of cases it is above 39°C (102°F). Inoculation within the confines of the eyelids or on the lids themselves causes a nonpainful palpebral conjunctivitis, preauricular lymphadenopathy, and fever, which characterizes the most common variant of cat-scratch disease (the oculoglandular syndrome of Parinaud).[89,90]

Severe systemic disease, including hepatosplenomegaly, osteolytic lesions, splenic abscesses and granulomas, mediastinal masses, encephalopathy, and neuroretinitis, are uncommon. The majority of patients recover without sequelae.

Parinaud oculoglandular syndrome

This is the most common ocular manifestation of this disease. It is characterized by unilateral conjunctivitis with polypoid granuloma, usually of the palpebral conjunctiva, and preauricular lymphadenopathy. Ask about contacts with cats in any atypical conjunctivitis accompanied by regional lymphadenopathy.

Neurologic complications

A large study characterized the neurologic complications of cat-scratch disease. Encephalopathy occurred in 80% of patients; 20% had cranial and peripheral nerve involvement with facial nerve paresis, neuroretinitis, or peripheral neuritis. The average age of encephalopathy patients was 10.6 years (range, 1 to 66 years). Almost twice as many males as females were affected. Fifty percent were afebrile and only 26% had temperatures higher than 39°C. Convulsions occurred in 46% and combative behavior in 40%. Lethargy with or without coma was accompanied by variable neurologic signs. Results of laboratory studies, including imaging of the CNS, were inconsistent and nondiagnostic. All patients recovered within 12 months; 78% recovered within 1 to 12 weeks. There were no neurologic sequelae. Treatment consisted of control of convulsions and supportive measures.

Bacillary angiomatosis

Bacillary angiomatosis is a vascular proliferative disease most commonly associated with long-standing human immunodeficiency virus (HIV) infection or other significant immunosuppression.[91] There is prolonged fever, arthralgia, weight loss, and splenomegaly of 2 or more weeks' duration. Multiple and widely distributed angiomatous nodules resembling Kaposi's sarcoma accompanied by symptoms of systemic cat-scratch disease were first reported in patients with acquired immunodeficiency syndrome (AIDS). There are three characteristic lesions: pyogenic granuloma-like papules, erythematous indurated plaques, and subcutaneous nodules. They vary from 1 mm to several centimeters in diameter and may be painful. The pyogenic granuloma-like papules bleed easily. Cutaneous and parenchymal lesions also occur in immunocompromised cardiac and renal transplant recipients. Immunocompetent persons can also develop cutaneous bacillary angiomatosis. Diagnosis often remains solely based on histologic findings.[92]

Diagnosis of cat-scratch disease

The diagnosis can be established by finding a primary lesion site in the presence of lymphadenopathy and a history of intimate exposure to cats. Lymph node biopsy may not be necessary if the above are present.

Serologic diagnosis using indirect fluorescence antibody (IFA) methods is made in either elevated titers of IgM (≥1:20) or IgG (≥1:256) antibodies or a fourfold increase in IgG titer between acute and convalescent sera.

Lymph node histopathology varies with time

A Warthin-Starry silver stain of lymph nodes and skin at the primary site of inoculation shows small pleomorphic bacilli.[93] The gram-negative pleomorphic bacilli are found within cells and are most abundant in areas of necrosis in skin and lymph nodes. The primary lesion should be carefully sought in young patients experiencing unilateral lymphadenopathy. It may be remembered as a bump or pimple, or it may be hidden on the scalp, within the earlobe, or between the fingers.

The bacillus can be cultured, but this is not routinely performed. The differential diagnosis includes nontuberculous mycobacterial disease.

Treatment

The bacillus is susceptible to several antibacterial agents in vitro, including penicillins, cephalosporins, aminoglycosides, tetracyclines, macrolides, quinolones, trimethoprim and sulfamethoxazole, and rifampin. In one study, azithromycin resulted in more rapid diminution in size of infected lymph nodes.[94] The majority of cases occurring in normal hosts do not require antibiotics.[95] By contrast, in immunocompromised patients, these infections are successfully treated with ciprofloxacin, trimethoprim-sulfamethoxazole, doxycycline, azithromycin, erythromycin, rifampin, and gentamycin.[94] Resistance to first-generation cephalosporins correlated with clinical failure of therapy. Many other commonly used antibiotics are not effective. Suppurating lymph nodes should be aspirated with a 16- to 18-gauge needle.

Animal and Human Bites

Animal bites, especially from dogs and cats, are common injuries.[96] Most wounds heal with conservative therapy designed to cleanse and disinfect the bite site. Some animal bites are serious or fatal.

Pasteurella species are the most common pathogen in dog and cat bites. Streptococci, staphylococci, *Moraxella*, *Corynebacterium*, and *Neisseria* are the next most common aerobic isolates. *Staphylococcus aureus* and *Streptococcus pyogenes* are found relatively infrequently. Anaerobes are rarely present alone; the majority of infections are mixed infections. *Fusobacterium*, *Bacteroides*, *Porphyromonas*, and *Prevotella* species are the predominant anaerobic isolates. Anaerobes were more often isolated from cat bites than from dog bites and from puncture wounds of the arms than from other parts of the body.

Anaerobic and aerobic bacteria infect human bite wounds. Humans harbors more pathogens than animals. Human bites have a higher incidence of serious infections and complications.[97] There are two types of human bites. Occlusional wounds occur when the teeth are sunk into the skin. Clenched-fist injuries occur when a tooth penetrates the hand. These require radiographic and surgical evaluation because severe complications result if a joint or bone is penetrated. Bacteria are carried beyond the penetration site beneath the skin when tendons are moved. The wound is usually 5 mm long. The hand becomes painful and swollen in 6 to 8 hours. *S. aureus*, *Eikenella corrodens*, *Haemophilus* species, and (in more than 50% of cases) anaerobic bacteria infect human bites. Residual disability and complications are frequent after clenched-fist injuries. Abscesses, osteomyelitis,[98] tendinitis, tendon rupture caused by infection, and residual stiffness of the joint may occur.

Management
Examination, irrigation, and debridement

Carefully examine all injuries. Bites that appear to be superficial may overlie fractures; involve lacerated tendons, vessels, or nerves; extend into body cavities; or penetrate joint spaces. Cultures taken at the time of injury are of little value because they cannot predict whether infection will develop or, if it does, the causative pathogens.

Copious irrigation at high pressure markedly decreases the concentration of bacteria in contaminated wounds.

Irrigation of the wound decreases the risk of infection. Tear wounds are copiously irrigated with sterile normal saline solution. Puncture wounds are irrigated using normal saline solution in a 20-mL syringe with an 18-gauge needle as a high-pressure jet.

Devitalized tissue in human bite wounds predisposes to infection. Elimination of the crushed devitalized tissue by debridement of wound edges is the key to control infection and to ensure a successful outcome following surgical reconstruction.[99]

Immunization for tetanus and rabies

Tetanus immunoglobulin and tetanus toxoid should be given to patients who have had two or fewer primary immunizations. Tetanus toxoid alone can be given to those who have completed a primary immunization series but who have not received a booster for more than five years.[100]

The bite of any mammal can transmit rabies. Rat bites pose a minimal risk. Cleaning a bite with soap is as effective as cleaning with quaternary ammonium compounds in lowering the risk of transmission of rabies.

Rabies prophylaxis is indicated for bites by carnivorous wild animals (skunks, raccoons), bats, and unvaccinated domestic dogs and cats. Vaccination is prophylactic, not therapeutic. Once signs of rabies occur, survival is rare.

All animals that behave wildly or erratically should be killed so that their brains can be evaluated for rabies. Quarantine healthy-appearing dogs, cats, and ferrets for 10 days and kill them if signs of illness occur. Rabies prophylaxis is indicated if laboratory tests confirm rabies in the dead animal or if the animal was not captured.

Patients who have not been vaccinated previously should receive both human rabies vaccine (a series of five doses administered intramuscularly in the deltoid area) and rabies immune globulin (20 IU/kg of body weight, with as much as possible infiltrated in and around the wound and the remainder administered intramuscularly at a site distant from that used for vaccine administration). Rabies prophylaxis is recommended after exposure to bats in a confined setting, particularly for children, even when no bites are visible.

When to suture the bite wound

Proper wound preparation with irrigation and debridement of devitalized tissue is the key to success. Wounds should be irrigated and left open if they are punctures rather than lacerations, are not potentially disfiguring, are inflicted by humans, involve the legs and arms (particularly the hands) as opposed to the face, or occurred more than 6 to 12 hours earlier in the case of bites to the arms and legs and 12 to 24 hours earlier in the case of bites to the face.

Facial lacerations from dog bites or cat bites are almost always closed. Foreign material in a contaminated wound increases the risk of infection; therefore subcutaneous sutures should be used sparingly.[100] Consider reevaluating wounds that were initially left open after 72 hours to determine whether delayed primary closure is indicated.

Antibiotics

Antibiotics are not given routinely. They are recommended for deep punctures (particularly if infected by cats), those that require surgical repair, wounds to the hands or near a bone, all moderate to severe wounds, crush injuries, and wounds that may have penetrated a joint.[101-104] Consider prophylactic therapy for patients who are bitten by those at risk for infection with the human immunodeficiency virus or hepatitis B virus.

Empirical therapy for dog and cat bites should be directed against *Pasteurella*, streptococci, staphylococci, and anaerobes. A combination of a (beta)-lactam antibiotic and a (beta)-lactamase inhibitor, a second-generation cephalosporin with anaerobic activity, or combination therapy with either penicillin and a first-generation cephalosporin or clindamycin and a fluoroquinolone are all likely to be effective. When given alone, azithromycin, trovafloxacin, and the new ketoside antibiotics may be useful.[105] Infection responds in most cases to amoxicillin/clavulanic acid, which is active against most potential bite pathogens.

Pasteurella species are usually susceptible to ampicillin, penicillin, second-generation and third-generation cephalosporins, doxycycline, trimethoprim-sulfamethoxazole, fluoroquinolones, clarithromycin, and azithromycin. Antibiotics typically used for routine infections of skin and soft tissue, such as antistaphylococcal penicillins, first-generation cephalosporins, clindamycin, and erythromycin, are less active against *Pasteurella*.[105]

Erythema and swelling in older wounds may indicate infection or a normal inflammatory response. Remove some or all of the sutures and drain pus. In most cases antibiotics should be administered intravenously. Elevate edematous body parts.

Stinging Insects

Honeybees, wasps, hornets, and yellow jackets sting when confronted. A wasp, for example, will vigorously pursue nest intruders. Insect repellents (e.g., DEET) offer no protection. A firm, sharp stinger is imbedded in the skin, followed immediately by secretion of venom. The honeybee stings once and dies. Its barbed stinger, glands, and viscera remain in the victim. Imbedded honeybee stingers should be flicked away with a knife or fingernail. If the stinger is grasped with fingertips, the venom glands will compress and make the sting worse. Stingers of other stinging insects are not barbed and remain intact, ready to be used again. The injected venom can cause a localized or generalized reaction. Reactions are classified as toxic or allergic.

Toxic reactions

Hymenoptera stings cause cutaneous local reactions of limited size and duration in most individuals. This nonallergic local reaction is a toxic response to venom constituents. There is a sharp, pinprick sensation at the instant of stinging, followed by moderate burning pain at the site. A red papule or wheal appears and enlarges if scratched (Figure 15-33). The reaction subsides in hours. Multiple stings can produce a systemic toxic reaction with vomiting, diarrhea, headache, fever, muscle spasm, and loss of consciousness. More than 500 stings at one time may be fatal.

Allergic reactions

Allergic reactions are mediated by IgE antibodies directed at venom constituents. Reactions are localized or generalized.

Localized reactions

Like the toxic reaction, the local allergic reaction begins with immediate pain, but the urticarial response is exaggerated. Swelling is thick and hard, as in angioedema. The urticarial plaque may be small or huge (Figure 15-34). Swelling lasts 1 to several days. Allergic local reactions greater than 10 cm in diameter are called large local reactions. They last for up to 5 days. Forty percent of patients with generalized allergic reactions have had large localized reactions.

Generalized reactions

The prevalence of generalized reactions to stings is approximately 0.4%. There are 40 fatalities from stings each year in the United States. Generalized reactions begin 2 to 60 minutes after the sting. Reactions vary from generalized itching with a few hives to anaphylaxis. Anaphylactic symptoms are typical of those occurring from any cause. They include generalized itching and hives, followed by shortness of breath, wheezing, nausea, and abdominal cramps. The reaction usually subsides spontaneously, but, in the unfortunate few, it

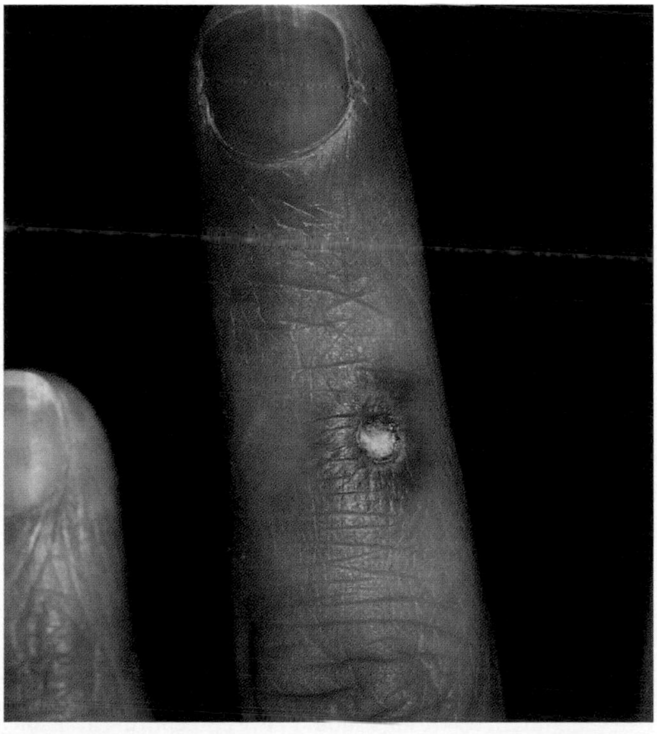

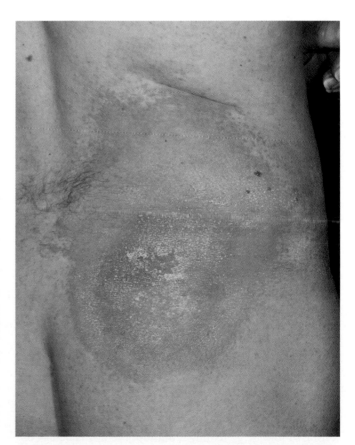

Figure 15-33 Bee sting. Severe local reaction with necrosis and ulceration at the sting site.

Figure 15-34 Bee sting. A huge, urticarial plaque occurred within hours in this patient with a known history of bee-sting allergy.

progresses, with edema of the upper airway causing obstruction and death. Following sting anaphylaxis, approximately 50% of patients continue to have allergic reactions to subsequent stings, but up to 42% have an improved response.[106]

Most reactions in children are mild, with just hives. Children with dermal reactions have only a benign course and are unlikely to have recurrent reactions. The more severe reactions, such as shock and loss of consciousness, are more common in adults. Adults whose reactions include urticaria, obstruction of the upper or lower airway, or hypotension, and children, whose reactions include obstruction of the upper or lower airway or hypotension, have an increased risk of future systemic reactions to stings.[107] Patients may develop delayed-onset allergic symptoms up to 1 week after the sting that range from typical anaphylaxis to serum sickness and are mediated by venom-specific IgE. Immunotherapy is recommended for patients with these reactions.[108] The possibility of a fatal insect sting should be considered in unwitnessed deaths occurring outdoors in summer.

The prognosis of patients with urticarial reactions to insect stings cannot be predicted by the immunologic tests presently available. One study found that 14% of patients with an urticarial reaction to previous insect stings had a systemic reaction with urticaria and angioedema with the next bite.[109]

Diagnosis

The diagnosis of *Hymenoptera* venom allergy is based on history, skin tests and determination of venom specific IgE-antibodies in the serum. Only rarely other tests are needed (specific IgG antibodies). To achieve a definite diagnosis, all findings have to be considered carefully, as "false-positive" and "false-negative" results can occur in all test systems. A diagnostic workup is not recommended for local reactions or for persons who have not experienced a systemic reaction. Patients who have large localized or generalized eruptions should be tested with venom extracts from honeybees, yellow jackets, yellow hornets, white-faced hornets, or wasps. Skin testing with species-specific, pure venom is the procedure of choice for determining sensitivity. Up to 15% of the general population may have positive results to such tests. The absolute titers of serum venom-specific IgE appear to be unrelated to a specific feature of stinging insect sensitivity. Negative RAST may have more clinical validity than a positive RAST. Low venom-specific IgG levels are associated with an elevated risk of treatment failure during the first 4 years of immunotherapy with yellow jacket or mixed vespid venoms.[110]

Indications for venom skin testing and immunotherapy

Hyposensitization is indicated in all patients with systemic IgE-mediated immediate type reactions. Venom testing should be deferred for 3 weeks or more after the sting. Skin testing should be done only if immunotherapy is being considered. Children younger than 16 years old with a history of a reaction limited to the skin do not require skin testing or immunotherapy. Anyone older than 16 years old with a history of a systemic reaction should have venom skin testing. It is desirable to test with all available venoms even if the stinging insect has been identified due to errors in identification and immunologic cross-reactions.

Various rush or conventional treatment protocols are used to reach the maintenance dose of usually 100 μg venom/4 weeks. Hyposensitization may be stopped if it lasted at least for 3 to 5 years, if systemic side effects did not occur, and if the patient has tolerated a sting challenge or a field-sting without systemic symptoms. In patients intensely exposed to *Hymenoptera* or in those with an increased risk of severe reactions, longer treatment has to be considered.

Immunotherapy leads to complete protection in more than 98% of patients with wasp (yellow jacket) venom allergy and in 75% to 80% of patients with bee venom allergy.[111] Serious adverse reactions to immunotherapy are rare. Immunotherapy lasts at least 3 to 5 years. After cessation of immunotherapy the frequency of systemic reactions to the sting of a wasp or bee is in the range of 5% to 15%. There are insufficient data on the long-term effect of immunotherapy.

A 2- to 5-hour regimen of rapid venom immunotherapy is a safe, alternative method of venom administration for patients who are at immediate risk for re-sting anaphylaxis.[112] Venom immunotherapy is effective in preventing recurrences of large local reactions but is not usually recommended for either adults or children.[113]

Treatment

Localized nonallergic stings are treated with ice or a paste made by mixing 1 teaspoon of meat tenderizer with 1 teaspoon of water. Localized allergic reactions are treated with cool, wet compresses and antihistamines.

Treatment of severe generalized reactions for adults includes aqueous epinephrine 1:1000 in a dosage of 0.3 to 0.5 mL administered subcutaneously and repeated once or twice at 20-minute intervals if needed. Epinephrine may be given intramuscularly if shock is imminent. If the patient is hypotensive, intravenous injections of 1:10,000 dilution may be necessary. If a severe reaction is feared, epinephrine should be administered immediately; to wait for symptoms to develop can be a dangerous practice.

Kits with preloaded epinephrine syringes are available (e.g., Epipen Auto-Injector, Anakit). Highly sensitive patients should have these kits available at home and during travel. For practice, one injection of physiologic saline should be self-administered under the supervision of a physician. Shortly after administration of epinephrine, antihistamines such as diphenhydramine (Benadryl 25 to 50 mg) are given orally or intramuscularly, depending on the severity of the reaction.

Patients with a history of insect sting anaphylaxis and positive venom skin test results should have epinephrine available.

Biting Insects

Biting insects such as fleas, flies, and mosquitoes do not bite in the literal sense; rather, they stab their victims with a sharp stylet covered with saliva. The sharp pain is caused by the stab; the reaction depends on the degree of sensitivity to the saliva. All of these insects are capable of transmitting infectious diseases. Biting insects seem to prefer some individuals to others. They are attracted by the warmth and moisture of humans. The patient's individual sensitivity determines the type and severity of the bite reaction. Patients who have not had previous exposure or those who have had numerous bites may show little or no response. Those who are sensitive develop localized urticarial papules and plaques immediately following the bite. The papules and plaques proceed to fade in hours and are replaced by red papules that last for days.

Papular urticaria

Papular urticaria refers to hypersensitivity bite reactions in children.[114,115] Young children who are left outside unattended in the summer months may receive numerous bites. They soon become sensitized, and subsequent bites show red, raised, urticarial papules that itch intensely (Figure 15-35). The young child who was initially indifferent to bites may

habitually excoriate newly evolved lesions, creating crusts and infection. Chronically excoriated lesions may last for months, eventually leaving white, round scars.

Fleas

Fleas are tiny, red-brown, hard-bodied, wingless insects that are capable of jumping approximately 2 feet. They have distinctive, laterally flattened abdomens that allow them to slip between the hairs of their hosts (Figure 15-36). They live in rugs and on the bodies of animals and may jump onto humans. Bubonic plague was spread throughout Europe in the Middle Ages by fleas that had fed on infected rats.

Flea bites occur in a cluster or group (Figure 15-37). A tiny, red dot or bite punctum may be seen at times. Most lesions are grouped around the ankles or lower legs, areas within easy leaping distance of the floor. Adult men are infrequently affected because their socks and pants protect them.

Control, elimination, and treatment

Fleas reside on cats, dogs, the animal's bedding, and in the entire house. All sources must be treated for effective flea control. Flea control involves eliminating the adult fleas on animals in the house and immature fleas in the environment. Carpets, pet bedding, and resting areas should be aggressively vacuumed. Wash pet bedding. Remove dead vegetation from animal resting areas outside. Many chemicals are available for control (pyrethrins, carbamates, organophosphate, imidacloprid, fipronil, sodium polyborate, insect growth regulators [methoprene], insect development inhibitors). There is no one best chemical. There are many formulations for the deliverance of the insecticides to the pet. Shampoos mechanically remove fleas but they have minimal residual effect.

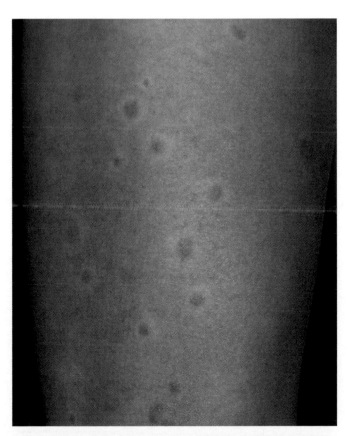

Figure 15-35 Papular urticaria. A hypersensitivity reaction to insect bites seen in children. A wheal develops at the site of each bite.

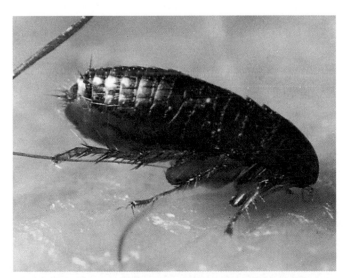

Figure 15-36 Flea. Thin wingless insects with very hard bodies and large hind legs adapted for jumping. *(Courtesy Ken Gray, Oregon State University Extension Services.)*

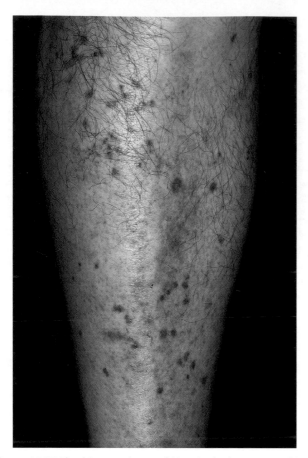

Figure 15-37 Flea bites. A cluster of bites in the knee area. This is a common site because a flea can jump no higher than approximately 2 feet.

Shampoos should be followed by a flea control rinse (dip) that contains an insecticidal product. Many flea sprays kill adult fleas, but their duration of action is short. Flea control powders, foams, concentrated solutions (spot treatments), and collars are all available. The indoor environment is best controlled by spraying either by a professional or the owner. This allows the product to be applied directly on the areas most frequented by the pets ("source points"). Large pieces of furniture must be moved to ensure that the spray reaches the areas of larval migration. The outdoor environment is controlled by sprays concentrated in areas frequented by the animals, (e.g., shaded areas that have a mild temperature and contain organic matter).[116]

Methoprene is an important new chemical for management of flea infestation. This is a synthetic equivalent of a natural insect hormone essential for growth regulation. Methoprene prevents flea larvae from maturing, and if used early in the year on carpets and animals' bedding should afford effective control. Methoprene (Siphotrol) is available in a spray and fogger. These products are claimed to protect against infestation for 4 months.[117]

Myiasis

The invasion of live human or animal tissue by fly larvae (maggots) is termed *myiasis*. Many organs can be involved[118] but the skin is the most common site.

Larvae species

Many species of flies around the world cause myiasis. Most cases are seen in returning travelers from Central or South America (*Dermatobia hominis*, the human botfly, a nonbiting insect) or from Africa (*Cordylobia anthropophaga*, the tumbu fly).[119,120]

Infestation

Females do not lay their eggs directly on their host but on the underside of a blood-sucking insect, such as a mosquito, biting fly, or tick. These insects transmit the larvae of the botfly via phoresis, a unique mechanism of egg deposition. Infection with the tumbu fly larvae occurs after direct contact with the eggs that are often deposited in clothes and towels. Young children who fall asleep outside are likely victims. Larvae may be acquired from petting or kissing dogs or cats contaminated with larvae. Larvae adhere and enter the nose, eyes, mouth, anus, or they penetrate skin. Larvae in the eyes, nose, or trachea of humans may attempt migration through deep organs. Those that penetrate skin develop at the site of penetration. Larvae enter the skin and reach the underlying subcutaneous tissue, where they feed and grow.[121] The time required for mature larvae to develop is species-specific (approximately 7 weeks). At maturity they enlarge the central pore and prepare to exit.

Clinical presentation

Most patients present in late August or early September. Lesions are found on the face, scalp, chest, arms, or legs. Clinically an abscess-like lesion develops. A red papule 2 to 4 mm in diameter appears (Figure 15-38). The lesion resembles a furuncle[122] or inflamed cyst and is called a warble; the maggot is called a bot. Flies that cause furuncular myiasis are called botflies. The head of the larva rises to the surface for air about once a minute through a small central pore. Movement of the larval spiracle (respiratory apparatus) may be observed. Serous or seropurulent exudate flows from the central punctum. Symptoms range from a mild itching or stinging to intense pain leading to agitation and insomnia. Sensation of movement in the lesion supports the diagnosis. An intense inflammatory reaction occurs in the tissue surrounding the larvae. Infection by *Tunga penetrans* may resemble myiasis. *T. penetrans* is a flea that invades the skin and produces a furuncular nodule. Tungiasis is almost always on the feet, whereas myiasis on the feet is rare. Tungiasis is acquired in South America and Africa.

MYIASIS

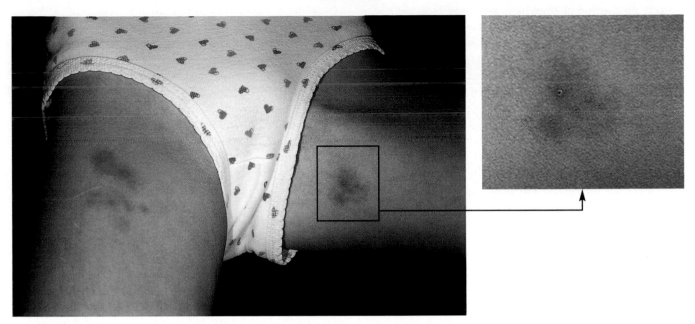

Figure 15-38 Myiasis. Fly larvae may be deposited on the skin and burrow into the host. They mature, induce skin surface erythema and rhythmically oscillate by rising to the surface to breath, then retracting back through the small orifice. Patients can feel this movement and may even see the worm as it rises through the orifice.

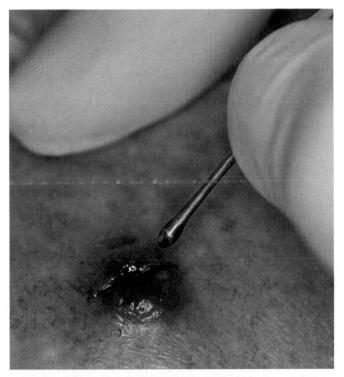

A, An incision is made across the central hole.

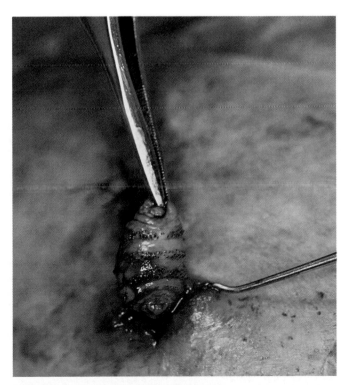

B, The larva is extracted intact with forceps.

Figure 15-39

Treatment

Correct diagnosis will prevent unnecessary treatment with antibiotics. In most cases the larva can be forced through the central hole with manual pressure. *D. hominis* is attached to the skin by hooklets. The larva's survival within its host is dependent upon the availability of oxygen. Obstruction of the breathing orifice with occlusive elements is effective. Apply an adhesive dressing such as tape and the larva becomes enmeshed within the dressing when it migrates toward the skin to get oxygen. Application of petroleum jelly over the pore may force the larva out for air. Another method involves the injection of lidocaine hydrochloride under the nodule. The pressure of the injection is sufficient to push the larva out.[123] Bacon therapy is another noninvasive technique. The fatty parts of raw bacon are placed over the opening of the skin lesion. The fly larva crawls far enough into the bacon and can be removed with forceps within 3 hours.[124] It is usually not necessary to enlarge the hole, but if the larva does not emerge, a no. 11 blade may be used to enlarge the hole slightly (see Figure 15-39). There is usually only one maggot in each mass. Rarely, a generalized reaction to fly bites may develop. Extracts are available for desensitization for a generalized reaction to fly bites.

Mosquitoes

Mosquito saliva is the source of antigens that produce the bite reactions in humans. Cutaneous reactions to mosquito bites are usually pruritic wheals and delayed papules. The rate of immediate reaction increases from early childhood to adolescence and decreases with age from adulthood. The appearance and intensity of the delayed reaction decreases with age. Arthus-type local and systemic symptoms can occur, but anaphylactic reactions are very rare.

A characteristic sequence of events takes place in all subjects exposed to mosquito bites over time. The initial bite causes no reaction, but with subsequent bites a delayed cutaneous lesion appears several hours after the bite and lasts 1 to 3 days or longer. After repeated bites for approximately 1 month, an immediate wheal develops that varies from 2 to 10 mm. Then, with further exposure for several months, the delayed reaction disappears. After repeated bites, the old bite sites may show flare-ups. Blisters can occur on the lower legs. In England, the condition known as seasonal bullous eruption was shown to be caused by mosquitoes. Patients with chronic lymphocytic leukemia may exhibit severe, delayed bite reactions that can appear before the malignancy has been diagnosed.[125] Patients with acquired immunodeficiency syndrome who had pruritus and chronic, nonspecific-appearing skin eruptions showed increased antibody titers to mosquito salivary gland antigens. This represents a form of chronic "recall" reaction. The increase may be a consequence of nonspecific B-cell activation, a feature of AIDS.[126]

No desensitization treatment is generally available for mosquito allergy.

Prevention and management

Biting insects are attracted to human body odor.

DEET. N,N-diethyl-3-methylbenzamide (DEET) is the most effective and best studied insect repellent currently on the market. This substance has a remarkable safety profile after 40 years of worldwide use. When DEET-based repellents are applied in combination with permethrin-treated clothing, protection against bites of nearly 100% can be achieved.[127] Plant-based repellents are generally less effective than DEET-based products.[128] DEET is especially active against mosquitoes, but it also repels biting flies, gnats, chiggers, ticks, and other insects. It does not repel stinging insects. DEET blocks the ability of some biting insects to track the victim's vapor trail. It is provided in most commercially available insect repellents, either alone or in combination with other chemicals that may enhance its effectiveness. Products containing DEET in concentrations above 75% are the most effective. Repellents are available as liquids, sticks, sprays, and saturated pads. The sprays contain the lowest concentration of DEET and are the most expensive. All exposed skin surfaces must be covered with repellent; insects seek out even small areas of skin that have not been covered. When insects begin to land on the skin, it is time for another application of DEET. Repellent may have to be applied every 2 hours in hot, humid weather, or it may protect up to 6 hours when the air is dry and cool.

OIL OF CITRONELLA. Oil of citronella has been used as an insect and animal repellent. It is found in many insect repellent products: candles, lotions, gels, sprays, and towelette wipes for use on clothing and people. These products repel mosquitoes, biting flies, and fleas but are not as effective as DEET.

ANTIHISTAMINES. In mosquito-sensitive subjects, prophylactically administered nonsedating antihistamines (e.g., Allegra 180 mg once daily, Zyrtec 10 mg), is an effective drug against both immediate and delayed mosquito-bite symptoms.[129]

PERMETHRIN. Permethrin, a pesticide used for the treatment of lice, is also effective as a clothing spray for protection against mosquitoes and ticks.

THIAMINE. A few reports claim that 75 to 150 mg of thiamine hydrochloride (Vitamin B-1) taken orally each day during the summer months protects against insect bites.[130] Others think that it is not effective. Thiamine hydrochloride is safe and may be worth trying, especially for children who are bitten often.

Insect bite symptoms are treated with cool, wet compresses, topical steroids, and oral antihistamines. A paste made of 1 teaspoon of meat tenderizer and 1 teaspoon of water provides symptomatic relief and discourages children from excoriating bites.

Creeping Eruption

Creeping eruption (cutaneous larva migrans) is a unique cutaneous eruption caused by the aimless wandering of the hookworm larvae through the skin. It is the most frequent skin disease among travelers returning from tropical countries. There was a history of exposure to a beach in 95% of patients.[131] *Ancylostoma braziliense* is the most common species. Infection is most frequent in warmer climates such as the Caribbean (especially Jamaica), Africa, Central and South America, Southeast Asia, and the Southeastern United States. Adult nematodes thrive in the intestines of dogs and cats, where they deposit ova that are carried to the ground in feces. The ova hatch into larvae and lie in ambush in the soil waiting for a cat or dog. In their haste to complete their growth cycle, these indiscriminate parasites may penetrate the skin of a human at the point where skin touches the soil. Workers who crawl on their backs under houses may acquire a diffuse infiltration with numerous lesions. The hookworms soon learn that they have preyed on the wrong host. The larva penetrates the skin in hopes of eventually reaching the intestines; however, physiologic limitations in humans prevent invasion deeper than the basal area of the epidermis. The trapped larva struggles a few millimeters to a few centimeters each day laterally through the epidermis in a random fashion, creating a tract reminiscent of the trail of a sea snail wandering aimlessly over the sand at low tide (Figure 15-40). Many larvae may be present in the same area, creating several closely approximated wavy lines.

Symptoms begin days to 3 weeks after exposure to infested soil. During larval migration, a local inflammatory response is provoked by release of larval secretions consisting largely of proteolytic enzymes. Itching is moderate to intense and secondary infection or eczematous inflammation occurs. Eosinophilia may approach 30% in some cases. The 1-cm larva stays concealed directly ahead of the advancing tip of the wavy, twisted, red-to-purple, 3-mm tract. If untreated, larvae usually die within 2 to 8 weeks, but occasionally persist for up to a year or more.[132] The dead worm is eventually sloughed away as the epidermis matures. Löffler's syndrome, which is a transitory, patchy infiltration of the lung, may develop with an accompanying eosinophilia of the blood and sputum.[133] This occurs with dermal penetration and subsequent larval invasion of the bloodstream. This is most common in patients with severe cutaneous infestation.

Management

Children are advised not to sit, lie, or walk barefoot on wet soil or sand. The ground should be covered with impenetrable material when sitting or lying on the ground. Complications (impetigo and allergic reactions), together with the intense pruritus and the significant duration of the disease, make treatment mandatory. Freezing the leading edge of the skin track rarely works and causes unnecessary tissue destruction. Topical treatment of the affected area with 10% to 15% thiabendazole solution or ointment has limited value for multiple lesions and hookworm folliculitis, and requires applications three times a day for at least 15 days. Oral thiabendazole 1.5 gm is not very effective when given as a single dose (cure rate, 68% to 84%) or once daily for 3 days and is not well tolerated. Treatment with a single 400-mg oral dose of albendazole gives cure rates of 46% to 100%. Albendazole 400 mg once daily for 3 to 5 days cured 77%,[131] but 400 mg/day for 7 days[134,135] is well tolerated and avoids no response and recurrence. Albendazole (Albenza) may be considered the first choice for treatment.[136] It is well tolerated and patient compliance is good. A single 12-mg oral dose of ivermectin gives cure rates of 81% to 100%.[137] Oral antibiotics and topical steroids are prescribed if secondary infection and eczematous inflammation are present.

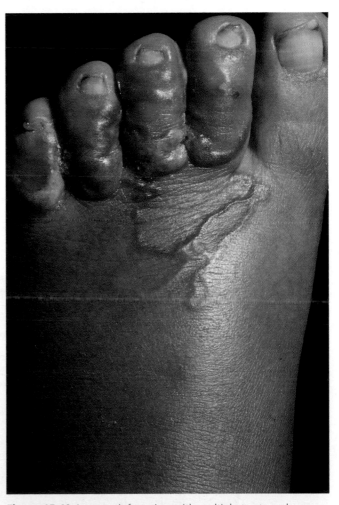

Figure 15-40 A severe infestation with multiple tracts and secondary infection of the toe webs.

Ants

Fire ants

The fire ant entered the United States from South America circa 1920 and spread quickly to several states in the southeast. There are four species of fire ants found in the United States in addition to the most common, *Solenopsis invicta*. Colonies have been found in Arizona, California, New Mexico, Virginia, and Puerto Rico. Invasion of buildings with sting attacks inside occupied dwellings, including health care facilities have been reported.[138] Fire ants can overwhelm their environment, causing destruction of land and animals. They cause a variety of health problems in humans, ranging from simple stings to anaphylaxis and death.

Between 30% and 60% of the population in infested areas are stung each year. Stings are most frequent during the summer; the legs of children are the most common target.

Fire ants are small ($\frac{1}{16}$- to $\frac{1}{4}$-inch long) and yellow-to-red or black with a large head containing prominent incurved jaws and a beelike stinger on the tail. They build large mounds (1 to 3 feet in diameter) in playgrounds, yards, and open fields in concentrations as high as 200 per acre. Colonies are formed at ground level in sandy areas. The grass at the periphery of the mound remains undisturbed and unharvested, unlike the mound of the harvester ant. The venom is made up almost entirely of piperidine alkaloids, in contrast to the venoms of other *Hymenoptera,* such as the wasp, which is up to one-half polypeptide proteins, measured by weight. The small fraction of proteins in fire-ant venom induces the IgE response. They have no natural enemies and may ultimately infest one quarter of the United States.[139]

The sting reaction

Sting reactions range from local pustules and large, late-phase responses to life-threatening anaphylaxis. The fire ant is aggressive and vicious. When provoked, they attack in numbers. In an instant, the fire ant grasps the skin with its jaws, which establishes a pivot point. It arches its body, injects venom through a distal abdominal stinger, then, if undisturbed, rotates and stings repeatedly, inflicting as many as 20 stings. This often results in a circle of stings with two tiny, red dots in the center where the jaws were attached. The pain is immediate and sharp, like a bee sting. Pain subsides in minutes and is replaced by a wheal and flare that resolves in 30 to 60 minutes[140]; 8 to 24 hours later a sterile vesicle forms and later becomes umbilicated. The contents of the vesicle rapidly become purulent (Figure 15-41). Pustules resolve in approximately 10 days. A large, local, late-phase reaction occurs in 17% to 56% of patients and lasts 24 to 72 hours. The plaque is red, edematous, indurated, and extremely pruritic. Eosinophils, neutrophils, and fibrin are present. Edema may be severe and compress nerves and blood vessels.

Patients who are allergic to fire ants may present with anaphylaxis.[141] This life-threatening reaction may occur hours after a sting. Check for stings on the lower extremity, especially between the toes, when a patient presents with anaphylaxis.

Treatment

The bite is treated with cool compresses, followed by application of a paste made with baking soda. Sarna lotion (0.5% camphor, 0.5% menthol) is soothing, especially if it is refrigerated. Application of meat tenderizer is of no value.[142] Oral antihistamines provide some relief. A short course of prednisone is used for severe local reactions.

IMMUNOTHERAPY. Sting reactions range from local pustules and large, late-phase responses to life-threatening anaphylaxis. Fire ant allergen-specific immunotherapy can reduce the risk of subsequent systemic reactions. Conventional and rush immunotherapy with fire ant whole body extract is effective, safe and efficacious; the rate of mild systemic reactions is low. Premedication is not necessary. Consider immunotherapy for patients with severe hypersensitivity to the venom or those who have had a previous anaphylactic reaction.[143] Skin test with whole body extract.

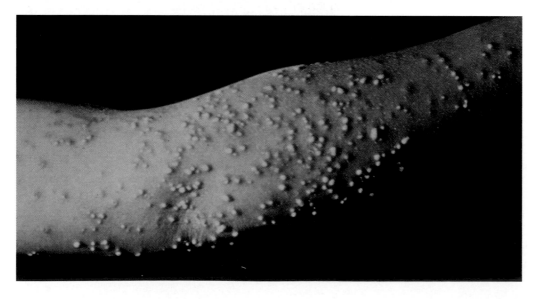

Figure 15-41 Fire ant stings. Multiple pustules in a cluster.

Dermatitis Associated with Swimming

There is increasing human contact with marine life. As more people travel to oceans for sports diving and other marine-related activities, the incidence of marine envenomations rises. Serious injury from a number of common sea creatures is possible.[144-146]

Swimmer's itch (fresh water)

Swimmer's itch (schistosome cercarial dermatitis) occurs on uncovered skin and is a transient, pruritic dermatitis caused by the epidermal penetration of cercariae, a larval form of animal schistosomes.[147] The microscopic larvae of the parasitic flatworm schistosomes, after being released from snails, swim in the water seeking a warm-blooded host, such as a duck. The indiscriminant larvae may accidentally penetrate a human and do not develop further. Schistosomes of humans cause systemic disease, but animal schistosome cercariae die after epidermal penetration, resulting in a rash. The disease is found throughout the world and restricted primarily to fresh water,[148] although salt water infestations have been reported.[149] In the United States, this disease is most common along bird migratory flyways, such as the Great Lakes or Long Island sound regions. Outbreaks are episodic and determined by snail maturation. Shedding occurs on bright, warm days in early or midsummer, with the highest incidence of infestation occurring near the shore.

Symptoms

The intensity of the eruption depends on the degree of sensitization. Some people do not develop a rash, whereas others swimming in the same water develop intense eruptions. Initial symptoms are minor after the first exposure, and papules occur only after sensitization is acquired, approximately 5 to 13 days later. The typical eruption occurs with subsequent exposures. It begins as bathing water evaporates from the skin surface and cercariae begin penetrating the skin.[150] Itching occurs for approximately 1 hour and is followed hours later by the development of discrete, highly pruritic papules and, occasionally, pustules surrounded by erythema at the points of contact. They reach maximum intensity in 2 to 3 days and subside in a week. Secondary infection occurs following excoriation.

Treatment

Treatment consists of relieving symptoms while the eruption fades. Itching is controlled with antihistamines, cool compresses, and shake lotions such as calamine lotion. Intense inflammation may be suppressed with group II through V topical steroids. Towel drying immediately after leaving the water is an effective preventative measure, since most larvae penetrate the skin as water is evaporating.

Nematocyst stings

Nematocysts are unique structures found on animals in the phylum Cnidaria. Nematocyst stings are responsible for the vast majority of skin problems in people who visit the reefs. Nematocysts are microscopic capsules used for both capturing prey and defense. They contain a toxin-covered, flexible, barbed whip that is uncoiled and discharged when touched (see the diagram below).

Cnidarians are either fixed to the reef or free swimming. Most are tiny individual animals that group together by the thousands to form fixed colonies, such as the corals and hydroids that make up most of a coral reef's structure. Jellyfish and anemones live as individuals. All of these animals have tentacles that contain nematocysts on their surfaces. The stings of most cnidarians are not harmful, but a few are quite toxic.

Vinegar

It is advisable to bring a plastic bottle of vinegar to the beach, because rubbing the affected area or washing with fresh water can cause nematocysts to discharge. Saturating the area with vinegar immobilizes unspent nematocysts.

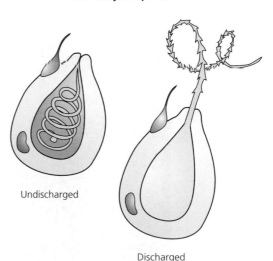

Nematocyst Capsules

Undischarged

Discharged

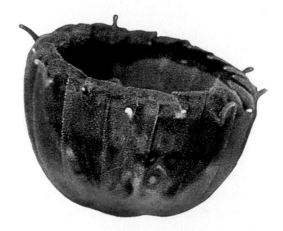

Figure 15-42 Sea thimble. The larva of this tiny jellyfish (½ to ¾ inches) is responsible for most cases of seabather's eruption in the Caribbean. *(Courtesy Reid E. McNeal, Grand Cayman, BWI.)*

Figure 15-43 Seabather's eruption. A common problem in the Caribbean. Nematocyst-bearing larvae may be trapped under the bathing suit and produce an intensely itching and painful papular eruption.

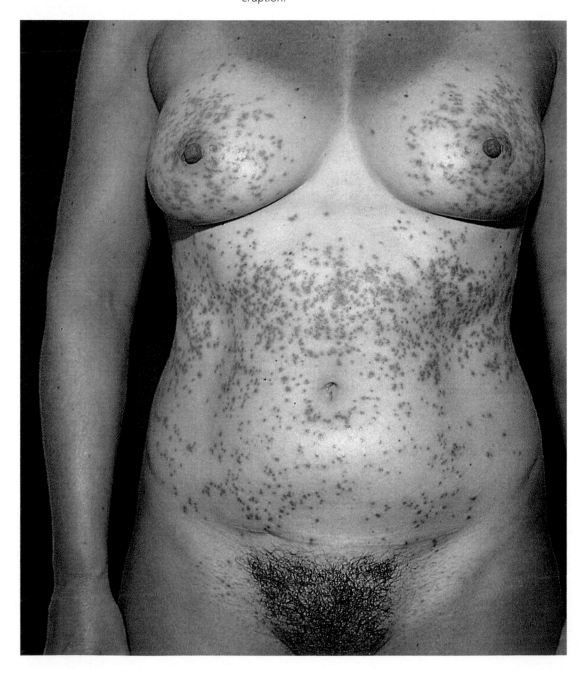

Seabather's eruption

Seabather's eruption occurs under bathing suits and is predominant in Mexico (Cancun and Cozumel), Bermuda, Florida, the Gulf states, and as far north as Long Island, New York. Larvae of members of the phylum Cnidaria (formerly Coelenterata), such as jellyfish,[151] and sea anemones,[152] have been implicated. Outbreaks occur when jellyfish or anemone larvae are transported to shore by ocean currents. The sea thimble (*Linuche unguiculata*) is the jellyfish responsible for seabather's eruption in the Caribbean[153] (Figure 15-42). Each sea thimble larva has more than 200 nematocysts, tiny organs that uncoil a threadlike, hollow stinger. When activated by skin contact, pressure, or contact with fresh water, the nematocysts are activated and toxin is forcefully injected into the swimmer's skin. Larvae are trapped under the bathing suit. Stinging is noted when the bather comes into shallow water or leaves the water. Prolonged wearing of a contaminated suit, strenuous exercise, and exposure to showers or freshwater pools activate nematocysts and make the symptoms much worse. Red, itchy papules or wheals resembling insect bites occur minutes to several hours later. The papules may coalesce to cover wide areas (Figure 15-43). The rash lasts for 3 to 7 days; severe cases last 6 weeks. Headache, chills, and fever are present in extensive cases. The rash may recur if a suit contaminated with nematocysts is reworn.

When the seasonal risk of seabather's eruption is present, children, people with a history of seabather's eruption, and surfers are at greatest risk. Many patients with seabather's eruption have specific IgG antibodies against thimble jellyfish antigen. The extent of the cutaneous eruption or sting severity correlates with antibody titer. This may explain why patients with a history of seabather's eruption are at greatest risk. Length of the time spent in water is not significantly associated with seabather's eruption.

Treatment is symptomatic, with cooling lotions (e.g., Sarna), antihistamines, topical steroids, and, in severe cases, prednisone. During the sea lice season, seabathers can minimize their risk by showering with their bathing suits off after seabathing.

Florida, Caribbean, Bahamas

Seabather's eruption (sea itch) is the most common marine-related problem in the waters south of the United States. Swimmers and divers are affected by the nematocyst-bearing tiny larvae of the sea thimble (a jellyfish). Itchy papules occur under or at the edge of bathing suits and wet suits. The eruption used to be seasonal but is now reported year-round. Areas with a high concentration of larvae change with the wind and tides.

Most sea animals are defensive. Divers who do not touch the fragile reef or handle fish are safe. Some of the sponges, corals, and anemones are toxic. Injuries to the feet caused by sea urchin spines are now uncommon because divers wear protective foot gear. Shuffling the feet in the water, rather than walking like on land, scares up sting rays buried in the sand. Stingrays are not aggressive, but stepping on a submerged ray's back can result in a deep, gaping wound. The floating Portuguese man-of-war is seen in Florida but is not common in the Caribbean. Becoming wrapped in its tentacles can result in severe swelling and blistering of an entire extremity. Box jellyfish (sea wasps) have a 2- to 3-inch cuboidal dome with 3-inch tentacles. These small creatures are occasionally seen in shallow water at night and are attracted to light. They are one of the most toxic animals on earth and can produce severe stings and shock. The erect dorsal spines of the odd-shaped, bottom-dwelling spotted scorpion fish are covered with a toxin that can penetrate rubber and skin.

Jellyfish and Portuguese man-of-war

There are two groups of stinging jellyfish found in the coastal waters of North America: the Portuguese man-of-war and the sea nettle (Figure 15-44). The dreaded Portuguese man-of-war has a large, purple air float up to 12 cm long that rides high out of the water and is carried by the wind across the ocean. Tentacles, with their attached stinging structure, the nematocysts, trail out several feet into the water. The red or white jellyfish seen floating in large groups or washed up on the beaches of the Atlantic coast are called sea nettles. They, too, have nematocyst-bearing tentacles, which measure up to 4 feet in length. Nematocysts are also found on the inferior surface of the body of the jellyfish. The Southeast Pacific box jellyfish contains the most potent marine venom known.

THE STING. When a small organism or a human brushes against an outstretched tentacle, the object is stung. Each tentacle has numerous rings of projecting stinging cells, and each cell contains a shiny oval body, the nematocyst. A tiny projecting trigger is on the outer surface of each nematocyst. On tactile stimulation, the nematocyst fires a threadlike whip with a hollow poisonous tip and recurved hooks on a node-like swelling at the base. The hooks hold the prey while the poisonous contents of the nematocyst are discharged through the thread into the body. The force of discharge is great enough to penetrate the upper dermis where the venom diffuses to enter the circulation.

Stings produce immediate burning, numbness, and paresthesias. Linear papules or wheals occur where a tentacle has brushed against the skin (Figure 15-45). Lesions either fade in hours or blister and become necrotic. Systemic toxic reactions (e.g., nausea, vomiting, headache, muscle spasms, weakness, ataxia, dizziness, low-grade fever) occur with severe or widespread stings. Movement of the envenomated part, such as a limb, leads to increased mobilization of the venom from the inoculation site. Fatalities may occur. It has been estimated that at least 50 feet of box jellyfish tentacles must touch the skin of an adult to deliver a fatal dose. Anaphylactic reactions may occur in victims who are allergic to jellyfish venom.

Recurrent linear eruptions after a sole primary envenomation have been reported. Most patients have only one recurrence, which takes place 5 to 30 days later, but some have multiple recurrences. In multiple recurrences, the duration of succeeding episodes become shorter, and the symptom-free intervals lengthen with successive recurrences. The recurrent eruption may be more severe. An immunologic reaction to intracutaneous sequestered antigen may explain this phenomenon.

TREATMENT. The envenomated part is immobilized to prevent mobilization of the venom. It is important to remove or inactivate the nematocysts as rapidly as possible. As long as the tentacles remain in contact with the skin, the nematocysts continue to discharge venom. If washed with fresh water or towel dried, unfired nematocysts on tentacles are activated. Tentacles and toxin are washed off by gently pouring sea water over the affected area. Remaining nematocysts and toxin on the skin are inactivated with alcohol (rubbing alcohol or liquor) or hot sea water. Any remaining tentacles are gently lifted off with a gloved hand. Remaining structures are removed after covering the area with a paste made of baking soda, flour, or talcum and sea water; this paste coalesces the tentacles. The dried paste is scraped off with a knife. Nematocysts of the Portuguese man-of-war can also be deactivated with vinegar. A good general rule for treatment is as follows: for areas on the East Coast north of North Carolina, baking soda should be used; for all other coastal areas of the continental United States, vinegar should be used. Moist beach sand is applied to soothe the irritation. Cool compresses and topical steroid creams suppress inflammation.

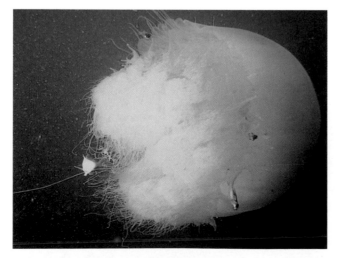

Figure 15-44 Jellyfish. Tentacles of varying lengths project from the base and trail in the water. Each tentacle contains hundreds of nematocysts. *(Courtesy Mike Nelson, South Africa.)*

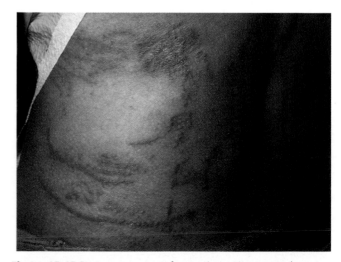

Figure 15-45 Portuguese man-of-war stings. Linear papules produced by nematocysts on tentacles that brushed against the skin.

Coral, hydroids, and anemones

CORAL. Coral is formed by limestone-secreting polyps that become fused, forming sharp, stonelike structures of various shapes and sizes. Coral is encountered in the Caribbean area, including Florida, Bermuda, the Bahamas, the West Indies, and in the Coral Sea extending from Australia to Hawaii and the Philippines. Like jellyfish, coral has nematocysts, but these are few and produce minor symptoms. The most important injuries are cuts (Figure 15-46). Itchy, red wheals ("coral poisoning") occur around the wound. Minor wounds are painful, slow to heal, and often become infected. Retained bits of calcium may cause a delayed, foreign-body reaction. Wounds should be cleansed thoroughly to remove bits of debris and treated with hydrogen peroxide.

Echinoderms (sea urchins and starfish)

Sea urchins are attached to rocks on the ocean floor. They are encased in a spheric hard shell with numerous brittle, sharp, calcified spines projecting from their surface (Figure 15-47). Pedicellaria are triple-jawed, pincerlike structures that are intermingled with the spines of some tropical species. Stepping or falling on the urchin results in penetrating wounds from spines or pedicellaria. The spines may break off and become imbedded in the wound. The spines or pedicellaria are venomous in some species (e.g., *Toxopneustes pileolus*). Venombearing spines are long, slender, and sharp, and are covered with a thin skin. Certain starfish produce wounds similar to those of sea urchins. Glandular tissue located beneath the skin produces slime that is released when the epidermal sheath is torn.

Reactions are immediate and delayed. Contact with spines produces an immediate burning sensation with redness and edema that may persist for hours. Wounds from venomous urchins cause immediate, excruciating pain and severe muscle aching. The wound area may be violet-black because of pigments located in the spines. Venomous species may cause the rapid onset of systemic symptoms such as paresthesias, muscular cramps and paralysis, hypotension, nausea, syncope, ataxia, and respiratory distress. Spines that enter joints may induce severe synovitis. Penetration over a metacarpal bone can cause a severe fusiform, reactive, distal swelling of the finger. Retained spines, if not spontaneously discharged or easily removed, may be dissolved with ammonia. An old native treatment is to pour hot wax on the skin and allow it to cool. The wax is then peeled off with the spines in it. Deep spines may have to be surgically excised. X-ray examination is important prior to surgical exploration. Delayed reactions are most commonly foreign-body granulomatous nodules that occur weeks or months later. They are less than 5 mm in diameter and are pink to purple. These may represent a hypersensitivity reaction. They respond to intralesional injections of triamcinolone acetonide (10 mg/mL) and to the surgical removal of spines. Chemicals present on the sea urchin's spines are apparently responsible for a delayed reaction that occurs in some individuals; this reaction consists of induration about the fingers and toes. It lasts for weeks, may cause joint deformity, and responds to systemic antibiotics and corticosteroids.

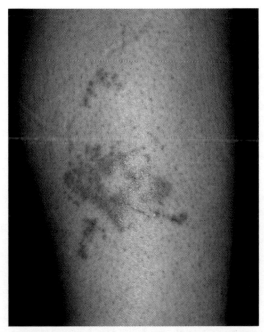

Figure 15-46 Coral poisoning. Calcareous material and protein may be forced into the skin after scraping against coral. Reaction to this foreign material may be intense and long lasting. Wounds become red and tender and may ulcerate. Linear streaks are characteristic.

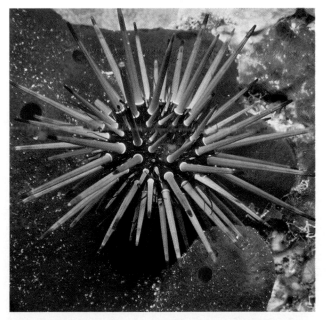

Figure 15-47 Reef urchin; body 1½ to 2 inches, spines 1 to 1½ inches. Pointed spines can cause puncture wounds. The spines crumble and remain lodged in the wound. (*Courtesy Steven F. Bennett, Grand Cayman, BWI.*)

References

1. Burkhart C, Burkhart C, Burkhart K: An epidemiologic and therapeutic reassessment of scabies, Cutis 2000; 65(4):233.

2. Chakrabarti A: Human notoedric scabies from contact with cats infected with Notoedres cati, Int J Dermatol 1986; 25:646.

3. Falk ES: Serum IgE before and after treatment for scabies, Allergy 1981; 36:167.

4. Arlian LG, Estes SA, Vyszenski-Moher DL: Prevalence of Sarcoptes scabiei in the homes and nursing homes of scabietic patients, J Am Acad Dermatol 1988; 19:806.

5. Liu HN, et al: Scabietic nodules: A dermatopathologic and immunofluorescent study, J Cutan Pathol 1992; 19:124.

6. Rasmussen JE: Lindane: A prudent approach, Arch Dermatol 1987; 123:1008.

7. Burkhart C, Burkhart C: Before using ivermectin therapy for scabies, Pediatr Dermatol 1999; 16(6):478; discussion 480.

8. Avila-Romay A, et al: Therapeutic efficacy, secondary effects, and patient acceptability of 10% sulfur in either pork fat or cold cream for the treatment of scabies, Pediatr Dermatol 1991; 8:64.

9. Maibach HI, Surber C, Orkin M: Sulfur revisited, J Am Acad Dermatol 1990; 23:154.

10. Taplin D, et al: Comparison of crotamiton 10% cream (Eurax) and permethrin 5% cream (Elimite) for the treatment of scabies in children, Pediatr Dermatol 1990; 7:67.

11. Holness DL, et al: Scabies in chronic health care institutions, Arch Dermatol 1992; 128:1257.

12. Yonkosky D, et al: Scabies in nursing homes: An eradication program with permethrin 5% cream, J Am Acad Dermatol 1990; 23:1133.

13. Wilson M, Philpott C, Breer W: Atypical presentation of scabies among nursing home residents, J Gerontol A Biol Sci Med Sci 2001; 56(7):M424.

14. Dannaoui E, et al: Use of ivermectin for the management of scabies in a nursing home, Eur J Dermatol 1999; 9(6):443.

15. Paasch U, Haustein U: Management of endemic outbreaks of scabies with allethrin, permethrin, and ivermectin, Int J Dermatol 2000; 39(6):463.

16. Miller RAW: Maculae ceruleae, Int J Dermatol 1986; 25:383.

17. Meinking T, et al: Comparative in vitro pediculicidal efficacy of treatments in a resistant head lice population in the United States, Arch Dermatol 2002; 138(2):220.

18. Burkhart C, Burkhart C, Burkhart K: An assessment of topical and oral prescription and over-the-counter treatments for head lice, J Am Acad Dermatol 1998; 38(6 Pt 1):979.

19. Burkhart C, Burkhart C: Oral ivermectin therapy for phthiriasis palpebrum, Arch Ophthalmol 2000; 118(1):134.

20. Bell T: Treatment of Pediculus humanus var. capitis infestation in Cowlitz County, Washington, with ivermectin and the LiceMeister comb, Pediatr Infect Dis J 1998; 17(10):923.

21. Shashindran CH, Gandhi IS, Krishnasamy S, et al: Oral therapy of pediculosis capitis with cotrimoxazole, Br J Dermatol 1978; 98:699-700.

22. Hipolito R, et al: Head lice infestation: Single drug versus combination therapy with one percent permethrin and trimethoprim/sulfamethoxazole, Pediatrics 2001; 107(3):E30.

23. Roberts R: Clinical practice. Head lice, N Engl J Med 2002; 346(21):1645.

24. Matthew M, DiSouza P, Mehta DK: A new treatment of phthiriasis palpebrarum, Ann Ophthalmol 1982; 14:439.

25. Allen VT, et al: Gypsy moth caterpillar dermatitis-revisited, J Am Acad Dermatol 1991; 24:979.

26. Pinson RT, Morgan JA: Envenomation by the puss caterpillar (Megalopyge opercularis), Ann Emerg Med 1991; 20:562.

27. Beaucher WN, Farnham JE: Gypsy-moth-caterpillar dermatitis, N Engl J Med 1982; 306:1301.

28. Shama SK, et al: Gypsy-moth-caterpillar dermatitis, N Engl J Med 1982; 306:1300.

29. Wong RC, Hughes SE, Voorhees JJ: Spider bites: Review in depth, Arch Dermatol 1987; 123:98.

30. Maretic Z: Latrodectism: Variations in clinical manifestations produced by Latrodectus species of spiders, Toxicon 1983; 21:457.

31. Miller TA: Latrodectism: Bite of the black widow spider, Am Fam Physician 1992; 45:181.

32. Zukowski CW: Black widow spider bite, J Am Board Fam Pract 1993; 6:279.

33. Schuman SH, Caldwell ST: 1990 South Carolina physician survey of tick, spider and fire ant morbidity, J S C Med Assoc 1991; 87:429.

34. O'Malley G, Dart R, Kuffner E: Successful treatment of latrodectism with antivenin after 90 hours, N Engl J Med 1999; 340(8):657.

35. Clark RF, et al: Clinical presentation and treatment of black widow spider envenomation: A review of 163 cases, Ann Emerg Med 1992; 21:782.

36. Key GF: A comparison of calcium gluconate and methocarbamol (Robaxen) in the treatment of lactrodectism (black widow spider) envenomation, Am J Trop Med Hyg 1981; 30:273.

37. Alario A, et al: Cutaneous necrosis following a spider bite: A case report and review, Pediatrics 1987; 79:618.

38. Sams H, et al: Necrotic arachnidism, J Am Acad Dermatol 2001; 44(4):561; quiz 573.

39. Cacy J, Mold J, for the Oklahoma Physicians Research Network: The clinical characteristics of brown recluse spider bites treated by family physicians: An OKPRN Study, J Fam Pract 1999; 48(7):536.

40. King LE, Jr, Rees R: Brown recluse spider bites: Keep cool, JAMA 1985; 254:2895.

41. Rees RS, et al: Brown recluse spider bites: A comparison of early surgical excision versus dapsone and delayed surgical excision, Ann Surg 1985; 202:659.

42. King LE, Rees RS: Dapsone treatment of a brown recluse bite, JAMA 1983; 250:648.

43. Futrell JM: Loxoscelism, Am J Med Sci 1992; 304:261.

44. Smith CW, Micks DW: The role of polymorphonuclear leukocytes in the lesion caused by the venom of the brown spider. Loxosceles reclusa, Lab Invest 1976; 22:90.

45. Anderson PC: Necrotizing spider bites, Am Fam Pract 1982; 26:198.

46. Sams H, et al: Nineteen documented cases of Loxosceles reclusa envenomation, J Am Acad Dermatol 2001; 44(4):603.

47. Anderson JF: Ecology of Lyme disease, Conn Med 1989; 53:343.

48. Lastavica CC, et al: Rapid emergence of a focal epidemic of Lyme disease in coastal Massachusetts, N Engl J Med 1989; 320:133.

49. Malane MS, et al: Diagnosis of Lyme disease based on dermatologic manifestations, Ann Intern Med 1991; 114:490.

50. Asbrink E: Cutaneous manifestations of Lyme borreliosis. Clinical definitions and differential diagnoses, Scand J Infect Dis Suppl 1991; 77:44.

51. Albrecht S, et al: Lymphadenosis benigna cutis resulting from Borrelia infection (Borrelia lymphocytoma), J Am Acad Dermatol 1991; 24:621.

52. Buechner SA, Rufli T, Erb P: Acrodermatitis chronica atrophicans: A chronic T-cell-mediated immune reaction against Borrelia burgdorferi? J Am Acad Dermatol 1993; 28:399.

53. Asbrink E, Hovmark A: Comments on the course and classification of Lyme borreliosis, Scand J Infect Dis Suppl 1991; 77:41.

54. Kristoferitsch W: Neurological manifestations of Lyme borreliosis: Clinical definition and differential diagnosis, Scand J Infect Dis Suppl 1991; 77:64.

55. Berger BW: Erythema chronicum migrans of Lyme disease, Arch Dermatol 1984; 120:1017.

56. Melski JW, et al: Primary and secondary erythema migrans in central Wisconsin, Arch Dermatol 1993; 129:709.

57. Halperin J: Nervous system Lyme disease, J Neurol Sci 1998; 153(2):182.

58. Steere A: Lyme disease, N Engl J Med 2001; 345(2):115.

59. Schlesinger PA, et al: Maternal-fetal transmission of the Lyme disease spirochete. Borrelia burgdorferi, Ann Inter Med 1985; 103:67.

60. Bunikis J, Barbour A: Laboratory testing for suspected Lyme disease, Med Clin North Am 2002; 86(2):311.

61. Berger BW, et al: Cultivation of Borrelia burgdorferi from blood of two patients with erythema migrans lesions lacking extracutaneous signs and symptoms of Lyme disease, J Am Acad Dermatol 1994; 30:48.

62. Sigal LH. Summary of the first 100 patients seen at a Lyme disease referral center, Am J Med 1990; 88:577.

63. Steere AC, et al: The overdiagnosis of Lyme disease, JAMA 1993; 269:1812.

64. Nadelman R, et al: Prophylaxis with single-dose doxycycline for the prevention of Lyme disease after an Ixodes scapularis tick bite, N Engl J Med 2001; 345(2):79.

65. Shapiro E: Doxycycline for tick bites—not for everyone, N Engl J Med 2001; 345(2):133.

66. Salazar JC, et al: Long-term outcome of Lyme disease in children given early treatment, J Pediatr 1993; 122:591.

67. Steere AC, Pachner AR, Malawista SE: Neurologic abnormalities of Lyme disease: Successful treatment with high dose intravenous penicillin, Ann Intern Med 1983; 99:767.

68. Steere AC, et al: Successful parenteral penicillin therapy of established Lyme arthritis, N Engl J Med 1985; 312:869.

69. Treatment of Lyme disease. Med Lett Drugs Ther 1988; 30(769):65.

70. Klempner M, et al: Two controlled trials of antibiotic treatment in patients with persistent symptoms and a history of Lyme disease, N Engl J Med 2001; 345(2):85.

71. Moore JA: Jarisch-Herxheimer reaction in Lyme disease, Cutis 1987; 39:397.

72. Berger BW: Treating erythema chronicum migrans of Lyme disease, J Am Acad Dermatol 1986; 15:459.

73. Shapiro ED, et al: A controlled trial of antimicrobial prophylaxis for Lyme disease after deer-tick bites, N Engl J Med 1992; 327:1769.

74. Couch P, Johnson CE: Prevention of Lyme disease, Am J Hosp Pharm 1992; 49:1164.

75. Piesman J, et al: Duration of tick attachment and Borrelia burgdorferi transmission, J Clin Microbiol 1988; 25:557.

76. Piesman J, et al: Duration of adult female Ixodes dammini attachment and transmission of Borrelia burgdorferi, with description of a needle aspiration isolation method, J Infect Dis 1991; 163:895.

77. Sexton DJ, Corey GR: Rocky Mountain "spotless" and "almost spotless" fever: A wolf in sheep's clothing, Clin Infect Dis 1992; 15:439.

78. Green WR, Walker DH, Cain BG: Fatal viscerotrophic Rocky Mountain spotted fever, Am J Med 1978; 64:523.

79. Conlon P, et al: Predictors of prognosis and risk of acute renal failure in patients with Rocky Mountain spotted fever, Am J Med 1996; 101(6):621.

80. Archibald L, Sexton D: Long-term sequelae of Rocky Mountain spotted fever, Clin Infect Dis 1995; 20(5):1122.

81. Bonawitz C, Castillo M, Mukherji S: Comparison of CT and MR features with clinical outcome in patients with Rocky Mountain spotted fever, AJNR Am J Neuroradiol 1997; 18(3):459.

82. Paddock C, et al; Hidden mortality attributable to Rocky Mountain spotted fever: Immunohistochemical detection of fatal, serologically unconfirmed disease, J Infect Dis 1999; 179(6):1469.

83. Welch KJ, et al: False-positive results in serologic tests for Rocky Mountain spotted fever during pregnancy, South Med J 1991; 84:307.

84. Cale D, McCarthy M: Treatment of Rocky Mountain spotted fever in children, Ann Pharmacother 1997; 31(4):492.

85. Kirkland K, Wilkinson W, Sexton D: Therapeutic delay and mortality in cases of Rocky Mountain spotted fever, Clin Infect Dis 1995; 20(5):1118.

86. Felz M, Smith C, Swift T: A six-year-old girl with tick paralysis [see comments], N Engl J Med 2000; 342(2):90.

87. Needham GR: Evaluation of five popular methods for tick removal, Pediatrics 1985; 75:997.

88. Carithers HA: Cat-scratch disease: An overview based on a study of 1,200 patients, Am J Dis Child 1985; 139:1124.

89. Jawad AS, Amen AA: Cat-scratch disease presenting as the oculoglandular syndrome of Parinaud: A report of two cases, Postgrad Med J 1990; 66:467.

90. Jackson MA, et al: Antimicrobial therapy for Parinaud's oculoglandular syndrome, Pediatr Infect Dis J 1992; 11:130.

91. Requena L, Sangueza O: Cutaneous vascular proliferation. Part II. Hyperplasias and benign neoplasms, J Am Acad Dermatol 1997; 37(6):887; quiz 920.

92. Gasquet S, et al: Bacillary angiomatosis in immunocompromised patients, AIDS 1998; 12(14):1793.

93. English CK, et al. Cat-scratch disease. Isolation and culture of the bacterial agent, JAMA 1988; 259:1347.

94. Bass J, et al: Prospective randomized double blind placebo-controlled evaluation of azithromycin for treatment of cat-scratch disease [see comments], Pediatr Infect Dis J 1998; 17(6):447.

95. Conrad D: Treatment of cat-scratch disease, Curr Opin Pediatr 2001; 13(1):56.

96. Griego R, et al: Dog, cat, and human bites: A review, J Am Acad Dermatol 1995; 33(6):1019.

97. Brook I: Human and animal bite infections, J Fam Pract 1989; 28:713.

98. Gonzalez MH, et al: Osteomyelitis of the hand after a human bite, J Hand Surg [Am] 1993; 18:520.

99. Agrawal K, et al: Primary reconstruction of major human bite wounds of the face, Plast Reconstr Surg 1992; 90:394.

100. Fleisher G: The management of bite wounds [editorial; comment]], N Engl J Med 1999; 340(2):138.

101. Dire DJ, et al: Prophylactic oral antibiotics for low-risk dog bite wounds, Pediatr Emerg Care 1992; 8:194.

102. Zubowicz VN, Gravier M: Management of early human bites of the hand: A prospective randomized study, Plast Reconstr Surg 1991; 88:111.

103. Goldstein EJC: Management of human and animal bite wounds, J Am Acad Dermatol 1989; 21:1275.

104. Anderson CR: Animal bites. Guidelines to current management, Postgrad Med 1992; 92:134.

105. Talan D, et al., for the Emergency Medicine Animal Bite Infection Study Group: Bacteriologic analysis of infected dog and cat bites [see comments], N Engl J Med 1999; 340(2):85.

106. Settipane GA, Boyd GK: Natural history of insect sting allergy: The Rhode Island experience, Allergy Proc 1989; 10:109.

107. Li JT, Yunginger JW: Management of insect sting hypersensitivity, Mayo Clin Proc 1992; 67:188.

108. Reisman RE, Livingston A: Late-onset allergic reactions, including serum sickness, after insect stings, J Allergy Clin Immunol 1989; 84:331.

109. Engel T, Heinig JH, Weeke ER: Allergy 1988; 43:289.

110. Golden DB, et al: Clinical correlation of the venom-specific IgG antibody level during maintenance venom immunotherapy, J Allergy Clin Immunol 1992; 90:386.

111. Graft D: Venom immunotherapy: When to start, when to stop, Allergy Asthma Proc 2000; 21(2):113.

112. Bernstein DI, et al: Clinical and immunologic studies of rapid venom immunotherapy in Hymenoptera-sensitive patients, J Allergy Clin Immunol 1989; 84:951.

113. Wright DN, Lockey RF: Local reactions to stinging insects (Hymenoptera), Allergy Proc 1990; 11:23.

114. Alexander JO: Papular urticaria and immune complexes, J Am Acad Dermatol 1985; 12:374.

115. Heng MCY, Kloss SG, Haberfelde GC: Pathogenesis of papular urticaria, J Am Acad Dermatol 1984; 10:1030.

116. Sousa C: Fleas, flea allergy, and flea control: A review, Dermatol Online J 1997; 3(2):7.

117. Burns DA: The investigation and management of arthropod bite reactions acquired in the home, Clin Exp Dermatol 1987; 12:114.

118. Singh I, et al: Myiasis in children: The Indian perspective, Int J Pediatr Otorhinolaryngol 1993; 25:127.

119. Schiff TA: Furuncular cutaneous myiasis caused by Cuterebra larva, J Am Acad Dermatol 1993; 28:261.

120. Baird JK, et al: North American cuterebrid myiasis. Report of seventeen new infections of human beings and review of the disease, J Am Acad Dermatol 1989; 21:763.

121. Arosemena R, et al: Cutaneous myiasis, J Am Acad Dermatol 1993; 28:254.

122. Gewirtzman A, Rabinovitz H: Botfly infestation (myiasis) masquerading as furunculosis, Cutis 1999; 63(2):71.

123. Loong PT, et al: Cutaneous myiasis: A simple and effective technique for extraction of Dermatobia hominis larvae, Int J Dermatol 1992; 31:657.

124. Brewer TF, et al: Bacon therapy and furuncular myiasis, JAMA 1993; 270:2087.

125. Weed RI: Exaggerated delayed hypersensitivity to mosquito bites in chronic lymphocytic leukemia, Blood 1993; 26:257.

126. Penneys NS, et al: Chronic pruritic eruption in patients with acquired immunodeficiency syndrome associated with increased antibody titers to mosquito salivary gland antigens, J Am Acad Dermatol 1989; 21:421.

127. Fradin MS, Day JF: Comparative efficacy of insect repellents against mosquito bites, N Engl J Med 2002; 347:13.

128. Fradin M: Mosquitoes and mosquito repellents: A clinician's guide, Ann Intern Med 1998; 128(11):931.

129. Reunala T, et al: Treatment of mosquito bites with cetirizine, Clin Exp Allergy 1993; 23:72.

130. Marks MB: Stinging insects: Allergy implications, Pediatr Clin North Am 1969; 16:177.

131. Blackwell V, Vega-Lopez F: Cutaneous larva migrans: Clinical features and management of 44 cases presenting in the returning traveller, Br J Dermatol 2001; 145(3):434.

132. Richey T, et al: Persistent cutaneous larva migrans due to Ancylostoma species, South Med J 1996; 89(6):609.

133. Ambrus J, Klein E: Loffler syndrome and ancyclostoma braziliense, N Y State J Med 1988; 88:498.

134. Veraldi S, Rizzitelli G: Effectiveness of a new therapeutic regimen with albendazole in cutaneous larva migrans, Eur J Dermatol 1999; 9(5):352.

135. Rizzitelli G, Scarabelli G, Veraldi S: Albendazole: A new therapeutic regimen in cutaneous larva migrans, Int J Dermatol 1997; 36(9):700.

136. Albanese G, Venturi C, Galbiati G: Treatment of larva migrans cutanea (creeping eruption): A comparison between albendazole and traditional therapy, Int J Dermatol 2001; 40(1):67.

137. Caumes E: Treatment of cutaneous larva migrans, Clin Infect Dis 2000; 30(5):811.

138. de SR, Williams D, Moak E: Fire ant attacks on residents in health care facilities: A report of two cases, Ann Intern Med 1999; 131(6):424.

139. de S RD, Soto-Aguilar M: Reactions to imported fire ant stings, Allergy Proc 1993; 14:13.

140. Ginsburg CM: Fire ant envenomation in children, Pediatrics 1984; 73:689.

141. Reisman RE: Stinging insect allergy, Med Clin North Am 1992; 76:883.

142. Ross EV, Jr, Badame AJ, Dale SE: Meat tenderizer in the acute treatment of imported fire ant stings, J Am Acad Dermatol 1987; 16:1189.

143. Moffitt J, Barker J, Stafford C: Management of imported fire ant allergy: Results of a survey, Ann Allergy Asthma Immunol 1997; 79(2):125.

144. Gurry D: Marine stings, Aust Fam Physician 1992; 21:26.

145. McGoldrick J, Marx JA: Marine envenomations; Part 1: vertebrates, J Emerg Med 1991; 9:497.

146. Auerbach PS: Marine envenomations, N Engl J Med 1991; 325:486.

147. Levy D, et al: Surveillance for waterborne-disease outbreaks—United States, 1995-1996, Mor Mortal Wkly Rep CDC Surveill Summ 1998; 47(5):1.

148. Loken B, Spencer C, Granath WJ: Prevalence and transmission of cercariae causing schistosome dermatitis in Flathead Lake, Montana, J Parasitol 1995; 81(4):646.

149. CDC: Cercarial dermatitis outbreak at a state park-Delaware, 1991, MMWR 1992; 41:225.

150. Mulvihill CA, Burnett JW: Swimmer's itch: A cercarial dermatitis, Cutis 1990; 46:211.

151. Tomchik RS, et al: Clinical perspectives on seabather's eruption, also known as 'sea lice,' JAMA 1993; 269:1669.

152. Freudenthal AR, Joseph PR: Seabathers' eruption, N Engl J Med 1993; 329:542.

153. Segura-Puertas L, et al : One Linuche mystery solved: All 3 stages of the coronate scyphomedusa Linuche unguiculata cause seabather's eruption, J Am Acad Dermatol 2001; 44(4):624.

Vesicular and Bullous Diseases

❏ **Blisters**
  Autoimmune blistering diseases
  Major blistering diseases
  Classification

❏ **Diagnosis of bullous disorders**

❏ **Dermatitis herpetiformis and linear IgA**
  bullous dermatosis
  Gluten-sensitive enteropathy
  Lymphoma
  Diagnosis of dermatitis herpetiformis

❏ **Bullae in diabetic persons**

❏ **Pemphigus**
  Pemphigus vulgaris
  Pemphigus foliaceus, IgA pemphigus, and
    pemphigus erythematosus
  Diagnosis of pemphigus
  Treatment
  Pemphigus in association with other diseases

❏ **The pemphigoid group of diseases**
  Bullous pemphigoid
  Localized pemphigoid
  Benign chronic bullous dermatosis of
    childhood
  Herpes gestationis (pemphigoid gestationis)

❏ **Pemphigoid-like disease**
  Epidermolysis bullosa acquisita

❏ **Benign familial chronic pemphigus**

❏ **Epidermolysis bullosa**

❏ **The newborn with blisters, pustules,**
  erosions, and ulcerations

Blisters

Vesicles and bullae are the primary lesions in many diseases. Some are of short duration and are quite characteristic, such as those in poison ivy and herpes zoster. In other diseases, such as erythema multiforme and lichen planus, a blister may or may not occur during the course of the disease. Finally, there is a group of disorders in which bullae are present almost continuously during the period of active disease. These autoimmune blistering diseases tend to be chronic, and many are associated with tissue-bound or circulating antibodies. This chapter deals with those disorders.

Autoimmune blistering diseases

Autoimmune blistering diseases cause impaired adhesion of the epidermis to epidermal basement membrane (e.g., the pemphigoid group of disorders [bullous, gestational, and mucous membrane]) or impaired adhesion of epidermal cells to each other (e.g., the pemphigus group of disorders). The autoantibodies target structural proteins that promote cell matrix (e.g., pemphigoid) or cell-to-cell (e.g., pemphigus) adhesion in skin. Autoimmune blistering diseases are characterized by substantial morbidity (pruritus, pain, disfigurement), and in some instances, mortality (secondary to loss of epidermal barrier function). Bullous pemphigoid is the most common autoimmune blistering disease. Treatment with systemic immunosuppressives has reduced morbidity and mortality in patients with these diseases.

Major blistering diseases

An overview of the major bullous diseases is presented in the diagram on p. 548. The differential diagnosis of all blistering diseases and the anatomy of the epidermis and epidermal basement membrane are shown in Figure 16-1, p. 549.

MAJOR BULLOUS DISEASES

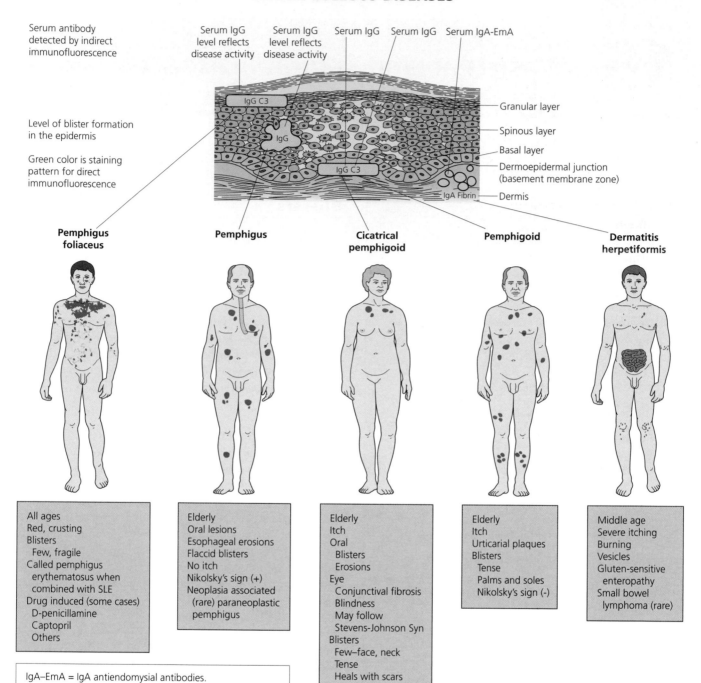

Serum antibody detected by indirect immunofluorescence

Serum IgG level reflects disease activity

Serum IgG level reflects disease activity

Serum IgG

Serum IgG

Serum IgA-EmA

Level of blister formation in the epidermis

Green color is staining pattern for direct immunofluorescence

IgG C3

IgG

IgG C3

IgA Fibrin

Granular layer

Spinous layer

Basal layer

Dermoepidermal junction (basement membrane zone)

Dermis

Pemphigus foliaceus

All ages
Red, crusting
Blisters
  Few, fragile
Called pemphigus
  erythematosus when
  combined with SLE
Drug induced (some cases)
  D-penicillamine
  Captopril
  Others

Pemphigus

Elderly
Oral lesions
Esophageal erosions
Flaccid blisters
No itch
Nikolsky's sign (+)
Neoplasia associated
  (rare) paraneoplastic
  pemphigus

Cicatrical pemphigoid

Elderly
Itch
Oral
  Blisters
  Erosions
Eye
  Conjunctival fibrosis
  Blindness
  May follow
  Stevens-Johnson Syn
Blisters
  Few—face, neck
  Tense
  Heals with scars

Pemphigoid

Elderly
Itch
Urticarial plaques
Blisters
  Tense
  Palms and soles
  Nikolsky's sign (-)

Dermatitis herpetiformis

Middle age
Severe itching
Burning
Vesicles
Gluten-sensitive
  enteropathy
Small bowel
  lymphoma (rare)

IgA–EmA = IgA antiendomysial antibodies.
Serum antibody–detected by indirect immunofluorescence.

BULLOUS DISEASES IN THE EPIDERMIS AND DERMOEPIDERMAL JUNCTION

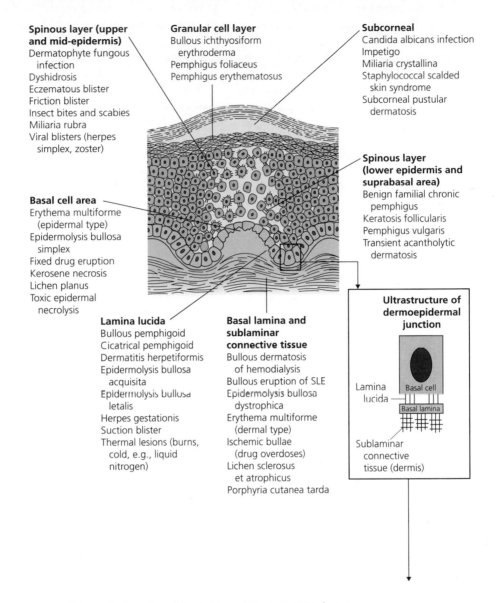

Spinous layer (upper and mid-epidermis)
Dermatophyte fungous infection
Dyshidrosis
Eczematous blister
Friction blister
Insect bites and scabies
Miliaria rubra
Viral blisters (herpes simplex, zoster)

Granular cell layer
Bullous ichthyosiform erythroderma
Pemphigus foliaceus
Pemphigus erythematosus

Subcorneal
Candida albicans infection
Impetigo
Miliaria crystallina
Staphylococcal scalded skin syndrome
Subcorneal pustular dermatosis

Spinous layer (lower epidermis and suprabasal area)
Benign familial chronic pemphigus
Keratosis follicularis
Pemphigus vulgaris
Transient acantholytic dermatosis

Basal cell area
Erythema multiforme (epidermal type)
Epidermolysis bullosa simplex
Fixed drug eruption
Kerosene necrosis
Lichen planus
Toxic epidermal necrolysis

Lamina lucida
Bullous pemphigoid
Cicatrical pemphigoid
Dermatitis herpetiformis
Epidermolysis bullosa acquisita
Epidermolysis bullosa letalis
Herpes gestationis
Suction blister
Thermal lesions (burns, cold, e.g., liquid nitrogen)

Basal lamina and sublaminar connective tissue
Bullous dermatosis of hemodialysis
Bullous eruption of SLE
Epidermolysis bullosa dystrophica
Erythema multiforme (dermal type)
Ischemic bullae (drug overdoses)
Lichen sclerosus et atrophicus
Porphyria cutanea tarda

Ultrastructure of dermoepidermal junction

Lamina lucida

Basal cell

Basal lamina

Sublaminar connective tissue (dermis)

Schematic Overview of the Epidermal Basement Membrane

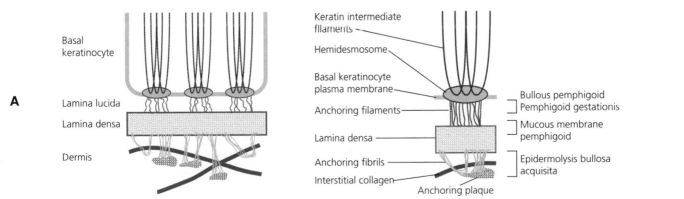

A

Basal keratinocyte

Lamina lucida

Lamina densa

Dermis

B

Keratin intermediate filaments

Hemidesmosome

Basal keratinocyte plasma membrane

Anchoring filaments

Lamina densa

Anchoring fibrils

Interstitial collagen

Anchoring plaque

Bullous pemphigoid
Pemphigoid gestationis

Mucous membrane pemphigoid

Epidermolysis bullosa acquisita

Figure 16-1 A, Electron microscopy studies of skin demonstrate that basal keratinocytes overlie the lamina lucida, which is in turn positioned just above the lamina densa (i.e., the basement membrane proper) and superficial dermis. **B,** Ultrastructurally, hemidesmosome-anchoring filament-attachment complexes bind the cytoskeleton of basal keratinocytes to the underlying lamina densa, anchoring fibrils, and fibrillar elements (e.g., interstitial collagen and elastin fibers) within the superficial dermis. The dominant regions within epidermal basement membrane that are targeted by IgG autoantibodies in patients with pemphigoid diseases and epidermolysis bullosa acquisita are indicated by brackets. *Adapted from Yancy KB, Egan CA: JAMA 2000; 284(3).*

Classification

A blister occurs when fluid accumulates at some level in the skin. The histologic classification of bullous disorders is based on the level in the skin at which that separation occurs (Figures 16-1 and the diagram on p. 548). Subcorneal blisters are not commonly seen intact; the very thin roof has little structural integrity and collapses. Intraepidermal blisters have a thicker roof and are more substantial, whereas subepidermal blisters have great structural integrity and can remain intact even when firmly compressed.

Epidermis

Desmosomes contribute to epidermal cell-cell adhesion. Desmosomal proteins (desmoglein 1, desmoglein 3) are the autoantigens of pemphigus foliaceus and pemphigus vulgaris (Table 16-1), respectively. Paraneoplastic pemphigus is associated with autoantibodies to desmosomal plaque protein, desmoplakin. These diseases have intraepidermal blistering.

The basement membrane zone (Figure 16-1)

The hemidesmosome is a membrane-associated protein complex that extends from the intracellular area of basal keratinocytes to the extracellular area. It links the cytoskeleton of the basal keratinocyte to the dermis. Hemidesmosomes are associated with anchoring filaments, threadlike structures traversing the lamina lucida. Anchoring fibrils, which consist of type VII collagen, extend from the lower portion of the lamina densa to anchoring plaques within the papillary dermis.

BASEMENT MEMBRANE ANTIGENS AND DISEASES. Different components of the basement membrane contain the autoantigens of several autoimmune bullous diseases (Table 16-2). Diseases of hemidesmosomes show subepidermal blisters and by direct immunofluorescence, linear deposits of IgG, C3, or IgA at the dermal epidermal junction. Bullous pemphigoid (BP) is a disease of hemidesmosomes. Two proteins, BP180 and BP230, are the targets of autoantibodies in BP. BP180 is the target of autoantibodies in herpes gestationis, cicatricial pemphigoid and linear IgA disease.[1] Laminin 5 is an anchoring filament-lamina densa component of hemidesmosomes. Autoantibodies to laminin 5 cause mucous membrane pemphigoid (cicatricial pemphigoid). Type VII collagen is the major structural component of anchoring fibrils. Type VII collagen is the autoantigen of epidermolysis bullosa acquisita.

Table 16-1 Molecular Classification of Pemphigus

Pemphigus type	Target desmosomal protein
Pemphigus vulgaris	Desmoglein 3 (and desmoglein 1)
Pemphigus foliaceus	Desmoglein 1
Paraneoplastic pemphigus	Desmoglein 3, desmoplakin 1, desmoplakin 2, BP 230, envoplakin, periplakin, other
IgA pemphigus	Desmocollin 1

From Mutasim DF, et al: J Am Acad Dermatol 2001; 45:803.

Table 16-2 Molecular Classification of Subepidermal Bullous Diseases

Bullous disease	Targeted molecule
Bullous pemphigoid (BP)	BP 180, BP 230 (hemidesmosome and lamina lucida)
Herpes gestationis	BP 180, BP 230 (hemidesmosome and lamina lucida)
Cicatricial pemphigoid	BP 180, laminin V (hemidesmosome and lamina lucida)
Epidermolysis bullosa acquisita	Type VII collagen (anchoring fibrils)
Bullous SLE	Type VII collagen (anchoring fibrils)
Linear IgA disease (adults and children)	LAD antigen (BP 180) (hemidesmosome and lamina lucida)
Dermatitis herpetiformis	Unknown

From Mutasim DF, et al: J Am Acad Dermatol 2001; 45:803.

Diagnosis of Bullous Disorders

The diagnosis of many chronic bullous disorders can often be made clinically. These diseases have such important implications that the diagnosis should be confirmed by histology and, in many instances, immunofluorescence (see Table 16-3, Figure 16-2, Tables 16-4 and 16-5).

BIOPSY

For light microscopy. A biopsy specimen must be taken from the proper area to demonstrate the level of blister formation and the nature of the inflammatory infiltrate (Figure 16-2 and Table 16-3). Small, early vesicles or inflamed skin provide the most diagnostic features. Ruptured or excoriated lesions are of little value and should not be sampled. A small portion of the intact skin should be included in the biopsy specimen. Punch biopsies done through the center of a large blister are of little value.

For immunofluorescence. In most cases, the first biopsy specimen should be taken from the edge of a fresh lesion. A second biopsy is often desirable to establish the diagnosis. One should sample skin near the lesion, preferably from a nonedematous, normal, or red area. The best site for obtaining a biopsy specimen is shown in Table 16-5 and Figure 16-2.

Table 16-3 Specimen Selection for Diagnosis of Vesiculo-Bullous Disorders

		Tissue (for direct immunofluorescence)		Serum	Tissue
		Normal tissue (mm from edge of lesion)	Perilesional tissue	Indirect immunofluorescence shows	Lesion—histology shows
SKIN	Pemphigus (all forms)	BX—3mm	BX	Pemphigus and pemphigoid antibodies Can differentiate various forms of pemphigus Levels have prognostic value	Acantholysis
	Pemphigoid (all forms) Epidermolysis bullosa acquisita Linear IgA disease	BX—3mm	BX	Pemphigus and pemphigoid antibodies Levels not of prognostic value	Subepidermal bulla
	Porphyria Pseudo-porphyria Bullous lichen planus Lichen planus	NN	BX	Serum porphyrin (positive only in porphyria)	Subepidermal bulla
	Dermatitis herpetiformis	BX—3-5 mm	NN	Endomysial IgA antibodies Levels have prognostic value	Subepidermal bulla
	Hailey-Hailey Darier's disease	NN	BX		Acantholysis
ORAL (mucosal biopsy)	Cicatricial pemphigoid Erosive lichen planus Pemphigus vulgaris	BX—10mm	BX	Pemphigus and pemphigoid antibodies (positive in only few cases with conventional techniques)	Same as skin biopsy
OCULAR (conjunctiva biopsy)	Ocular cicatricial pemphigoid	NN	BX	Pemphigus and pemphigoid antibodies (positive in only few cases with conventional techniques)	Same as skin biopsy

Modified from Immunopathologic studies of the skin, Buffalo, NY, Beutner Laboratories.
BX, Biopsy; *NN,* not needed.

LEVEL OF BLISTER FORMATION. For blisters occurring above the basement membrane zone, the level of blister formation can be determined easily with routine studies. Blisters occurring in the dermoepidermal junction (basement membrane zone) area (see Figure 16-1) were once considered subepidermal in location. With the electron microscope, it has been shown that blisters may occur at different levels in that complex area. Electron microscopy is not routinely used; adequate diagnostic information can be obtained from sections stained with hematoxylin and eosin and from immunofluorescence studies.

IMMUNOFLUORESCENCE. Immunofluorescence is a laboratory technique for demonstrating the presence of tissue-bound and circulating antibodies.[2] Most chronic bullous disorders have specific antibodies that either are fixed to some component of skin or are circulating. Many laboratories around the country provide this testing service and supply transport media and mailing containers for tissue specimens. (Examples are Beutner Laboratories, Buffalo, NY, 1-716-838-0549; IMMCO Diagnostics, Buffalo, NY, 1-800-537-TEST;

and Mayo Medical Laboratories, Rochester, MN, 1-800-533-1710.) Freezing of specimens is no longer required.

Direct immunofluorescence (skin). Direct immunofluorescence is designed for demonstration of tissue-bound antibody and complement. Sectioned biopsy specimens are treated with fluorescein-conjugated antisera to human immunoglobulins (IgG, IgA, IgM, IgD, and IgE), C3, and fibrin; they are then examined with a microscope equipped with a special light source.

Indirect immunofluorescence (serum). Indirect immunofluorescence is used for demonstration of circulating antibodies directed against certain skin structures. Thin sections of animal squamous epithelium (monkey esophagus, etc.) are first incubated with the patient's serum. Skin-reacting antibodies in the serum attach to specific components of the animal epithelium. Fluorescein-labeled anti–human IgG antiserum is then added for specific identification of the circulating antibody. The circulating antibody responsible for the IgA deposition has not yet been identified, and indirect immunofluorescence is negative.

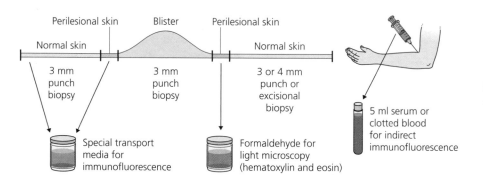

Figure 16-2 Specimen selection for diagnosis of vesiculo-bullous disorders.

Table 16-4 Diagnosis of Autoimmune Bullous Diseases

Histopathology	Direct immunofluorescence	Indirect immunofluorescence	Diagnosis
Suprabasal	1. IgG ± C3 at ICS 2. IgG ± C3 at ICS + BMZ	IgG at ICS, monkey esophagus IgG at ICS, rat bladder	Pemphigus vulgaris > paraneoplastic pemphigus
Subcorneal	1. IgA at ICS 2. IgG ± C3 at ICS 3. IgG ± C3 at ICS, Ig ± C3 at BMZ	IgA at ICS IgA at ICS IgG at ICS + ANA	IgA pemphigus Pemphigus foliaceus Pemphigus erythematosus
Subepidermal noninflammatory	1. IgG, C3 ± IgM, IgA at BMZ 2. IgG, IgA ± IgM, C3 in blood vessel walls	1. Dermal side of SSS 2. Epidermal side of SSS Negative	Epidermolysis bullosa acquisita Bullous pemphigoid Porphyria cutanea tarda, Pseudo-PCT
Subepidermal with eosinophil-rich infiltrate	C3, IgG at BMZ	Epidermal side of SSS	Bullous pemphigoid Herpes gestationis Mucosal pemphigoid

Subepidermal with neutrophil-rich infiltrate	1. Granular IgA in dermal papillae and BMZ
	2. Linear IgA ± C3, BMZ
	3. IgG, IgM, C3, IgA, fibrinogen
		Negative on epithelium
		    (+antiendomysial antibodies)
		IgA at BMZ
		1. Dermal side of SSS
		
		2. Dermal side of SSS and positive lupus serology
			Dermatitis herpetiformis
			
			Linear IgA disease
			Epidermolysis bullosa acquisita,
			    rare antiepiligrin disease
			Bullous systemic lupus
			    erythematosus

From Mutasim DF, et al: J Am Acad Dermatol 2001; 45:803.
BMZ, Basement membrane zone; *ICS,* intercellular space; *SSS,* salt-split skin; ±, with or without; >, more likely than.

Table 16-5 Bullous and Vasculitic Disorders—Immunofluorescence Tests

Disorder	Selection of biopsy site for direct immunofluorescence*	Biopsy findings: direct immunofluorescence	Serum findings: circulating antibody detected by indirect immunofluorescence
Bullous pemphigoid	Erythematous perilesional skin or mucosa	IgG and/or C3, also other Ig in BMZ; linear—about 50%-80%; deposits disappear as disease subsides. Biopsy normal forearm skin for this study. Biopsy split in 1M NaCl: IgG is in BMZ of roof (and less often in the floor) or split	IgG class BMZ antibodies—about 70%; level does not correlate with disease activity
Cicatricial pemphigoid	Erythematous perilesional skin or mucosa	IgG and/or C3, also other Ig in BMZ; linear—about 10%-80%. Biopsy split in 1M NaCl: IgG is in BMZ of roof (and less often in the floor) of split	IgG and IgA class BMZ antibodies—10% routine preparation; 82% on salt-split human skin substrate
Epidermolysis bullosa acquisita†	Erythematous perilesional skin or mucosa	Ig and/or C3 in BMZ; linear—almost 100%. Biopsy split in 1M NaCl: IgG is in BMZ of floor of split	IgG class BMZ antibodies—about 25%
Dermatitis herpetiformis Classic	Perilesional skin	IgA, also F and C in dermal papillae; granular or fibrillar—more than 90% in normal skin	IgA class EMA in about 70% AGA in about 60% ARA in about 36%
Linear IgA disease	Perilesional skin	IgA—100%, also F, rarely C, at BMZ; linear	IgA class BMZ antibodies—about 10% incidence
Henoch-Schönlein purpura	Lesions no older than 24-48 h	Granular IgA in vessels	None
Herpes gestationis	Erythematous perilesional skin	C (100%), Ig (30%-50%) in BMZ; linear	HG factor—about 50%; IgG class BMZ antibodies—about 20%
Pemphigus, all forms except Hailey-Hailey disease	Erythematous perilesional skin	IC deposits of IgG—about 80%; deposits disappear as disease subsides.	IC antibodies—more than 90%; level correlates with disease activity
Erythema multiforme	Edge of involved skin Lesions no older than 24-48 h	Granular IgG and C3 deposits in blood vessels	None
Leukocytoclastic vasculitis	Lesions no older than 24-48 h	Granular Ig (mostly IgM), C3, and F in vessels	None
Lichen planus	Edge of involved skin; avoid old lesions or ulcers	Ig, C and F in cytoid bodies in epidermis, F around rete pegs	None
Porphyria cutanea tarda and other forms of porphyria	Edge of involved skin, sun-exposed	Strong, homogeneous IgG in and around vessel walls, also immunofluorescent band at BMZ	Vascular IgG (IgA and fibrin); IgG in BMZ in lesional skin only
Benign chronic bullous dermatosis of childhood	Erythematous perilesional skin	Same as for dermatitis herpetiformis or pemphigoid	Same as for dermatitis herpetiformis or pemphigoid

Modified from Handbook of clinical relevance of tests, IMMCO Diagnostics, Buffalo, NY.

IC, Intercellular area of stratum spinosum; *BMZ,* basement membrane zone; *Ig,* immunoglobulin; *F,* fibrin or fibrinogen; *C,* complement; *HG,* herpes gestationis factor; *EMA,* endomysial antibodies; *AGA,* antigliadin antibodies; *ARA,* antireticulin antibodies.

*For most bullous diseases two biopsies are recommended: (1) from edge of a fresh lesion and (2) from adjacent normal skin.

†To differentiate epidermolysis bullosa acquisita from bullous pemphigoid, further direct immunofluorescence studies on lesional biopsy specimens and on normal skin split at the lamina lucida by NaCl are required to demonstrate the location of immunoreactants, laminin, and type IV collagen.

Dermatitis Herpetiformis and Linear IgA Bullous Dermatosis

Dermatitis herpetiformis is a rare, chronic, intensely burning, pruritic vesicular skin disease associated in most instances with a subclinical gluten-sensitive enteropathy and IgA deposits in the upper dermis. The reported prevalence in northern Europe is 1.2 to 39.2 per 100,000. The prevalence in Utah in 1987 was 11.2 per 100,000. The average age of onset was 41.8 years, patients having symptoms for an average of 1.6 years before diagnosis.[3]

Dermatitis herpetiformis is rare in children. There is a strong association with specific human histocompatibility leukocyte antigens: HLA-B8 (60%), HLA class II antigens HLA-DR3 (95%), and HLA-DQw2 (100%).[4,5]

Linear IgA bullous dermatosis has clinical features similar to those of dermatitis herpetiformis, but has a different histologic and immunofluorescence pattern and there is no associated small bowel disease. Drug-induced linear IgA bullous dermatosis is rare but increasing in frequency.

Sulfones produce a dramatic response within hours, but without drugs, some patients have chosen suicide as the only means of relief.

CLINICAL PRESENTATION. Dermatitis herpetiformis usually begins in the second to fifth decade, but many cases have been reported in children.[6] The disease is rarely seen in African Americans or Asians. Dermatitis herpetiformis presents initially with a few itchy papules or vesicles that are a minor annoyance; they may be attributed to bites, scabies, or neurotic excoriation, and they sometimes respond to topical steroids. In time the disease evolves into its classic presentation of intensely burning urticarial papules, vesicles, and, rarely, bullae, either isolated or in groups such as in herpes simplex or zoster (therefore the term *herpetiformis*).

The vesicles are symmetrically distributed and appear on the elbows, knees, scalp and nuchal area, shoulders, and buttocks (Figures 16-3 to 16-5).

The distribution may be more generalized. Destruction of the vesicles by scratching provides relief but increases the difficulty of locating a primary lesion for biopsy. Intact lesions for biopsy may be found on the back.

The symptoms vary in intensity, but most people complain of severe itching and burning. One should always think of dermatitis herpetiformis when the symptom of burning is volunteered. The symptoms may precede the onset of lesions by hours, and patients can frequently identify the site of a new lesion by the prodromal symptoms. Treatment does not alter the course of the disease. Most patients have symptoms for years, but approximately one third are in permanent remission.

The vesicular-bullous form is confused with bullous erythema multiforme and bullous pemphigoid. A strong association between dermatitis herpetiformis and diverse thyroid abnormalities has been reported and most likely represents a grouping of immune-mediated disorders. Hypothyroidism was the most common, occurring in 14% of patients. There were clinical or serologic abnormalities in 50% of patients with dermatitis herpetiformis.[7]

Oral symptoms occur in 63% of patients. Oral dryness and recurrent oral mucosal ulceration are the most commonly reported findings.

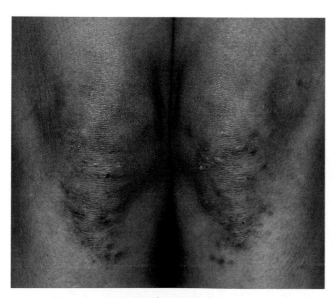

Figure 16-3 Dermatitis herpetiformis. Vesicles are symmetrically distributed on the knees. Most have been excoriated.

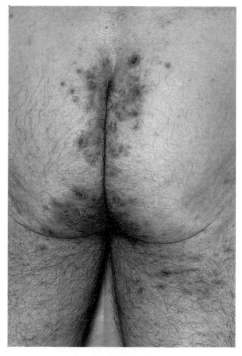

Figure 16-4 Dermatitis herpetiformis. Vesicles and erosions are commonly found on the buttocks.

DERMATITIS HERPETIFORMIS

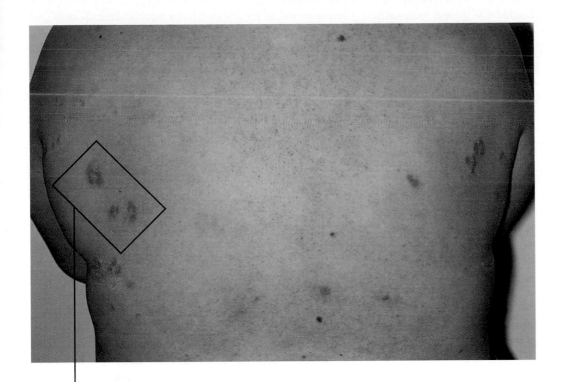

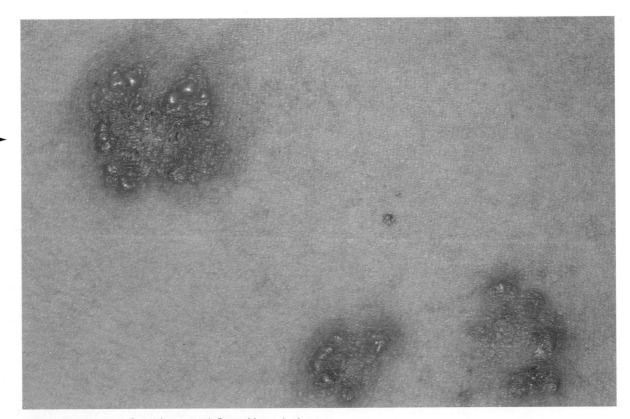

Figure 16-5 Groups of vesicles on an inflamed base. Lesions are not usually as numerous as in pemphigus or pemphigoid. Enlargement of inset shows vesicles that resemble a herpes virus infection; therefore the designation *herpetiformis*.

Celiac-type dental enamel defects. Celiac-type permanent-tooth enamel defects were found in 53% of patients with dermatitis herpetiformis. The grades of these defects were milder than those described for severe celiac disease. This finding suggests that these patients were already suffering from subclinical gluten-induced enteropathy in early childhood, when the crowns of permanent teeth develop.[8,9]

Linear IgA bullous dermatosis. Linear IgA bullous dermatosis (LABD) may present clinically as typical dermatitis herpetiformis, typical bullous pemphigoid, cicatricial pemphigoid or in an atypical morphologic pattern, and it has histologic features similar to dermatitis herpetiformis. Drugs such as vancomycin are responsible for some cases. Lesions develop within 24 hours to 15 days after the first dose.[10] The diagnosis of LABD is confirmed by direct immunofluorescence, which shows the presence of linear deposition of IgA at the epidermal basement membrane zone (BMZ). Some patients demonstrate both IgA and IgG BMZ autoantibodies. There is no gluten-sensitive enteropathy. Some patients have a circulating-IgA class anti-BMZ antibody on indirect immunofluorescence. Circulating IgA autoantibodies to tissue transglutaminase are detectable in DH but not in linear IgA disease or other subepidermal autoimmune bullous diseases.[11]

Gluten-sensitive enteropathy

A gluten-sensitive enteropathy with patchy areas of villous atrophy and mild intestinal wall inflammation is found in the majority of patients with dermatitis herpetiformis. The changes in the small intestine are similar to but less severe than those found in ordinary gluten-sensitive enteropathy; symptoms of malabsorption are rarely encountered. Fewer than 20% of patients have malabsorption of fat, D-xylose, or iron. A significant correlation was found between IgA antiendomysial antibodies (IgA-EmA) and the severity of gluten-induced jejunum damage. Serum IgA-EmA was present in approximately 70% of patients with dermatitis herpetiformis on a normal diet. IgA-EmA was positive in 86% of dermatitis herpetiformis patients with subtotal villous atrophy, and 11% of dermatitis herpetiformis patients with partial villous atrophy or mild abnormalities. IgA-EmA antibodies disappear after 1 year of a gluten-free diet with the regrowth of jejunal villi. The relationship between IgA-EmA and villous atrophy is a useful diagnostic marker because the enteropathy present in dermatitis herpetiformis is usually without symptoms and therefore difficult to identify.[12]

Lymphoma

Small bowel lymphoma and nonintestinal lymphoma have been reported in patients with dermatitis herpetiformis and celiac disease. All lymphomas occurred in patients whose dermatitis herpetiformis had been controlled without a gluten-free diet (GFD) or in those who had been treated with a GFD for less than 5 years.[13] Therefore patients are advised to adhere to a strict GFD for life. One study showed that the incidence of non-Hodgkin's lymphoma was significantly increased in patients with dermatitis herpetiformis.[14] That study also confirmed that the patients with dermatitis herpetiformis treated mainly with a GFD have no increased general mortality.

Diagnosis of dermatitis herpetiformis

SKIN BIOPSY. Figure 16-6 is an example of new red papular lesions that have not blistered. Subepidermal clefts of evolving vesicles, and neutrophils and eosinophils in microabscesses within dermal papillae, are demonstrated. Linear IgA bullous dermatosis histologically resembles dermatitis herpetiformis or bullous pemphigoid.[15]

IMMUNOFLUORESCENCE STUDIES. IgA is not uniformly distributed throughout the skin, and IgA is present in greater amounts near active lesions. Therefore the preferred biopsy site for immunofluorescence studies is normal appearing or faintly erythematous skin that is adjacent to an active lesion.[16] The diagnostic Ig deposits are usually destroyed in an active lesion during the blistering process. More than 90% of patients with dermatitis herpetiformis have granular or fibrillar IgA deposits in the dermal papillae; patients with linear IgA bullous dermatosis have linear deposits of IgA in the BMZ. This includes patients treated with sulfones. Multiple speci-

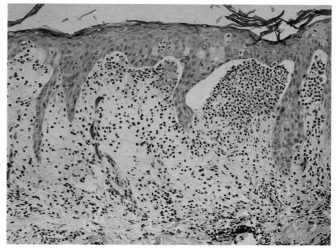

Figure 16-6 Dermatitis herpetiformis. Subepidermal clefts with microabscesses of neutrophils and eosinophils in the dermal papilla.